KANDARPA HANDBOOK OF INTERVENTIONAL RADIOLOGIC PROCEDURES

6th EDITION

KANDARPA HANDBOOK OF INTERVENTIONAL RADIOLOGIC PROCEDURES

Robert Lewandowski, MD
Lindsay Machan, MD
Parag J. Patel, MD, MS
Krishna Kandarpa, MD, PhD

6TH EDITION

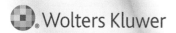

Wolters Kluwer

Philadelphia • Baltimore • New York • London
Buenos Aires • Hong Kong • Sydney • Tokyo

Acquisitions Editor: Nicole Dernoski
Development Editor: Eric McDermott
Editorial Coordinator: Christopher Rodgers/Vinodhini Varadharajalu
Marketing Manager: Kirsten Watrud
Production Project Manager: Kirstin Johnson
Manager, Graphic Arts & Design: Stephen Druding
Manufacturing Coordinator: Beth Welsh/Lisa Bowling
Prepress Vendor: Aptara, Inc.

Sixth Edition

9 8 7 6 5 4 3 2 1

Printed in Singapore

Library of Congress Cataloging-in-Publication Data

Names: Kandarpa, Krishna, editor. | Machan, Lindsay, editor. | Patel, Parag
   J., editor. | Lewandowski, Robert (Robert J.), editor.
Title: Kandarpa handbook of interventional radiologic procedures / [edited
   by] Krishna Kandarpa, Lindsay Machan, Parag J. Patel, Robert
   Lewandowski.
Other titles: Handbook of interventional radiologic procedures
Description: Sixth edition. | Philadelphia : Wolters Kluwer, [2023] |
   Preceded by Handbook of interventional radiologic procedures / [edited
   by] Krishna Kandarpa, Lindsay Machan, Janette D. Durham. Fifth edition.
   [2016]. | Includes bibliographical references and index.
Identifiers: LCCN 2022031416 (print) | LCCN 2022031417 (ebook) | ISBN
   9781975146269 (paperback) | ISBN 9781975146283 (ebook)
Subjects: MESH: Radiography, Interventional—methods | Handbook
Classification: LCC RC78.2 (print) | LCC RC78.2 (ebook) | NLM WN 39 |
   DDC 616.07/572–dc23/eng/20220801
LC record available at https://lccn.loc.gov/2022031416
LC ebook record available at https://lccn.loc.gov/2022031417

shop.lww.com

Dedicated to the innovative spirit
of interventional radiologists.

CONTRIBUTORS

Hani H. Abujudeh, MD, MBA, FSIR, FACR, FASER
Director of Quality Assurance
Chairman Clinical Quality Committee
Radiology, Envision Physician Services
Detroit, Michigan

Osman Ahmed, MD
Associate Professor of Vascular and
    Interventional Radiology
Radiology
University of Chicago
Chicago, Illinois

Sun Ho Ahn, MD, FSIR
Assistant Professor of Radiology
The Warren Alpert Medical School of
    Brown University
Providence, Rhode Island

Mohammed T. Alshammari, MD
Consultant Interventional Radiologist
Security Forces Hospital Program
Riyadh, Saudi Arabia

Parag Amin, MD
Assistant Professor of Radiology
Loyola University Medical Center
Maywood, Illinois

Ronald S. Arellano, MD, FSIR
Associate Professor of Radiology
Massachusetts General Hospital/
    Harvard Medical School
Boston, Massachusetts

David R. Bamshad, MD
Resident Physician
Diagnostic, Molecular, and
    Interventional Radiology
Mount Sinai Health System
New York, New York

Debra Barnes, BS, RT(R), CV
Interventional Radiology Supervisor
Interventional Radiology, The Froedtert
    & the Medical College of Wisconsin
Milwaukee, Wisconsin

James F. Benenati, MD
Clinical Professor of Radiology
Miami Cardiac and Vascular Institute
Herbert Wertheim College of Medicine
Florida International University
Miami, Florida

Zachary Berman, MD
Assistant Clinical Professor of
    Interventional Radiology
University of California, San Diego
San Diego, California

Michael A. Bettmann, MD, FSIR, FACR, FAHA
Professor of Radiology Emeritus
Wake Forest University School of
    Medicine
Winston-Salem, North Carolina

Shivank Bhatia, MD
Chairman of Interventional Radiology
The University of Miami Miller School
    of Medicine
Miami, Florida

Peter R. Bream, Jr., MD, FSIR
Clinical Professor of Radiology
Department of Radiology
The University of North Carolina at
    Chapel Hill
Chapel Hill, North Carolina

William F. Browne, MD
Assistant Professor of Clinical Radiology
Department of Radiology, Division
    of Vascular and Interventional
    Radiology
Weill Cornell Medicine/NewYork-
    Presbyterian Hospital
New York, New York

Elena Bozzi, MD
Interventional Radiologist
Division of Interventional Radiology
University of Pisa - Azienda Ospedaliero
    Universitaria Pisana
Pisa, Italy

Leonardo A. Campos, MD
Post Ddoc Research Scholar
Charles T. Dotter Department of
    Interventional Radiology
Oregon Health and Sciences University
Portland, Oregon

Leandro Cardarelli-Leite, MD
Adult and Pediatric Interventional
    Radiologist
Assistant Professor, Department of
    Medical Imaging
Western University
London, Canada

Leigh Casadaban, MD
Assistant Professor
Department of Radiology
University of Colorado, Anschutz
    Medical Center
Aurora, Colorado

Francisco Cesar Carnevale, PhD
Chief of the Vascular Interventional
    Radiology
Radiology Institute
University of Sao Paulo Medical School
    Sao Paulo, Brazil

Arais Cavada, ARNP, RN
Miller School of Medicine
University of Miami
Miami, Florida

Matthew D. Cham, MD
Associate Professor of Radiology
Icahn School of Medicine at Mount Sinai
New York, New York

Danny Chan, MD
Precision Vascular
Dallas, Texas

Maye M. Chan, PA-C
Division of Abdominal Imaging and
    Intervention
Brigham and Women's Hospital
Boston, Massachusetts

Danny Cheng, MD
Assistant Clinical Professor of Radiology
UC Davis Medical Center
Sacramento, California

Jared D. Christensen, MD
Assistant Professor of Radiology
Duke University Medical Center
Durham, North Carolina

John Chung, MD, FRCPC
Clinical Instructor of Radiology
The University of British Columbia
Vancouver, British Columbia, Canada

Roberto Cioni, MD
Interventional Radiologist, Chief
Division of Interventional Radiology
University of Pisa - Azienda Ospedaliero
    Universitaria Pisana
Pisa, Italy

Timothy W.I. Clark, MD, FSIR
Associate Professor of Clinical
    Radiology and Surgery
Perelman School of Medicine at the
    University of Pennsylvania
Philadelphia, Pennsylvania

Meghan R. Clark, MD
Interventional Radiology Resident
Division of Vascular and Interventional
    Radiology
Department of Radiology and Medical
    Imaging
University of Virginia Health System
Charlottesville, Virginia

Shannon Coleman, RN, BSN
Clinical Nurse Educator
Interventional Radiology
Vancouver General Hospital
Vancouver, British Columbia, Canada

Joshua Cornman-Homonoff, MD
Assistant Professor
Radiology and Biomedical Imaging
Yale School of Medicine
New Haven, Connecticut

Anne M. Covey, MD, FSIR
Associate Professor of Radiology
Memorial Sloan Kettering Cancer
    Center
Weill Cornell Medical Center
New York, New York

Laura Crocetti, MD, PhD, EBIR, FCIRSE
Associate Professor of Radiology
Interventional Radiologist
Division of Interventional Radiology
University of Pisa - Azienda Ospedaliero
    Universitaria Pisana
Pisa, Italy

John Crowe, MD
Assistant Professor of Anesthesiology
College of Medicine
University of Cincinnati
Cincinnati, Ohio

Michael D. Dake, MD
Senior Vice-President for Health
    Sciences and Professor
Medical Imaging, Medicine, and Surgery
University of Arizona
Tucson, Arizona

Michael Darcy, MD
Professor of Radiology
Mallinckrodt Institute of Radiology
Washington University in St. Louis
St. Louis, Missouri

André Moreira de Assis, MD
Vascular Interventional Radiology
    Radiology
University of São Paulo
São Paulo, Brazil

Kush R. Desai, MD, FSIR
Associate Professor of Radiology,
    Surgery, and Medicine
Director, Deep Venous Interventions
Division of Interventional Radiology
Feinberg School of Medicine
Northwestern University
Chicago, Illinois

Elizabeth H. Dibble, MD
Assistant Professor of Diagnostic Imaging
The Warren Alpert Medical School of
    Brown University
Providence, Rhode Island

Josée Dubois, MD, MSc, FRCPC
Interventional Radiologist
Department of Medical Imaging
CHU Sainte-Justine
Montreal, Quebec, Canada

Pouya Entezari, MD
Department of Radiology
Division of Interventional Radiology
Northwestern Memorial Hospital
Chicago, Illinois

Jeremy J. Erasmus, MD
Professor of Diagnostic Radiology
MD Anderson Cancer Center
Houston, Texas

Joseph P. Erinjeri, MD, PhD
Vice Chairman
Department of Radiology
Memorial Sloan Kettering Cancer Center
New York, New York

Khashayar Farsad, MD, PhD
Assistant Professor
Dotter Interventional Institute
Oregon Health and Science University
Portland, Oregon

Dimitrios K. Filippiadis, MD, PhD, MSc, EBIR
Associate Professor of Diagnostic and
    Interventional Radiology
2nd Department of Radiology, University
    General Hospital "ATTIKON"
Medical School, National and
    Kapodistrian University of Athens
Attikon, Greece

Siobhan M. Flanagan, MD
Assistant Professor of Radiology
Division of Interventional Radiology
    and Vascular Medicine
University of Minnesota
Minneapolis, Minnesota

Michael G. Flater, RN
Territory Manager
ZOLL LifeVest
Pittsburgh, Pennsylvania

Brian Funaki, MD
Professor of Radiology
University of Chicago
Chicago, Illinois

Ahmed Gabr, MD
Radiology Resident
Department of Radiology
Northwestern University
Chicago, Illinois

Ripal T. Gandhi, MD, FSVM
Associate Clinical Professor
Miami Cardiac and Vascular Institute
Herbert Wertheim College of Medicine
Florida International University
Miami, Florida

Joseph J. Gemmete, MD, FACR, FSIR, FCIRSE, FAHA
Professor of Radiology, Neurosurgery, Neurology, and Otolaryngology
Program Director, Neurointerventional Radiology Fellowship
Department of Radiology
Divisions of Neuroradiology and Vascular/Interventional Radiology
Michigan Medicine
Ann Arbor, Michigan

Christos S. Georgiades, MD, PhD, FSIR, FCIRSE
Associate Professor of Radiology and Surgery
Johns Hopkins University
Baltimore, Maryland

Patrick Gilbert, MD
Interventional Radiologist
Department of Radiology
Centre Hospitalier de l'Université de Montréal (CHUM)
Université de Montréal
Montreal, Quebec, Canada

Marie France Giroux, MD
Interventional Radiologist
Department of Radiology
Centre Hospitalier de l'Université de Montréal (CHUM)
Université de Montréal
Montreal, Quebec, Canada

Daniel I. Glazer, MD
Medical Director of CT
Radiology
Brigham and Women's Hospital
Boston, Massachusetts
Medical Director of Cross-Sectional Interventional Radiology
Radiology
Harvard Medical School
Boston, Massachusetts

Jafar Golzarian, MD
Professor Interventional Radiology
Radiology
University of Minnesota Medical School
Minneapolis, Minnesota

Karen Marshall-Grace, RN, MSN, CRN
Program Manager
Northwestern Memorial Hospital
Lombard, Illinois

Alexey Gurevich, MD
Interventional Radiology Resident
Hospital of the University of Pennsylvania
Philadelphia, Pennsylvania

Zuhal Haidari, MPH
Director of Quality and Performance Improvement
Society of Interventional Radiology
Fairfax, Virginia

Carolyn Hammen, MS, RT(R), PA-C
Physician Assistant
Department of Radiology
Medical College of Wisconsin
Milwaukee, Wisconsin

Rulon L. Hardman, MD, PhD
Assistant Professor of Radiology
University of Utah
Salt Lake City, Utah

Ziv J. Haskal, MD, FSIR, FAHA, FACR, FCIRSE
Professor of Radiology
University of Virginia School of Medicine
Charlottesville, Virginia

Peter B. Hathaway, MD
Utah Imaging Associates
Utah Vascular Clinic
Salt Lake City, Utah

Denise Hegemann, BSN, RN, CRN
Staff RN
Interventional Radiology
Froedtert Hospital
Milwaukee, Wisconsin

Michael B. Heller, MD
Assistant Professor
Department of Radiology and Biomedical Imaging
University of California, San Francisco
San Francisco, California

Katharine J. Henderson, MS
Genetic Counselor
Radiology and Biomedical Imaging
Yale University School of Medicine
New Haven, Connecticut

Claudia I. Henschke, PhD, MD
Professor of Radiology
Icahn School of Medicine at Mount Sinai
New York, New York

Manraj K.S. Heran, MD, FRCPC
Associate Professor of Radiology
University of British Columbia
Vancouver, British Columbia, Canada

Stephen G.F. Ho, MD, FRCPC
Clinical Professor
Department of Radiology
University of British Columbia
Vancouver, British Columbia, Canada

David M. Hovsepian, MD
Clinical Professor of Radiology
Stanford University School of Medicine
Stanford, California

Maxim Itkin, MD
Associate Professor of Radiology and
    Surgery
University of Pennsylvania Medical Center
Philadelphia, Pennsylvania

Hamed Jalaeian, MD
Assistant Professor of Clinical
    Interventional Radiology
Interventional Radiology
University of Miami
Miami, Florida

**Michele H. Johnson, MD, FACR,
    FASER**
Professor of Radiology and Biomedical
    Imaging
Department of Radiology and
    Biomedical Imaging
Yale University School of Medicine
New Haven, Connecticut

Kyle Jones, PhD
Professor
Imaging Physics
The University of Texas MD Anderson
    Cancer Centre
Houston, Texas

Rathachai Kaewlai, MD
Department of Diagnostic and
    Therapeutic Radiology
Mahidol University
Bangkok, Thailand

John A. Kaufman, MD, MS
Professor of Interventional Radiology
Department of Interventional Radiology
School of Medicine
Oregon Health and Science University
Portland, Oregon

Alexios Kelekis, MD, PhD
Professor of Diagnostic and
    Interventional Radiology
National and Kapodistrian University
    of Athens
2nd Dpt of Radiology, University
    Hospital Attikon
Athens, Greece

Andrew Kesselman, MD, RPVI
Assistant Professor of Vascular and
    Interventional Radiology
Department of Radiology
Weill Cornell Medicine
New York, New York

Brandon M. Key, MD
Assistant Professor of Radiology
Vascular and Interventional Radiology
Medical College of Wisconsin
Milwaukee, Wisconsin

Neil M. Khilnani, MD, FSIR, FAVLS
Associate Professor of Clinical Radiology
Weill Cornell Medicine
New York, New York

Jin Hyoung Kim, MD, PhD
Professor of Radiology
Department of Radiology
Asan Medical Centre
Seoul, South Korea

Ye Joon Kim, MD
Resident Physician
Department of Radiology
Section of Vascular and Interventional
    Radiology
University of Chicago
Chicago, Illinois

Sirish A. Kishore, MD
Assistant Professor
Department of Radiology
Weill Cornell Medical Center
New York, New York

Darren Klass, MBChB, MD, MRCS, FRCR, FRCPC
Interventional Radiologist
University of British Columbia and Cleveland Clinic London
Vancouver, Canada and London, United Kingdom

Maureen P. Kohi, MD, FSIR, FCIRSE, FAHA
Ernest H. Wood Distinguished Professor and Chair
Department of Radiology
University of North Carolina at Chapel Hill
Chapel Hill, North Carolina

Andrew R. Kolarich, MD
Diagnostic and Interventional Radiology Resident
Department of Radiology
The Johns Hopkins Hospital
Baltimore, Maryland

K. Pallav Kolli, MD
Assistant Professor of Clinical Radiology
University of California, San Francisco
San Francisco, California

Sebastian Kos, EBIR, FCIRSE
Chairman
Institute of Radiology and Nuclear Medicine
Hirslanden Klinik
St. Anna, Luzern, Switzerland

Alexander H. Lam, MD, RPVI
Assistant Professor
Department of Radiology
Weill Cornell Medicine
New York, New York

Marcus A. Lehman, MD, MBA
Assistant Professor of Anesthesiology
Anesthesiology
University of Cincinnati
Cincinnati, Ohio

Evan Lehrman, MD
Assistant Professor of Radiology and Biomedical Imaging
University of California, San Francisco
San Francisco, California

Jeffrey Leichter, MD
Assistant Professor of Clinical Interventional Radiology
University of Miami
Miami, Florida

David M. Liu, BSc, MD, FRCPC
Clinical Associate Professor
MultiCare Tacoma General Hospital
Tacoma, Washington

Robert Lookstein, MD, MHCDL, FSIR, FAHA, FSVM
Professor
Department of Diagnostic, Molecular and Interventional Radiology
Icahn School of Medicine at Mount Sinai
New York, New York

David C. Madoff, MD, FSIR, FACR, FCIRSE
Professor of Radiology, Medicine (Oncology) and Surgery (Oncology)
Vice Chair for Clinical Research
Section Chief, Interventional Radiology
Co-Director, Yale Interventional Oncology Research Lab
Department of Radiology and Biomedical Imaging
Yale School of Medicine
New Haven, Connecticut

Katherine Marchak, MD
Resident
Interventional Radiology
University of Colorado Anschutz
Aurora, Colorado

Miklos Marosfoi, MD
Assistant Professor
Tufts University School of Medicine
Division of Neurointerventional Radiology
Lahey Hospital and Medical Center
Burlington, Massachusetts

Michael L. Martin, BMSc, MD, FRCPC
Clinical Associate Professor of Radiology
University of British Columbia
Vancouver, British Columbia, Canada

Mesha L. Martinez, MD
Director of Pediatric Neurointerventional Radiology
Indiana University School of Medicine
Indianapolis, Indiana

John T. Matson, MD
Resident Physician
Vascular and Interventional Radiology
University of Virginia Health System
Charlottesville, Virginia

Alan H. Matsumoto, MD, FACR, FSIR, FAHA
Chair and Theodore E. Keats Professor of Radiology
University of Virginia Health System
Charlottesville, Virginia

DéAnn O. McNamara, MS, ACNP-BC, CRN
Clinical Educator
Division of Interventional Radiology
Brigham and Women's Hospital
Boston, Massachusetts

Donald L. Miller, MD, FSIR, FACR
Chief Medical Officer
Office of Radiological Health
Center for Devices and Radiological Health, U.S. Food and Drug Administration
Silver Spring, Maryland

Robert J. Min, MD, MBA, FSIR, FACR
Chair of Radiology
Medicine
Weill Cornell Medicine
New York, New York

Heather Molina, PA-C, MMS
Physician Assistant
Interventional Radiology
Northwestern Memorial Hospital
Chicago, Illinois

Airton Mota Moreira, MD, PhD
Interventional Radiologist
Hospital Sirio-Libanes
Sao-Paulo, Brazil

Timothy P. Murphy, MD
Chief Executive Officer
Summa Therapeutics, LLC
Providence, Rhode Island

Rakesh Navuluri, MD, FSIR
Associate Professor
IR Residency Program Director
Director, IR Clinic
Vascular and Interventional Radiology
The University of Chicago
Chicago, Illinois

Andrew S. Niekamp, MD
Vascular Interventional Radiologist
Radiology Associates of South Florida
Miami, Florida

Emanuele Orrù, MD
Assistant Professor
Tufts University School of Medicine
Division of Neurointerventional Radiology
Lahey Hospital and Medical Center
Burlington, Massachusetts

Johanna M. Ospel, MD, PhD
Radiologist
University Hospital Basel
Basel, Switzerland

Siddharth A. Padia, MD
Professor of Radiology
Interventional Radiology
David Geffen School of Medicine at UCLA
Los Angeles, California

Aneeta Parthipun, MBBS, FRCR
International Radiology Consultation
Guy's and St Thomas' NHS Foundation Trust
London, United Kingdom

Neil V. Patel, MD
Assistant Professor
Tufts University School of Medicine
Division of Neurointerventional Radiology
Lahey Hospital and Medical Center
Burlington, Massachusetts

Sheena Patel, MPH
Senior Manager
Guidelines and Standards
Society of Interventional Radiology
Fairfax, Virginia

Aalpen A. Patel, MD, MBA
Chair, Department of Radiology:
Medical Director of AI
Professor of Radiology, School of Medicine
Geisinger Medical Center
Danville, Pennsylvania

Edward F. Patz Jr, MD
James and Alice Chen Professor of Radiology
Professor of Pharmacology and Cancer Biology
Duke University Medical Center
Durham, North Carolina

Joseph F. Polak, MD, MPH, FAIUM, FACR
Professor of Radiology
Tufts University School of Medicine
Adjunct Professor of Radiology
Boston University School of Medicine
Boston, Massachusetts

Jeffrey S. Pollak, MD
The Robert I. White, Jr. Professor of Interventional Radiology
Yale University School of Medicine
New Haven, Connecticut

Suraj Prakash, MD, MBA
Interventional Radiology Resident
Medical College of Wisconsin
Milwaukee, Wisconsin

Martin R. Prince, MD, PhD, FACR
Professor of Radiology
Cornell and Columbia Universities
New York, New York

Bradley B. Pua, MD
Assistant Professor of Radiology
New York-Presbyterian Hospital
Weill Cornell Medicine
New York, New York

Tracy Puttre, MSN, APNP, AGPCNP-C
Manager of Advanced Practice Providers
Department of Radiology
Vascular and Interventional Radiology
Diagnostic Radiology
Medical College of Wisconsin
Milwaukee, Wisconsin

Lawlor Quinlan, BA, JD
Attorney
Connors & Vilardo, LLP
Orchard Park, New York

Crystal Razavi, MD
University of Arizona
College of Medicine
Tucson, Arizona

Mahmood K. Razavi, MD, FSIR, FSVM
Director
Centre for Clinical Trials and Research
Heart and Vascular Centre
Providence St. Joseph Hospital Orange
Orange, California

Shilpa Reddy, MD
Assistant Professor of Clinical Radiology and Surgery
Radiology
Perelman School of Medicine at the University of Pennsylvania
Philadelphia, Pennsylvania

Sidney Regalado, MD
Clinical Assistant Professor of Radiology
NorthShore University HealthSystem
University of Chicago Hospitals
Evanston, Illinois

Stephen P. Reis, MD, MBA, FSIR
Assistant Professor of Radiology
Division of Interventional Radiology
Columbia University Irving Medical Center
New York, New York

Ahsun Riaz, MD
Associate Professor of Radiology
Co-Director
Complex Hepatobiliary Interventions and Portal Hypertension
Interventional Radiology
Northwestern University
Chicago, Illinois

William S. Rilling, MD, FSIR
Professor
Interventional Radiology
Medical College of Wisconsin
Milwaukee, Wisconsin

Anne Roberts, MD
Professor of Radiology
Interventional Radiology
University of California, San Diego
La Jolla, California

Arthur Oliver Romero, MD, MSC, FCCP
Assistant Professor
Department of Internal Medicine
Kirk Kerkorian School of Medicine
University of Nevada
Las Vegas, Nevada

David A. Rosenthal, MHP, PA-C, DFAAPA
Chief Physician Assistant
Division of Interventional Radiology
Brigham and Women's Hospital
Boston, Massachusetts

Wael E. A. Saad, MD, FSIR
Professor and Director of Vascular &
    Interventional Radiology
Vice Chair of Image-guided Procedures
Department Radiology & Imaging
    Sciences
University of Utah
Salt Lake City, Utah

Tarun Sabharwal, MBBCh, FRCSI,
    FRCR, FSIR, FCIRSE, EBIR
Consultant Interventional Radiologist
Department of Interventional Radiology
Guy's and St. Thomas' Hospitals
London, United Kingdom

Riad Salem, MD, MBA
Professor of Radiology, Medicine, and
    Surgery
Northwestern University
Chicago, Illinois

Matthew J. Scheidt, MD
Assistant Professor of Radiology
Associate Program Director of
    Interventional Radiology Residency
Vascular Interventional Radiology
Medical College of Wisconsin
Milwaukee, Wisconsin

Kimberly L. Scherer, DO
Assistant Professor of Radiology
Division of Interventional Radiology
Weill Cornell Medicine
New York, New York

Todd Schlachter, MD
Assistant Professor
Department of Radiology and
    Biomedical Imaging
Yale University School of Medicine
New Haven, Connecticut

Kristofer Schramm, MD
Radiology, INC
Mount Carmel Health System
Columbus, Ohio

Beth A. Schueler, PhD
Medical Physics Division
Department of Radiology
Mayo Clinic
Rochester, Minnesota

Eric J. Seeley, MD
Interventional Pulmonologist
Bronchoscopy and Interventional
    Pulmonary Medicine
University of California, San Francisco
San Francisco, California

J. Anthony Seibert, PhD, FAAPM,
    FACR
Professor
Department of Radiology
University of California Davis Health
    System
Sacramento, California

Daniel P. Sheeran, MD
Interventional Radiologist
Department of Radiology and Medical
    Imaging
The University of Virginia
Charlottesville, Virginia

Ji Hoon Shin, MD
Section Director
Professor of Radiology
Interventional Radiology
Asan Medical Center
University of Ulsan
Seoul, South Korea

Andrew Sideris, MD
Resident
Interventional Radiology
New York-Presbyterian Columbia
    University
New York, New York

Stuart G. Silverman, MD, FACR
Professor of Radiology
Brigham and Women's Hospital
Harvard Medical School
Boston, Massachusetts

Ajay K. Singh, MD
Assistant Professor of Radiology
Massachusetts General Hospital
Harvard Medical School
Boston, Massachusetts

Akhilesh K. Sista, MD, FSIR, FAHA
Associate Professor
Vascular and Interventional Radiology
Radiology
NYU Grossman School of Medicine
New York, New York

Stephen B. Solomon, MD
Chief of Interventional Radiology
Memorial Sloan Kettering Cancer Center
New York, New York

Ho-Young Song, MD, PhD
Professor of Radiology
Asan Medical Center
University of Ulsan
Seoul, South Korea

Michael C. Soulen, MD, FSIR, FCIRSE
Professor of Radiology and Surgery
University of Pennsylvania
Philadelphia, Pennsylvania

Gilles Soulez, MD, MSc, FRCPC, FSIR
Professor of Radiology
Centre Hospitalier de l'Université de Montréal
Montreal, Quebec, Canada

James B. Spies, MD, MPH
MPH Professor of Radiology
Georgetown University School of Medicine
Washington, DC

Brian Stainken, MD
Interventional Radiologist
Stamford Hospital
Stamford, Connecticut

Keith J. Strauss, MSc, FAAPM, FACR
Assistant Professor of Radiology
University of Cincinnati School of Medicine
Cincinnati, Ohio

Reza Talaeie, MD
Associate Professor and Associate Program Director IR/DR Residency
Department of Radiology
University of Minnesota
Minneapolis, Minnesota

Alda Tam, MD, MBA
Professor
Interventional Radiology
The University of Texas MD Anderson Cancer Center
Houston, Texas

Ashraf Thabet, MD
Radiologist
Radiology
Massachusetts General Hospital
Boston, Massachusetts

Iakovos Theodoulou, BSc (Hons), MBBS, FHEA
Interventional Radiologist
Guy's and St Thomas' NHS Foundation Trust
London, United Kingdom

Nanda Deepa Thimmappa, MD
Assistant Professor of Clinical Radiology
University of Missouri School of Medicine
Columbia, Missouri

Lindsay Marie Thornton, MD
Assistant Professor
Clinical Interventional Radiology
University of Miami Miller School of Medicine
Miami, Florida

Scott O. Trerotola, MD
Stanley Baum Professor of Radiology and Professor of Radiology in Surgery
Vice Chair for Quality, Radiology
Associate Chair and Chief, Interventional Radiology
Director, Penn HHT Center of Excellence
Perelman School of Medicine at the University of Pennsylvania
Philadelphia, Pennsylvania

David W. Trost, MD
Associate Professor of Clinical Radiology
New York-Presbyterian Hospital/ Weill Cornell Medical Center
New York, New York

Sean M. Tutton, MD, FSIR, FCIRSE
Professor of Radiology and Orthopedics
University of California
San Diego, California

Alexander Ushinsky, MD
Assistant Professor of Interventional Radiology
Department of Radiology
Washington University in St. Louis
St. Louis, Missouri

Venu Vadlamudi, MD, RPVI, FSIR, FSVM, FASA, FACC
Associate professor
Department of Radiology
The University of Tennessee Health Science Centre
Memphis, Tennessee

Thuong G. Van Ha, MD
Professor of Radiology
University of Chicago Medicine
Chicago, Illinois

Emily Vande Slunt, BSRT (R)(VI)
Interventional Radiology Technologist
Froedtert Hospital
Milwaukee, Wisconsin

Suresh Vedantham, MD
Professor of Radiology and Surgery
Washington University School of Medicine
St. Louis, Missouri

Vibhor Wadhwa, MD, EBIR
Interventional Radiology Fellow
Department of Radiology
NewYork-Presbyterian/Weill Cornell Medical Center
New York, New York

Ajay K. Wakhloo, MD, PhD, FAHA
Professor
Tufts University School of Medicine
Chief
Division of Neurointerventional Radiology
Lahey Hospital and Medical Center
Burlington, Massachusetts

David S. Wang, MD
Clinical Assistant Professor of Radiology
Stanford University School of Medicine
Stanford, California

Shantanu Warhadpande, MD
Assistant Professor, Interventional Radiology
University of Michigan Medical Center
Ann Arbor, Michigan

Joshua L. Weintraub, MD, FSIR
Professor of Radiology
New York-Presbyterian Hospital/Columbia University Medical Center
New York, New York

Evelyn P. Wempe, MBA, MSN, ARNP, ACNP-BC, AOCNP, CRN
Director of Nursing, Interventional Radiology
University of Miami Miller School of Medicine
Miami, Florida

Luke R. Wilkins, MD
Assistant Professor of Radiology
University of Virginia
Charlottesville, Virginia

Zachary M. Wilseck, MD
Fellow, Neuroradiology and Neurointerventional Radiology
Division of Neuroradiology
Department of Radiology
Michigan Medicine
Ann Arbor, Michigan

Ronald S. Winokur, MD, FSIR, RPVI
Assistant Professor of Radiology
Weill Cornell Medicine
New York, New York

David F. Yankelevitz, MD
Professor of Radiology
Icahn School of Medicine at Mount Sinai
New York, New York

Don C. Yoo, MD
Associate Professor of Radiology (Clinical)
The Warren Alpert Medical School of Brown University
Providence, Rhode Island

Chang Jin Yoon, MD
Professor
Department of Radiology
Seoul National University College of Medicine
Seoul, South Korea

Jessica H. Yoon, MD, MBA
Interventional Radiology Resident
Department of Diagnostic Imaging
Brown University
Providence, Rhode Island

Joseph Zikri, MD
Assistant Professor
Department Interventional Radiology
University of Miami Miller School of Medicine
Miami, Florida

ABOUT THE EDITORS

ROBERT J. LEWANDOWSKI, MD

Professor of Radiology, Medicine, and Surgery in the Feinberg School of Medicine at Northwestern University. He serves as the Director of Interventional Oncology at the Northwestern University Robert H. Lurie Comprehensive Cancer Center. Dr. Lewandowski joined the staff at Northwestern in 2006 upon completion of his fellowship training in Vascular and Interventional Radiology. Dr. Lewandowski received his medical degree from Michigan State University College of Human Medicine in 1999, and he completed a Diagnostic Radiology Residency at William Beaumont Hospital in Royal Oak, Michigan in 2005.

LINDSAY MACHAN, MD

Associate Professor of Radiology, University of British Columbia and Interventional Radiologist, Vancouver Hospital, Vancouver, Canada. Previously served as regional lead, Interventional Radiology Vancouver Coastal Health, and interventional radiologist at the Hammersmith Hospital in London, United Kingdom, and the Hospital of the University of Pennsylvania in Philadelphia, Pennsylvania. He received his MD from the University of Alberta, Edmonton, Canada. Diagnostic Radiology residency and Interventional fellowship were completed at the University of British Columbia. He is a past President of the Western Angiographic and Interventional Society and a founding member of the Canadian Interventional Radiology Association. He was a co-founder of Angiotech Pharmaceuticals, Inc., and Ikomed Medical, Vancouver, Canada, both medical device companies.

PARAG J. PATEL, MD, MS

Professor of Radiology & Surgery, Medical College of Wisconsin, Froedtert Hospital, Milwaukee, Wisconsin. He received his MD, MS, and Diagnostic Radiology training at Loyola University Stritch School of Medicine in Maywood, Illinois. He completed his Vascular & Interventional Radiology fellowship training at the Miami Cardiac & Vascular Institute in Miami, Florida. He is the Program Director of the Interventional Radiology residency at the Medical College of Wisconsin and was the Graduate Medical Education Councilor for the Society of Interventional Radiology before serving as the President of the Society of Interventional Radiology.

KRISHNA KANDARPA, MD, PhD

Director, Research Sciences and Strategic Directions, National Institute of Biomedical Imaging and Bioengineering, National Institutes of Health, Bethesda, Maryland. Previously, he served as Chief Medical and Scientific

Officer, Delcath Systems, Inc., New York, New York; Professor and Chair of Radiology at the University of Massachusetts Medical School and Radiologist-in-Chief, UMass Memorial Medical Center, Worcester, Massachusetts; Professor of Radiology, Cornell Medical School, and Chief of Service, Cardiovascular & Interventional Radiology, New York-Presbyterian Hospital, New York, New York; Associate Professor of Radiology, Harvard Medical School; and Co-Director, Cardiovascular & Interventional Radiology, Brigham and Women's Hospital, Boston, Massachusetts. He received a doctorate in Engineering Science from Pennsylvania State University, State College, Pennsylvania, and a doctorate in medicine from the University of Miami, Miami, Florida. He was past President and Chair of the SIR Research & Education Foundation and on the Board of Directors, Academy of Radiology Research.

FOREWORD

The field of interventional radiology continues to grow and to change. The scope of care provided by this critical medical discipline has advanced rapidly over the three decades since the very first edition of this *Handbook* in 1989. There are few other disciplines that have changed so much in this brief amount of time. The scope of this change is represented by the table of contents that has expanded to over 100 chapters, and more important, the *Handbook* continues to emphasize not only procedures that have been described in previous editions but also the important expanding roles of endovascular and nonvascular interventional therapies for a multitude of disease states.

In this edition, reflecting changes in the health care delivery, important chapters on quality assurance and improvement, risk management, as well as safety—including radiation and infection control—have been expanded, commensurate with the maturation of the field and its role in organized medicine. Clinical practice of interventional radiology has continued to grow and there are sections that focus on patient management, both during the procedure of course, but also on the management pre- and postprocedure, providing the reader with a complete compendium of necessary information in a concise and easy to navigate format.

It is hard to imagine how the *Handbook of Interventional Radiologic Procedures* could possibly improve over prior editions. Since its initial publication, this *Handbook* has become an essential reference for interventionalists at all levels of experience. It will undoubtedly be essential for residents and fellows during their training and should remain an important reference for practitioners who will benefit from the valuable practical information contained in this volume.

The field of interventional radiology continues to evolve as both a clinical and a procedural discipline. The challenges of creating a comprehensive handbook of practical information in a volume that can actually be carried around has become more difficult with continued expansion of the scope and numbers of interventional procedures. Yet the editors and authors have amassed a volume that remains brisk and focused in style, extremely well organized and catalogued to make it easy for the reader to get critical information when necessary, in both hard copy and electronic format, in the treatment of specific patients. This handbook is a tool in the hands of interventionalists, which is as helpful as any of the devices that may be used in specific procedures. In keeping with the times, an updated electronic version for handheld devices is once again provided.

As in the past, I'm certain that the sixth edition of the *Handbook of Interventional Radiologic Procedures* will become an indispensable tool and resource in the lab coat of all interventional radiologists and staff performing these procedures.

Barry T. Katzen, MD, FACC, FACR, FSIR

PREFACE

From inability to let well alone; from too much zeal for the new and contempt for what is old; from putting knowledge before wisdom, science before art, and cleverness before common sense, from treating patients as cases, and from making the cure of the disease more grievous than the endurance of the same, Good Lord, deliver us.

Sir Robert Hutchinson

Correspondence regarding modern treatment in the *British Medical Journal*, March 12, 1953, p. 671.

Interventional radiology is a vibrant and growing field. It has evolved rapidly due, in large part, to the ingenuity of its practitioners. Although it is true that necessity may have mothered many inventions, for IR, scientific and technologic advances and competitive pressures have done much to motivate an innovational spirit. Future success will depend not only on the continued innovations by practitioners but, more importantly, for them to proactively embrace the clinical management of patients. Fortunately, the pace of innovations and the specialty's acquisition of clinical management skills have necessitated this 6th *Handbook of Interventional Radiologic Procedures*. In fact, the number and variety of IR procedures has increased to such a degree, that the printed version, originally intended to be carried in the pocket, was soon to become a doorstop. But, fortunately, advances in information technology and publication trends have pushed us into electronic versions. For this edition, as for the last one, we have a portable printed version and provide access to an e-Book, which includes important ancillary information that is not immediately necessary for day-to-day practice. These ancillary chapters remain an important part of the practitioners' armamentarium.

The book is designed to serve as a resource for practicing interventional radiologists, IR fellows, radiology residents in training, and for those skilled general radiologists who continue to perform IR procedures. This book has served similarly for nurses and special procedure technologists, complementing their own vital knowledge and skills which they bring to the suite.

We realize that there is no single way to perform a procedure and do not intend to be rigidly prescriptive. We intend rather to provide a framework that the interventionalist can use and build upon as experience is gained. As in prior editions, each chapter has been organized in a consistent outline format to facilitate easy access to specific sections on indications and contraindications, preprocedure preparation, procedural protocol, postprocedure care, and expected outcomes—all toward *improving patient safety* by preventing complications, or managing them appropriately when they do occur. This latter information is especially useful while the procedure is being discussed with the patient before obtaining informed consent. We have—to the best of our ability—corrected mistakes and oversights from prior editions.

We are eternally grateful to all of the contributors worldwide for their generosity and painstaking efforts in creating what we hope will be another successful handbook. We thank Dr. Barry Katzen for kindly writing the foreword. We thank Eric McDermott of Wolters Kluwer for guiding us through the process.

K. K.
L. M.
P. P.
R. L.

CONTENTS

ABBREVIATIONS

A	Ankle	APTT	Activated partial thromboplastin time
AAA	Abdominal aortic aneurysm	ARDS	Adult respiratory distress syndrome
AASLD	American Association for the Study of Liver Diseases	ARNP	Advanced registered nurse practitioner
ABI	Ankle-brachial index	ASA	Acetylsalicylic acid
ACA	Anterior cerebral artery	ASA	American Society of Anesthesiologists
ACAS	Asymptomatic Carotid Atherosclerosis Trial	ASD	Atrial septal defect
ACD	Advance care directives	ASPECTS	Alberta Stroke Program early computed tomography scan
ACE	Angiotensin-converting enzyme	AT	Anterior tibial
ACLS	Advanced cardiac life support	ATIII	Antithrombin III
ACR	American College of Radiology	ATM	Atmospheres
		AV	Arteriovenous
ACT	Activated clotting time	A-V	Atrioventricular
ADC	Analog-to-digital converter	AVF	Arteriovenous fistula
		AVG	Arteriovenous graft
ADH	Antidiuretic hormone	AVM	Arteriovenous malformation
ADP	Adenosine diphosphate		
AE	Adverse events	AVP	Amplatzer vascular plug
AECD	Automatic external cardioverter-defibrillator	BAC	Bronchioloalveolar carcinoma
AF	Atrial fibrillation	BAE	Bronchial artery embolization
AFB	Acid-fast bacilli		
AFP	α-Fetoprotein	BCLC	Barcelona clinic liver cancer
AGIH	Acute gastrointestinal hemorrhage	BE	Balloon expandable
AHRQ	Agency for Healthcare Research and Quality	β-hCG	Beta human chorionic gonadotropin hormone
AK	Above-knee	BGC	Balloon-guiding catheter
ALS	Amyotrophic lateral sclerosis	bid	Two times per day
AMFPI	Active matrix flat-panel imager	BIPAP	Bi-level positive airway pressure
AMI	Acute mesenteric ischemia	BLS	Basic life support
		BMI	Body mass index
AML	Angiomyolipoma	BMS	Bare-metal stents
Ao	Aorta	BMT	Bone marrow transplant
AP	Anteroposterior	BOT	Balloon occlusion tolerance
APD	All-purpose drainage		
APF	Arterioportal fistula	BP	Blood pressure

BPH	Benign prostatic hyperplasia	CLI	Critical limb ischemia
BRTO	Balloon-occluded retrograde transvenous obliteration	CMS	Centers for Medicare and Medicaid Services
BTK	Below-the-knee	CNS	Central nervous system
BUN	Blood urea nitrogen	COPD	Chronic obstructive pulmonary disease
BW	Bandwidth	COX	Cyclooxygenase
CABG	Coronary artery bypass graft	CP	Cerebral protection
CAD	Coronary artery disease	CPAP	Continuous positive airway pressure
CAS	Carotid artery stenting	CPAS	Congenital pulmonary artery stenosis
CASH	Chemotherapy-associated steatohepatitis	CPOE	Computerized physician order entry
CAVATAS	Carotid and Vertebral Artery Transluminal Angioplasty Study	CPR	Cardiopulmonary resuscitation
CaVenT	Catheter-directed venous thrombolysis	CPRF	Curved planar reformats
CBC	Complete blood count	CPT	Current procedural terminology
CBCT	Cone-beam computed tomography	Cr	Creatinine (serum)
CBF	Cerebral blood flow	CQI	Continuous quality improvement
CBV	Cerebral blood volume	CR-BSI	Catheter-related bloodstream infections
CC	Cisterna chyli	CRC	Colorectal cancer
CCA	Common carotid artery	CREST	Carotid Revascularization Endarterectomy versus Stenting Trial
CCD	Charge-coupled device		
CCS	Canadian Cardiovascular Society	CRP	C-reactive protein
CDC	Centers for Disease Control and Prevention	CSF	Cerebrospinal fluid
		CsI	Cesium iodide
CDT	Catheter-directed thrombolysis	CT	Computed tomography
		CTA	Computed tomographic angiography
CEA	Carcinoembryonic antigen; carotid endarterectomy	cTACE	Conventional transarterial chemoembolization
CFA	Common femoral artery	CTO	Chronic total occlusion
CFV	Common femoral vein	CTP	CT perfusion
CHA	Common hepatic artery	CTV	Computed tomography venography
CHF	Congestive heart failure		
CIA	Common iliac artery	CV	Central venous
CIN	Contrast-induced nephropathy	CVA	Cerebral vascular accident
		CVC	Central venous catheter
CIWA	Clinical Institute Withdrawal Assessment	CVD	Chronic venous disease
		CXR	Chest radiograph; chest x-ray
CKD	Chronic kidney disease		
CLABSI	Central line–associated bloodstream infection	D5½NS	5% dextrose, half-normal saline solution

D5W	5% Dextrose solution	EIA	External iliac artery
DAP	Dose–area product	ENT	Ear, nose, and throat
DAVF	Dural arteriovenous fistula	EPD	Embolic protection device
DCI	Delayed cerebral ischemia	ERCP	Endoscopic retrograde
DEB	Drug-eluting bead;		cholangiopancreatography
	drug-eluting balloon	ERF	Esophagorespiratory
DER	Dual-energy radiography		fistula
DES	Drug-eluting stent	ESBL	Extended-spectrum
DH	Degree of hypertrophy		beta-lactamase
DIC	Disseminated intra-	ESCAPE	Endovascular Treatment
	vascular coagulopathy		for Small Core and Ante-
DICOM	Digital imaging and com-		rior Circulation Proximal
	munication in medicine		Occlusion with Emphasis
DIPS	Direct intrahepatic		on Minimizing CT to
	portosystemic shunt		Recanalization Times
DLGJ	Double-lumen gastrojeju-	ESI	Epidural steroid injection
	nostomy	ESWL	Extracorporeal shock
DIR	Dose Index Registry;		wave lithotripsy
	double inversion recovery	EUS	Endoscopic ultrasound
DM	Diabetes mellitus	EVA-3S	Endarterectomy versus
DMSO	Dimethyl sulfoxide		angioplasty in patients
DNI	Do not intubate		with symptomatic severe
DNR	Do not resuscitate		carotid stenosis
DOQI	Disease Outcomes	EVAR	Endovascular aortic
	Quality Initiative		aneurysm repair
DQE	Detective quantum	EVLT	Endovenous laser
	efficiency		treatment
DSA	Digital subtraction	EVOH	Ethylene vinyl alcohol
	angiography	EXTEND-	Extending the time for
DTPA	Diethylenetriamine	IA	thrombolysis in emer-
	pentaacetic acid		gency neurological
DUS	Doppler ultrasound;		deficits–intra-arterial
	duplex ultrasound	FB	Foreign body
DVT	Deep vein thrombosis	FDA	U.S. Food and Drug
E&M	Evaluation and		Administration
	Management	FDG-PET	Positron emission
EASL	European Association for		tomography
	the Study of the Liver	^{18}F-FDG	^{18}F-fluorodeoxyglucose
ECG	Electrocardiogram	FFP	Fresh frozen plasma
ECOG	Eastern Cooperative	FHVP	Free hepatic venous
	Oncology Group		pressure
ECST	European Carotid	FLR	Future liver remnant
	Surgery Trial	FNA	Fine-needle aspiration
ED	Emergency department	FNH	Focal nodular hyperplasia
EDV	End-diastolic velocity	FOV	Field-of-view
EGFR	Epidermal growth factor	GA	General anesthesia
	receptor	GABA	γ-Aminobutyric acid
eGFR	Estimated GFR	Gd	Gadolinium

GDA	Gastroduodenal artery
GDC	Gugliemi detachable coil
Gd-MRA	Gadolinium enhanced MRA
GFR	Glomerular filtration rate
GI	Gastrointestinal
GJ	Gastrojejunostomy
GP	Glycoprotein
GSV	Greater saphenous vein
GU	Genitourinary
GW	Guidewire
HA	Hepatic artery
HAP	Hepatic artery pseudoaneurysm
HAS	Hepatic artery stenosis
HASTE	Half-Fourier acquisitions with single-shot turbo-spin echo
HAT	Hepatic artery thrombosis
HCC	Hepatocellular carcinoma
HCFMEA	Health Care Failure Mode and Effects Analysis
hCG	Human chorionic gonadotropin
HCl	Hydrochloride
Hct	Hematocrit
HD	Hemodialysis
Hgb	Hemoglobin
HHT	Hereditary hemorrhagic telangiectasia
HIFU	High-intensity focused ultrasound
HIT	Heparin-induced thrombocytopenia
HITT	Heparin-induced thrombocytopenia with thrombosis syndrome
HMPAO	Hexamethylpropylene-amine oxime
HMW	High-molecular-weight
HOCA	High-osmolality contrast agents
HPS	Hepatopulmonary syndrome
HR	Hazard ratio; heart rate
HSG	Hysterosalpingogram
HT	High thigh
HTN	Hypertension

HU	Hounsfield unit
HV	Hepatic venous
HVPG	Hepatic venous pressure gradient
IA	Intra-arterial
IC	Intracranial
ICA	Internal carotid artery
ICBT	Intercostobronchial trunk
ICD-10	International Classification of Diseases, 10th revision
ICH	Intracerebral hemorrhage
ICP	Intracranial pressure
ICSS	International Carotid Stenting Study
ICU	Intensive care unit
ID	Internal diameter
IFU	Instructions for use
IHI	Institute for Healthcare Improvement
IHSS	Idiopathic hypertrophic subaortic stenosis
II	Image intensifier
IIA	Internal iliac artery
IIEF	International Index of Erectile Function
IJ	Internal jugular
IJV	Internal jugular vein
IM	Intramuscular
IMA	Inferior mesenteric artery; internal mammary artery
IMS III	Interventional Management of Stroke III
IMV	Inferior mesenteric vein
INR	International normalized ratio
IO	Interventional oncology
IOM	Institute of Medicine
IPSS	International Prostate Symptom Score
IQR	Interquartile range
IR	Interventional radiology; interventional radiologist
IRE	Irreversible electroporation
ISAT	International Subarachnoid Aneurysm Trial

ISV	Internal spermatic vein	MAO	Monoamine oxidase
ITT	Intention to treat	MAP	Mean arterial pressure
IV	Intravenous; intravenously	MBB	Medial branch block
IVA	Inferior vesical artery	MC	Manual compression
IVC	Inferior vena cava	MCA	Middle cerebral artery
IVUS	Intravascular ultrasound	mCRC	Metastatic colon cancer
J-tube	Jejunostomy	mCTA	Multiphase CTA
KAP	Kerma–area product	MD	Medical doctor
KGR	Kinetic growth rate	MI	Myocardial infarction
KP	Kyphoplasty	MIP	Maximum intensity projection
K-RAS	Kirsten Rat Sarcoma Viral Oncogene Homolog	MODS	Multiple organ dysfunction syndrome
KTS	Klippel–Trenaunay syndrome	MPA	Multipurpose shape
kVp	Kilovolt peak	MPR	Multiplanar reformations
KVO	Keep vein open	MR	Magnetic resonance
LA	Left atrial; left atrium	MRA	Magnetic resonance angiography
LAD	Left anterior descending		
LAO	Left anterior oblique	MR CLEAN	Multicenter Randomized Clinical Trial of Endovascular Treatment for Acute Ischemic Stroke in the Netherlands
LCD	Liquid crystal display		
LDCT	Low-dose CT		
LDH	Lactate dehydrogenase		
LDL	Low-density lipoprotein		
LFT	Liver function test	MRCP	Magnetic resonance cholangiopancreatography
LGIB	Lower GI bleeding		
LM	Lymphatic malformations	MRDSA	Magnetic resonance digital subtraction angiography
LMA	Laryngeal mask airway		
LMWH	Low–molecular-weight heparin		
		mRECIST	Modified Response Evaluation Criteria in Solid Tumors
LOCA	Low-osmolality contrast agents		
		MR RESCUE	Mechanical Retrieval and Recanalization of Stroke Clots Using Embolectomy
LOCM	Low osmolar contrast medium		
LSCA	Left subclavian artery		
LSF	Lung shunt fraction	MRI	Magnetic resonance imaging
LSN	Last seen normal		
LUTS	Lower urinary tract symptoms	MRV	Magnetic resonance venogram; magnetic resonance venography
LV	Left ventricle; left ventricular		
		mTICI	Modified thrombolysis in cerebral infarction
LVEDP	Left ventricular end-diastolic pressure		
		MTT	Mean transit time
LVEDV	Left ventricular end-diastolic volume	MWA	Microwave ablation
		nAC	n-Acetyl cysteine
LVO	Large vessel occlusion	$NaHCO_3$	Sodium bicarbonate
MAA	Macroaggregated albumin	NASCET	North American Symptomatic Carotid Endarterectomy Trial
MAC	Monitored anesthesia care		

nBCA	*n*-Butyl cyanoacrylate
NCCT	Noncontrast computed tomography
NG	Nasogastric
NG-tube	Nasogastric tube
NIH	National Institutes of Health
NIHSS	National Institutes of Health Stroke Scale
NINDS	National Institute of Neurological Disorders and Stroke
NKF-KDOQI	National Kidney Foundation Kidney Disease Outcomes Quality Initiative
NLST	National Lung Screening Trial
NOHAH	Nonocclusive hepatic artery hypoperfusion syndrome
NOMI	Nonocclusive mesenteric ischemia
NPH	Neutral protamine Hagedorn
NPO	Nil per os
NS	Normal saline
NSAID	Nonsteroidal anti-inflammatory drug
NSCLC	Non–small cell lung cancer
NSF	Nephrogenic systemic fibrosis
NTG	Nitroglycerin
NYHA	New York Heart Association
OD	Outer diameter
OP	Outpatient
OPSI	Overwhelming post-splenectomy infection
OR	Operating room
OSA	Obstructive sleep apnea
PA	Physician's assistant; pulmonary artery
PACS	Picture archiving and communication system
PAD	Peripheral arterial disease; pulmonary artery diastolic
PAE	Prostate artery embolization
PAP	Pulmonary arterial pressure
PARTO	Plug-assisted retrograde transvenous obliteration
PAVM	Pulmonary arteriovenous malformation
PBD	Percutaneous biliary drainage
PCA	Patient-controlled analgesia; posterior cerebral artery
PCC	Prothrombin complex concentrate
PCDT	Pharmacomechanical catheter-directed thrombolysis
PCI	Percutaneous coronary intervention
PC-MRA	Phase contrast-MRA
PCN	Percutaneous nephrostomy
PCORI	Patient-Centered Outcomes Research Institute
PCSA	Patient-controlled sedation
PCW	Pulmonary capillary wedge
PCWP	Pulmonary capillary wedge pressure
PD	Peritoneal dialysis
PDCA	Plan–Do–Check–Act
PE	Peroneal; pulmonary embolism/embolus
PEEP	Positive end-expiratory pressure
PEG	Polyethylene glycol
PEM	Polidocanol endovenous microfoam
PERP	Patient entrance reference point
PET	Positron emission tomography
PFO	Patent foramen ovale
PGA	Polyglycolic acid
PGJ	Percutaneous gastrojejunostomy

PIAA	Physician Insurers Association of America	QA	Quality assurance
PICC	Peripherally inserted central catheter	qEASL	Quantitative European Association for the Study of the Liver
PIOPED	Prospective Investigation of Pulmonary Embolism Diagnosis	qid	Four times per day
		QISS	Quiescent interval single shot
PJ	Percutaneous jejunostomy	QOL	Quality of life
PMMA	Polymethylmethacrylate	RA	Right atrium
PMT	Percutaneous mechanical thrombectomy	RAO	Right anterior oblique
		RAPTURE	Radiofrequency Ablation of Pulmonary Tumors Response Evaluation
PO	By mouth		
PPH	Postpartum hemorrhage		
P-PS	Power-pulse spray	RAS	Renal artery stenosis
pr	Per rectum	RBBB	Right bundle branch block
PRBC	Packed red blood cell	RBC	Red blood cell
PRG	Percutaneous radiologic gastrostomy	RCA	Root cause analysis
		RCC	Renal cell carcinoma
PSA	Pseudoaneurysm	RCT	Randomized controlled trial
PSA	Prostate-specific antigen		
PSD	Peak skin dose	RF	Radiofrequency
PSV	Peak systolic velocity	RFA	Radiofrequency ablation
PT	Prothrombin time; posterior tibial	RHV	Right hepatic vein
		RI	Renal insufficiency; resistive index
PTA	Percutaneous transluminal (balloon) angioplasty	RIJ	Right internal jugular
PTC	Percutaneous transhepatic cholangiography	RIM	Rösch inferior mesenteric
PTD	Percutaneous thrombolytic device	RN	Registered nurse
		ROBOT	Rotational bidirectional thrombectomy
PTFE	Polytetrafluoroethylene		
PTRA	Percutaneous transluminal renal angioplasty	ROI	Region of interest
		ROSE	Rapid on site evaluation
PTS	Postthrombotic syndrome	RPO	Right posterior oblique
PTT	Partial thromboplastin time	RR	Respiratory rate
		RT	Respiratory therapist
PTX	Pneumothorax	rt-PA	Recombinant tissue plasminogen activator
PV	Percutaneous vertebroplasty; portal vein/venous	RV	Right ventricle
PVA	Polyvinyl alcohol	RVEDP	Right ventricular end-diastolic pressure
PVC	Premature ventricular contraction		
		RVR	Renal vein renin
PVE	Portal vein embolization	SAH	Subarachnoid hemorrhage
PVR	Pulmonary vascular resistance; pulse volume recording		
		SAP	Superabsorbent polymer
		SBP	Systolic blood pressure
PVS	Portal vein stenosis	SBRT	Stereotactic body radiotherapy
PVT	Portal vein thrombosis		

SC	Subcutaneous; subclavian
SEER	Surveillance, Epidemiology, and End Results
SEMS	Self-expanding metallic stents
SEV	Superficial epigastric vein
SFA	Superficial femoral artery
sFLR	Standardized future liver remnant
SI	Sacroiliac
SICH	Symptomatic intracranial hemorrhage
SIN	Salpingitis isthmica nodosa
SIR	Society of Interventional Radiology
SIRS	Systemic inflammatory response syndrome
SK	Streptokinase
SMA	Superior mesenteric artery
SMV	Superior mesenteric vein
SNMMI	Society of Nuclear Medicine and Molecular Imaging
SNR	Signal-to-noise ratio
SNRB	Selective nerve root block
SPACE	Stent-supported percutaneous angioplasty of the carotid artery versus endarterectomy
SPECT	Single-photon emission computed tomography
SPGR	Spoiled gradient echo
SPN	Solitary pulmonary nodules
SQ	Subcutaneous
SSFP	Steady-state free precession
SSFSE	Single-shot fast spin echo
SSI	Surgical site infection
SSV	Short saphenous vein
STIR	Short T1 inversion recovery
STS	Sodium tetradecyl sulfate
SUV	Standardized uptake value
SVC	Superior vena cava
SVR	Systemic vascular resistance
SVS	Society of Vascular Surgery

SVT	Superficial venous thrombosis
SWIFT PRIME	Solitaire with the Intention for Thrombectomy as Primary Endovascular Treatment
TA	Tumescent anesthesia
TAA	Thoracic aortic aneurysm
TACE	Transarterial chemoembolization
TAE	Transarterial embolization
TCD	Transcranial Doppler
TcPO$_2$	Transcutaneous oxygen pressure
TD	Thoracic duct
TDE	Thoracic duct embolization
TEE	Transesophageal echo
TELV	Total estimated liver volume
TEVAR	Thoracic endovascular aortic repair
TFT	Thin-film transistor
TIA	Transient ischemic attack
TIPS	Transjugular intrahepatic portosystemic shunt
TLR	Target lesion revascularization
TLV	Total liver volume
TNB	Transthoracic needle biopsy
TNK	Tenecteplase
TNM	Tumor, node, metastasis
TOF	Time-of-flight
TOPAS	Thrombolysis or peripheral arterial surgery
TPN	Total parenteral nutrition
TR	Repetition time
TRICKS	Time resolved imaging of contrast kinetics
TTP	Thrombotic thrombocytopenic purpura; time to peak
TTS	Time to start
TURP	Transurethral resection of prostate
UAE	Uterine artery embolization

UFE	Uterine fibroid embolization	VIPR	Vastly undersampled isotropic projection reconstruction
UK	Urokinase	VM	Venous malformations
UR	Urinary retention	V̇/Q̇	Ventilation/perfusion
US	Ultrasound	VS	Vital signs
UTI	Urinary tract infection	VT	Ventricular tachycardia
VAA	Visceral arterial aneurysms	VTE	Venous thromboembolism
VB	Vertebral body	WBC	White blood cell
VCD	Vascular closure device	WHO	World Health Organization
VEGF	Vascular endothelial growth factor	WHOL	Worst headache of life
VENC	Velocity encoding value	WHVP	Wedged hepatic venous pressure
VIP	V-Twist Integrated Platform		

SECTION I
VASCULAR ACCESS

1 Gaining Vascular Access
Khashayar Farsad, MD, PhD

All endovascular procedures, no matter how simple or complex, begin with gaining vascular access. It is easy to take this critical step for granted; however, when Sven Seldinger had his self-proclaimed "severe attack of common sense" in 1953 with the sequence of needle access, wire through the needle, and exchange of the needle for a catheter, reproducible success at gaining vascular access laid the foundation for what would ultimately become the field of Interventional Radiology. Vascular access options have continued to evolve with advanced image guidance and small access devices.

Retrograde Common Femoral Artery Access and Initial Catheterization

Preparation and Puncture

1. Sterile puncture-site preparation (shave off inguinal area if necessary, followed by antiseptic iodine or chlorhexidine solution scrub) and draping of the supine patient.
2. Locate the femoral artery and inguinal ligament (which runs from the anterior superior iliac spine to the pubic tubercle) by palpation (Fig. 1.1). The true position of the inguinal ligament is about 1 to 2 cm below the location estimated by palpation or fluoroscopy. The common femoral artery should be palpable approximately 1 to 2 cm below and medial to a point halfway along the inguinal ligament.
3. Identify the inferior femoral head by fluoroscopy using a metal clamp to mark the skin entry site (Fig. 1.1). The artery should be entered over the middle of the medial third of the femoral head to enable adequate compression of the artery against the femoral head at the end of the procedure. A skin entry site over the inferior femoral head allows the arterial puncture to be directly over the femoral head after the needle has passed through the subcutaneous tissues. A thinner patient can have a skin entry site more directly overlying the middle of the femoral head, and a patient with more subcutaneous tissue may require a skin entry site further inferior. A puncture window of only 3 to 5 cm is available for safe common femoral artery puncture (Fig. 1.1).
4. Localizing the puncture site by fluoroscopy over the femoral head or with specific palpation techniques for anatomical localization is important to:
   a. Prevent high arterial entry (cephalad to the inguinal ligament) that cannot be adequately compressed and therefore may lead to uncontrollable internal bleeding.
   b. Prevent low arterial entry (e.g., superficial femoral or profunda femoral artery) that may result in a pseudoaneurysm due to difficulty with manual compression.
5. Induce local anesthesia with 1% or 2% lidocaine (without epinephrine). Consider the addition of 1-mL sodium bicarbonate 8.4% in the syringe with each 10 mL of lidocaine to minimize the burning sensation during injection.

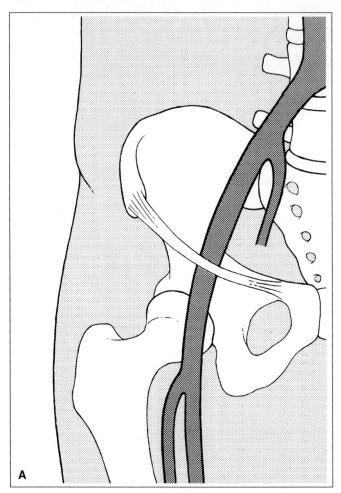

FIGURE 1.1 • Anatomical relationships of the femoral artery. **A:** Shows the common femoral artery crossing over the medial third of the femoral head. The vein (not shown) is approximately 0.5 to 1.5 cm medial to the femoral artery. Arterial and venous puncture sites should be over the femoral head and well below the inguinal ligament, which is shown crossing diagonally from the anterior superior iliac spine to the superior pubic tubercle. A hemostat is positioned to define the femoral head and proper position is checked fluoroscopically. (*continued*)

a. Create a skin wheal at the entry site (using 25-gauge, 5/8-in needle) and perform deeper injection on each side of the artery.
b. Gently aspirate as the needle is advanced and inject anesthetic upon needle withdrawal to avoid intravascular lidocaine injection. Slow, gentle injection will minimize associated pain. Onset of anesthesia occurs within 2 minutes after injection.
c. Make a superficial skin incision (3 mm long × 3 mm deep) with a no. 11 blade scalpel. Use a curved 5-in mosquito forceps to spread the subcutaneous tissues. Adequate dissection of subcutaneous tissues in this

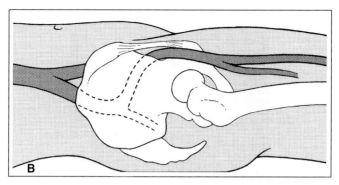

FIGURE 1.1 • (Continued) **B:** A lateral view of the same region illustrates how the external iliac artery and vein (not shown) dive deep into the pelvis above the inguinal ligament. A puncture site above the ligament cannot be compressed and could result in a large pelvic hemorrhage. Skin entry at the inferior femoral head enables the arterial access to be directly over the femoral head.

manner facilitates subsequent passage of catheters and sheaths, enables egress of blood at the skin rather than internally, and is also important when considering use of an arterial closure device to allow the device to track easily to the arteriotomy site and not get bound by the subcutaneous tissues.

6. **Puncture guided by palpation (Fig. 1.2)**
   a. Place two fingers (e.g., middle and index fingers) to palpate the artery above and below the anticipated puncture site. Apply local anesthetic, create the dermatotomy, and spread the subcutaneous tissues as described above. Advance the access needle parallel to the course of the femoral artery and at approximately 45 degrees with respect to the skin, until the arterial pulsations are felt transmitted through the needle. Enter the artery with a steady forward thrust.
   b. In obese patients and in those with prior local surgery, the anatomical landmarks may be markedly different from those expected.
   c. If difficulty is encountered in puncturing the artery, fluoroscopy may be used to direct the needle along anticipated landmarks. Alternatively, use ultrasound guidance (see below).
   d. Arterial wall calcification will occasionally provide a target by fluoroscopy.
7. Single-wall punctures are preferred and important when directly accessing vascular grafts, when the patient has abnormal clotting parameters, or for prevention of puncture-site bleeding. Careful single-wall, single-stick entry is also important if one is considering using a percutaneous arterial closure device. Improper technique can result in vessel wall trauma regardless of the type of needle used. (For available needles, see Chapter e-94.)
8. Once there is good pulsatile blood return through the needle, a guidewire should be *gently* advanced up the femoral artery without resistance, through the iliac arteries, and into the aorta under fluoroscopic guidance.
   a. Assessment if the blood return is nonpulsatile: venous puncture (puncture more laterally if necessary), needle partially intramural (reposition), and severe occlusive disease. Gentle hand injection of contrast before proceeding further can identify potential occlusive disease (Fig. 1.3).
   b. If difficulty is experienced in passing the wire out the tip of the needle, **do not force the wire.** Gentle manipulation is permissible, but it is better to pull the wire and needle out, hold pressure on the puncture site for 3 to 5 minutes, and start again.

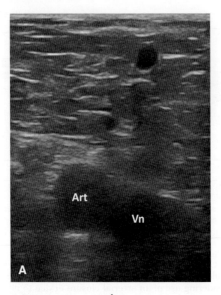

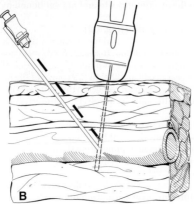

FIGURE 1.2 • A: Transverse grayscale ultrasound view of the common femoral artery (*Art*) using a linear transducer. **B:** Orientation of the transducer and needle during ultrasound-guided puncture. (*continued*)

    c. If the guidewire cannot be advanced through the iliac arteries, a 5-Fr dilator can be introduced into the femoral artery over the wire, and if brisk back-bleeding is noted, contrast may be gently injected by hand to evaluate the problem.

    d. Knowledge of the wires available and their uses will be helpful in negotiating tortuous or difficult iliac arteries (see Chapter e-94).

9. Ultrasound guidance: Routine use has demonstrated decreased frequency of access site–related complications in large retrospective and prospective series (1,2), and is recommended for all punctures. This technique allows precise identification of the common femoral artery and allows for direct single-pass puncture.

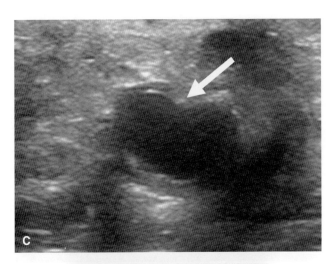

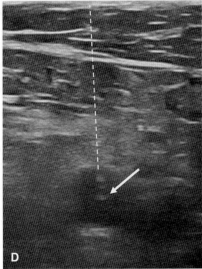

FIGURE 1.2 • (*Continued*) **C:** Artery being tented by the needle (*arrow*). **D:** Needle tip (*arrow*) seen in the artery. (*continued*)

Ultrasound guidance is ideal for patients with poorly palpable pulses and patients who are obese or who have higher bleeding risks. The technique is as follows (Fig. 1.4):

a. Localize the femoral head under fluoroscopy as described earlier.

b. Use a high-frequency linear transducer draped with a sterile probe cover.

c. Identify the common femoral artery and vein. The common femoral vein is identified by the confluence with the great saphenous vein and will be easily compressible in the absence of thrombus. The common femoral artery is directly lateral to the common femoral vein and will be pulsatile and not easily

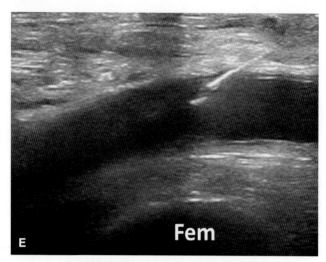

FIGURE 1.2 • (*Continued*) **E:** Longitudinal view used to illustrate the subcutaneous track and needle puncture directly over the femoral head (*Fem*).

compressible. The common femoral artery bifurcation should be identified by grayscale or color Doppler to confirm a common femoral artery puncture above the bifurcation. Acoustic shadowing from calcified plaque may obscure the artery lumen. Color Doppler can be used in this instance to confirm patency and to target for puncture if needed.

d. Puncture the artery with the ultrasound probe in transverse orientation and the needle positioned along the middle of the transducer. Standard or echogenic vascular access needles (thin-walled, 18- to 19-gauge, 2.75-in long) or 21-gauge micropuncture needles can be used. Care should be taken to puncture the anterior arterial wall and not the side of the artery due to poor visualization of the needle trajectory by ultrasound.

e. Micropuncture access kits comprise a 21-gauge echogenic needle, a 0.018-in platinum-tipped microwire, and a 4- or 5-Fr micropuncture dilator with a stiff inner stylet and an outer sheath capable of transitioning to a standard 0.035-in or 0.038-in working wire after the microwire and inner stylet are removed.

f. After confirmation of arterial puncture by blood return and, ideally, by visualization of the needle tip in the artery, a guidewire is advanced through the needle. Contrast injection can also be used to confirm common femoral artery access (Fig. 1.5).

Catheterization

1. Once the wire is advanced into the aorta, an appropriate dilator may be introduced over the wire if needed, and the dilator subsequently exchanged for the desired catheter. If a micropuncture needle is used, the 4- or 5-Fr micropuncture transitional dilator is advanced over the 0.018-in wire, the inner stylet and microwire are removed, and exchange is made for a larger (0.035-in or 0.038-in) working wire for subsequent catheters or sheaths.

   a. Advancing the catheter may be difficult if the entry angle is acute or if subcutaneous tissues have not been adequately spread.

   b. In patients who are obese, who have diseased arteries, or who have had scarring from prior vascular procedures, a stiff wire can reduce subcutaneous

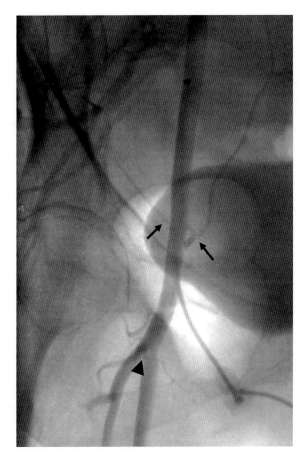

FIGURE 1.3 • Contrast injection confirming common femoral artery access. Angiographic land-marks for the common femoral artery include the deep inferior epigastric artery (medial) and deep circumflex iliac artery (lateral) above (*arrows*), and the femoral bifurcation below to the superficial femoral and profunda femoral arteries (*arrowhead*).

buckling. A guidewire with a diameter matching the inner lumen diameter of the angiographic catheter often works best by creating a smoother transition between the wire and catheter. Taping a large abdominal pannus back away from the groin is also useful for advancing catheters.

c. An appropriately sized introducer sheath may be used to minimize risk of arterial trauma if multiple catheter exchanges are anticipated. If a sheath is used, it is important to frequently flush the sheath or connect it to a pressure bag with heparinized saline to prevent thrombus from forming within the sheath.

2. Always confirm the position of the tip of the catheter fluoroscopically prior to power injection.

a. Check for free backflow, aspirate, and flush.

b. Inject a small amount of contrast by hand to confirm vessel location.

c. Avoid power injection into the intercostal and lumbar arteries.

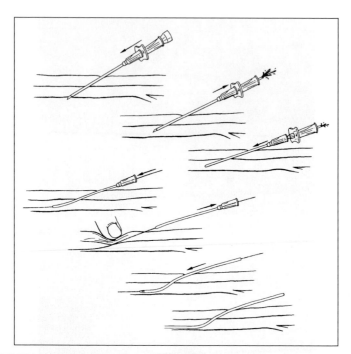

FIGURE 1.4 • Schematic of the Seldinger puncture technique using an open beveled needle. Top to bottom: (1) Needle is introduced into the artery until brisk pulsatile backflow of blood is noted; (2) a wire is introduced through the needle; (3) wire is fixed and needle removed with compression over the puncture site; (4) the track is dilated over the wire (or the micropuncture dilator set is advanced if using the micropuncture system); and (5) a catheter is placed over the working wire. (Reprinted with permission from Johnsrude IS, Jackson DS, Dunnick NR. *A Practical Approach to Angiography.* 2nd ed. Little, Brown; 1987:36.)

    d. Injection and imaging: Determine desired contrast volume and flow rate based on catheter location and select the appropriate filming sequence (see subsequent tables for suggested angiography protocols).

Antegrade Common Femoral Artery Puncture
1. **Procedure (Fig. 1.6):** The skin incision (not the arterial puncture site) may have to be above the inguinal ligament in some patients. Just as in retrograde puncture, the goal is to have the arteriotomy directly over the femoral head after passing through the subcutaneous tissues. A good landmark for the skin incision is the acetabulum. Arterial puncture site, angle of entry, and technique are otherwise similar to the retrograde approach. In obese patients, the abdominal pannus should be upwardly retracted and secured; however, an antegrade approach may prove impractical in many obese patients due to the challenge of passing through the lower abdominal pannus to appropriately access the artery over the femoral head.
2. **Converting a retrograde to an antegrade femoral artery puncture:** A reverse-curve or "shepherd's crook"–shaped catheter–guidewire combination can be used to pass the guidewire antegrade caudal to the puncture site, carefully withdrawing the catheter–guidewire combination until the orientation angle is favorable to advance the catheter down the leg, followed by catheter advancement over the

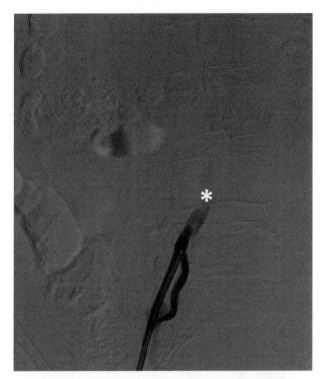

FIGURE 1.5 • Occlusion of the common iliac artery (*asterisk*) noted with contrast injection. If smooth guidewire passage is obstructed, contrast injection may reveal an occlusion as the underlying cause. (Image courtesy of Dr. Jesse Liu)

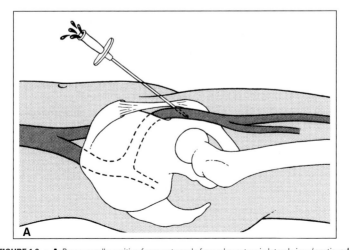

FIGURE 1.6 • **A:** Proper needle position for an antegrade femoral puncture in lateral view. (*continued*)

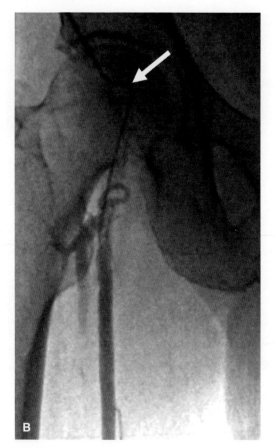

FIGURE 1.6 • (*Continued*) **B:** Angiogram after antegrade access and placement of a micropuncture sheath showing puncture site over the femoral artery (*arrow*).

guidewire. If this technique is anticipated, a more vertical puncture through the subcutaneous tissues directly over the femoral head may be considered to facilitate catheterization in both retrograde and antegrade fashion.

Vascular Access for Arterial Grafts and Patch Angioplasty

1. Gaining access into arterial bypass grafts and arteries treated with prior patch angioplasty is acceptable for diagnostic angiography and therapeutic procedures (Fig. 1.7). A single-wall puncture should be performed using either palpation or US guidance, accessing the graft or hood of the patch angioplasty directly. Due to scarring from prior surgery, use of dilators and potentially stiffer wires may be needed to facilitate catheter or sheath passage.
2. Protocol for hemostasis after access to a graft or vessel treated with patch angioplasty is standard manual compression as for conventional arterial access.

Tibiopedal Artery Access

1. Tibiopedal artery access has expanded therapeutic options for complex arterial revascularization procedures. Access to tibiopedal arteries can be part of

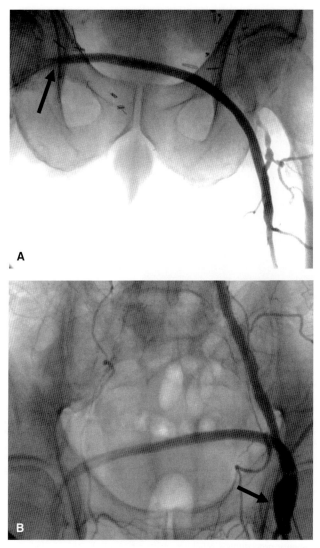

FIGURE 1.7 • A: Puncture of a femoral–femoral bypass graft over the right groin (*arrow*) for left lower extremity runoff angiography. (Image courtesy of Dr. Kenneth J. Kolbeck) **B:** Puncture of the anastomotic "hood" from patch angioplasty of the left common femoral artery for angiography. *Arrows* show access points.

a combination antegrade–retrograde revascularization whereby a guidewire advanced retrograde to recanalize a tibiopedal vessel is snared from an antegrade approach for subsequent angioplasty or stenting via larger access sheaths.

2. Dedicated micropuncture kits for pedal access have been developed to enable access and intervention directly from the tibiopedal approach.

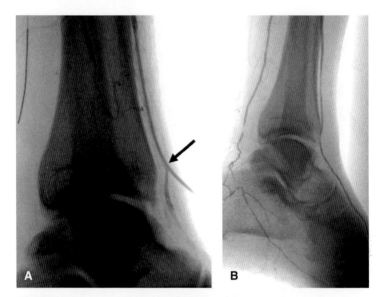

FIGURE 1.8 • Tibial artery access. **A:** Retrograde US-guided access to the distal anterior tibial/dorsalis pedis artery (*arrow*) with contrast injection through the access sheath. **B:** Angiogram from antegrade access (not shown) after removal of pedal access sheath.

3. Access options include the distal anterior tibial or dorsalis pedis artery (Fig. 1.8), posterior tibial artery, peroneal artery, as well as various pedal vessels directly. US guidance is typically used (1), although with calcified vessels, some operators choose fluoroscopic guidance. Intraluminal passage of the guidewire can be monitored using US or fluoroscopy. A cocktail of a calcium channel blocker (e.g., verapamil 2.5 mg), vasodilator (e.g., nitroglycerine 0.25 mg), and heparin (e.g., 2,500 to 5,000 IU) can be administered after access to minimize vasospasm and vessel thrombosis.

4. Hemostasis after tibiopedal arterial access can be performed via direct manual compression, inflation of an angioplasty balloon from a separate antegrade access during tibiopedal sheath/catheter withdrawal, or potential use of a compression band (see below for radial artery access).

Upper Extremity Arterial Access

1. **Radial artery access.** Transradial artery access (TRA) has rapidly become standard for many cardiac interventions, and is increasingly used for diagnostic and therapeutic procedures in other vascular territories. Indications include aortoiliac occlusive disease, infections or irritation in the inguinal regions, operator preference based on intended catheterizations, a desire for early ambulation, need for anticoagulation and antiplatelet agents, or patient preference.

   a. Radial artery access kits are commercially available. These typically includes a 1.5-in 20- to 22-gauge access needle with a short bevel, a 0.018- to 0.025-in microwire, and 4- to 6-Fr hydrophilic introducer sheaths with a tapered transition between the introducer and sheath.

   b. Optimal patients—radial artery diameter larger than intended access catheter/sheath, evidence of an intact palmar arch (Allen test or Barbeau test), no vasospasm (e.g., Raynaud), and no present or planned same-arm AV fistula for dialysis. The ulnar artery may be used, but achieving adequate hemostasis

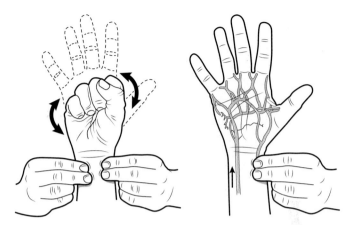

FIGURE 1.9 • Allen test. Compression over both radial and ulnar arteries is performed while the hand is clenched in a fist, causing blanching of the skin. The hand is then opened, and compression over the ulnar artery is released to see whether ulnar arterial flow is sufficient to reperfuse the hand.

with compression may be trickier due to the relationship of the ulnar artery to the carpal bones.

c. Allen test is performed by manual compression of both radial and ulnar arteries while the patient clenches their fist until the hand becomes blanched (Fig. 1.9). The hand is opened and compression of the ulnar artery released, observing for the presence of capillary refill in the hand. A normal Allen test demonstrates reperfusion within 7 seconds, whereas an abnormal test takes over 10 seconds. Waveform plethysmography with a pulse oximeter on the thumb (Barbeau test) is a more objective method to monitor reperfusion, and allows for continuous monitoring during the procedure. It is uncertain whether abnormal Allen or Barbeau tests are relative contraindications for transradial access as risks of hand ischemia and loss of function have not been associated with radial artery occlusion (3).

d. The hand is placed supine on an arm board and taped in a dorsiflexed position with a rolled towel or dedicated support under the wrist (Fig. 1.10). Access is achieved using either palpation or ultrasound guidance, and a 45- to 70-degree needle angle. The guidewire is gently advanced using US or fluoroscopy, over which the radial access sheath is advanced and flushed. A cocktail of a calcium channel blocker (e.g., verapamil 2.5 mg), vasodilator (e.g., nitroglycerine 0.25 mg), and heparin (e.g., 2,500 to 5,000 IU) is administered immediately via the radial artery sheath to minimize vasospasm and vessel thrombosis. The cocktail is typically mixed with blood or saline to minimize pain from vessel irritation.

e. Operators need to be aware of radial artery anatomic variants, most important of which is the radial loop, a tortuosity that can be found near the origin of the radial artery (Fig. 1.11). This can be identified ahead of time with US or with injection of contrast after initial access. If a radial loop is identified, it can often be reduced simply by gentle passage of a hydrophilic guidewire across the segment.

f. Postprocedure, the sheath can be promptly removed, even with the patient fully anticoagulated. Radial compression devices with an inflatable bladder are designed to maintain hemostasis without obliterating blood flow (Fig. 1.12). The compression devices restrict wrist flexion and are worn between 1 and 4 hours, during which the patient may sit up or ambulate.

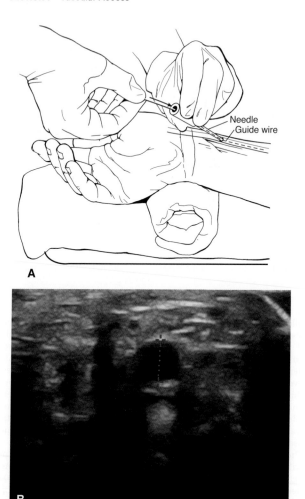

FIGURE 1.10 • A: The hand is placed supine and in slight dorsiflexion with a towel or dedicated splint. Palpation or ultrasound guidance is then used to get micropuncture access to the radial artery. US image of the radial artery in (**B**) axial and (**C**) longitudinal views. **D:** Using the Seldinger technique, a sheath is advanced over the wire for stable access into the artery. (*continued*)

    g. Complications are rare but include spasm, dissection, radial artery occlusion, digital ischemia, nerve injury, traumatic AV fistula, hematoma, and compartment syndrome. Complications are more frequent when there are anatomical variations.

2. **Distal radial artery access.** Distal radial artery access (dTRA) involves access to the radial artery in the region of the anatomic snuffbox (Fig. 1.13).

    a. Rather than being in a supinated position, the patient's hand is positioned prone, often laid over the lower abdomen.

    b. Using US guidance or palpation, the artery is punctured over the anatomic snuffbox using the same radial access kit.

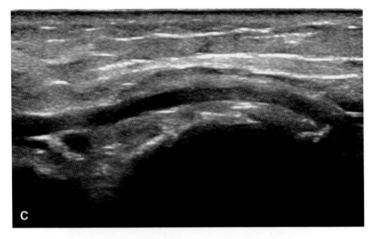

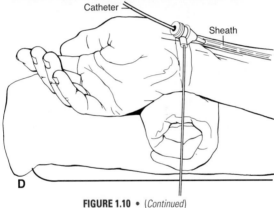

FIGURE 1.10 • (*Continued*)

c. Hemostasis is achieved with manual compression, or using a dedicated distal transradial artery access compression device.

d. Purported advantages to dTRA over TRA: Patient and operator comfort since the hand can be neutral or pronated and operator and equipment positioning may be similar to femoral access; access is distal to the superficial palmar branch of the radial artery supplying the superficial palmar arch, theoretically reducing risk of hand ischemia with distal radial artery occlusion (4).

3. **Brachial artery access.** Prior to TRA, brachial artery access was often used when indicated. Brachial artery access remains a viable option if TRA/dTRA is contraindicated due to vessel size, spasm, or lack of suitable device catheter lengths (Fig. 1.14). Bilateral blood pressures and pulse exams are performed. The arm is supinated and the antecubital fossa is prepared and draped. Micropuncture access and US guidance are recommended for safety and to avoid direct nerve injury, although access with palpation alone may also be used. If the patient feels an electric shock sensation going down the arm, the needle may have encroached on a nerve and should be withdrawn and carefully advanced more caudal or cephalad along the artery.

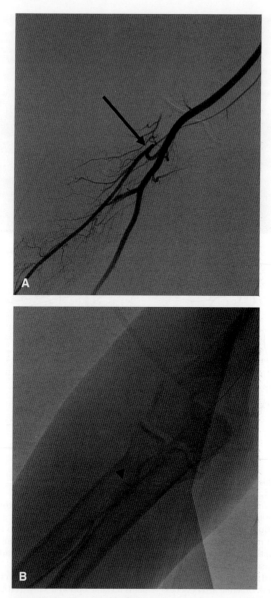

FIGURE 1.11 • **A:** Angiogram after achieving radial access shows a radial artery loop (*arrow*).
B: A hydrophilic guidewire (*arrowhead*) is gently advanced across the loop to reduce the loop and
enable desired catheterization. (Image courtesy of Dr. Jesse Liu)

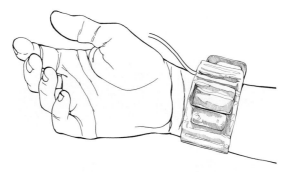

FIGURE 1.12 • A soft air-filled bladder provides compression to the radial artery when inflated to the mean arterial blood pressure to provide hemostasis while preserving blood flow, termed patent hemostasis.

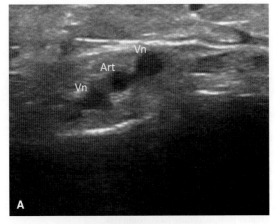

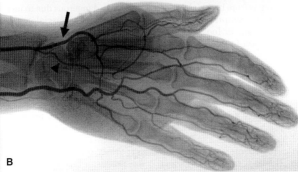

FIGURE 1.13 • Distal radial artery access (dTRA). **A:** US image of the radial artery (*Art*) and paired veins (*Vn*) in the anatomic snuffbox. **B:** Angiogram of the hand showing the radial artery in the anatomic snuffbox (*arrow*) distal to the origin of the superficial palmar branch (*arrowhead*) providing collateral flow to the palmar arch. (Image courtesy of Dr. John A. Kaufman).

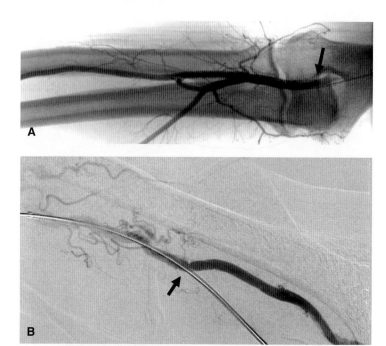

FIGURE 1.14 • **A:** Low brachial artery access near the distal humerus. (Image courtesy of Dr. Robert E. Barton). **B:** High brachial artery access along the mid humerus. (Image courtesy of Dr. Ramsey Al-Hakim). *Arrows* mark sites of arterial access.

a. Low brachial artery access, just cephalad to the antecubital fossa, can facilitate postprocedure hemostasis by enabling compression against the distal humerus.

b. High brachial artery access can be performed when necessary, with potentially greater postprocedure hematoma risk.

c. Hematomas from brachial artery access can be dangerous due to median and ulnar nerve compression within the medial brachial fascial compartment with potential for long-term injury if not immediately decompressed. This risk is greater for high brachial artery access and axillary artery access (see below).

d. It is important to note that compressive nerve injury may not be from a visible hematoma, can occur in the presence of maintained distal pulses, and can be delayed in presentation by days. Patient symptoms should guide escalation of care.

4. **Axillary artery access.** Axillary artery access was the first upper extremity artery used for percutaneous angiography, but lost favor due to risks of brachial plexus compression injury from hematomas. More recently, there has been increased interest in using the axillary artery as an upper extremity access site, particularly for large-bore devices unsuitable for brachial or radial arterial access sites. In this case, preprocedural planning with CT angiography (CTA) may be very helpful to delineate anatomy and exclude occlusive disease that may impair the procedure.

a. The arm is abducted and hand placed under the head. The axillary region is prepared and draped.

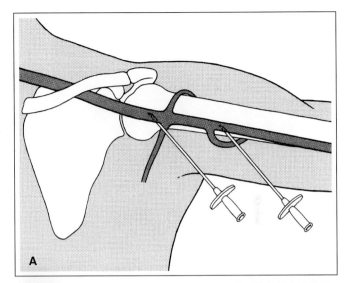

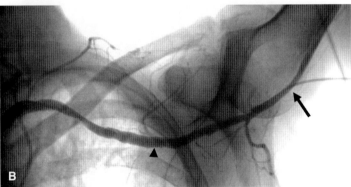

FIGURE 1.15 • A: Anatomic relationship of the axillary artery to the humeral head and location of axillary and low brachial artery puncture sites. **B:** Example of peripheral axillary artery access near the humeral head (*arrow*) for compression postprocedure. A more central access (*arrowhead*) would require compression against the second rib. (Image courtesy of Dr. Robert E. Barton).

b. US guidance and micropuncture access are recommended for safety and to avoid direct brachial plexus nerve injury. Administer local anesthesia carefully and avoid deep penetration because of the proximity of the brachial plexus.

c. The proximal segment of the axillary artery, along the deltopectoral groove, can facilitate compression against the second rib; a more peripheral segment, along the lateral axillary fold, would require compression against the humeral head (Fig. 1.15).

d. The axillary (and brachial) arteries are relatively mobile and can roll during access. Stabilizing the artery at the intended puncture site with fingers on either side may help.

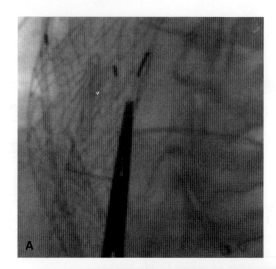

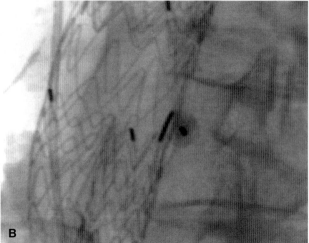

FIGURE 1.16 • A–C: Translumbar aortogram for embolization of endoleak after endovascular aneurysm repair (EVAR) using angulation and fluoroscopy. (Images courtesy of Dr. John A. Kaufman). (*continued*)

    e. Use of a sheath can facilitate catheter exchanges and provide a means for infusion of vasodilators and calcium channel blockers if needed.

    f. Use of closure devices has also been described with axillary artery access.

Direct Aortic Access

1. Translumbar diagnostic aortography has largely been replaced by upper extremity access options. Translumbar aortic access, however, remains a valuable technique for embolization of endoleaks (Fig. 1.16) after endovascular aortic aneurysm repair (EVAR, see Chapter 18).

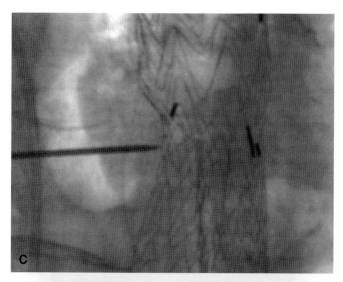

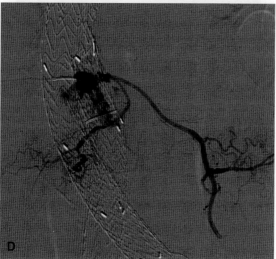

FIGURE 1.16 • (*Continued*) **D:** Translumbar angiogram showing endoleak and communicating lumbar arteries.

2. Direct aortic access from a transcaval approach has also been described for percutaneous cardiac interventions and embolization of endoleaks. When large-bore devices have been used, as for transcatheter aortic valve repair (TAVR), the aortocaval communication has been closed with a cardiac occluder device. For access, a transjugular intrahepatic portosystemic shunt (TIPS) set or a radiofrequency wire may be used to puncture the aorta via a transfemoral or transjugular approach, with intravascular ultrasound (IVUS) guidance from an alternative venous access site (Fig. 1.17).

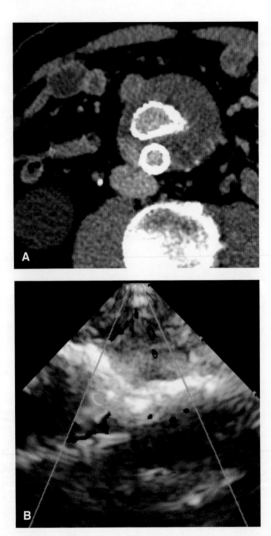

FIGURE 1.17 • **A:** Contrast-enhanced CT and (**B**) intravascular US image from a probe in the IVC of abdominal aortic aneurysm endoleak. (*continued*)

Abdominal and Lower Extremity Venous Access
1. Common femoral vein access
   a. The common femoral vein is located about 0.5 to 1.5 cm medial to the femoral artery (see Fig. 1.1). A landmark of the common femoral vein by US is the confluence of the great saphenous vein (Fig. 1.18).
   b. **Single-wall needle technique:** Ultrasound guidance enables direct visualization of the puncture and minimizes the chance of arterial trauma. A 21-gauge micropuncture needle is commonly used for access. Some operators like to attach a half-filled syringe with heparinized saline to the needle with short connection tubing to confirm intraluminal access with aspiration

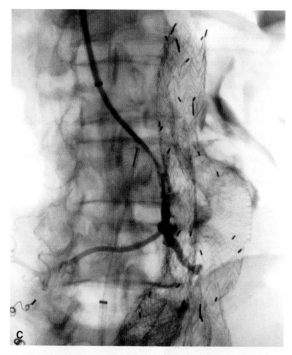

FIGURE 1.17 • (*Continued*) **C:** Angiogram of endoleak after transcaval access. (Images courtesy of Dr. Ramsey Al-Hakim).

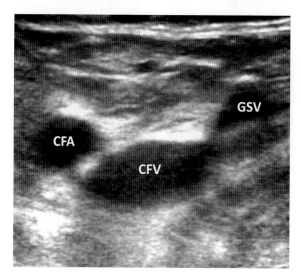

FIGURE 1.18 • Common femoral vein (CFV) lies medial to the common femoral artery (CFA) below the inguinal ligament. The confluence with the great saphenous vein (GSV) is a landmark by US.

of blood with all venous access. A Valsalva maneuver can help to distend the vein during which time the needle–syringe assembly is advanced toward the femoral vein with gentle intermittent suction. When the anterior wall of the vein has been crossed, dark venous blood will be noted in the syringe with aspiration. Gently detach the syringe while keeping the position of the needle firmly fixed. If nonpulsatile venous blood is noted exiting from the needle hub, the appropriately sized wire is advanced into the femoral vein. Subsequent dilation and catheter placement using the Seldinger technique is similar to the arterial technique described earlier.

    c. Postprocedure manual compression for 5 to 10 minutes is usually sufficient.

2. Popliteal vein access

    a. The popliteal vein typically lies lateral and superficial to the popliteal artery in the popliteal fossa, between the heads of the gastrocnemius muscle.

    b. A landmark of the popliteal vein by US is the confluence with the short saphenous vein (Fig. 1.19).

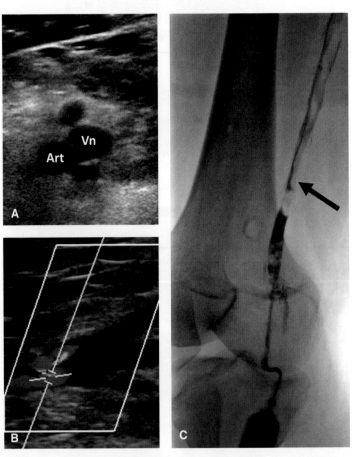

FIGURE 1.19 • **A:** Popliteal vein (*Vn*) lies superficial to the popliteal artery (*Art*) in the popliteal fossa. **B:** US can be used to access a patent portion of the vein in the setting of thrombus. **C:** Venogram shows filling defects consistent with thrombus (*arrow*).

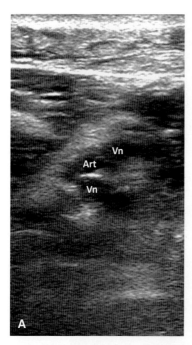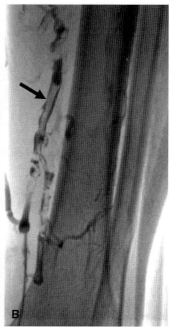

FIGURE 1.20 • A: Paired posterior tibial veins (*Vn*) adjacent to the posterior tibial artery (*Art*) at the level of the ankle. **B:** Venogram shows filling defects consistent with thrombus (*arrow*).

    c. As with common femoral vein access, US and a micropuncture access set are commonly used. Take care to avoid puncture of the tibial nerve, which lies posterior (superficial by US from the popliteal fossa) to the popliteal vein.

    d. Postprocedure manual compression for 5 to 10 minutes is usually sufficient.

3. Tibial vein access

    a. Useful for potential access to thrombosed segments more centrally for venography or intervention. The posterior tibial veins are the most common sites for access (Fig. 1.20).

    b. Paired posterior tibial veins lie superficially on either side of the posterior tibial artery along the medial ankle.

    c. The foot is laterally rotated, and US and micropuncture access are used.

    d. Intervention can be performed directly via tibial vein access, or a guidewire can be snared from a second access in a larger vein centrally for subsequent intervention.

4. Translumbar IVC access

    a. Translumbar IVC access is a valuable option in patients with otherwise occluded cervical and upper extremity central veins requiring long-term venous access (Fig. 1.21).

    b. A guidewire or pigtail catheter via a common femoral vein approach may be initially placed in the IVC with the patient supine to serve as a landmark by fluoroscopy. The catheter is secured and the patient then positioned prone.

    c. The skin insertion site is 8 to 10 cm lateral to midline on the right, and above the iliac crest.

    d. A 15- to 20-cm 18- to 22-gauge needle is advanced toward the L3 vertebral body, angling medially and superiorly from the skin entry site toward the indwelling wire/catheter landmark previously placed. If a vertebral body is contacted, the needle is slightly backed out and redirected and advanced anteriorly.

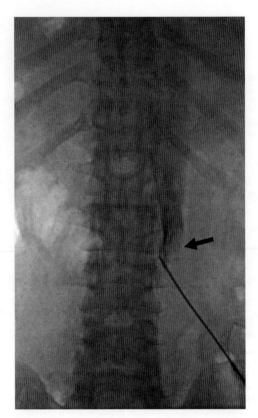

FIGURE 1.21 • Translumbar inferior vena cava (IVC) access. With the patient prone, an 18- to 22-gauge needle is advanced from a point 8- to 10-cm right lateral to midline above the iliac crest, aiming superiorly and centrally at approximately 45-degree angles toward the L3 vertebral body. If contact with the vertebral body is made, the needle is backed out slightly and redirected anteriorly. A wire or pigtail catheter positioned in the IVC from a common femoral vein approach may also be used as a target. Contrast injection confirms IVC access (*arrow*).

    e. After confirmation of caval access with contrast injection through the needle, a guidewire is advanced to the inferior cavoatrial junction for completion of the procedure.

Upper Extremity Venous Access
1. Cephalic or basilic vein access
    a. These are superficial veins of the upper extremity commonly used for venography or placement of a peripherally inserted central venous catheter (PICC). The cephalic vein lies superficial to the biceps along the lateral aspect of the arm and drains into the axillary vein by the shoulder, while the basilic vein courses along the medial aspect of the arm and drains into the brachial vein or directly into the axillary vein.
    b. Because of their superficial location, these veins can roll and collapse easily. A more centrally placed tourniquet facilitates vein distension for puncture with a micropuncture access kit, after which the tourniquet is released for guidewire passage.

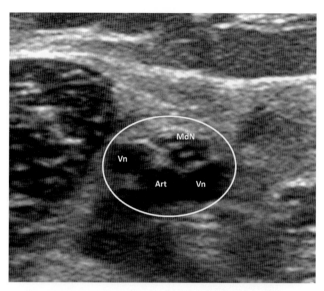

FIGURE 1.22 • US image of the left upper extremity demonstrates the paired brachial veins (*Vn*) adjacent to the brachial artery (*Art*) in the neurovascular bundle (*circle*). Note the location of the median nerve (*MdN*) anterior to the artery.

2. Brachial vein access
   a. The brachial vein is a deep vein, lies deeper in the subcutaneous tissues, and is in closer approximation to the neurovascular bundle, increasing potential risks for access (Fig. 1.22).
   b. Brachial vein access can be an alternative if the superficial veins are inaccessible.
3. Subclavian vein access
   a. Although palpation and landmarks have traditionally been used for subclavian vein access, US allows direct visualization and avoidance of the artery, nerves, and pleura.
   b. The US transducer is positioned transversely relative to the course of the vein and artery just caudal to the mid portion of the clavicle, or slightly more peripherally. The subclavian vein lies anterior to the artery. The pleural edge will be seen as a thin echogenic line by US (Fig. 1.23).
   c. After instilling local anesthetic, a micropuncture needle is used to directly puncture the subclavian vein from a subclavicular approach, and a guidewire is passed centrally under fluoroscopy.

Cervical Venous Access
1. Internal jugular vein access
   a. The internal jugular vein (IJV) is commonly used as an access point for central lines, the superior or inferior vena cava, the iliac veins, and hepatic or renal veins.
   b. The vein is superficial and lateral to the common carotid artery near the level of the thyroid gland (Fig. 1.24).
   c. US guidance and micropuncture access are typically used as described above.
   d. The US transducer is positioned transversely relative to the orientation of the vessels. A position just above the clavicle is important for a smooth course of tunneled central venous catheters, with orientation of the needle along the

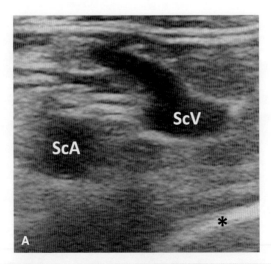

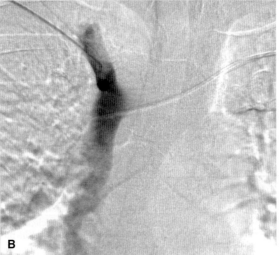

FIGURE 1.23 • A: Transverse subclavicular US image showing the location of the subclavian vein (*ScV*) at the confluence with the external jugular vein and the subclavian artery (*ScA*), relative to the pleural edge in the far field (*asterisk*). **B:** Contrast venography after access confirms patency to the superior vena cava. (Image courtesy of Dr. Masahiro Horikawa).

long access of the US transducer to facilitate the lateral entry of the catheter. A direct anterior puncture is appropriate when the IJV is used as an access site for other procedures.

2. External jugular vein access
   a. The external jugular vein (EJV) is a superficial vein lying along the sternocleidomastoid muscle in the supraclavicular fossa, and draining into the central subclavian vein.
   b. The EJV is an alternative access site when the IJV is occluded. US guidance and micropuncture access are used for IJV access.

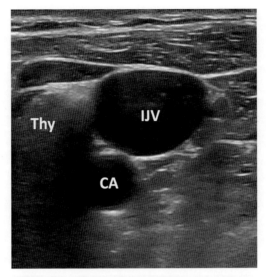

FIGURE 1.24 • US image of the internal jugular vein (*IJV*) in relation to the common carotid artery (*CA*) deep and medially, and the thyroid gland (*Thy*) medially.

   c. Central wire passage may be more challenging with an EJV approach due to a relatively acute angle at the confluence with the subclavian vein (Fig. 1.25).

Postprocedure Management (1)

1. **Compression of arterial puncture** (15 minutes): If the patient has been heparinized during the procedure, make sure the coagulation parameters have normalized (partial thromboplastin time [PTT] close to control value or activated clotting time [ACT] of approximately 150 seconds) before the catheter is removed and the puncture site is compressed.

   a. Make sure the patient is comfortable because cooperation is essential during compression. Administer additional lidocaine around the puncture site as needed.

   b. Remove the catheter as you are about to compress the artery. If a pigtail or reverse-curve catheter has been used, a wire should be placed to straighten the catheter before it is removed to reduce the risk of vessel injury.

   c. No sponges or towels should be used while compressing the access site so that any bleeding is visible. Remove drapes to make sure a developing hematoma is not obscured.

   d. Compress at, above, and below the actual puncture site to maximize hemostasis (Fig. 1.11). Do not obliterate the pulse. Distal pulses should be faintly palpable.

   e. Apply steady moderate pressure for 10 minutes. Then gently reduce pressure over the next 5 minutes. Never remove compression abruptly.

   f. If rebleeding occurs, repeat compression for 15 minutes.

   g. Devices for unattended prolonged groin compression (e.g., C-clamp, pneumatic compression cuffs) are labor-saving for selected cooperative patients but require familiarity by personnel. Utilize a protocol for management.

   h. At termination of compression, palpate all distal pulses and compare with baseline examination.

   i. Bed rest with legs extended should be ordered for 4 to 6 hours (the head of the bed may be elevated slightly); patient may be allowed to "log roll" with assistance.

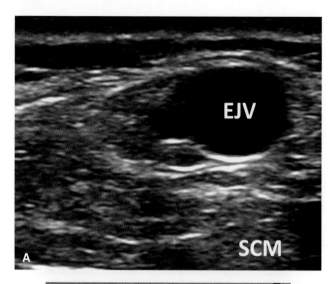

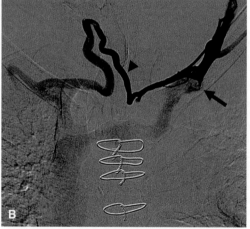

FIGURE 1.25 • **A:** US of the external jugular vein (*EJV*) superficial to the sternocleidomastoid muscle (*SCM*) in the subcutaneous tissues. **B:** Venogram after access shows the angle at the confluence with the subclavian vein (*arrow*) and collateral filling of the anterior jugular vein (*arrowhead*). (Image courtesy of Dr. Teodora Bochnakova).

    j. Check groin for bleeding or hematoma every 15 minutes for 1 hour, then every 30 minutes for 1 hour, and then every hour for 4 hours.

    k. Check blood pressure and pulse every 30 minutes for 2 hours and then every hour for 4 hours.

    l. IV fluids may be given until the patient can take oral food and liquid. Adjust fluid administration according to the patient's cardiopulmonary and renal status.

    m. If the patient is unable to void and is in urinary distress, a urinary catheter may be placed until the patient is able to ambulate.

2. **Arterial puncture closure devices**: See Chapter 3.

3. **Compression of venous puncture** (5 to 10 minutes): Apply steady pressure as described earlier, easing off gently toward the end. For uncomplicated, small French-size venous punctures, bed rest may be limited to 1 to 2 hours, while for larger access sizes 4 to 6 hours may be needed.

Prevention and Management of Complications

1. The incidence of complications (Table 1.1) may increase with the severity of the underlying clinical status of the patient and the duration of the procedure (5,6).
2. Thrombosis
   a. Catheter factors include size (relative to arterial lumen), type of material, and length of intravascular dwell time.
   b. Patient factors include extent of intimal vessel damage, vasospasm, and coagulation status.
   c. Systemic heparinization reduces risk of thrombosis.
3. Hemorrhage (puncture-site hematoma)
   a. Locate puncture site accurately over the femoral head because compression of the artery is best at that site; arterial punctures above and below the femoral head are difficult to compress adequately.
   b. Compress above and below skin entry site to prevent antegrade and retrograde bleeding.
   c. Using smaller sized access (5 Fr and below) may reduce the risk of complications.
   d. Reversal of anticoagulation by monitoring ACT can minimize risk of hemorrhage.
   e. Management of puncture-site hematoma or uncontrollable bleeding
      (1) If a groin hematoma is present, trace its margins with ink and monitor size.
      (2) Notify a vascular surgeon in cases of uncontrollable puncture-site bleeding, diminution or loss of pulses, neurologic symptoms in the extremity, or suspicion of a retroperitoneal hematoma (in this case, obtain an abdominal CT scan to confirm or rule out the diagnosis quickly).
4. Pseudoaneurysm: Avoid superficial femoral artery puncture (low puncture); adequate groin compression becomes difficult without support of the femur underneath. See Chapter 3 for treatment.

Table 1.1	Complication Rates and Thresholds for Diagnostic Angiography (5,6)	
Complication	**Rates (%)**	**Adverse Event Thresholds (%)**
Access site hematoma (requiring escalation of care)	0.0–1.7	0.5–3.0
Access site occlusion	0.0–0.76	0.2–1.0
Pseudoaneurysm or arteriovenous fistula	0.04–0.30	0.2
Vessel dissection	0.43	0.5–1.0
Subintimal contrast injection	0.0–0.44	0.5–1.0
Distal embolism	0.0–0.10	0.2–0.5
Major contrast media reaction	0.0–3.58	0.5–5.0
Postcontrast nephropathy	0.2–3.0	0.2–5.0

ACR–SIR–SPR Practice Parameter for the Performance of Arteriography Revised 2017 (Resolution 14) 2017 [updated 2017. Available from: https://www.acr.org/-/media/ACR/Files/Practice-Parameters/Arteriog.pdf. Dariushnia SR, Gill AE, Martin LG, Saad WE, Baskin KM, Caplin DM, et al. Quality improvement guidelines for diagnostic arteriography. *J Vasc Interv Radiol.* 2014;25(12):1873–81.

5. Embolization: To prevent sequelae of distal embolization, consider:
   a. Immediate percutaneous or surgical thrombectomy
   b. Selective catheter-directed thrombolysis, depending on the severity and progression of symptoms
6. Contrast-induced nephropathy: See Chapter 65.

Injection Rates and Image-Acquisition Programs

Catheter Angiography

Injection rates and image-acquisition programs should be tailored for the patient when indicated; however, for the vast majority of studies, routine programs are useful (Tables 1.2 to 1.5). The suggested injection volumes and rates are applicable for

Table 1.2   **Visceral and Peripheral Angiography (General Guidelines)**

Study (Injection Site)	Total Volume and Rate[a]	Image-Acquisition Program[b]
Abdominal aortogram (above celiac axis)	40 mL at 20 mL/s	3/s × 2 s 1/s × 3 s
Arch aortogram	50 mL at 25 mL/s	3/s × 3 s 1/s × 3s
Bilateral lower extremity runoff (distal aorta)	96 mL at 8 mL/s	1/s × 3 s = pelvis 1/s × 2 s = thigh 1/s × 4 s = knee Delays = calf/foot
Pelvic arteriogram (distal aorta)	30 mL at 15 mL/s	2/s × 3 s 1/s × 3 s
Unilateral lower extremity runoff (ipsilateral common iliac artery)	60 mL at 6 mL/s	1/s × 3 s = pelvis 1/s × 2 s = thigh 1/s × 3 s = knee Delays = calf/foot
Renal transplant (iliac fossa; ipsilateral common iliac artery)	12 mL at 6 mL/s	3/s × 2 s 2/s × 2 s Delays as needed
Renal transplant (iliac fossa; selective ipsilateral hypogastric artery)	10 mL at 4 mL/s	3/s × 2 s 2/s × 2 s Delays as needed
Unilateral renal arteriogram (proximal ipsilateral renal artery)	12 mL at 4–6 mL/s	3/s × 2 s 1/s × 2 s Delays as needed
Celiac arteriogram (selective)	30 mL at 4–6 mL/s	2/s × 3 s Delays for portal venous phase
Hepatic arteriogram (selective)	5–20 mL at 1–3 mL/s	2/s × 3 s 1/s × 3 s Delays as needed
Gastroduodenal arteriogram (selective)	10–15 mL at 2–3 mL/s	2/s × 2 s 1/s × 3 s Delays as needed

(*continued*)

Table 1.2   Visceral and Peripheral Angiography (General Guidelines) (*Continued*)

Study (Injection Site)	Total Volume and Rate[a]	Image-Acquisition Program[b]
Splenic arteriogram (selective)	10–20 mL at 2–4 mL/s	2/s × 3 s Delays as needed
Left gastric arteriogram (selective)	10–15 mL at 2–3 mL/s	1/s × 4 s Delays as needed
Superior mesenteric arteriogram (selective)	30 mL at 4–6 mL/s	1/s × 4 s Delays for portal venous phase
Inferior mesenteric arteriogram (selective)	15 mL at 3 mL/s	2/s × 2 s 1/s × 3 s Delays as needed
Lumbar arteriogram (selective)	5 mL hand	1/s
Inferior phrenic arteriogram (selective)	8–12 mL at 1–3 mL/s	1/s × 8 s
Subclavian arteriogram (distal to cephalic arteries)	18 mL at 6 mL/s	1/s stations to hand
Hand arteriogram (midbrachial artery)	16 mL at 4 mL/s	1/s until venous phase

[a]Based on digital subtraction angiography (DSA) with isosmolar contrast.
[b]Delays = one image every second or every other second for parenchymal and venous phases.

Table 1.3   Venous Angiography

Study (Injection Site)	Total Volume and Rate	Image-Acquisition Program
Inferior venacavogram (from iliac vein confluence)	40 mL at 20 mL/s	4/s × 4 s
Common femoral vein	24 mL at 6 mL/s	2/s × 4 s
Renal venogram (selective)	25 mL at 10 mL/s after injecting epinephrine into renal artery	2/s × 4 s 1/s × 2 s
Adrenal venogram (selective)	Left: 8 mL by hand Right: 5 mL by hand	2/s 2/s
Superior venacavogram (unilateral or bilateral antecubital vein)	30 mL at 15 mL/s	0 × 3 s 1/s × 12 s
Wedge hepatic venogram	5 mL by hand	2/s

Table 1.4 **Pulmonary Angiography**

Study (Injection Site)	Total Volume and Rate	Image-Acquisition Program
Unilateral pulmonary arteriogram	50 mL at 25 mL/s	4/s × 3 s 1/s × 3 s
Lobar pulmonary arteriogram	18 mL at 6 mL/s	4/s × 3 s 1/s × 3 s
Right ventriculogram (intracavitary)	50 mL at 15 mL/s	Cine
Right atriogram (intracavitary)	50 mL at 25 mL/s	Cine

digital angiography if sufficiently diluted contrast medium is used. When using non-diluted contrast, both rates and volumes may be adjusted down significantly, especially for selective injections into smaller vessels (e.g., visceral, renal, and extremity arteries). Injection should be at a sufficient rate and volume to adequately visualize the segment of interest (usually the length of the vessel included within the acquisition frame) while accounting for washout and dilution by the incoming blood.

Cone-Beam CT

Cone-beam CT can be used for rotational angiography to define vascular supply and anatomy as well as for soft tissue tomography to assess tissue perfusion. Applications include identification of arterial supply and assessment of tumor embolization during transarterial chemoembolization, identification of arterial supply to aneurysms or vascular malformations, identification of the adrenal vein during adrenal vein sampling, and identification and treatment of endoleaks related to endovascular abdominal aortic aneurysm repair. After catheterization, the patient and C-arm are appropriately positioned for acquiring cone-beam

Table 1.5 **Useful Obliquities for Peripheral Angiography**

Anatomy of Interest	Projection
Carotid bifurcation	Lateral and AP (with head turned opposite)
Carotid siphon	Lateral
Circle of Willis	Variable AP views in different craniocaudal projections
Aortic arch (to open arch)	AP and steep (70 degrees) LAO
Aortic arch (for brachiocephalic vessels)	45-degree LAO with head true lateral, chin raised, and shoulders dropped down
Selective pulmonary artery	AP and lateral; left 45–60-degree LAO; right 45–60-degree RAO Opposite obliques for lower lobe branches
Origins of mesenteric vessels	Lateral aorta
Hepatic artery branches	Left: RAO 30–45 degrees Right: LAO 30–45 degrees
Origin of renal arteries	10–15-degree LAO
Common iliac bifurcation	Contralateral oblique 45 degrees
Common femoral bifurcation	Ipsilateral oblique 45 degrees

AP, anteroposterior; LAO, left anterior oblique; RAO, right anterior oblique.

Table 1.6 Sample Cone-Beam CT Protocol for Hepatic Angiography (7)

Catheter Location	Contrast Volume	Injection Rate	Dilution	Scan Time	Acquisition Delay	Findings
Proper or selective hepatic artery	12–64 mL	1–3 mL/s	100–370 mg iodine/mL	5–10 s	2–10 s arterial phase followed by 20–40 s parenchymal/venous phase	Tumor supply in first phase; parenchymal enhancement or pseudocapsule in delayed phases

Tacher V, Radaelli A, Lin M, Geschwind JF. How I do it: Cone-beam CT during transarterial chemoembolization for liver cancer. *Radiology*. 2015;274(2):320–34.

CT (CBCT). Often, power injection is used with nondiluted versus diluted contrast depending on the indication and manufacturer recommendations. Depending on catheter location, injection rates are between 1 mL and 12 mL per second, and an initial 2- to 10-second acquisition delay is selected for the arteriographic phase, followed by various delayed phases to highlight parenchymal and venous structures. A sample protocol for imaging the liver during transarterial chemoembolization is provided in Table 1.6 (7). Once the images are acquired, dedicated software processes the imaging data from the various projections on a reconstruction workstation to provide multiplanar and three-dimensional (3D) rendered images. The technology for this application continues to evolve to improve soft tissue contrast resolution, greater field of view, faster acquisition, and decreased radiation.

Considerations for Preprocedure Preparation Prior to Gaining Arterial or Venous Access

1. **Bleeding and thrombosis risks**. Consensus management guidelines can be found through clinical standards of practice published by the Society of Interventional Radiology (SIR), and endorsed by the Cardiovascular and Interventional Radiology Society of Europe (CIRSE) and the Canadian Association for Interventional Radiology (CAIR) (8). Procedures have been categorized as low bleeding risk versus high bleeding risk. Recommendations for monitoring coagulation parameters, use of blood products, and management of anticoagulation and antiplatelet medication are related to the risks of the procedure and access site.
2. **Renal dysfunction** (see Chapter 66)
3. **Prior documented reaction to iodinated contrast media** (see Chapter 65)
4. **Lidocaine hypersensitivity (local infiltration)** (see Chapter 63)

R e f e r e n c e s

1. Mustapha JA, Diaz-Sandoval LJ, Jaff MR, et al. Ultrasound-guided arterial access: outcomes among patients with peripheral artery disease and critical limb ischemia undergoing peripheral interventions. *J Invasive Cardiol*. 2016;28(6):259–264.
2. Seto AH, Abu-Fadel MS, Sparling JM, et al. Real-time ultrasound guidance facilitates femoral arterial access and reduces vascular complications: FAUST (Femoral Arterial Access With Ultrasound Trial). *JACC Cardiovasc Interv*. 2010;3(7):751–758.
3. van Leeuwen MAH, Hollander MR, van der Heijden DJ, et al. The ACRA anatomy study (assessment of disability after coronary procedures using radial access): a comprehensive anatomic and functional assessment of the vasculature of the hand and relation to outcome after transradial catheterization. *Circ Cardiovasc Interv*. 2017;10(11):e005753.

4. Koury A Jr, Monsignore LM, de Castro-Afonso LH, et al. Safety of ultrasound-guided distal radial artery access for abdominopelvic transarterial interventions: a prospective study. *Diagn Interv Radiol.* 2020;26(6):570–574.

5. ACR–SIR–SPR Practice Parameter for the Performance of Arteriography. Revised 2017 (Resolution 14) [updated 2017]. Available from https://www.acr.org/-/media/ACR/Files/Practice-Parameters/Arteriog.pdf

6. Dariushnia SR, Gill AE, Martin LG, et al. Quality improvement guidelines for diagnostic arteriography. *J Vasc Interv Radiol.* 2014;25(12):1873–1881.

7. Tacher V, Radaelli A, Lin M, et al. How I do it: cone-beam CT during transarterial chemoembolization for liver cancer. *Radiology.* 2015;274(2):320–334.

8. Patel IJ, Rahim S, Davidson JC, et al. Society of Interventional Radiology Consensus Guidelines for the periprocedural management of thrombotic and bleeding risk in patients undergoing percutaneous image-guided interventions-Part II: Recommendations: Endorsed by the Canadian Association for Interventional Radiology and the Cardiovascular and Interventional Radiological Society of Europe. *J Vasc Interv Radiol.* 2019;30(8):1168–1184.e1.

2   Vascular Closure Devices

Evan Lehrman, MD, Andrew Sideris, MD
Stephen P. Reis, MD, MBA, FSIR, and Joshua L. Weintraub, MD, FSIR

Introduction

Arterial access is required for a wide range of procedures ranging from interventional oncology and peripheral arterial disease to aneurysm repair and trauma. The sheaths used in such procedures range from approximately 4 Fr for diagnostic angiography to 12 to 25 Fr for endograft delivery. The subsequent safe and effective arterial access site closure and hemostasis is the goal for interventional radiologists. Although manual compression (MC) has been the gold standard for achieving hemostasis for smaller arteriotomies since the inception of interventional radiology, vascular closure devices (VCDs) were introduced in the early 1990s to help achieve hemostasis for larger arteriotomies. The primary benefits of these devices include decreased time to hemostasis and ambulation, as well as improvement in patients' comfort and satisfaction. More recently, entirely external VCD devices have also been developed for transradial access (TRA) site closure and hemostasis. While there have been concerns regarding the failure or complication rate of VCDs versus MC, a large body of evidence and experience has now accumulated to support their common usage. Advantages and disadvantages exist for both methods of arteriotomy closure (Table 2.1).

Indications

VCDs have been approved for arterial access site closure and hemostasis after retrograde common femoral artery (CFA) or radial artery puncture.

1. In the CFA, VCDs are most often employed for the closure of arteriotomies of size 6 Fr or greater, but may also be used for smaller arteriotomies.
2. In the radial artery, the only VCDs employed are entirely external (such as mechanical compression aids or hemostatic patches) due to smaller vessel size.

Off-Label Uses for Vascular Closure Device
Many VCD instructions for use (IFU) manuals will not include these situations, but there is an improving evidence base for use outside of retrograde CFA or radial access (1).
1. High puncture—external iliac artery
   a. MC likely to be ineffective—risk for retroperitoneal hematoma that can be life threatening

Table 2.1 **Advantages/Disadvantages of Manual Compression and Vascular Closure Devices**

Method	Advantages	Disadvantages
Manual Compression	–Gold standard –No device cost –Limited learning curve	–Delayed time to hemostasis –Delayed time to ambulation –Patient discomfort –Anticoagulation must be reversed (ACT <180) –Decreased workflow and longer length of patient stay
Vascular Closure Devices	–Immediate hemostasis –Decreased time to ambulation –Improved patient comfort and satisfaction –Hemostasis possible with anticoagulation	–Device cost –Learning curve for each device –Immediate repuncture not recommended for all devices –Potential for device-related complications

  b. Reports of using Angio-Seal in this clinical scenario when patient characteristics are favorable
  c. Surgical treatment may be necessary
2. Low puncture—SFA
  a. SFA puncture closure okay if >5 mm
3. Antegrade puncture
  a. Several reports support VCDs after antegrade puncture (CFA or SFA)
4. Nonfemoral artery puncture closure using VCDs has been described
  a. Brachial artery
  b. Popliteal artery
  c. Axillary artery

Contraindications

The only absolute contraindication to VCD use is patient hypersensitivity/allergy to the device material. If any of the below conditions exist, consider an alternative strategy or MC:
1. General conditions
  a. Contaminated field (infected VCD needs to be treated surgically with high morbidity and not insignificant mortality)
  b. Uncontrolled hypertension systolic blood pressure (SBP) >180 mm Hg
  c. Morbid obesity—body mass index (BMI) >40
  d. Severe calcified atherosclerotic peripheral artery disease (some reports suggest VCD may be safe in this population)
2. CFA conditions
  a. CFA is tortuous, small (less than 5 mm), or there is a high femoral bifurcation (above the femoral head)
    (1) Consider contralateral CFA or ipsilateral superficial femoral artery (SFA) access
  b. If there is prior angioplasty, or presence of stent or bypass graft
    (1) Consider contralateral CFA or ipsilateral SFA access
  c. Large atherosclerotic plaque on the anterior wall of the access site
    (1) Consider using ultrasound-guided puncture technique to avoid plaque
  d. Back wall puncture or multiple puncture attempts required for initial access

Procedure

The following general steps should be taken prior to device deployment as part of the VCD procedure:

1. Perform an ipsilateral CFA angiogram to assess puncture site location and vessel caliber (Fig. 2.1)
   a. 5 to 10 mL contrast hand injection through the sheath
   b. Can be documented at the start of the case through a micropuncture sheath prior to upsizing to the procedural sheath
   c. Oblique projections often necessary to separate sheath and CFA for clear identification of the access entry site
2. Consider reprepping the dermatotomy with a ChloraPrep and fresh sterile towels
3. Consider glove change or removal of outer gloves if double gloved
4. Consider readministration of subcutaneous lidocaine into the soft tissues for anesthesia
5. Consider blunt dissection of the soft tissue tract between the skin and the arteri-otomy
   a. Crucial for successful delivery of several of the VCDs
   b. Helps alert operator to incomplete hemostasis, readily seen as bleeding from the puncture site
6. Exchange the existing sheath over a wire for the VCD or insert the VCD into the sheath depending on the device being used
7. Deploy the device—see following sections for specific instructions and diagrams for several of the commonly used devices from each category

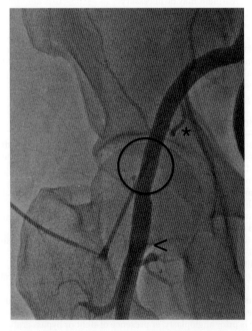

FIGURE 2.1 • Common femoral angiogram, performed through the indwelling sheath. The puncture (*black circle*) is appropriate for device closure, between the takeoff of the inferior epigastric artery (*asterisk*) and the femoral bifurcation (<), in a vessel >5 mm in caliber. Please note this puncture could also be closed with MC as it enters the CFA directly over the femoral head. (Angiogram courtesy of San Francisco General Hospital, San Francisco, CA.)

8. Bed rest for 1 to 2 hours, followed by ambulation trial
9. Assess arteriotomy site for evidence of delayed hematoma or pseudoaneurysm (PSA) prior to discharge

Steps specific to TRA closure:
1. Deploy the device—see following sections for specific instructions and diagrams of the most commonly used mechanical compression aid
2. Device worn for 1 to 2 hours, during which time the patient may ambulate
3. Assess wrist for evidence of delayed hematoma or PSA prior to discharge

Types of Devices

Several categories of VCD are currently manufactured, each with their own mechanism of action, applications, and learning curves.

1. **Active approximators (mechanical suture-mediated or clip devices) (Table 2.2)**

   These devices physically close the arteriotomy with suture- or nitinol clip-based material that is fixed to the vessel wall to achieve a limited form of surgical closure. With these devices, the arteriotomy is cinched closed. Active approximators are considered the most secure form of VCD for large arteriotomies. Adjunctive MC is theoretically unnecessary.

2. **Passive approximators (mechanical plug devices) (Table 2.3)**

   These devices deploy a sealant, gel, or plug onto the arteriotomy site that creates a mechanical barrier to achieve hemostasis. With some of these devices, hemostasis is augmented through use of a collagen-based plug to promote clot formation. Adjunctive MC is often held for 1 to 3 minutes.

3. **Compression assist devices (Table 2.4)**

   This heterogeneous group of devices mechanically promote hemostasis, but do not leave any material behind at the end of the procedure. With these devices, there is theoretical lower risk of infection or embolization/arterial occlusion given lack of implanted material. Adjunctive MC must be held, but for a shorter duration than expected with MC alone.

4. **Hemostatic patches (Table 2.5)**

   These patches are placed externally over the dermatotomy at the end of the procedure. With these products, substances interact with blood products to augment hemostasis. Adjunctive MC must be held, but for a shorter duration than expected with MC alone.

5. **Mechanical compression aids (Table 2.6)**

   These entirely external devices allow MC to be performed by the device rather than an operator. Routine duration of MC is required with these devices.

Table 2.2	Active Approximators (Mechanical Suture-Mediated and Clip Devices)			
Device	**Manufacturer**	**Mechanism**	**Sheath Size (Fr)**	**Comments**
Starclose SE	Abbott Vascular	Clip	5, 6	Extravascular nitinol clip cinches arteriotomy closed
Perclose–ProGlide	Abbott Vascular	Suture	5–8 (up to 21 with preclose technique)	Monofilament polypropylene suture
Prostar XL	Abbott Vascular	Suture	8.5–10	Braided polyester suture, used for larger sheaths

Table 2.3 Passive Approximators (Mechanical Plug Devices)

Device	Manufacturer	Mechanism	Sheath Size (Fr)	Comments
Mynx —Grip —Control	Cordis	Sealant	5–7	Extraluminally deployed polyethylene glycol plug while intravascular balloon creates temporary hemostasis
EXOSEAL	Cordis	Sealant	5–7	Extraluminally deployed polyglycolic acid plug
FISH	Morris Innovative	Sealant	5–8	Bioabsorbable matrix patch premounted on procedural sheath
VASCADE	Cardiva Medical	Collagen plug	5–7	Collagen plug deployed while intravascular disc creates temporary hemostasis
Angio–Seal	Terumo	Collagen Plug/ implanted anchor	5–8	Collagen plug secured by implanted intraluminal footplate

Selected Device Profiles

1. **Angio-Seal** (Terumo, Somerset, NJ) passive approximator
   a. **Mechanism:** An intravascular footplate and extravascular collagen plug are sandwiched around the arteriotomy and anchored with a suture.
   b. **Features**
      (1) Hemostasis is augmented through use of a collagen-based plug to promote clot formation.
      (2) All components, including the intravascular anchor, are fully absorbed at 60 to 90 days.
      (3) If reentry is necessary within 90 days, access is recommended to be at least 1 cm from the previous site.
   c. **Angio-Seal deployment (V-Twist Integrated Platform [VIP] model) (Fig. 2.2)**
      (1) Exchange the procedure sheath with the Angio-Seal locator system.
      (2) Blood flow through the locator visually confirms proper sheath position in the artery.
      (3) Insert the Angio-Seal VIP device into the sheath until you hear a "click."
      (4) Gently pull back on the locking cap until you hear another "click."

Table 2.4 Compression Assist Devices

Device	Manufacturer	Mechanism	Sheath Size (Fr)	Comments
CATALYST —CATALYST II —CATALYST III	Cardiva Medical	Drug-coated temporary occlusive disc		Intravascular disc left in place under tension until hemostasis achieved and then disc removed. CATALYST II coated in kaolin/chitosan. CATALYST III adds protamine sulfate.

Table 2.5 Hemostatic Patches

Device	Manufacturer	Mechanism	Comments
Syvek Excel	Marine Polymer Technologies	Patch	Poly-N-acetyl glucosamine activates platelets
Clo-Sur PAD	Merit Medical Systems	Patch	Positively charged polyprolate acetate biopolymer attracts red blood cells
D-Stat Dry	Teleflex	Patch	Thrombin activates clotting factors and platelets
Chitoclot Pad	Anscare	Patch	Positively charged chitosan molecules attract red blood cells and platelets
Statseal disc	Biolife	Patch	Biopolymer concentrates clotting factors, and potassium ferrate binds red blood cells
Quikclot	Z-Medica	Patch	Kaolin activates clotting factors

(5) The anchor is now locked in place and device is ready to be deployed.
(6) Gently pull back on the Angio-Seal VIP device until the suture has stopped spooling.
(7) Maintain upward tension on the device and gently advance the compaction tube until resistance is felt.
(8) Cut the suture and remove the device.

2. **StarClose SE** (Abbott Vascular, Abbott Park, IL) active approximator
   a. **Mechanism:** A nitinol clip is deployed around the arteriotomy, cinching it closed.
   b. **Manual release:** If the device cannot be retracted after clip deployment, a manual release will need to be performed. A small dilator is inserted into the manual release hole on the side of the device (see the IFU for exact location).
   c. **Features**
      (1) Secure mechanical closure
      (2) Immediate reaccess possible
      (3) Check for known hypersensitivity to nickel-titanium (nitinol clip) prior to usage

Table 2.6 Mechanical Compression Aids

Device	Manufacturer	Mechanism	Access Site	Comments
Femostop	Abbott Vascular	Balloon compression	Femoral	Device positioned around patient and then balloon inflated.
CompressAR ExpressAR	Advanced Vascular Dynamics	Disc compression	Femoral	Device positioned around patient, then disc tightened.
Safeguard	Merit Medical Systems	Balloon compression	Femoral/radial	Device positioned around patient and then balloon inflated.
TR Band	Terumo	Balloon compression	Radial	Device positioned around patient and then balloon inflated.

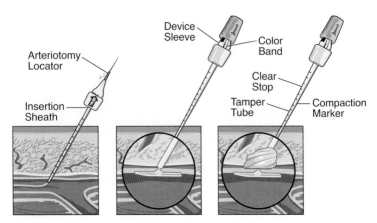

Arteriotomy Locator

Insertion Sheath

Device Sleeve

Color Band

Clear Stop

Tamper Tube

Compaction Marker

FIGURE 2.2 • Angio-Seal deployment—see Section 1.c for detailed instructions. (Courtesy of St. Jude Medical.)

   d. StarClose deployment (Fig. 2.3)
     (1) Exchange the procedural sheath for a StarClose sheath over a 0.035-in guidewire.
     (2) Remove the inner dilator and wire.
     (3) Insert the StarClose device until it clicks into the sheath.
     (4) Deploy the locator wing by pressing down on the blue plunger at the back of the device—a click will be heard.
     (5) Pull the device back until resistance is met at the vessel wall.
     (6) Shuttle the thumb advancer forward splitting the sheath—a click will be heard.
     (7) Deploy the clip by increasing the angle of the device and pressing the blue button—a click will be heard.
3. Perclose (Abbott Vascular, Abbott Park, IL) active approximator
   a. Mechanism: Sutures are deployed on either side of the arteriotomy site with a preformed knot. The knot is tightened then locked using the provided knot pusher.

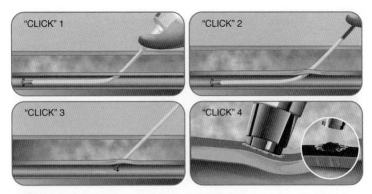

"CLICK" 1

"CLICK" 2

"CLICK" 3

"CLICK" 4

FIGURE 2.3 • StarClose deployment—see Section 2.d for detailed instructions. (Courtesy of Abbott Vascular. © 2010 Abbott Laboratories. All rights reserved.)

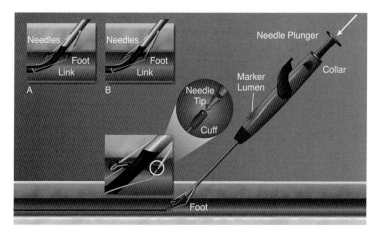

FIGURE 2.4 • Perclose deployment—see Section 3.c for detailed instructions. (Courtesy of Abbott Vascular. © 2010 Abbott Laboratories. All rights reserved.)

b. **Features**
   (1) Wire access can be maintained throughout the entire deployment. If hemostasis is not achieved, another Perclose or different device can be deployed.
   (2) Two devices can be utilized for preclosure of large arteriotomies up to 21 Fr.
   (3) Immediate reaccess possible.
   (4) Simplified knot delivery with pre-tied knot.
c. **Perclose ProGlide deployment (Fig. 2.4)**
   (1) Exchange the procedural sheath for a Perclose device over a 0.035-in guidewire.
   (2) When the wire exit hole nears the dermatotomy, remove the wire.
   (3) Advance the device until pulsatile blood flow is seen from the marker lumen.
   (4) Deploy the footplate and pull pack until resistance is met.
   (5) Depress the plunger until a click is heard, deploying the needles (Fig. 2.4A,B).
   (6) Pull back on the plunger until the suture exiting the back of the device is taut.
   (7) Cut the suture using the trimming tool on the front of the device.
   (8) Collapse the footplate.
   (9) Retract the device (optional: reinsert the wire through the wire exit hole).
   (10) Use the knot pusher to advance the knot along the blue suture as the device is removed.
   (11) Lock the knot by pulling on the white suture.
4. **Prostar XL** (Abbott Vascular, Abbott Park, IL) active approximator
   a. **Mechanism:** Two braided polyester sutures and four nitinol needles are deployed from the arterial lumen and pulled out through the tissue tract then tied by hand.
   b. **Features**
      (1) Can be used to close larger arteriotomies—IFU up to 10 Fr.
      (2) Sutures can be tied with wire in place—if hemostasis not achieved, second Prostar or other device can be deployed.
      (3) Immediate reaccess possible.
      (4) Steepest learning curve.

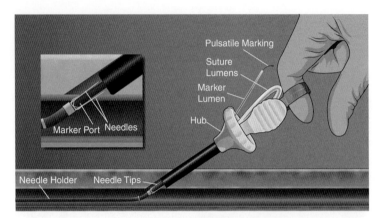

FIGURE 2.5 • Prostar XL deployment—see Section 4.c for detailed instructions. (Courtesy of Abbott Vascular. © 2010 Abbott Laboratories. All rights reserved.)

c. **Prostar XL deployment (Fig. 2.5)**
   (1) Slightly extend the skin incision and blunt dissect the tissue tract.
   (2) Exchange the sheath for a Prostar XL device over a 0.035-in guidewire.
   (3) Advance the device until the wire exit port reaches the dermatotomy and then remove the wire and advance the device to the skin.
   (4) Squeeze the white interlocks together with thumb and forefinger unlocking the barrel.
   (5) Advance the barrel while rotating back and forth until pulsatile blood returns.
   (6) Turn the ring-shaped handle 90 degrees clockwise and then pull it out of the back hub of the barrel—this deploys the needles.
   (7) Retrieve the four needles/suture tails from the back of the device using a Kelly clamp.
   (8) Cut the needles off the end of each suture tail and discard.
   (9) Retract the device until the sutures can be seen along the device shaft and harvest the suture tails from the device hub.
   (10) Pair up the suture tails across from each other (green with green and white with white).
   (11) Tie a sliding self-locking knot with one suture and set it to the side.
   (12) Tie a sliding self-locking knot with the second suture and advance it to the arteriotomy while removing the Prostar device from the vessel then tighten the suture.
   (13) Advance and tighten the knot that was previously tied and set to the side.
5. **Mynx** (Cordis, Santa Clara, CA) passive approximator
   a. **Mechanism:** A polyethylene glycol (PEG) sealant plug is delivered to the extravascular surface of the artery while an intravascular balloon is inflated for temporary hemostasis. The balloon is then deflated and removed. Two models are available—MynxControl and MynxGrip.
   b. **Features**
      (1) Grip technology—PEG tip adheres to outer surface of vessel wall.
      (2) Device is used through the indwelling procedural sheath.
      (3) Balloon can be inflated with contrast for fluoroscopic visualization during SFA and antegrade puncture closures.
      (4) Immediate reaccess possible.
      (5) All components are fully absorbed within 30 days.

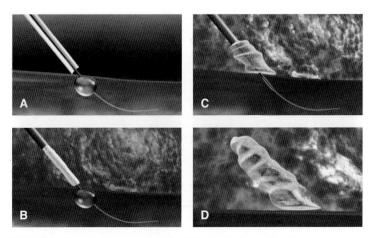

FIGURE 2.6 • Mynx deployment—see Section 5.c for detailed instructions. (Courtesy of AccessClosure.)

c. **MynxGrip deployment (Fig. 2.6)**
   (1) Insert the device through the indwelling sheath up to the white shaft marker.
   (2) Inflate the balloon and close the stopcock; check the inflation indicator.
   (3) Retract the device until the balloon is against the arteriotomy (Fig. 2.6A).
   (4) Open the stopcock on the procedural sheath to confirm temporary hemostasis.
   (5) Advance the green shuttle delivering the PEG to the arteriotomy (Fig. 2.6B).
   (6) Withdraw the sheath and green shuttle to the back of the device.
   (7) Move the advancer tube forward two notches.
   (8) Lay the device down for a moment.
   (9) Deflate the balloon and remove it through the advancer tube (Fig. 2.6C).
   (10) Remove the advancer tube and apply light pressure for 2 minutes (Fig. 2.6D).
6. **EXOSEAL** (Cordis, Santa Clara, CA) passive approximator
   a. **Mechanism:** A bioabsorbable polyglycolic acid (PGA) plug is deployed into the extravascular tract overlying the arteriotomy. The plug is held in place within the tract by the overlying fascia.
   b. **Features**
      (1) Used through indwelling sheath.
      (2) Bioabsorbable material completely resorbed at 60 to 90 days.
      (3) Lockout mechanism prevents intravascular deployment.
      (4) Not for use with sheaths greater than 12 cm in length.
   c. **EXOSEAL Deployment (Fig. 2.7)**
      (1) The device is inserted through the indwelling procedural sheath (Fig. 2.7A) until pulsatile blood return is visualized from the indicator port (Fig. 2.7B).
      (2) The sheath and device are retracted together until the pulsatility of blood diminishes (Fig. 2.7C,D).
      (3) The indicator window is then checked (Fig. 2.7E)—the device is in proper extravascular position at the arterial surface when the indicator switches from black/white to black/black.
      (4) If the indicator switches to black/red, it has been retracted too far and tension should be released.

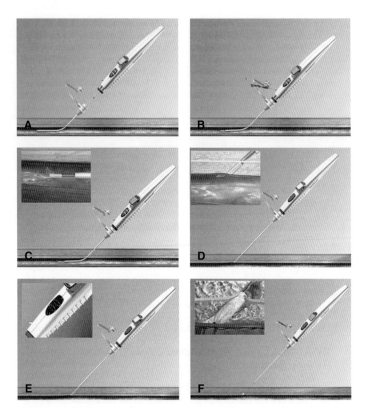

FIGURE 2.7 • EXOSEAL deployment—see Section 6.c for detailed instructions. (Reprinted with permission from Treitl M, Eberhardt K, Maxien D, et al. Arterielle Verschlusssysteme. *Radiologe.* 2013;53:230–245.)

    (5) With a black/black indicator window, the plug is deployed by pressing the green switch on the handle (Fig. 2.7F).

        The device and sheath are removed and MC is held for 2 minutes.

7. Catalyst III (Cardiva, Santa Clara, CA) compression assist devices

  a. Mechanism: A drug-coated intravascular disc is temporarily deployed and kept under tension at the end of the procedure until hemostasis is achieved and then the disc is removed. Adjunctive MC must be held, but for a shorter duration than expected with MC alone.

  b. Features

    (1) Used through indwelling sheath.

    (2) Immediate reaccess is possible.

    (3) No deposition of material eliminates implant-related complications.

    (4) Catalyst III disc is coated with kaolin/chitosan, as well as protamine sulfate, to promote hemostasis.

    (5) Check for known allergy to protamine sulfate or shellfish prior to usage.

  c. Catalyst III deployment (Fig. 2.8)

    (1) The device wire is inserted through an 11-cm length indwelling procedural sheath until the white gripper reaches, but does not enter the hub of the sheath (modified technique possible on 15- or 25-cm sheath).

    (2) The disc is deployed by pulling the actuator back until it locks in place and 7 mm of green mark is visible.

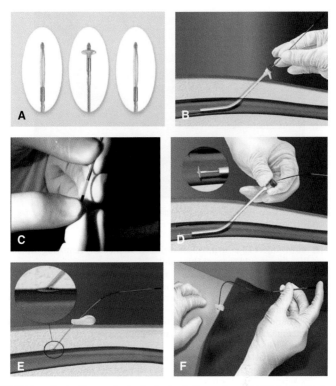

FIGURE 2.8 • Catalyst III—see Section 7.c for detailed instructions. (© 2020 Cardiva Medical, Santa Clara, CA)

    (3) Retract sheath over the device wire and grasp the white gripper when it appears at the distal end of the introducer sheath.

    (4) Gently lift upward and apply tension on the white gripper until white coating on the wire is visible at skin level.

    (5) Attach clip to the wire at skin level to continue tension until hemostasis achieved (recommended minimum 15 minutes).

    (6) For device removal, collapse disc by pressing on the actuator and then remove while maintaining proximal MC.

8. **TR Band** (Terumo, Somerset, NJ) mechanical compression aid

    a. **Mechanism:** An entirely external device that achieves radial artery hemostasis by means of a titratable balloon/strap construct that is fastened to the patient's wrist. The balloon is positioned over the arteriotomy site and inflated until bleeding stops.

    b. **Features**

        (1) Immediate reaccess is possible.

        (2) No deposition of material eliminates implant-related complications.

        (3) Relatively easy to use.

    c. **TR Band deployment (Fig. 2.9)**

        (1) Withdraw procedural sheath 2 to 3 cm.

        (2) Apply the device by aligning the green marker (located on the center of the compression balloon) 1 to 2 mm proximal to the puncture site, and fasten the strap to the patient's wrist.

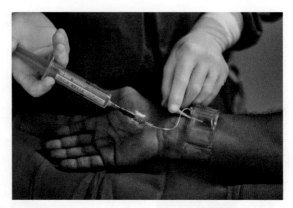

FIGURE 2.9 • TR Band—see Section 8.c for detailed instructions. (© 2020 Terumo, Somerset, New Jersey, United States.)

(3) Slowly inject 15 to 18 mL of air while simultaneously removing the sheath. Bleeding should cease at this point.

(4) Begin removing air from the balloon until rebleeding occurs. Reinject 1 to 2 mL of air. Bleeding should again stop.

(5) Confirm radial pulse or evaluate radial artery patency by using the reverse Barbeau's test.

(6) TR Band deployed for 60 minutes (heparin 50 units per kg or less), or 120 minutes (heparin greater than 50 units per kg).

(7) Remove 3 to 5 mL air every 10 to 15 minutes or slow deflation in one step (accelerated) per operator preference.

(8) If bleeding occurs during removal, reinflate the balloon and wait 15 to 30 minutes.

Advanced Techniques

1. **Preclose technique for large arteriotomies**
   a. Suture-mediated VCD used to close large arteriotomies.
   b. Used for percutaneous endovascular aneurysm repair.
   c. Access initially obtained with 6-Fr sheath and 0.035-in guidewire.
   d. Two Perclose ProGlide devices are deployed in succession each rotated 30 degrees in opposite directions (10 o'clock and 2 o'clock).
   e. Sutures left untightened and secured to the side.
   f. Serial dilatation of the arteriotomy and completion of the repair.
   g. The sheath is removed over a 0.035-in guidewire with MC and the preformed knots are cinched tight in sequential order of their placement.
   h. MC released
      (1) If hemostasis confirmed—remove guidewire.
      (2) If pulsatile blood flow persists—deploy another Perclose or Angio-Seal.
      (3) If hemostasis still not achieved, reinsert sheath; surgical repair needed.
   i. MC reapplied for 5 to 10 minutes after hemostasis confirmed.
   j. Bed rest for 6 hours

2. **Treatment of CFA pseudoaneurysm (PFA)**
   a. Percutaneously access PSA with a micropuncture needle and navigate the mandril wire through neck into the parent artery
   b. Exchange for 0.035-in guidewire and deploy active approximator Angio-Seal or active approximator VCD.
   c. Consider in patients with coagulopathy who fail thrombin injection.

3. **Inadvertent subclavian artery catheter placement (2)**
   a. Case reports during attempted central venous access.
   b. Angio-Seal, StarClose, Mynx, and Perclose use reported for arterial closure after catheter removal over a wire.
   c. An arterial occlusion balloon can be inserted from groin access and used adjunctively while the indwelling catheter is exchanged for the VCD.
4. **Venous closure (3)**
   a. Angio-Seal and Perclose have been used for venous closure both at completion or as preclosure before dilation to a large sheath size.

Complications (Table 2.7)

1. Access-site complications are rarely life threatening, but even minor complications may result in longer hospital stays and increased 1-year mortality rates (4). Complications are often multifactorial with potential contributions from:
   a. Initial access quality/location/size
   b. Anticoagulant/antiplatelet/thrombolytic medications
   c. Choice of device and technique used for deployment or MC
2. Major complications
   a. Result from damage to the vessel during device deployment, dislodgment of atherosclerotic plaque during deployment, or device embolization.
   b. Vessel damage is most likely to occur with use of active approximator devices that mechanically cinch the arteriotomy closed, but device embolization can occur with active or passive approximators.
   c. Major complications usually require open surgical or endovascular repair.
   d. Overall, these complications are quite rare with decreased incidence after evolution of devices and cumulative operator experience.
3. Minor complications
   a. Minor complications usually result from device failure or ineffective MC.
   b. Hematomas are usually managed conservatively but may require transfusion.
   c. PSA is usually managed with thrombin injection or compression with stent-graft coverage or VCD closure reserved for refractory cases.
   d. Injury to superficial cutaneous branches of the femoral nerve with otherwise unremarkable Angio-Seal deployment has been reported.

Results

1. Early case reports and trial data of coronary catheterization patients in the 1990s and 2000s demonstrated increased complications with the use of VCDs, however legitimacy issues have been raised regarding extrapolation of these early findings to procedures performed in patients at higher risk of vascular complications (5).
2. A meta-analysis specific to interventional radiology reviewed 34 studies with a pooled analysis of VCDs (Angio-Seal, StarClose, Perclose, and Duett). It showed a nonsignificant decrease in complications versus MC (6).

Table 2.7 Major and Minor Complications of Vascular Closure Device Deployment

Major Complications	Minor Complications
Limb ischemia	Hematoma
Device embolization	Pseudoaneurysm
Artery occlusion	Arteriovenous fistula
Arterial laceration	Nerve injury
Retroperitoneal hematoma	
Access site infection	

3. A data registry specific to interventional radiology collected data from across 10 European countries, with a total enrollment of 1,107 patients. It showed device deployment was successful in 97.2% of cases. The complication rate was 2.4% (7).
4. A meta-analysis of 34 studies with a pooled analysis of VCDs (VasoSeal, Angio-Seal, ProGlide, Prostar, StarClose, Exoseal, Catalyst, Femoseal, EVS, X-PRESS, EpiClose-T, and FISH) showed reduced time to hemostasis and ambulation compared to MC (8).
5. A 2016 Cochrane systematic review found no difference in the incidence of vascular injury of VCDs compared to MC, as well as no difference in efficacy or safety of VCDs with different mechanisms of action (9).
6. A 2018 meta-analysis of 12 studies with 7,961 coronary catheterization patients showed significantly lower major bleeding and vascular complications associated with TRA compared to CFA VCDs (suture devices or vessel plugs) (10).

Key Take-Home Points

1. The literature has firmly established that VCDs decrease time to hemostasis and ambulation, when compared to the gold standard of MC.
2. After 20 years of device evolution and collective operator experience, data now suggest that the devices are not different from MC in terms of efficacy, safety, or vascular complications.
3. With dozens of devices to choose from, the key to successful VCD deployment is familiarity with the concept, mechanism, and instructions for each device used in one's practice. Knowing the steps of deployment is insufficient; the operator must be able to visualize what is happening inside and around the artery as each button is pushed and each plunger depressed.
4. Some devices are better suited than others for certain clinical applications and patient populations. The key is to become comfortable with multiple devices that can be deployed with confidence in a predictable fashion.

References

1. Barbetta I, van den Berg JC. Access and hemostasis: femoral and popliteal approaches and closure devices—why, what, when, and how? *Semin Intervent Radiol.* 2014;31(4):353–360.
2. Mousa AY, Abu-Halimah S, Nanjundappa A, et al. Inadvertent subclavian artery cannulation and options for management. *Vascular.* 2015;23(2):132–137.
3. Mylonas I, Sakata Y, Salinger M, et al. The use of percutaneous suture-mediated closure for the management of 14 French femoral venous access. *J Invasive Cardiol.* 2006;18(7):299–302.
4. Ortiz D, Jahangir A, Singh M, et al. Access site complications after peripheral vascular interventions: incidence, predictors, and outcomes. *Circ Cardiovasc Interv.* 2014;7(6):821–828.
5. Sheth RA, Walker TG, Saad WE, et al. Quality improvement guidelines for vascular access and closure device use. *J Vasc Interv Radiol.* 2014;25(1):73–84.
6. Das R, Ahmed K, Athanasiou T, et al. Arterial closure devices versus manual compression for femoral haemostasis in interventional radiological procedures: a systematic review and meta-analysis. *Cardiovasc Intervent Radiol.* 2011;34(4):723–738.
7. Reekers JA, Müller-Hülsbeck S, Libicher M, et al. CIRSE vascular closure device registry. *Cardiovas Intervent Radiol.* 2011;34(1):50–53.
8. Cox T, Blair L, Huntington C, et al. Systematic review of randomized controlled trials comparing manual compression to vascular closure devices for diagnostic and therapeutic arterial procedures. *Surg Technol Int.* 2015;27:32–44.
9. Robertson L, Andras A, Colgan F, et al. Vascular closure devices for femoral arterial puncture site haemostasis. *Cochrane Database Syst Rev.* 2016;3:CD009541.
10. Chugh Y, Bavishi C, Mojadidi MK, et al. Safety of transradial access compared to transfemoral access with hemostatic devices (vessel plugs and suture devices) after percutaneous coronary interventions: a systematic review and meta-analysis. *Catheter Cardiovasc Interv.* 2020;96(2):285–295.

3 Management of Vascular Complications

John Chung, MD, FRCPC and
Darren Klass, MBChB, MD, MRCS, FRCR, FRCPC

Introduction

Access site complications are relatively rare, ranging from small hematomas to transection of the access artery with exsanguination (1). Common complications and their occurrence rates are listed in Tables 3.1 and 3.2.

Pseudoaneurysms

The most common vascular access site complication requiring intervention is pseudoaneurysm formation. Surgical repair has surprisingly high complication rates, from 19% to 32% (2), including inadequate wound healing, femoral neuralgias, and lymphatic leaks; thus, ultrasound-guided procedures have revolutionized their treatment (3).

Indication
1. Identification of an arterial access site pseudoaneurysm. Conservative, observational management has largely been abandoned.

Contraindications
Absolute
1. Hemodynamically unstable patient
2. Active hemorrhage (retroperitoneal or percutaneous); expanding hematoma
3. Impending skin necrosis due to size of hematoma/pseudoaneurysm
4. Acute distal limb ischemia due to compression effects of hematoma/pseudoaneurysm
5. Active infection at the site of percutaneous access

Relative
1. Width of pseudoaneurysm neck >8 mm
2. Lack of any discernible pseudoaneurysm neck
3. Pseudoaneurysm sac diameter <10 mm (increased risk of arterial thrombosis)

Preprocedure Preparation
1. Detailed imaging, most commonly with ultrasound, or alternatively computed tomographic angiography (CTA) or magnetic resonance angiography (MRA). The extent and morphology of the pseudoaneurysm should be identified, including the number of lobes the pseudoaneurysm has as well as the width and length of its neck. If performing ultrasound, the Doppler waveform pattern of the outflow artery should also be assessed.
2. Recent laboratory data should be obtained, including complete blood count (CBC), platelets, and international normalized ratio (INR).
3. Doppler or palpation assessment of ipsilateral foot arteries (dorsalis pedis, tibialis posterior) immediately prior to percutaneous therapy.

Procedure
Ultrasound-Guided Compression (3)
1. The first described ultrasound-guided management of iatrogenic pseudoaneurysms. It remains the preferred treatment option for pseudoaneurysms <1 cm and is still an acceptable therapy when thrombin is not available.

Table 3.1   **Common Complications Following Percutaneous Femoral Arterial Access**

Complication	Incidence (%)
Hematoma	5–23
Pseudoaneurysm	0.2–9
Arteriovenous fistula	0.1–2.1
Hemorrhage	0.15–0.44
Dissection/occlusion	<0.5
Neuropathy	0.21
Infection	<0.1

2. Inject copious amounts of local anesthetic. Consider intravenous sedation. Due to extensive bruising, these patients are often exquisitely tender.
3. A linear array (4 to 7 MHz) ultrasound transducer is placed on the affected groin with direct visualization of the pseudoaneurysm neck and body (or lobe closest to the neck in a multilobed, complex pseudoaneurysm) as well as the artery from which the pseudoaneurysm arises.
4. With real-time color Doppler sonographic guidance, pressure is applied on the pseudoaneurysm via the probe to eliminate flow through the pseudoaneurysm while maintaining flow through the parent artery.
5. Pressure is slowly alleviated at 10-minute intervals to assess for any persistent flow through the pseudoaneurysm.
6. At the first instance persistent flow is identified, step 4 is repeated until the pseudoaneurysm internal flow remains obliterated when transducer pressure is fully released.
7. Limitations of this technique include the relatively long time required, patient discomfort with possible need for sedation, and higher failure rates relative to other ultrasound-guided treatment methods.

Ultrasound-Guided Thrombin Injection (2,3)

1. This method is the standard of care in most institutions.
2. Standard sterile preparation and draping of the affected site and a sterile cover is applied to an ultrasound transducer (most commonly a 4 to 7 MHz linear array probe).
3. Subcutaneous local anesthesia is administered as needed. Due to extensive bruising, these patients are often exquisitely tender.
4. Preparation of thrombin solution. Multiple thrombin formulations are available. Typically, it is reconstituted with sterile saline. Use of bovine or human thrombin in concentrations of 100 to 1,000 IU per mL has been described, all with equal efficacy.
   a. In some institutions, thrombin is only available as part of a kit (e.g., Tisseel [Baxter, Deerfield, IL]) containing various doses of dehydrated human thrombin. The provided 2-mL calcium chloride solution is injected into a 1,000 IU thrombin vial. The mixture is vigorously swirled to reconstitute the thrombin into solution. The resultant 2-mL thrombin solution is further added to a 10-mL syringe containing 8 mL of sterile saline, resulting in a 10-mL solution with a concentration of 100 IU per mL.
5. Ultrasound-guided insertion of a 21- or 22-gauge needle into the pseudoaneurysm is performed, preferentially into the proximal most lobe in direct communication with the pseudoaneurysm neck in complex pseudoaneurysms.
6. The thrombin solution is injected slowly in increments of 0.1 to 0.2 mL (10 to 20 IU) under real-time sonographic color Doppler visualization of the

pseudoaneurysm, *only* until there is complete cessation of internal color Doppler flow.
7. Sonographic grayscale and color Doppler assessment of the pseudoaneurysm is performed 10 minutes after thrombin injection to ensure it remains thrombosed; if any residual flow has returned, additional thrombin is injected as per steps 4 and 5.

Postprocedure Management
1. Doppler or palpation assessment of ipsilateral foot circulation immediately after percutaneous therapy.
2. Bed rest for a minimum of 2 hours after ultrasound-guided therapy.
3. Follow-up ultrasound Doppler assessment of the pseudoaneurysm in 24 hours is essential.

Results (2,3)
1. Ultrasound-guided compression
   a. Technical success ranges from 63% to 88%.
   b. Mean compression times are 30 to 44 minutes; thus patient discomfort and need for sedation/analgesia are frequent.
   c. Failure rates increase significantly if the patient is anticoagulated (≤70%) or if the pseudoaneurysm size is >4 cm.
2. Ultrasound-guided thrombin injection
   a. Primary technical success rates 90% to 94%, with overall success rates ranging from 93% to 100%. Mean injected thrombin dose ranges from 225 to 425 IU.
   b. Procedural times are significantly shorter than ultrasound-guided compression. Patient sedation is typically not necessary.
   c. Failures usually in pseudoaneurysms >6 cm in diameter.

Complications (1–3)
1. Groin pain (41%)
2. Pseudoaneurysm reperfusion (2.1%)
3. Thromboembolism (0.8%)
4. Allergic reaction, if bovine thrombin is used
5. Blood-borne infections, if human thrombin is used
6. Acute expansion and/or rupture of the pseudoaneurysm after therapy necessitating emergency surgery (2.1%); this has only been described with ultrasound-guided compression

Management of Complications (1,3)
1. Groin pain—analgesia is typically sufficient.
2. Pseudoaneurysm reperfusion—repeat ultrasound-guided therapy is the first recourse in most cases.
3. Thromboembolism—management depends on severity. If nonocclusive, it can be managed with systemic anticoagulation. If occlusive and/or extensive, surgical thrombectomy or endovascular pharmacomechanical thrombolysis should be performed.
4. Allergic reaction—avoid use of bovine-derived thrombin in patients with allergy to bovine products. If allergic reaction occurs, start standard treatment of anaphylaxis.
5. Acute pseudoaneurysm expansion/rupture—limit use of the ultrasound-guided compression technique to pseudoaneurysms <4 cm in size and in patients who are not actively anticoagulated.

Other Access Site Complications (1–5)

1. *Hematoma*—this is the most common minor complication.
   a. Typically managed conservatively. The hematoma can be outlined with a marking pen and inspected at regular intervals (such as when vital signs are taken) to ensure no expansion.

   b. If the hematoma is massive and symptomatic (e.g., causing femoral neuralgia or acute limb ischemia), surgical evacuation may be required.

2. *Arteriovenous fistula*—the use of ultrasound guidance to ensure single-wall arterial access greatly minimizes this complication.

   a. Surgical repair is usually necessary.

   b. If asymptomatic, it can be initially managed conservatively as up to one-third will spontaneously resolve.

   c. Endovascular treatment could be considered if the patient is not a surgical candidate. If the fistulous tract is of sufficient length, it can be embolized with coils. Fistula occlusion with a nitinol-covered stent within the arterial segment is possible but not considered ideal given the downsides of stenting across a moving joint.

3. *Arterial dissection*—treatment depends on the severity.

   a. If focal and non–flow-limiting, it could be managed conservatively with imaging surveillance, typically via CTA.

   b. If flow-limiting, prolonged endovascular balloon inflation across the dissection should be performed to reappose the dissected intima with the vessel media.

   c. If the dissection extends into the iliac arteries, placement of self-expanding nitinol stents within the iliac arteries may be necessary to maintain luminal patency.

4. *Arterial thrombosis*—therapy depends on the extent of thrombus.

   a. Thrombosis not complicated by dissection, if nonocclusive can be managed medically with systemic anticoagulation.

   b. If occlusive, surgical thrombectomy is the treatment of choice because the arteriotomy can be repaired at the same time. If thrombosis was induced by a vascular closure device, any intravascular component can be definitively removed.

   c. If the patient is not a surgical candidate, endovascular access can be achieved from a second arterial access site (typically the contralateral common femoral artery), and endovascular pharmacomechanical thrombolysis can be performed.

5. *Retroperitoneal hematoma/uncontrollable puncture site bleeding*—may result from a high arterial puncture above the inguinal ligament with retroperitoneal bleeding, or failure to achieve primary hemostasis after appropriately placed puncture.

   a. Retroperitoneal bleeding is usually not immediately clinically obvious and can be devastating. Early clues before pain or hypotension can be decreased urine output or tachycardia. Urgent noncontrast pelvic computed tomography (CT) is the diagnostic method of choice and is recommended even when there is slight suspicion.

   b. The standard of therapy is urgent surgical repair.

      (1) If there is intraarterial access when discovered, angioplasty balloon can be inflated at, or a temporary occlusion balloon proximal to, the site of injury while the patient awaits surgery.

   c. If vascular surgery is not readily available or the patient is not a surgical candidate, placement of a covered stent across the vascular injury can be performed. The stent graft should be nitinol-based, sized 1 mm larger than the vessel diameter in which it is to be placed (remember that the artery may be contracted if the patient is hypotensive), be as short as possible, and should not be landed across the common femoral bifurcation if possible (1).

Considerations Specific to Radial Access

1. *Radial artery occlusion (RAO)* (6,7)—this is the most common complication and, in the vast majority of cases, is asymptomatic.

   a. Mitigation is most important:

Table 3.2 Common Complications Following Percutaneous Radial Arterial Access	
Complication	**Incidence (%)**
Hematoma	<1
RAO	<1
Pseudoaneurysm	<0.1
Compartment syndrome	<0.01
Arterial perforation	<0.03
Neuropathy/vasculitis	<0.1

(1) Adopting the practice of nonocclusive radial artery hemostasis and concomitant prophylactic ulnar artery compression reduces occurrence rates to <1%.

(2) Heparinization and use of lowest profile devices appropriate for the case also further reduce rates of RAO.

(3) Practicing strict catheter and sheath hygiene, including aspirating before flushing devices.

(4) Appropriate use of heparin for cases. Weight-based heparin should be utilized for all cases. 50–75 IU per kg is used for 4- and 5-Fr cases and 100 IU per kg for 6-Fr and above and for complex cases in our institution.

b. If the patient is asymptomatic, do nothing.

c. 4 weeks of LMWH has been shown to facilitate RAO recanalization in 87% of patients.

d. In rare instances of RAO causing distal ischemia, more aggressive measures can be undertaken. There are no established guidelines, but treatment can include admission with therapeutic heparinization to more aggressive measures such as pharmacomechanical thrombolysis or thrombectomy.

e. If RAO is recognized during or immediately following the procedure, attempts should be made to recanalize the vessel and preserve it for future use. If the sheath is still in situ, suction thrombectomy can be performed. If the sheath has been removed, the patient can be placed on a therapeutic weight-based heparin infusion for an hour. This has been shown to recanalize radial artery occlusions when combined with transient ulnar artery compression. Transient ulnar artery compression increases the flow of blood through the radial artery as it recanalizes (8).

The steps are as follows:

(1) Apply radial hemostasis band and inflate balloon to allow for patent hemostasis.

(2) Apply hemostatic band to ulnar artery and inflate balloon to occlude the ulnar artery.

(3) Begin a peripheral heparin infusion for 1 hour with a loading dose of heparin prior to the infusion.

(4) Remove the ulnar compression and heparin infusion at 1 hour, but leave the radial hemostatic band in place until hemostasis is achieved, ensuring patent hemostasis.

2. *Radial artery spasm (RAS)* (9)—this manifests as acute, focal arm pain.

a. Mitigation is most important; with proper precautions, RAS can be reduced to 1%.

(1) Application of EMLA patch and nitroglycerin cream to skin overlying the radial artery.

(2) Use ultrasound guidance and single-wall puncture technique rather than blind double-wall technique.

(3) Apply tumescent anesthesia (mixture of 9 mL 1% lidocaine and 100-mcg nitroglycerin) along sides of the radial artery prior to access.

(4) Use sheaths designed specifically for the radial artery, which are lower profile, hydrophilic, and have smooth tapering between dilator and sheath tip.

(5) Use IA spasmolytic cocktail upon sheath introduction but prior to catheter/wire advancement. 5-mg verapamil alone or 1.25 to 5 mg of verapamil + 100 to 200 mcg of nitroglycerin has been shown to significantly reduce RAS. Our institution employs 2.5 to 5 mg of verapamil and 200 mcg of nitroglycerin in our cocktail. Younger females are more prone to spasm so consider 5-mg verapamil for UFE.

(6) Recognize variant radial artery anatomy, as high origin radial arteries and radial artery loops are much more prone to RAS. Preprocedure ultrasound assessment of the radial artery can identify these variants, which can help the operator proceed more cautiously.

b. When encountered, the first step is to readminister another dose of the initial spasmolytic cocktail.

c. If the above fails, the next step is to localize the site of spasm on angiography/ultrasound and administer high-dose tumescent anesthesia (15 mL 1% lidocaine and 1,000-mcg nitroglycerin) locally in the subcutaneous space around the spasmed segment.

d. Finally, further sedating the patient will result in smooth muscle relaxation with undoing of the spasm. Very rarely, general anesthesia is required.

3. Hematoma formation (10)
  a. Mitigation is most important:
    (1) Ensure appropriate use of hemostatic devices – operators should ensure they have full knowledge of how to apply hemostatic bands specific to their institution.
    (2) Have established post-procedural care orders, including monitoring of the puncture site at set intervals (for example q15 minutes for the first hour) and what to do in the event bleeding or a hematoma is seen (for example, re-inflate compression device, apply pressure, notify IR).
  b. If a hematoma has formed, the EASY Hematoma Classification (10) is an established guideline for grading radial access hematomas, including treatment recommendations:
    (1) Grades I and II – give analgesia, apply additional compression, apply local ice.
    (2) Grades III and IV (very rare with appropriate post-procedural monitoring) – give analgesia, apply additional compression, apply local ice, inflate a blood pressure cuff around the forearm.
    (3) Grade V (compartment syndrome; should almost never occur with appropriate post-procedural monitoring) – surgery to evacuate hematoma/repair arterial defect.

4. Perforation/dissection of radial artery—rare occurrence.
  a. Mitigation is most important:
    (1) Avoid use of hydrophilic guidewires as they more often inadvertently course into small branches. Use atraumatic tipped, nonhydrophilic guidewires such as Bentson or Wholey wires.
    (2) If resistance is met, **do not** attempt to continue advancing guidewire.
  b. If vessel injury occurs, crossing the injured segment with a wire and catheter will often tamponade the injury. Focal pressure/blood pressure cuff inflation can also be applied if extravasation is present. At the end of the case, check angiography can determine if the injury has resolved.

5. *Pseudoaneurysm formation*—rare occurrence.
  a. Compression therapy:

(1) Apply ultrasound-guided spot compression to site at 15- to 30-minute intervals, similar to as described above for femoral pseudoaneurysms.

(2) Reapply radial band at pseudoaneurysm with prolonged compression (1 to 3 hours) followed by ultrasound reassessment.

   b. Ultrasound-guided thrombin injection, similar to as described above for femoral pseudoaneurysms. Note that the majority of radial artery pseudoaneurysms will not have a morphology considered safe for thrombin injection; therefore, this treatment technique is much less frequently employed.

   c. Tincture of time. On short-term 1- to 2-week follow-up, these can been found to have spontaneously thrombosed.

   d. Primary surgical repair if the above have all failed.

6. *Neuralgia*—exceedingly rare, likely due to a reactive vasculitis as the sensory alterations often do not follow a single-nerve distribution.

   a. Mitigation is most important:

   (1) Avoid overextending the patient's wrist during the procedure.

   (2) Avoid excessive/aggressive compression hemostasis.

   b. As the condition is predominantly self-limiting, conservative therapy such as nonsteroidal antiinflammatory drug analgesia is often sufficient.

References

1. Tsetis D. Endovascular treatment of complications of femoral arterial access. *Cardiovasc Intervent Radiol.* 2010;33(3):457–468.

2. Krueger K, Zaehringer M, Strohe D, et al. Postcatheterization pseudoaneurysm: results of US-guided percutaneous thrombin injection in 240 patients. *Radiology.* 2005;236(3):1104–1110.

3. Morgan R, Belli AM. Current treatment methods for postcatheterization pseudoaneurysms. *J Vasc Interv Radiol.* 2003;14(6):697–710.

4. Stone PA, Campbell JE, AbuRahma AF. Femoral pseudoaneurysms after percutaneous access. *J Vasc Surg.* 2014;60(5):1359–1366.

5. Vlachou PA, Karkos CD, Bains S, et al. Percutaneous ultrasound-guided thrombin injection for the treatment of iatrogenic femoral artery pseudoaneurysms. *Eur J Radiol.* 2011;77(1):172–174.

6. Pancholy SB, Bernat I, Bertrand OF, et al. Prevention of radial rtery occlusion after transradial catheterization: the PROPHET-II randomized Trial. *JACC Cardiovasc Interv.* 2016;9(19):1992–1999.

7. Hahalis GN, Leopoulou M, Tsigkas G, et al. Multicenter randomized evaluation of high versus standard heparin dose on incident radial arterial occlusion after transradial coronary angiography: the spirit of artemis study. *JACC Cardiovasc Interv.* 2018;11(22):2241–2250.

8. Bernat I, Bertrand OF, Rokyta R, et al. Efficacy and safety of transient ulnar artery compression to recanalize acute radial artery occlusion after transradial catheterization. *Am J Cardiol.* 2011;107(11):1698–1670.

9. Kwok CS, Rashid M, Fraser D, et al. Intra-arterial vasodilators to prevent radial artery spasm: a systematic review and pooled analysis of clinical studies. *Cardiovasc Revasc Med.* 2015;16(8):484–490.

10. Bertrand OF, Larose E, Rodés-Cabau J, et al. Incidence, predictors, and clinical impact of bleeding after transradial coronary stenting and maximal antiplatelet therapy. *Am Heart J.* 2009;157(1):164–169.

SECTION II
TRANSARTERIAL PROCEDURES

4 Endovascular Management of Acute Ischemic Stroke

**Zachary M. Wilseck, MD, Johanna M. Ospel, MD, PhD,
Joseph J. Gemmete, MD, FACR, FSIR, FCIRSE, FAHA, and
Venu Vadlamudi, MD, RPVI, FSIR, FSVM, FASA, FACC**

Introduction

Stroke is a sudden neurologic change and is the leading cause of severe disability and fifth leading cause of death in the United States with enormous health care and societal costs. There are two main forms of stroke: ischemic stroke (85% to 87%) and hemorrhagic stroke (13% to 15%). In acute ischemic stroke (AIS), thromboembolic occlusion of an artery interrupts perfusion of brain parenchyma. The goal of AIS treatment is to recanalize the occluded vessel and thereby avoid progression to infarction, limit disability, and return the patient to functional independence.

The two treatment options for AIS are (1) intravenous (IV) thrombolytic therapy (alteplase or tenecteplase) and (2) endovascular thrombectomy (EVT). IV alteplase is a proven medical revascularization therapy for AIS indicated in selected patients up to 4.5 hours after symptom onset and in some cases, with advanced imaging, up to 9 hours after symptom onset. However, IV alteplase is often ineffective in large vessel occlusion (LVO) stroke which often carries higher morbidity and mortality. IV tenecteplase has been studied including in the setting of EVT and has shown good effect but is not yet standard of care. Multiple prospective randomized controlled trials (RCTs) have demonstrated that EVT is highly effective in reducing disability in selected patients with acute LVO anterior circulation stroke and is currently recommended broadly in LVO patients presenting up to 6 hours from symptom onset and in selected patients up to 24 hours from symptom onset (1–10).

The statement that "time is brain" cannot be overemphasized when treating stroke. An estimated 1.9 million neurons are lost per minute in untreated acute LVO strokes. Every 30-minute delay is associated with a 10% decrease in functional outcome at 90 days. Time can be saved across every level of stroke care from prehospital care to intraprocedural technique to optimize patient outcomes. Identification of appropriate patients with noninvasive imaging, an emphasis on rapid and complete revascularization with modern thrombectomy devices and techniques, and a multidisciplinary commitment to process improvement are critical factors for improving patient outcomes.

Background for EVT

In 2015, five landmark RCTs were published which demonstrated efficacy of endovascular therapy in the setting of anterior circulation AIS (1–5). These RCTs not only demonstrated improvements in functional independence and modified Rankin Score (mRS) at 90 days but also showed there were no statistical differences in mortality or symptomatic intracranial hemorrhage (sICH) between the intervention and control groups. In 2016, the HERMES meta-analysis pooled patient data from the RCTs published in 2015, including a total of 1,287 patients, and established the number needed to treat with EVT was 2.6 to reduce disability by at least 1 point on the mRS. HERMES also demonstrated benefit of EVT across virtually all patient subgroups (8).

In 2018, the DAWN and DEFUSE-3 trials evaluated the role of EVT in patients with symptom onset between 6 and 16 hours (DEFUSE-3) and 6 and 24 hours (DAWN) (6,7). Patients were carefully selected using advanced imaging including computed tomography perfusion (CTP), magnetic resonance diffusion-weighted imaging (MRI-DWI), or perfusion imaging (MRI-PWI) (6,7). Both trials demonstrated superior functional outcomes with EVT compared to the control group (6,7). In summary, these 7 RCTs and subsequent meta-analysis support thrombectomy in selected patients up to 24 hours from symptom onset (1–8). Additional trials and registries have added to the body of evidence in support of EVT for LVO stroke.

Indications

Patient selection for EVT is based on the location of the occlusion, time from symptom onset, and imaging findings that confirm LVO and presence of salvageable brain tissue.
1. Presence of a target occlusion: The strongest data for EVT are in patients with occlusions of the intracranial internal carotid artery and/or proximal middle or anterior cerebral artery (ICA/M1/A1). There are also data demonstrating benefit of EVT in M2 segment middle cerebral artery occlusions and posterior circulation occlusions, but the evidence is less robust.
2. Time window: Within 6 hours from symptom onset, EVT can be performed without advanced imaging beyond CT head and CTA. In the 6- to 24-hour time window, advanced imaging such as perfusion imaging (CTP or MRP) or multiphase CTA is recommended in order to ensure the presence of salvageable brain tissue.
3. Evidence of salvageable brain tissue on imaging: Various strategies exist to confirm the presence of salvageable brain tissue (penumbra). In the 6-hour time window, the extent of hypodensity on noncontrast CT (ASPECTS) can provide an estimate of tissue viability while in the extended time window (6 to 24 hours), some form of advanced imaging (e.g., perfusion imaging) is recommended.

Contraindications

Absolute
1. Anaphylactic reaction to iodinated contrast.
2. Intracranial hemorrhage (either primary hemorrhagic stroke or gross hemorrhagic conversion of an ischemic stroke).

Relative
1. Minimal clinical deficit or rapidly improving stroke symptoms after IV thrombolytic therapy.
2. Lack of salvageable tissue. This will depend on the imaging strategy used and it is sometimes hard to completely determine whether salvageable tissue is present or not.
3. Poor baseline functional status. The majority of RCTs excluded patients with poor baseline functional status (i.e., mRS > 3). Clinical judgment should guide decision making because some patients who are high functioning may not be independent

at baseline (such as those with lower extremity amputations) and may benefit substantially from reperfusion therapy.
4. Limited life expectancy or other severe medical comorbidities.
5. Coagulopathy. Some patients presenting with LVO stroke may be on anticoagulation or have other coagulopathies that may preclude use of IV thrombolytic therapy but generally does not preclude EVT.

Preprocedural Preparation

1. **Triage, History and Physical Examination**
    a. Patients with AIS should be rapidly evaluated in the emergency room in consultation with a neurologist. Clinical stroke patterns and syndromes are important for the interventionalist to understand and discuss with the neurologist (Tables 4.1 and 4.2). The NIHSS (NIH Stroke Scale) should be documented as it is a standardized method of determining stroke severity and monitoring changes over time.
    b. Establishing the time of symptom onset is critical to determine eligibility for IV thrombolytic therapy and EVT. If the exact time of onset is unknown, the last time the patient was seen normal is used as the onset.
    c. Review of medications, allergies, and comorbidities.
    d. A documented peripheral pulse examination is important during physical examination. Most EVT interventions are performed from a femoral approach. In case femoral pulses are absent, if there is a known occlusion of the abdominal aorta, or if the vessel occlusion is in the posterior circulation, radial artery access or carotid access can serve as an alternate access site.

Table 4.1 **Large Vessel Occlusion (LVO) Stroke Patterns**

Anterior Circulation	
ACA occlusion	• Contralateral hemiparesis: leg > arm • Contralateral sensory loss: leg > arm • Confusion, personality changes
MCA occlusion	• Contralateral hemiparesis: arm/face > leg • Contralateral sensory loss: arm/face > leg • Aphasia • Spatial neglect • Homonymous hemianopia on opposite side of the infarct • Gaze deviation toward side of stroke
Posterior Circulation	
PCA occlusion	• Contralateral homonymous hemianopia • Contralateral sensory loss • Possible aphasia • Disconjugate gaze (uncommon)
Vertebrobasilar occlusion	• Ataxia, vertigo, diplopia, dysarthria, hiccups, nausea, vomiting • Disconjugate gaze • Crossed signs • Decreased level of consciousness

ACA, anterior cerebral artery; MCA, middle cerebral artery; PCA, posterior cerebral artery.

Table 4.2 Lacunar Stroke Patterns

Pure motor	Equal weakness in the contralateral face, arm, and leg
Pure sensory	Equal numbness or paresthesia in the contralateral face, arm, and leg
Mixed sensory motor	Numbness and weakness equally distributed in the contralateral face, arm, and leg
Clumsy hand dysarthria	Incoordination and weakness of one hand with slurred speech and facial weakness
Ataxic hemiparesis	Cerebellar ataxia and weakness on the same side of the body, with the ataxia out of proportion to weakness

2. Preprocedural Evaluation

a. Laboratory evaluation ideally includes complete blood count; international normalized ratio (INR); and serum electrolytes including creatinine, finger-stick glucose, and troponin. These labs are important for overall care of patient presenting with stroke but they should not delay EVT.

b. Imaging evaluation (see below).

c. IV thrombolytic therapy: All patients who are eligible should receive full-dose IV alteplase (0.9 mg per kg). Currently, IV tenecteplase is not yet standard of care for thrombolytic therapy but has been studied in several trials and shows promise. Table 4.3 further outlines inclusion/exclusion criteria for IV thrombolytic therapy.

d. Consent: Consent should be obtained when possible depending on clinical circumstance (including stroke syndrome) and availability of family/power-of-attorney. If none are available, emergency consent may be required.

e. IV access: IV access is critical for administration of IV thrombolytic therapy and additional medications such as for anesthetic and blood pressure management. Ideally, at least two large-bore IVs should be placed.

f. Blood pressure management: Collateral circulation maintains perfusion to the ischemic penumbra through leptomeningeal collaterals. Prior to revascularization, permissive hypertension is acceptable. If the patient has not received IV thrombolytic therapy, a blood pressure of up to 220/110 mm Hg is acceptable unless there are signs of end-organ injury. If IV thrombolytic therapy has been administered, the pressure should be brought to less than 180/105 mm Hg for 24 hours.

g. Foley catheter placement: Foley catheter placement can be considered (ideally in the emergency department) but should not delay the procedure.

h. Groin preparation: Rapid groin preparation in the angiography suite should be employed. Data have suggested no significant increase in groin access infection rates without shaving in the setting of EVT.

3. Imaging Evaluation

Urgent imaging should occur for patient triage and guidelines suggest that radiologic imaging should begin within 25 minutes and be interpreted within 45 minutes of arrival in at least 80% of cases (9). Imaging in acute AIS needs to answer four questions: (1) Is there evidence of intracranial hemorrhage?; (2) Is there a vessel occlusion and, if so, where is it located?; (3) Is there evidence of salvageable brain tissue?; and (4) How can the occlusion be accessed when EVT is performed? Because of wide availability and speed of CT, most centers rely on CT imaging (noncontrast CT [NCCT], CT angiography [CTA], and CTP when appropriate) in the neuroimaging workup of acute stroke.

Table 4.3   **Inclusion/Exclusion Criteria for Intravenous Tissue Plasminogen Activator**

Inclusion Criteria: Arrival within 4.5 h of onset or "last known well"
- Ischemic stroke causing a measurable neurologic deficit
- Onset <4.5 h before beginning treatment
- Age >18 y

Exclusion Criteria
- Intracranial hemorrhage
- History of previous intracerebral hemorrhage
- Head trauma or prior stroke within the last 3 mo
- Arterial puncture in noncompressible site in last 7 days
- Recent intracranial or spinal surgery
- Blood pressure >185 mm Hg systolic or 110 mm Hg diastolic
- Blood glucose <50 mg/dL
- Large area of infarction on CT head (hypodensity >1/3 of cerebral hemisphere)
- Active internal bleeding
- Acute bleeding diathesis, including, but not limited to
  - Platelets less than 100,000/μL
  - Anticoagulant use with INR >1.7 or PT >15
  - Current use of direct thrombin or Xa inhibitors with elevated sensitive laboratory tests
  - Heparin use within 48 h with elevated APTT above the upper limit of normal

Relative Exclusion Criteria for patients arriving within 3 h of onset or "last known well"
Under some circumstances, patients can receive alteplase despite one or more relative contraindications. Careful weighing of risks and benefits is required.
- Minor or rapidly improving symptoms
- Pregnancy
- Seizure at the onset with residual neurologic deficits
- Major surgery or trauma within previous 14 days
- GU or GI tract hemorrhage within the last 21 days
- Acute MI within last 3 mo

Additional Exclusion Criteria for patients presenting within 3–4.5 h
- Age >80 y
- Severe stroke (NIHSS >25)
- Current/recent oral anticoagulant use regardless of INR
- History of both diabetes and a previous stroke

PT, prothrombin time; APTT, activated partial thromboplastin time; GU, genitourinary; GI, gastrointestinal; MI, myocardial infarction.

1. *Is there evidence of intracranial hemorrhage?*
   Intracranial hemorrhage can easily be identified on NCCT as hyperdensity in the parenchyma and/or extraaxial spaces.
2. *Is there a vessel occlusion and, if so, where is it located?*
   Accurate localization of the vascular occlusion confirms the diagnosis and is crucial to decide whether the occlusion can be targeted with EVT or not. Anterior circulation LVOs (i.e., intracranial ICA, A1, and M1 occlusions) should always be treated with EVT if possible. Medium vessel occlusions (e.g., M2 and M3 segments) have a higher probability to recanalize with IV thrombolytic therapy but they are increasingly treated with EVT as well. Posterior circulation LVOs, especially basilar LVO, should be considered for EVT given poor outcomes.

3. *Is there evidence of salvageable brain tissue?*
   Multiple imaging techniques can be used to determine the presence of salvageable brain tissue, including NCCT, CTA, and mCTA. Based on current level 1 evidence, perfusion imaging (CTP and MRP) is recommended only in the late time window (6 to 24 hours from symptom onset).
   a. Noncontrast computed tomography (NCCT)
      The Alberta Stroke Program Early CT Score (ASPECTS) is a 10-point scale for defining early ischemic changes on NCCT. A normal NCCT scan yields a score of 10 with 1-point deducted for every area of ischemic change in a defined segment. EVT is currently not recommended (level of evidence 1a) in patients with a large ischemic core (ASPECTS <6), although several ongoing trials are investigating whether certain patients with ASPECTS <6 can benefit from EVT.
   b. Computed tomographic angiography (CTA)
      CTA can be rapidly acquired and is highly accurate at localizing vessel occlusions. CTA can estimate the collateral supply of the affected brain parenchyma. Patients with poor collaterals may not benefit from EVT. However, since standard CTA images demonstrate the intracranial vasculature at a single time point only, and collateral filling may occur with delay, standard CTA tends to underestimate collateral status.
   c. Multiphase CTA (mCTA)
      mCTA utilizes additional venous phases to assess collaterals and evaluate patients with a large core infarct who may not benefit from EVT. A standard CTA is performed in late arterial phase from the aortic arch through the vertex, and then two additional acquisitions are immediately performed in venous and late venous phases through the brain only. Poor collaterals, defined as collateral filling of <50% of the MCA territory on the three phases, indicates little or no salvageable tissue and correlates well with ASPECTS ≤5.
   d. CTP
      CTP involves an additional contrast bolus with continuous scanning of either a segment of brain or whole brain imaging (based on scanner type). The data from the CTP examination are postprocessed by software used to calculate various parameters such as time to start (TTS), time to peak (TTP), mean transit time (MTT), cerebral blood volume (CBV), and cerebral blood flow (CBF). Color-coded maps are generated. Brain at risk is best quantified by areas where TTP is >6 seconds. Areas where CBV or CBF falls below specified thresholds are used to estimate the core infarct (e.g., rCBV <30%).
   e. Magnetic resonance imaging (MRI/MRP)
      DWI on MRI is the most sensitive modality for early detection of irreversibly injured brain. MRI alone is also highly sensitive for blood products. The disadvantages of MRI mainly involve lack of 24/7/365 availability, slower acquisition times, additional time required to screen patients for implants and metallic foreign bodies, increased sensitivity to patient motion, and patient claustrophobia. MR perfusion-weighted images can be used to determine the ischemic penumbra of brain at risk similar to CTP, but is less often used because of above contraindications, access, and availability issues.

4. *How can the occlusion be accessed when EVT is performed?*
   CTA (or MRA if an MR-based protocol is used) covers the arterial vasculature from the aortic arch to the vertex and provides useful information about extracranial and intracranial vessel anatomy (e.g., caliber, vessel tortuosity, stenosis or occlusion, and anatomical variants) which is important for procedural planning and choice of access and catheters/thrombectomy devices.

Procedure

1. General considerations
   a. Airway protection and anesthetic considerations

      Anesthetic management of EVT patients remains controversial. In most cases, conscious sedation will be sufficient unless the patient is very agitated. General anesthesia may be performed for airway protection, if the patient is uncooperative, or if the target occlusion is a medium/distal vessel occlusion in which case the vessel size is smaller and even small patient movements can lead to complications. Ideally, an anesthesiologist is available by default in the angiography suite to keep time delays at a minimum.

   b. Angiographic equipment

      Stroke intervention is ideally performed utilizing biplane imaging and digital subtraction angiography. This allows for easier identification of emboli, increased safety navigating intracranial anatomy, and lower contrast use.

   c. Vascular access

      Access can be obtained in standard fashion although some patients may be receiving concurrent IV thrombolytic therapy and are at higher risk for bleeding complications. Ultrasound-guided micropuncture access can mitigate many of these complications and requires little extra time when used routinely. Most EVT procedures are performed via femoral access, although radial access is increasingly used as well, particularly if the LVO is in the posterior circulation. In rare cases of severely tortuous or occluded iliac arteries and/or aorta, direct carotid access may be considered.

2. Target vessel access and initial angiography

   The majority of EVT access devices (balloon guide catheters [BGCs] and distal access sheaths) are intended for femoral access and, therefore, will be addressed with this in mind. Following femoral arterial access, an 8- or 9-Fr sheath can be placed which accommodate all currently available access systems. Alternatively, a distal access sheath can be used directly in the femoral artery without need for a larger introducer sheath. BGCs should ideally be placed through a sheath as the deflated balloon may cause injury at the arteriotomy site at the conclusion of the procedure.

   Initial angiography provides information on the state of the occlusion (i.e., resolved vs. continued) and additional opportunity for selection of thrombectomy device(s) and technique. Direct selection of the target vessel can be performed utilizing the access catheter/sheath in combination with a long 125-cm 5-Fr/6-Fr diagnostic angiography catheter of various shapes. Alternatively, initial selection of the target vessel using a diagnostic angiography catheter can be performed followed by placement of an exchange-length wire and exchanging for the desired access catheter/sheath. Given that patients will have antecedent noninvasive vascular imaging, extracranial angiography may not be necessary unless there is concern/plan for tandem lesion pathology (i.e., concomitant extracranial carotid stenosis/occlusion with intracranial LVO).

3. Mechanical thrombectomy

   Currently, there are three dominant techniques for mechanical thrombectomy: stent-retriever thrombectomy, aspiration thrombectomy, and primary combined approaches utilizing both stent-retriever and aspiration. All of the above approaches can be combined with a BGC utilizing compatible equipment.

   a. Stent-retrievers

      Stent-retrievers are self-expandable stents with an attached delivery wire and delivered via a microcatheter. Once the microcatheter has been placed beyond the occlusion site with the help of a microwire, the microwire is removed and the stent-retriever inserted and advanced to the tip of the microcatheter and unsheathed. After 3 to 5 minutes, the stent-retriever is usually fully opened and the thrombus has incorporated through the stent struts into the stent lumen, with the struts now contacting the vessel wall. After it has fully opened and incorporated with thrombus, the operator

Table 4.4	Assessing Reperfusion Quality with the Expanded Thrombolysis in Cerebral Infarction (eTICI) Score
eTICI Score	**Description**
0	No Reperfusion
1	Antegrade reperfusion past the initial occlusion, but limited distal branch filling with little or slow distal reperfusion
2a	Antegrade reperfusion of <50% of the occluded target artery previously ischemic territory (e.g., in 1 major division of the MCA and its territory)
2b	Antegrade reperfusion of 50–90% of the previously occluded target artery ischemic territory (e.g., in 2 major divisions of the MCA and their territories)
2c	Near complete perfusion except for slow flow/occlusion in a few distal cortical vessels, i.e. reperfusion of at least 90% of the territory
3	Complete antegrade reperfusion of the previously occluded target artery ischemic territory

removes the stent-retriever with the captured thrombus by pulling the delivery wire with flow arrest/reversal via the inflated BGC under suction. If the clot has been removed, the check angiogram will show completely restored blood flow. Stent-retriever thrombectomy was used in all major thrombectomy trials, most commonly with use of a BGC, and therefore is a technique recommended by current guidelines.

b. Contact aspiration

In aspiration thrombectomy, a large-bore aspiration catheter is navigated to the occlusion site, and the catheter tip is positioned as close as possible to the proximal end of the thrombus. Aspiration is then applied either manually with a large-volume syringe or via use of an aspiration pump for a minimum of 60 to 90 seconds. The thrombus is either completely aspirated or the proximal entailed by the catheter and withdrawn with the catheter, thereby restoring blood flow. Recent trials have shown that contact aspiration seems to be similarly effective compared to stent-retriever thrombectomy.

c. Combined approaches

Primary combined approaches use both stent-retriever and contact aspiration, thereby potentially minimizing the risk of distal embolization and improving chances of complete first-pass reperfusion.

4. Assessing Thrombectomy Success

Reperfusion speed and quality are the two key prognostic factors in AIS. Thus, the overarching goal of thrombectomy is to open the occluded blood vessel quickly and completely. Reperfusion quality is measured with the expanded Thrombolysis in Cerebral Infarction Score (Table 4.4), while reperfusion speed is reflected by the time from groin puncture to reperfusion. First-pass reperfusion (i.e., eTICI 2b/2c/3 after the first retrieval attempt) is another important angiographic outcome measure and higher eTICI scores are associated with improved clinical outcomes.

5. Vascular Access Management

After thrombectomy, common femoral arteriography should be performed to ensure that there is no access sheath-related complication (e.g., dissection, thrombosis, occlusive sizing) and anatomy is appropriate for possible closure device placement. Closure device placement including for larger access sheaths (8- or 9-Fr) and/or concomitant/antecedent IV thrombolytic therapy has been shown safe and effective. Manual pressure for hemostasis can be performed but may be more challenging with increased bleeding risks/complications especially in the above scenarios. If necessary, a short (11 to 25 cm) femoral access sheath can be sutured in and left in place postoperatively. If the sheath is left in place, it should be connected to a pressurized heparinized saline infusion to prevent sheath/vessel thrombosis and can be connected to a transducer for invasive blood pressure measurement.

Postprocedural Management

Following thrombectomy, patients should be directed to an intensive care unit with nursing staff and physicians and are best managed in a dedicated neurointensive care unit. Factors increasing the risk of requiring critical care interventions in patients with an AIS can be determined by the Intensive Care after Thrombolysis (ICAT) score. About one in four patients with AIS will need critical care interventions as systemic complications in the setting of an AIS can pose significant secondary brain injury (10).

Besides monitoring and stabilization of vital parameters, postthrombectomy care specifically aims to prevent, detect, and treat thrombolytic and/or thrombectomy-related complications such as access site complications, allergic reactions, intracranial hemorrhage, and reperfusion injury. Since the latter two occur more often with elevated blood pressures, current guidelines recommend blood pressure ≤180/105 mm Hg as a target during thrombectomy and in the first 24 hours after the procedure. If successful reperfusion was achieved, one may consider lowering blood pressure levels further. The access site should be carefully checked for any hematoma. Blood glucose levels should be monitored and hyperglycemia be treated (target blood glucose level: <180 mg per dL). Body temperature should be kept euthermic, as to date, there is no proven neuroprotective effect of hypothermia in humans with AIS. Finally, a swallowing test should be performed, and if the risk of aspiration is considered high, early feeding tube use may be considered (10).

Mobilization, physical and occupational therapy, and speech therapy should be initiated as early as possible. Detailed diagnostic workup of AIS etiology in the postacute phase should be performed (e.g., EKG, echocardiography, carotid duplex ultrasound, lipid panel, coagulation profile, cardiac biomarkers, erythrocyte sedimentation rate, antinuclear antibody, rheumatoid factor, homocysteine level, and hemoglobin A1c) and appropriate secondary stroke prevention therapy should be initiated (10).

EVT Procedural Steps for M1 MCA LVO with Primary Combined Approach

1. Under ultrasound guidance utilizing a micropuncture access set, access the right common femoral artery and place an 0.035-in × 75-cm Amplatz super stiff wire (Boston Scientific, Marlborough, MA).
2. Over the wire, place a 9-Fr × 23-cm BriteTip sheath (Cordis, Santa Clara, CA) positioned in the lower abdominal aorta and connected to heparinized saline flush. The side arm of the sheath can be used for intraoperative invasive blood pressure measurements.
3. All wires and catheters should be flushed/prepped with heparinized saline. In addition, prepare the 8-Fr × 95-cm Walrus BGC (Q'Apel Medical, Fremont, CA) with dilute (50%) contrast to remove air to prevent intracranial air embolism should the balloon rupture intraoperatively.
4. Load a coaxial system with a 5-Fr × 125-cm Vitek catheter (Cook Medical, Bloomington, IN) within the BGC and over an 0.035-in × 180-cm Glidewire

Advantage (Terumo, Somerset, NJ) with a heparinized saline drip attached to a rotating hemostatic valve on the BGC.

5. Advance the coaxial system in the aorta and aortic arch and manipulate to select the common carotid artery and advance the BGC over the 5-Fr catheter and wire (can be done under roadmap guidance if needed).

6. Following removal of the wire, obtain large field-of-view cervicocerebral angiography to assess the extracranial vasculature and confirm presence of the intracranial LVO. Intracranial imaging should go through the delayed venous phase to assess collaterals and potentially identify the distal aspect of the occlusion.

7. Reintroduce the 0.035-in wire and over the wire and 5-Fr catheter, advance the BGC to as high a position in the cervical internal carotid artery as reasonable. Tortuosity, loops, and resistance should be carefully assessed.

8. Following removal of the wire and 5-Fr catheter, introduce a Sofia Plus large-bore aspiration catheter (MicroVention, Alisa Viejo, CA) over a Trevo Trak 21 microcatheter (Stryker Neurovascular, Fremont, CA) and 0.014-in × 215-cm Synchro-2 Support microwire (Stryker Neurovascular, Fremont, CA). The large-bore aspiration catheter and microcatheter should be connected to heparinized saline flushes on rotating hemostatic valves.

9. Manipulate the microwire and microcatheter through and beyond the LVO, ideally into the inferior division M2 branch.

10. Advance the large-bore aspiration catheter over the microcatheter/microwire system as high into the ICA as possible without losing access.

11. Remove the microwire and deliver Trevo NXT 4-mm × 41-mm stent-retriever (Stryker Neurovascular, Fremont, CA). Push-and-fluff technique during unsheathing of the stent-retriever can help better incorporate clot. In addition, it is recommended to place a significant portion of the stent-retriever (50% or more) beyond the LVO so that if the clot slips or migrates on retrieval there is more distal stent to continue to engage the clot.

12. With the stent-retriever fully deployed, further advance the large-bore aspiration catheter over the microcatheter and stent-retriever system into the distal ICA.

13. Remove the microcatheter. The stent-retriever will act as an anchor to preserve intracranial access.

14. Connect the side arm of the large-bore aspiration catheter to an aspiration pump/tubing.

15. Connect the side arm of the BGC to a 60-mL VacLok syringe (Merit Medical, South Jordan, UT).

16. After 5 minutes of the stent-retriever in place, slowly advance the large-bore aspiration catheter under continuous suction to the face of the LVO/stent-retriever to "cork" the clot.

17. Inflate the BGC. Inflation should be performed until the edges of the balloon begin to achieve a rectangular shape with rounded edges.

18. With aspiration on the BGC via the 60-mL VacLok syringe and continuous suction on the large-bore aspiration catheter via the pump, remove the aspiration catheter and stent-retriever en bloc using a slow and steady pulling motion. Be careful not to pull the stent-retriever all the way into the large-bore aspiration catheter which could shear off clot to distal or new territories.

19. Remove the rotating hemostatic valve off the back of the BGC before pulling the stent-retriever/large-bore aspiration catheter out completely to prevent embolization. Once out of the patient, hand the large-bore aspiration catheter/stent-retriever to a back table team member to help re-prep and reload for a potential additional pass.

20. Vigorously aspirate the BGC to remove embolic debris and waste that blood.

21. Deflate the BGC and perform a diagnostic angiogram to assess reperfusion.
22. Attach a new rotating hemostatic valve (connected to heparinized saline flush) to the BGC.
23. If carotid spasm is present from manipulation, consider administration of intra-arterial verapamil (2.5 to 5 mg) or nitroglycerine (50 to 100 µg) if the blood pressure permits.
24. Repeat steps as needed to reasonably maximize revascularization.
25. Remove the BGC.
26. Withdraw the groin access sheath into the external iliac artery and perform a femoral arteriogram. If reasonable, achieve hemostasis with a closure device.
27. Document a brief operative note/operative note which includes findings and relevant time and data metrics (e.g., groin access, revascularization time, eTICI, etc.).
28. Discuss the case/procedure with the neurologist/ICU team and transfer the patient to the ICU for postprocedural management.

Postprocedural Complications

Access Site Complications (2% to 11%)

Access site complications include access site hematoma, peripheral nerve injury, acute limb ischemia, distal arterial embolization, arterial dissection, pseudoaneurysm formation, infection, and retroperitoneal hemorrhage. In the arm, compartment syndrome, arteritis, and hand ischemia are possible. For direct carotid puncture, safely achieving hemostasis may be more problematic with the risk of airway obstruction. Management ranges from conservative management (sufficient in most cases), initiating blood transfusion, to emergent or semiurgent surgical or endovascular repair.

Neurologic
Embolization to a New Vascular Territory (1% to 8.6%)

During retrieval of the clot, it may embolize to a proximal previously unaffected territory or distally within the target artery. This may put other areas of the brain at risk for an AIS. Potential contributing factors to distal embolization may be related to the procedure technique and clot type. Distal embolizaton is less common with BGCs. Large emboli can be removed using standard thrombectomy techniques. For distal embolization, intraarterial thrombolytic infusion can be used if appropriate; however these are not approved by the FDA for intraarterial use. Smaller suction thrombectomy catheters and stent-retrievers have also been utilized.

Symptomatic Intracranial Hemorrhage (1.6% to 9.3%)

sICH is defined as a hemorrhage with an NIHSS score increase of greater than or equal to 4 points. Low ASPECT, large ischemic core, very low cerebral blood flow, thrombus length >14 mm, baseline stroke severity, and diabetes have been shown to be associated with increased risk of sICH. Reversal of recombinant tissue plasminogen can be performed with cryoprecipitate, platelet transfusion, recombinant factor VIIa, aminocaproic acid, or tranexamic acid. Coagulopathy can be reversed with platelets, fresh-frozen plasma, prothrombin complex concentrate, and vitamin K. Postprocedural MRI of the brain or a dual-energy CT can be useful to differentiate contrast staining from a disrupted blood–brain barrier versus ICH. Optimizing blood pressure management postoperatively is important, although the optimal blood pressure range following thrombectomy is still unclear.

Cerebral Edema

Cerebral edema is commonly seen in patients with AIS, particularly with large, extensive infarcts (i.e., low ASPECTS). Treatment options for cerebral edema include head of bed elevation, hyperventilation, hyperosmotic therapy, and surgical decompression.

Seizures (<1%)

Clinical seizures following an AIS are rare occurring in about 1% of cases. Males with an NIHSS score greater than 10 are at a higher risk. A seizure is an independent risk factor for a poor outcome.

Intracranial Arterial Perforation (1% to 2%)

Intracranial arterial perforation is a serious complication which may occur during thrombectomy and may result in significant morbidity and mortality and most commonly occurs when navigating the intracranial circulation in a blind manner or during stent-retriever withdrawal. This complication was reported in 12/868 (1.3%) patients in the seven stroke EVT RCTs. In a large case series, 16 perforations occurred in 1,599 patients, of which 56% (9/16) died and 25% (4/16) had a good functional outcome. If an arterial perforation is identified by extravasation of contrast material this should be treated similar to any procedural vessel rupture by reducing the blood pressure, reversing any anticoagulation, and inflating an intracranial balloon. If bleeding persists, occlusion of the damaged arterial segment with liquid embolic agents (*n*-butylcyanoacrylate or ethylene vinyl alcohol copolymer) or detachable coils may be necessary but is associated with poor outcomes.

Arterial Dissection (0.6% to 3.9%)

Dissection can involve the puncture site, or extracranial or intracranial vessels. It appears on angiography as a localized contrast pocket, intimal flap, or double lumen. Treatment options include anticoagulation or dual antiplatelet therapy if the dissection is nonflow limiting to balloon angioplasty or stent placement for a lesion that is severely flow-limiting.

Cardiac

Cardiac complications can commonly be seen following AIS and may not be a direct result of EVT.

Myocardial Infarction

Acute myocardial infarction (AMI) is seen in 2% of all patients with an AIS with an increased cumulative risk over 10 years. AMI is the setting of AIS is associated with poor outcomes and increased mortality.

Cardiac Arrhythmias

The most common arrhythmias following an AIS include atrial fibrillation and atrial flutter, reported in up to 10% of patients. This can result in hemodynamic compromise requiring immediate management.

Congestive Heart Failure

Left ventricular systolic dysfunction is reported in up to 28% of the patients with an AIS and diastolic dysfunction in 18%. Congestive heart failure is an independent marker of poor outcome in patients with an AIS and is associated with cardiac and pulmonary complications.

Respiratory

Respiratory complications are also common in patients suffering an AIS and may not be a direct result of EVT.

Airway Management/Mechanical Ventilation

The inability to maintain a patent airway because of altered mental status is the most common indication for admitting a patient with an AIS to the ICU. Approximately 1% of patients with stroke will require mechanical ventilation. Patients requiring ventilation have associated poorer outcomes and a longer hospital stay.

Pneumonia

Stroke associated pneumonia has been reported in up to 56% of patients in stroke units. Dysphagia and altered level of consciousness can contribute to development of pneumonia. Pneumonia confers a poor functional outcome and mortality as high as 50%.

References

1. Berkhemer OA, Fransen PS, Beumer D, et al. A randomized trial of intraarterial treatment for acute ischemic stroke. *N Engl J Med*. 2015;372(1):11–20.
2. Campbell BC, Mitchell PJ, Kleinig TJ, et al. Endovascular therapy for ischemic stroke with perfusion-imaging selection. *N Engl J Med*. 2015;372(11):1009–1018.
3. Goyal M, Demchuk AM, Menon BK, et al. Randomized assessment of rapid endovascular treatment of ischemic stroke. *N Engl J Med*. 2015;372(11):1019–1030.
4. Saver JL, Goyal M, Bonafe A, et al. Stent-retriever thrombectomy after intravenous t-PA vs. t-PA alone in stroke. *N Engl J Med*. 2015;372:2285–2295.
5. Jovin TG, Chamorro A, Cobo E, et al. Thrombectomy within 8 hours after symptom onset in ischemic stroke. *N Engl J Med*. 2015;372:2296–2306.
6. Nogueira RG, Jadhav AP, Haussen DC, et al. Thrombectomy 6 to 24 hours after stroke with a mismatch between deficit and infarct. *N Engl J Med*. 2018;378(1):11–21.
7. Albers GW, Marks MP, Kemp S, et al. Thrombectomy for stroke at 6 to 16 hours with selection by perfusion imaging. *N Engl J Med*. 2018;378(8):708–718.
8. Goyal M, Menon BK, van Zwam WH, et al. Endovascular thrombectomy after large-vessel ischaemic stroke: a meta-analysis of individual patient data from five randomised trials. *Lancet*. 2016;387(10029):1723–1731.
9. Powers WJ, Rabinstein AA, Ackerson T, et al. Guidelines for the Early Management of Patients With Acute Ischemic Stroke: 2019 Update to the 2018 Guidelines for the Early Management of Acute Ischemic Stroke: A Guideline for Healthcare Professionals From the American Heart Association/American Stroke Association. *Stroke*. 2019;50: e344–e418.
10. Turc G, Bhogal P, Fischer U, et al. European Stroke Organisation (ESO) and European Society for Minimally Invasive Neurological Therapy (ESMINT) guidelines on mechanical thrombectomy in acute ischemic stroke. *J Neurointerv Surg*. 2019;11(6): 535–538.

5 Carotid Artery Stenosis

Neil V. Patel, MD, Emanuele Orrù, MD, Miklos Marosfoi, MD,
and Ajay K. Wakhloo, MD, PhD, FAHA

Introduction

Approximately 87% of all new strokes are ischemic in nature, with an estimated 20% to 30% due to atherosclerotic disease of the extracranial internal carotid artery (ICA). The primary mechanism of stroke in patients with atherosclerotic disease of the ICA, which sometimes extends to the common carotid artery (CCA), is the embolization of atherosclerotic debris or thrombotic material from the plaque into the more distal cerebral vasculature. Though stroke has been associated with both stenotic and nonstenotic ipsilateral carotid diseases, there seems to be a synergistic effect between thromboembolism to the cerebral vasculature and diminished downstream flow to the ipsilateral brain from concomitant carotid stenosis.

It was early in the 1900s that some of the first observations of a relationship between stroke and extracranial carotid artery disease were made. However, it took almost another 50 years for the understanding of this relationship to lead to the development of carotid endarterectomy (CEA). CEA is now a widely available, broadly accepted therapy for carotid revascularization with proven efficacy and low procedural morbidity. Carotid balloon angioplasty was first performed in 1980, and a stent in the carotid artery was first used in 1989 to treat an intimal flap after angioplasty. Since those early days, carotid artery stenting (CAS) has evolved to become a widely accepted, minimally invasive alternative to CEA with similar benefits and procedural risk as indicated by a number of large-scale randomized controlled trials (RCTs) comparing the two techniques. These trials are summarized in the last section of this chapter.

CAS is routinely performed to treat symptomatic patients with stenosis greater than 70% on duplex ultrasonography (US) (1). As technology and techniques for CAS evolve, indications for CAS may expand to a broader subset of patients requiring carotid artery revascularization.

Also, though atherosclerotic stenosis exceeding 50% is the most established risk factor for arteriogenic stroke, there are several features of plaques (e.g., ulceration, active inflammation) that are associated with higher rates of stroke, independent of the degree of stenosis (2). As an understanding of this symptomatic nonstenotic carotid disease (SyNC) evolves, patient selection guidelines for CAS may change.

Indications

According to the 2011 guidelines on the management of patients with extracranial carotid and vertebral artery disease, patients meeting the following criteria are candidates for carotid revascularization (1).

1. Patients at average or low surgical risk who experience nondisabling ischemic stroke or transient cerebral ischemic symptoms, including hemispheric events or amaurosis fugax, within 6 months (symptomatic patients) should undergo CEA if the diameter of the lumen of the ipsilateral ICA is reduced more than 70% as documented by noninvasive imaging or more than 50% as documented by catheter angiography and the anticipated rate of perioperative stroke or mortality is less than 6%.

2. CAS is indicated as an alternative to CEA for symptomatic patients at average or low risk of complications associated with endovascular intervention when the diameter of the lumen of the ICA is reduced by more than 70% as documented by noninvasive imaging or more than 50% as documented by catheter angiography and the anticipated rate of periprocedural stroke is less than or equivalent to CEA.
3. Patients who are at high risk for CEA are considered to benefit particularly from the reduced procedural risks of CAS. Note that many of the major high-risk criteria pertain to cardiac factors; the Carotid Revascularization Endarterectomy versus Stenting Trial (CREST) trial (3) showed a significant reduction in the risk of myocardial infarction (MI) in patients undergoing stenting versus endarterectomy (1.1% vs. 2.3%), at the cost of higher stroke risk (4.1% vs. 2.3%). Subgroup analysis of the CREST data indicates that the increased periprocedural stroke risk for CAS versus CEA may exist in women, but not in men (4). Patients have been considered "high risk for CEA" when they have the following major comorbidities and/or anatomic conditions (or two minor criteria in some investigations) (5,6).
   a. High-risk comorbidities
      (1) Major criteria
         (a) Congestive heart failure (New York Heart Association functional class III/IV)
         (b) Left ventricular ejection fraction <30%
         (c) Chronic obstructive pulmonary disease with forced expired volume <30%
         (d) Recent open-heart surgery (within 6 weeks)
         (e) Dialysis-dependent renal failure
         (f) Uncontrolled diabetes (fasting glucose >400 mg per dL, urine ketones >2)
         (g) Patients under evaluation for or awaiting major organ transplantation
      (2) Minor criteria
         (a) Age >75 years
         (b) Unstable angina (Canadian Cardiovascular Society class III/IV)
         (c) Recent MI (<30 days)
         (d) Major diseased coronary arteries (>2) with >70% stenosis (patients with angina)
         (e) Planned peripheral vascular surgery, or other major surgeries postcarotid intervention
   b. Anatomic high-risk conditions
      (1) Major criteria
         (a) Tandem stenosis (hemodynamically significant carotid artery stenosis with one or more ipsilateral intracranial stenoses)
         (b) Carotid dissection
         (c) Previous neck or head radiation therapy/surgery including area of stenosis
         (d) Surgically inaccessible lesions at or above C2 or below clavicle
         (e) Spinal immobility of the neck
         (f) Laryngeal palsy or laryngectomy
         (g) Tracheostomy
         (h) Tumor-encased carotid arteries
         (i) Markedly irregular, ulcerated plaque
      (2) Minor criteria
         (a) Contralateral total occlusion, contralateral carotid disease requiring revascularization, or other limitation of cross-flow circulation
         (b) Restenosis post-CEA or attempted CEA with arteriotomy, at least 31 days prior

(c) Planned coronary artery bypass graft or valve replacement postcarotid revascularization procedure

In addition to patients selected according to these guidelines, there is a distinct population of patients who suffer embolic strokes related to carotid webs. These fibrous septa, which occur at the ICA ostia, are believed to reflect a variant of fibromuscular dyplasia. Affected individuals tend to be young, presenting with nonlacunar infarcts. Untreated or on medical management alone, these lesions are associated with an approximately 30% risk of recurrent strokes, therefore making treatment indicated in all cases of symptomatic carotid web. CAS has been shown to be safe and effective in this population (7).

Contraindications

In addition to absolute and relative contraindications applicable to all angiographic and interventional procedures, the following considerations apply to CAS:

1. Absolute contraindications
   a. Chronic carotid artery occlusion
   b. Allergy or nonresponsiveness to sufficient antiplatelet medications
   c. Allergy to metals in the stent (nickel, titanium, cobalt, chromium, and others depending on the stent chosen)
   d. Uncorrectable bleeding diathesis
   e. Anatomic configurations that prohibit navigation of the devices to their target locations
2. Relative contraindications
   a. Fresh clot within stenosis
   b. Recent stroke (<4 to 6 weeks old) or prior disabling stroke (modified Rankin scale >3)
   c. Recent intracranial hemorrhage
   d. Positive blood cultures/sepsis
   e. Immunologically compromised state
   f. Circumferential or near-circumferential calcification

Preprocedure Workup

1. Baseline history and physical examination
   a. Consider obtaining consultation for cardiac and/or pulmonary risk assessment prior to procedure.
   b. Patients with any potential impairment of renal function should be assessed for the risk of contrast-induced nephropathy. Dialysis should be coordinated as necessary for patients with end-stage renal disease.
2. Comprehensive neurologic evaluation by an independent neurologist, including assessment with the National Institutes of Health Stroke Scale, modified Rankin scale, and Barthel index of activities of daily living
3. Serum electrolytes including blood urea nitrogen and creatinine, complete blood count, prothrombin time/international normalized ratio (INR)/partial thromboplastin time
4. Urine human chorionic gonadotropin for women of childbearing age

Imaging

1. US with Doppler analysis is the mainstay of screening for carotid stenosis. It is widely available and shown to accurately depict a flow-limiting stenosis in the carotid arteries. A qualified technologist in a certified laboratory should perform the examination. The primary parameters evaluated are peak systolic

velocity (PSV) and a direct estimation of plaque thickness. Secondary parameters include end-diastolic velocity and ICA/CCA ratio (ratio of PSV in the ICA to PSV in the ipsilateral CCA). US may provide details on plaque composition and surface characteristics, but it is an operator-dependent modality with sensitivity and specificity that may vary greatly for the detection of features of a vulnerable plaque. The mean sensitivity across several studies for the detection of plaque ulcerations has been estimated to be close to 60% with a specificity of 74%.

2. Computed tomography angiography (CTA) is useful for evaluating the degree of stenosis and calcifications of the aortic arch and carotid arteries and should be considered a part of routine evaluation before carotid revascularization procedures. An accurate evaluation of the type of aortic arch, tortuosity of the CCA, and course and caliber of the vessel proximal and distal to the stenosis can also be obtained via this method for procedural planning As the resolution of newer generation of multiple detector CT improves, so does the detection of ulceration in an atherosclerotic plaque in the carotid arteries. This information is useful in planning the procedural approach and in device selection. CTA has also a high sensitivity and specificity to diagnose intracranial stenosis, which can be very relevant when planning an intervention on a patient with extracranial carotid stenosis. CTA is also useful if US/magnetic resonance angiography (MRA) results are discordant, or if MRA is contraindicated. CTA of the craniocervical carotid arteries is continuously evolving with the development of newer bone subtraction algorithms which allow for much improved visualization of the ICA at the skull base/clinoidal region.

3. MRI can be utilized for both anatomical and pathophysiologic characterization of carotid plaques. MRA can be used to exclude stenosis but is limited in quantifying the degree of stenosis and is susceptible to a wide variety of artifacts. Multiple techniques are available:
   a. Time-of-flight—does not require intravenous contrast
   b. Phase-contrast—allows quantification of blood flow, flow velocity, and blood volume
   c. Contrast-enhanced—improves image quality and lowers artifacts related to nonlaminar flow. Multiple studies have demonstrated a strong association between findings on dedicated MRI sequences without and with contrast and histologic morphologic measurements. Data from these and other studies support the notion that features of plaque composition alone may provide value in the assessment of risk of future events. This is still considered by some of limited value for the characterization of plaque calcification

4. Digital subtraction angiography (DSA) remains the gold standard for the evaluation of carotid and intracranial atherosclerosis. A complete cerebral and cervical DSA may be considered in selected cases to assess hemodynamics across the circle of Willis, to assess collateral supply, to better characterize atherosclerotic lesions seen on noninvasive imaging, or to distinguish between occlusion and subocclusive stenosis. A complete DSA can be performed in the same setting as a planned CAS.

Procedure Preparation

1. CAS may be performed under moderate sedation, monitored anesthesia care (MAC), or general anesthesia (GA), with continuous monitoring during the procedure of the electrocardiogram (ECG), blood pressure (BP), and pulse oximetry. An arterial line for continuous BP measurement is recommended, especially when a carotid lesion is located at the carotid bifurcation.

2. Correct hypo/hyperglycemia preprocedurally and monitor intraprocedurally.
3. Correct INR to <1.5. Utilize a bridging strategy with unfractionated heparin when medically indicated, keeping the PTT two to three times baseline.
4. Patients should continue their home medications except for β-blockers (due to potential bradycardia during manipulation at the carotid bulb) and metformin. Metformin should be halted 24 hours prior to and 48 hours after the procedure to minimize the risk of lactic acidosis, should renal damage occur after contrast administration.
   a. The American College of Radiology has adopted a more relaxed policy for metformin management that varies according to renal dysfunction and presence of comorbidities. Given the substantial complexity and challenges in implementing the new guidelines, the authors consider continuing with the standard protocol of suspending metformin, as highlighted above, as a more practical approach with little to no significant impact on patients.
5. Premedication for elective cases should be started at least 5 days prior to procedure (1,8).
   a. Antiplatelet therapy: Before and for a minimum of 30 days after CAS, dual-antiplatelet therapy with aspirin (81 to 325 mg daily) plus clopidogrel (75 mg daily) is recommended. Aspirin should be continued indefinitely after the procedure. Clopidogrel (Plavix) is usually continued for a minimum of 6 weeks and up to 12 months following the procedure. In patients unable to take clopidogrel, ticagrelor (Brilinta) 60 to 90 mg by mouth (PO) two times per day (bid) can be substituted.
   b. Antihypertensive therapy: Administration of antihypertensive medications is recommended to control BP before and after CAS.
   c. Statins: Treatment with a statin medication is recommended for all patients with extracranial carotid atherosclerosis to reduce low-density lipoprotein (LDL) cholesterol below 100 mg per dL or below 70 mg per dL when there is a history of associated ischemic stroke and/or diabetes mellitus. Statin therapy should be continued indefinitely.
6. Emergent cases (less than 72 hours from onset of ischemic stroke). At present, there is no consensus on medical or endovascular management of patients with acute ischemic stroke presenting with severe clinical symptoms due to atherosclerotic stenosis/occlusion of the extracranial ICA. The authors recommend a loading dose of clopidogrel 300 mg PO and aspirin 650 mg PO or PR 3 to 4 hours prior to procedure. If ticagrelor is being used instead of clopidogrel, the patient should receive a loading dose of 180 mg prior to an emergent procedure.

Intraprocedural Medications

Blood Thinners

1. Anticoagulation—The procedure is performed with anticoagulation for all indications using either unfractionated heparin or a direct thrombin inhibitor.
   a. Unfractionated heparin with a target activated clotting time (ACT) of 250 to 300 seconds. Start with a 50 to 80 IU per kg IV bolus. Frequently, the stenting is accomplished within 20 to 30 minutes of this bolus. If the case is prolonged past 30 minutes, check the ACT and titrate appropriately.
   b. Direct thrombin inhibitors can be indicated in patients with heparin-induced thrombocytopenia. Standardized regimens of bivalirudin and argatroban are yet to be established.
      (1) Suggested dosing regimen for argatroban is 15 to 30 μg/kg/min IV infusion that can be achieved with a 350 μg per kg IV bolus, followed by 25 μg/kg/min IV infusion.

(2) Suggested dosing regimen for bivalirudin is 0.75 mg per kg IV bolus, followed by infusion at 1.75 mg/kg/h IV × 4 hours. ACT should be monitored 5 minutes after bolus and may give an additional 0.3 mg per kg IV bolus if needed.

2. Glycoprotein IIb/IIIa (GPIIb/IIIa) inhibitors in case of acute in-stent platelet-rich clot formation after deployment. Baseline ACT should be lower than 200 seconds prior to administration to reduce the risk of intracranial hemorrhage. This can be achieved by blocking part of the heparin activity with IV infusion of protamine.
   a. Eptifibatide (Integrilin)—2 µg/kg/min IV. Start with 180 µg per kg bolus (up to 22.6 mg total), with a maximum maintenance infusion of 15 mg per hour.
   b. Abciximab (ReoPro)—0.125 µg/kg/min IV × 12 hours. Start 0.25 mg per kg IV bolus 10 to 60 minutes prior the start of the procedure. Maximum infusion dose is 10 µg per minute.

Management of Intraprocedural Bradycardia

1. Glycopyrrolate—0.2 to 0.4 mg IV. This drug is administered prophylactically in cases where the target lesion is close to the carotid bulb, as pressure on the baroreceptors during percutaneous transluminal angioplasty or stent placement may trigger bradycardia; may repeat dose if there is a long interval before angioplasty.
2. Atropine—0.6 to 1.0 mg IV bolus.
3. Rarely, dopamine is used.

Intra-Arterial Antihypertensive Medications and Vasospasm Treatment

1. Nicardipine is useful in the treatment of vasospasm related to cerebral protection device (CPD) placement, angioplasty, and stent placement. This can be given preventatively after access to the target vessel, prior to endovascular intervention. The dose is 2 to 10 mg IV bolus at a slow rate of approximately 1 mg per minute. Monitor BP closely.
2. Verapamil has the same benefits, dose, and administration rate as nicardipine.

Management of Hypotension

1. Colloid (20% albumin) solution can be useful in managing periprocedural hypotension by expanding intravascular volume. Additionally, albumin is considered beneficial for improving cerebral microcirculation independent of increased BP.
   a. Albumin should be administered slowly, 50 mL over 20 minutes and may be repeated every 4 to 6 hours.

Equipment

1. Guidewires
   a. A torqueable, hydrophilic 0.035-in guidewire with a shapeable tip is used to facilitate selective catheterization of the CCA (e.g., GlideWire, Terumo Medical Corp, Somerset, NJ).
   b. A stiff, exchange-length 0.035-in wire is used when needed to exchange the diagnostic catheter for the guide catheter (e.g., Amplatz Extra Stiff 260 cm or 300 cm, Cook Medical Inc, Bloomington, IN).
   c. Hybrid wires, such as the Advantage Glidewire (Terumo), provide a hydrophilic distal segment fused to a stiff proximal shaft. These can be useful in providing support for both sheath placement and selective catheterization.
   d. In cases where a CPD cannot be used, a 0.014-in or 0.018-in wire is navigated beyond the stenotic lesion to support positioning of a PTA balloon for predilatation. An exchange-length wire may be necessary if non–rapid-exchange catheters or balloons are to be used for this.
2. Catheters
   a. A 6-Fr or, occasionally, 7/8-Fr guide catheter is typically used for CAS. The guide sheath diameter is dictated by the specifications of the stent system being used, and often varies with the stent diameter. A short access sheath

Table 5.1 Carotid Stents and Cerebral Embolic Protection Devices

Manufacturer	Stent System	Filter Device
Abbott Vascular (Santa Clara, CA)	RX Acculink	AccuNet
Abbott Vascular (Santa Clara, CA)	xACT	Emboshield BareWire
Boston Scientific Corp (Natick, MA)	WALLSTENT	FilterWire EZ
Cordis Corp (Miami, FL)	Precise RX	Angioguard RX
Covidien (Plymouth, MN)	PROTÉGÉ RX	SpiderFX

is typically necessary only if a balloon guide is being used to obtain proximal flow control.
  b. 4- or 5-Fr catheters of different shapes (e.g., Bernstein II, Sidewinder II, Multipurpose, Vertebral, Headhunter), are used to cannulate the CCA of interest and, if needed, other cervical vessels. To minimize the need for exchanges, we recommend using a long (125-cm) diagnostic catheter placed coaxially within the guide sheath.
3. Cerebral protection devices
  a. Current practice advocates for the use of a CPD when performing carotid stenting (4). CPDs mitigate the risk of stroke during CAS from emboli generated during traversal and manipulation of the diseased vessel segment.
  b. Filters are the most commonly used CPDs (Table 5.1). These consist of collapsible meshes mounted at the ends of 0.014-in guidewires. The guidewire is navigated beyond the stenosis and the filter is deployed. The filter traps embolic debris, which is removed along with the device after stent placement and PTA.
  c. The MO.MA Ultra Device (Medtronic Vascular Inc, Santa Rosa, CA) is a proximal protection device that consists of a catheter exchanged over a stiff 0.035-in wire in the external carotid artery. The distal balloon is inflated in the external carotid artery, the stiff guidewire is retracted, and the proximal balloon is inflated in the CCA. While on flow arrest through the ICA, a 0.014-in guidewire is navigated across the stenosis to support angioplasty and stenting. After stent deployment and, if needed, postplasty, aspiration through the MO.MA Ultra device is performed, retrieving debris. The distal and proximal balloons are then deflated and antegrade flow is restored. The MO.MA Ultra device is withdrawn. This protection device has a distal tip profile of 5 Fr and requires an introducer sheath of at least 9 Fr.
  d. Transcarotid artery revascularization (TCAR) is a hybrid surgical/endovascular approach to providing cerebral protection by flow reversal. An open surgical access is obtained to the ipsilateral CCA. A specialized access sheath is placed into the CCA and connected to a circuit that shunts blood through a second sheath that is inserted into a femoral vein. Once the circuit is in place, the proximal CCA is clamped, providing flow reversal in the carotid artery and return of blood to the circulation via the femoral vein. Angioplasty and stenting are then performed through the CCA sheath under continuous flow reversal. At the conclusion of the procedure, the sheath is removed. The arteriotomy and CCA cutdown are closed surgically. Prospective, single-arm registry data indicates that this is an effective approach for minimizing stroke risk during carotid intervention (9).
4. PTA balloons
  a. For predilatation (if required prior to stent placement), choose a 3–4-mm × 20–30-mm noncompliant PTA balloon. If unable to navigate the lesion, predilatation can be performed using a low-profile cerebral or coronary

angioplasty balloon, such as the Gateway (Stryker Neurovascular, Fremont, CA) or Maverick (Boston Scientific Corp, Natick, MA).

b. For dilatation after stent placement, choose a 4–7-mm × 20–30-mm noncompliant PTA balloon. As a guideline, the diameter should match that of the normal artery distal to the target lesion. In cases of immediate restenosis due to recoil, a 1- to 2-mm larger postdilatation balloon may be needed.

5. Stents

  a. Self-expandable stents are used for the majority of CAS due to their superior crush resistance and their ability to regain their shape when deformed (see Table 5.1). These advantages are important due to the mobility of the neck. Balloon expandable stents offer more precise placement and still have a role in the treatment of CCA ostial lesions, where the segment of artery being treated remains protected by the thoracic cage.

  b. Landing zones should be at least 5 to 10 mm distal and proximal to the atherosclerotic plaque. It is preferable to cover the entire target lesion using a single stent. Lesions located in tortuous carotid segments may be treated by overlapping two shorter stents, which avoids the arterial kinking and pseudo-occlusion that generally occurs distal to a stented segment due to straightening of the ICA.

  c. Stents should be oversized 1 to 2 mm above the diameter of the vessel in the landing zones. In contradistinction to PTA balloons, stents are sized with reference to the larger, more proximal host vessel. Tapered stents are available and may be useful in cases where there is a particularly large discrepancy between proximal and distal landing zone diameters.

Procedure in Detail

1. Access

  a. CAS has typically been performed via common femoral artery access. Recently radial access has been used with good effectiveness and safety profiles. Radial access can be particularly advantageous in certain configurations of aortic arch anatomy, and may carry a lower risk of access site morbidity than femoral access in patients on DAPT. Final determination of access site and materials used to cannulate the carotid of interest should always be based on a thorough review of preoperative cross-sectional imaging.

  b. US-guided femoral arterial access has been shown to reduce the risk of vascular access complications versus fluoroscopic guidance alone. Therefore, we recommend that access should be obtained in all cases by US-guided micropuncture technique. To avoid retroperitoneal hemorrhage from femoral access, fluoroscopy should be used to ensure that the puncture is below the inguinal ligament.

  c. After placement of the femoral sheath (and an arterial line, if needed), initiate anticoagulation (see **Intraprocedural medications**, above).

2. Diagnostic angiography

  a. Using a selective diagnostic catheter and a hydrophilic guidewire, perform selective catheterization of the target CCA. Avoid traversing the carotid bifurcation with the wire or catheter in these cases.

  b. Presenting angiographic acquisitions should include frontal, oblique, and lateral views of the neck; frontal and lateral views of the intracranial circulation; and any additional projections needed to clarify the anatomy. Three-dimensional rotational angiography (3DRA) of the carotid bulb may be helpful in evaluating high-grade stenosis and calcified lesions. 3DRA can also be helpful to illustrate the best projection for navigation across the stenosis and the optimal projection for stent deployment, though these projections can often be determined preoperatively on cross-sectional imaging.

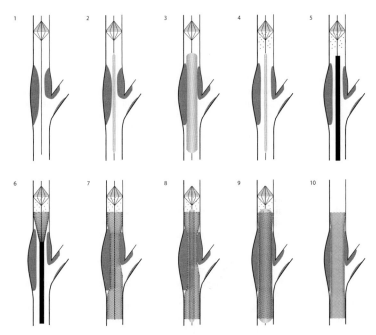

FIGURE 5.1 • The carotid stenting procedure step-by-step.

   c. Key points to assess:
      (1) Define the lesion extent (length, degree of stenosis) and regional anatomy (landing zone diameters; relationships of the lesion to the carotid bulb; degree of calcification, tortuosity, ulceration, and thrombus).
      (2) Assess the circle of Willis and intracranial collateral blood supply. External carotid artery injections may also be necessary to evaluate for collateral supply to the intracranial circulation.
      (3) Identify potential dangerous anastomoses to the internal carotid circulation from the external carotid circulation and the vertebrobasilar system.
3. Carotid stenting procedure
   a. Prepare equipment. Having the stent, balloon, and (if applicable) CPD recapture catheter ready will help you to limit the time that the CPD is deployed. Be sure to choose a guide catheter that can accommodate the stent(s) you are likely to use.
   b. Advance the guide catheter into the CCA, either over the selective catheter or by exchange. Ideally, the guide is positioned so that its tip is distal enough to provide sufficient support but proximal enough to permit complete deployment of the stent. In some circumstances, it may be necessary to position the guide more distally and withdraw it during the stent deployment.
   c. Consider prophylactic administration of glycopyrrolate to prevent bradycardia (see **Intraprocedural medications**, above).
   d. Obtain CCA angiograms at working projections determined during the diagnostic angiography.
   e. If using a filter-type CPD, carefully navigate the CPD through the stenosis and deploy it in a straight distal segment of the ICA (Fig. 5.1, step 1). Remove the CPD sheath. If flow arrest is being used, the balloons are inflated at this step.

f. In cases predilatation is needed, advance a PTA balloon over the wire until its markers are placed across the stenotic segment of the ICA, covering it completely, and perform angioplasty (Fig. 5.1, steps 2 to 4). Remove the PTA balloon. Before any angioplasty maneuver, particularly at the ICA bifurcation, the anesthesiology team should be notified, as stimulation of the carotid bulb could cause unexpected and significant bradycardia.

g. Over the wire, position the stent delivery system so that the stent covers the entire target lesion, including plaque adjacent to the stenotic segment (Fig. 5.1, step 5). Bony features can serve to landmark the extent of the lesion and guide the stent placement prior to deployment; however, because the stent systems are stiff and can distort the anatomy, a new roadmap or DSA is the most accurate way to ensure that the stent is precisely positioned. The stent should be deployed slowly but steadily, starting slightly more distal to the intended landing point, as it is possible to pull back the construct during controlled deployment (Fig. 5.1, steps 6 to 7).

h. Once the stent is deployed, remove the delivery catheter, obtain a follow-up angiogram, and assess for residual stenosis.

i. If needed, perform poststent PTA (if residual stenosis >10% to 15%). Balloon size should match or slightly exceed the distal normal artery diameter (Fig. 5.1, steps 8 and 9).

j. Remove the PTA balloon and obtain a follow-up angiogram of the CCA in multiple views.

k. Remove the CPD using the included resheathing catheter (Fig. 5.1, step 10), or aspirate blood and deflate the occlusion balloons.

l. Obtain follow-up angiograms of the CCA and of the intracranial circulation. It is important to assess for vasospasm, dissection, and distal emboli. Administer verapamil or nicardipine, as indicated.

4. The femoral sheath should be removed in accordance with the access closure method selected.

Postprocedure Management

1. If the patient is stable, admit to a step-down unit for 24-hour (overnight) observation.
   a. Check vital signs and neurologic examination every hour.
   b. Keep systolic BP between 100 mm Hg and 160 mm Hg.
   c. If placed, keep the Foley catheter to gravity until a few hours before discharge.
   d. Start PO fluids and advance to regular diet as tolerated.
   e. Hydrate the patient with normal saline solution at 150 mL per hour for a total of 400 mL.
   f. Initiate deep vein thrombosis prophylaxis.
   g. Time of bedrest and mobility privileges depend on arteriotomy location, closure modality, and institutional policies. Ideally, the head of bed should be raised as soon as possible to avoid reperfusion injury.

Follow-Up

1. Continue clopidogrel 75 mg PO daily and aspirin 81 mg PO daily for 6 weeks. After 6 weeks, patients remain on aspirin 81 mg PO daily for life.
2. Obtain carotid US at 3 months, 6 months, 1 year, and 2 years postprocedure.

Complications and Management

1. Allergic contrast reaction, renal damage, and access site hemorrhagic or ischemic events are managed similarly to any other angiographic examination.

2 Anticoagulation and antiplatelet therapy may increase the frequency and severity of bleeding complications.

3. Bradycardia is sometimes observed if the target lesion is calcified and in the proximity of the carotid bulb. It is usually transient and resolves spontaneously. Bradycardia can be avoided by slow inflation of the PTA balloon under ECG monitoring and/or by pretreatment with glycopyrrolate. Atropine may be needed, albeit infrequently, as discussed previously. Rarely, the patient may require a temporary transvenous ventricular pacemaker.

4. Arterial hypotension should be managed with colloid infusion, dopamine, or Neo-Synephrine as necessary. In a small number of cases, CAS can result in several days of hypotension, necessitating a longer admission. This is likely secondary to injury to carotid bulb baroceptors at the time of PTA/stenting.

5. Arterial vasospasm generally resolves spontaneously. Otherwise, treat with nicardipine or verapamil as discussed previously.

6. Arterial dissection, if flow limiting, might necessitate treatment with acute stenting. If the dissection is not flow limiting, single- or dual-antiplatelet therapy is favored for prevention of embolic phenomena.

7. Acute thromboembolism. Consult a stroke interventionalist for the most appropriate approach. Depending on the size and location of the embolic occlusion, a number of treatments are available to manage acute thromboembolism, including intra-arterial ReoPro or Integrilin, intra-arterial tPA, thrombectomy with a stent retriever, aspiration thrombectomy. Ancillary treatment may include colloid infusion and induction of arterial hypertension.

8. Plaque rupture with immediate vessel occlusion after PTA can be treated by stenting to reopen the lesion. This underlines the utmost importance of keeping a wire across the diseased segment until stenting is complete.

9. In case of incomplete coverage of the target lesion, a second stent should be placed.

10. Neck hematoma may occur during PTA/CAS due to venous or arterial rupture. It generally occurs in patients who have undergone prior CEA and usually self-containing. In case of vessel rupture, immediately reverse heparinization with IV protamine (10 mg of protamine per every 1,000 units of heparin administered). If there is major vessel rupture, immediately occlude the vessel with a balloon catheter. Reconstructive methods could include emergent placement of a covered stent (currently off-label). Permanent endovascular occlusion of the entire carotid artery with coils should be considered. Transfer patient for emergency surgery if needed.

11. Reperfusion brain edema can be managed with mannitol and corticosteroids.

12. Intracerebral hemorrhage may be reperfusion-related or due to delayed transformation of a small ischemic insult. In very rare cases, subarachnoid hemorrhage can occur. Patients that experience these complications usually have had long-standing, subocclusive stenosis. Depending on the significance of the injury, the patient should be evaluated by the neurosurgery team and admitted to the ICU. Consider a period of single-antiplatelet therapy.

13. MI is a very rare complication during CAS; consult a cardiologist.

Data from Randomized Controlled Trials

1. The North American Symptomatic Carotid Endarterectomy Trial (NASCET) was the first to demonstrate that symptomatic patients with carotid stenosis benefited from surgical revascularization over medical therapy, with significant reduction in the rates of stroke and mortality in populations with stenosis ≥50% (10). These findings were corroborated by the European Carotid Surgery Trial (ECST) (11). The results of the Asymptomatic Carotid Atherosclerosis Study (ACAS) showed that CEA is superior to medical management for asymptomatic

patients with ≥60% stenosis and serve as the basis for performing revascularization procedures in this population (12).

2. The Carotid and Vertebral Artery Transluminal Angioplasty Study (CAVATAS) was the first large RCT to demonstrate the feasibility and safety of endovascular carotid interventions (13). Despite the use of stents in only 26% of the patients in the endovascular arm and the absence of CPDs, the CAVATAS showed similar major risks and effectiveness between CEA and CAS at 3 years. The subsequent proliferation of CAS devices was accompanied by the enrollment of patients into a number of manufacturer-supported trials.

3. The Stenting and Angioplasty with Protection in Patients at High Risk for Endarterectomy (SAPPHIRE) trial was an RCT comparing CAS versus CEA in high-risk patients who had symptomatic or asymptomatic carotid artery diseases (5,11). SAPPHIRE showed that, in a population at high risk for CEA, CAS was noninferior to CEA in the 30-day risk of stroke, death, or MI. Furthermore, SAPPHIRE showed that CAS was noninferior to CEA in the risk of reaching a composite end point at 3 years. The results of several manufacturer supported trials then showed that, in patients at high risk for CEA, CAS was noninferior to objective performance criteria derived from historical CEA studies. The results of these trials supported the U.S. Food and Drug Administration (FDA) approval of the variety of devices now available and have supported the continued use of CAS in the high-risk population.

4. The results of two more RCTs casted doubt over the safety of CAS. The Endarterectomy versus Angioplasty in Patients with Symptomatic Severe Carotid Stenosis (EVA-3S) and Stent-supported Percutaneous Angioplasty of the Carotid Artery versus Endarterectomy (SPACE) trials were both terminated early after failing to prove the noninferiority of CAS to CEA for periprocedural complications (14–17). It is important, however, to highlight that these studies had concerns about operator inexperience in the CAS arm and nonuniform use of CPDs. The EVA-3S trial was a multicenter study that required only limited operator experience (five prior CAS procedures, or no CAS procedures, if supervised). The SPACE trial was conducted without the now mandatory use of CPDs, which were employed in only 27% of the cases. These factors likely resulted in a higher periprocedural event rate, leading to premature study termination due to safety and futility issues.

5. The initial early results of the International Carotid Stenting Study (ICSS) suggested that CEA was superior to CAS at 120-day follow-up, the risk of stroke, death, or procedural MI was 8.5% in the CAS group versus 5.2% in the CEA group ($P = .006$) (18). The initial conclusion was that CEA should remain the treatment of choice for patients requiring carotid revascularization. However, the results of the long-term data from this same study have recently been made available (19). Regarding these long-term outcomes of the ICSS study, 1,713 patients were assigned to stenting ($n = 855$) or endarterectomy ($n = 858$) and followed up for a median of 4.2 years (interquartile range [IQR] 3.0–5.2, maximum 10.0). Three patients withdrew immediately, and therefore, the intention to treat population comprised 1,710 patients. The number of fatal or disabling strokes (52 vs. 49) and cumulative 5-year risk did not differ significantly between the stenting and endarterectomy groups (6.4% vs. 6.5%; hazard ratio [HR] 1.06, 95% CI 0.72–1.57, $P = .77$). Strokes were more frequent in the stenting group than in the endarterectomy group but were mainly nondisabling. As a result, the ICSS long-term functional outcome and risk of fatal or disabling stroke were ultimately found to be similar for stenting and endarterectomy for symptomatic carotid stenosis.

6. The largest RCT comparing CAS versus CEA for the treatment of carotid artery stenosis and for the prevention of stroke was an NIH-sponsored CREST study (3,20). This study included low- and medium-risk patients. The primary end point in CREST was a composite including any stroke, MI, or death in the periprocedural period, and all ipsilateral strokes thereafter. In 2,502 patients followed for

up to 4 years, there was no significant difference between the rates of reaching the primary end point in the CAS and CEA groups (7.2% vs. 6.8%, $P = .51$). CAS was associated with a higher risk of periprocedural stroke (4.3% vs. 2.3%, $P = .01$); CEA was associated with a higher risk of periprocedural MI (1.1% vs. 2.3%, $P = .03$). The risk of major periprocedural stroke was not significantly different (0.9% vs. 0.7%, $P = .52$), indicating that the excess strokes attributable to CAS were nondisabling or minor. In those patients undergoing CAS, four angiographic variables were associated with more periprocedural strokes: severe distal tortuosity, sequential lesions, lesion length greater than 20 mm, and a narrow mouth ulcer in the carotid plaque. Attention to these characteristics may help in patient selection. Furthermore, the CREST data demonstrated an interaction between age and treatment efficacy, with CAS showing greater efficacy than CEA in patients below 70 years of age. In patients above age 70, CEA showed greater efficacy.

7. The ongoing CREST-2 trial is running at 120 clinical centers across the United States and Canada. The study is funded by the NIH National Institute of Neurological Disorders and Stroke (NINDS) and is fundamentally designed to comprise two parallel RCTs that build on the data collected by the CREST team but diverges in one crucial way. Instead of comparing one procedure to the other (CEA vs. CAS), CREST-2 compares a combination of CEA and intensive medical management to intensive medical management alone, and CAS combined with intensive medical management to intensive medical management alone, in two separate arms. Both arms will randomize 600 patients to each group for a total of 2,480 patients, all of whom have at least 70% or higher blockage of one of their carotid arteries but have not suffered a stroke from it. The trial began enrolling patients in early 2014, and is expected to be completed by the end of 2022. The results of this study may provide a more definitive answer regarding the roles of CEA versus CAS and whether asymptomatic ≥70% carotid stenosis should be managed medically.

The results of RCTs comparing CEA with CAS in patients with symptomatic carotid stenosis are summarized in Table G.1; trials comparing CEA with CAS in patients with asymptomatic carotid stenosis are summarized in Table G.2.

References

1. Brott TG, Halperin JL, Abbara S, et al. ASA/ACCF/AHA/AANN/AANS/ACR/ASNR/CNS/SAIP/SCAI/SIR/SNIS/SVM/SVS guideline on the management of patients with extracranial carotid and vertebral artery disease: executive summary: a report of the American College of Cardiology Foundation/American Heart Association Task Force on Practice Guidelines, and the American Stroke Association, American Association of Neuroscience Nurses, American Association of Neurological Surgeons, American College of Radiology, American Society of Neuroradiology, Congress of Neurological Surgeons, Society of Atherosclerosis Imaging and Prevention, Society for Cardiovascular Angiography and Interventions, Society of Interventional Radiology, Society of NeuroInterventional Surgery, Society for Vascular Medicine, and Society for Vascular Surgery. Developed in collaboration with the American Academy of Neurology and Society of Cardiovascular Computed Tomography. *J Am Coll Cardiol*. 2011;57(8):1002–1044.

2. Goyal M, Singh N, Marko M, et al. Embolic stroke of undetermined source and symptomatic nonstenotic carotid disease. *Stroke*. 2020;51(4):1321–1325. doi:10.1161/STROKEAHA.119.028853

3. Brott TG, Hobson RW II, Howard G, et al. Stenting versus endarterectomy for treatment of carotid-artery stenosis. *N Engl J Med*. 2010;363(1):11–23.

4. Howard VJ, Lutsep HL, Mackey A, et al. Influence of sex on outcomes of stenting versus endarterectomy: a subgroup analysis of the Carotid Revascularization Endarterectomy versus Stenting Trial (CREST). *Lancet Neurol*. 2011;10(6):530–537. doi:10.1016/S1474-4422(11)70080-1

5. Yadav JS, Wholey MH, Kuntz RE, et al. Protected carotid-artery stenting versus endarterectomy in high-risk patients. *N Engl J Med*. 2004;351(15):1493–1501.

6. Massop D, Dave R, Metzger C, et al. Stenting and angioplasty with protection in patients at high-risk for endarterectomy: SAPPHIRE Worldwide Registry first 2,001 patients. *Catheter Cardiovasc Interv.* 2009;73(2):129–136.

7. Haussen DC, Grossberg JA, Bouslama M, et al. Carotid web (intimal fibromuscular dysplasia) has high stroke recurrence risk and is amenable to stenting. *Stroke.* 2017;48(11): 3134–3137. doi:10.1161/STROKEAHA.117.019020

8. Amarenco P, Bogousslavsky J, Callahan A III, et al. High-dose atorvastatin after stroke or transient ischemic attack. *N Engl J Med.* 2006;355(6):549–559.

9. Kashyap VS, Schneider PA, Foteh M, et al. Early outcomes in the ROADSTER 2 Study of transcarotid artery revascularization in patients with significant carotid artery isease. *Stroke.* 2020;51(9):2620–2629. doi:10.1161/STROKEAHA.120.030550

10. Barnett HJ, Taylor DW, Eliasziw M, et al. Benefit of carotid endarterectomy in patients with symptomatic moderate or severe stenosis. *N Engl J Med.* 1998;339:1415–1425.

11. European Carotid Surgery Trialists' Collaborative Group. Randomised trial of endarterectomy for recently symptomatic carotid stenosis: final results of the MRC European Carotid Surgery Trial (ECST). *Lancet.* 1998;351:1379–1387.

12. Walker MD, Marler JR, Goldstein M, et al. Endarterectomy for asymptomatic carotid artery stenosis. Executive Committee for the Asymptomatic Carotid Atherosclerosis Study. *JAMA.* 1995;273:1421–1428.

13. Ederle J, Bonati LH, Dobson J, et al. Endovascular treatment with angioplasty or stenting versus endarterectomy in patients with carotid artery stenosis in the carotid and vertebral artery transluminal angioplasty study (CAVATAS): long-term follow-up of a randomised trial. *Lancet Neurol.* 2009;8(10):898–907.

14. Mas JL, Chatellier G, Beyssen B, et al. Endarterectomy versus stenting in patients with symptomatic severe carotid stenosis. *N Engl J Med.* 2006;355(16):1660–1671.

15. Mas JL, Trinquart L, Leys D, et al. Endarterectomy versus angioplasty in patients with symptomatic severe carotid stenosis (EVA-3S) trial: results up to 4 years from a randomised, multicentre trial. *Lancet Neurol.* 2008;7(10):885–892.

16. Ringleb PA, Allenberg J, Brückmann H, et al. 30 Day results from the SPACE trial of stent-protected angioplasty versus carotid endarterectomy in symptomatic patients: a randomised non-inferiority trial. *Lancet.* 2006;368(9543):1239–1247.

17. Eckstein HH, Ringleb P, Allenberg JR, et al. Results of the stent-protected angioplasty versus carotid endarterectomy (SPACE) study to treat symptomatic stenoses at 2 years: a multinational, prospective, randomised trial. *Lancet Neurol.* 2008;7(10): 893–902.

18. Ederle J, Dobson J, Featherstone RL, et al. Carotid artery stenting compared with endarterectomy in patients with symptomatic carotid stenosis (International Carotid Stenting Study): an interim analysis of a randomised controlled trial. *Lancet.* 2010;375(9719): 985–997.

19. Bonati LH, Dobson J, Featherstone RL, et al. Long-term outcomes after stenting versus endarterectomy for treatment of symptomatic carotid stenosis: the International Carotid Stenting Study (ICSS) randomised trial. *Lancet.* 2015;385(9967): 529–538.

20. Gurm HS, Yadav JS, Fayad P, et al. Long-term results of carotid stenting versus endarterectomy in high-risk patients. *N Engl J Med.* 2008;358(15):1572–1579.

6 Vascular Emergencies of the Head and Neck

Mesha L. Martinez, MD, Joshua Cornman-Homonoff, MD, and Michele H. Johnson, MD, FACR, FASER

Introduction

Vascular emergencies of the head and neck may require predominantly neurosurgical or otorhinolaryngologic management, although there is considerable overlap (trauma, carotid blow out). In either case, angiography plays a central role in therapy, with protocols varying by indication and selectivity essential to safe and successful endovascular diagnosis and intervention (1,2).

Neurologic and Neurosurgical Disorders

Intracranial Subarachnoid Hemorrhage (SAH) (3)

Etiology and Differential Diagnosis

1. Trauma is the most common cause of SAH and is uncommonly associated with major vascular injury. The distribution of blood and associated intracranial and soft tissue injury permits differentiation from aneurysmal SAH in most cases.
2. Rupture of saccular ("berry") aneurysm is the second most common cause. The incidence of ruptured aneurysm varies by location (Table 6.1). Giant, fusiform, and dissecting intracranial aneurysms represent a smaller subset of aneurysms and rarely present with SAH.
3. Other less common causes of subarachnoid hemorrhage include reversible vasoconstriction syndrome (RCVS), pial and mixed pial-dural arteriovenous malformation (AVM), dural arteriovenous fistula (DAVF), vasculitis, and moyamoya circulation patterns.

Clinical Presentation

1. Symptoms include headache, classically described as worst headache of life (WHOL), syncope, emesis, neck pain/stiffness, and photophobia.
2. Onset is usually acute, although some may present later following sentinel headache or after several days of intractable headache.

Noninvasive Imaging

1. Noncontrast computed tomography (CT) demonstrates hyperdense blood within the subarachnoid spaces, basal cisterns, sulci, and ventricles. The distribution of blood varies with the location of the aneurysm (Table 6.2).
2. Computed tomographic angiography (CTA) at the time of initial CT often permits identification of the aneurysm and characterization sufficient for triage and planning for endovascular treatment or open surgery. CTA may not circumvent the need for digital subtraction angiography (DSA) but may reduce the number of injections required for diagnosis prior to treatment.

Indications for Cerebral Angiography (DSA)

1. Clinical and imaging criteria for suspected nontraumatic SAH for triage and treatment
2. Negative or nondiagnostic CTA or to clarify uncertain CTA findings
3. In lieu of CTA when renal function is impaired

Contraindications to Cerebral Angiography

1. Hemodynamic instability

Table 6.1	Incidence of Ruptured Aneurysms by Location
Location	**Incidence (%)**
Anterior communicating artery	30.3
Posterior communicating artery	25.0
Middle cerebral artery bifurcation	13.1
Internal carotid artery bifurcation	4.5
Anterior choroidal artery	4.3
M1 segment of middle cerebral artery	3.9
Basilar bifurcation	2.0
A1 segment of anterior cerebral artery	1.5
Distal middle cerebral artery	1.4
Distal posterior cerebral artery	0.9
Vertebrobasilar junction	0.9
Midbasilar artery	0.8
Posterior inferior cerebral artery	0.8

2. Relative contraindications include renal failure, uncontrolled hypertension, iodinated contrast allergy

Preprocedural Preparation

Standard preangiographic workup includes routine labs, appropriate intravenous access, and continuous monitoring of hemodynamics and intracranial pressure (ICP) as dictated by the patient's clinical condition.

Procedure

1. Heparin bolus immediately following access, either as a standard dose (approximately 2,000 units intravenously [IV]) or weight-based dose, to achieve an activated clotting time (ACT) of 200 to 250 seconds. This may be omitted in the setting of intracranial hemorrhage.
2. Femoral or radial access routes are most common for cerebral angiography. When radial access is utilized, a "radial cocktail" (author's preference consists of

Table 6.2	Distribution of Subarachnoid Hemorrhage (SAH) by Aneurysm Location
Anterior communicating artery	SAH in anterior interhemispheric fissure or septum pellucidum Hematoma in anteromedial frontal lobe
Posterior communicating artery	SAH in suprasellar cistern, ambient (perimesencephalic) cistern Hematoma in anteromedial frontal lobe, basal ganglia
Middle cerebral artery	SAH in ipsilateral sylvian fissure Hematoma in temporal lobe
Basilar artery	SAH in interpeduncular cistern Hematoma in midbrain
Posterior inferior cerebellar artery	SAH in prepontine cistern, fourth ventricle Cerebellar hematoma

400-mcg nitroglycerine, 5-mg verapamil (2.5 cc), and 2,000 units heparin) should be administered slowly through the sheath to reduce the risk of local vasospasm.

3. Vascular interrogation—initially directed to the suspected aneurysm location. Complete cerebral angiography should include bilateral common/internal/external carotid arteries (or bilateral common carotid arteries; the latter only when catheterization is difficult or when significant disease of the carotid bifurcation precludes safe distal catheterization). Bilateral vertebral arteries (or one vertebral artery with reflux into the contralateral vertebral artery proximal to the origin of the posterior inferior cerebellar artery).

4. Conventional angiography utilizes planar imaging in frontal, lateral, and oblique projections to facilitate visualization of the vessel branch points where aneurysms usually arise.

5. Digital rotational angiography with three-dimensional (3D) reconstruction images is the standard of care, providing multiple projection images for working projection delineation with reduction of contrast and radiation as compared to conventional angiography.

6. Adjunctive maneuvers to improve visualization of communicating arteries such as carotid cross-compression and Alcock's test, vertebral injection with carotid compression, are rarely necessary since the introduction of rotational angiography.

Other Considerations

1. Negative DSA: Traditionally, angiography is repeated 7 to 10 days later to exclude the possibility of missing an aneurysm secondary to vasospasm or intraaneurysmal thrombus. Current practice is repeat CTA, performed within 1 week and prior to discharge. Magnetic resonance imaging (MRI) with magnetic resonance angiography (MRA) using black blood techniques (vessel wall imaging) has been helpful in diagnosis of blister aneurysms as well as for identification of which aneurysm has ruptured when there are multiple. Follow-up DSA remains the reference standard.

2. Spinal subarachnoid hemorrhage
   a. Spinal subarachnoid hemorrhage often presents with headache or cervical pain. SAH frequently at the skull base and upper cervical region.
   b. MRI/MRA and CTA may be useful in identification of the level of pathology and may allow for more limited spinal angiography.
   c. Additions to the cerebral angiographic protocol include injection of both cervical vertebral arteries, the costocervical and thyrocervical trunks and intersegmental arteries. Contrast load may be large so volume should be closely monitored.

Postprocedure Management

1. Hemostasis achieved at the puncture site in standard fashion with manual compression, femoral vascular closure device or radial TR band.

2. Neurologic and vascular checks are included in the postprocedural nursing order set.

Results

1. CTA demonstrates ruptured aneurysm in the majority and aids in triage of patients to endovascular treatment or surgical clipping.

2. DSA sensitivity is >85%. Imaging (repeat DSA or CTA) following negative DSA, increases sensitivity to greater than 95%.

3. MRI/MRA of the brain and spine may be adjunctive, when initial arterial imaging is unrevealing. Black blood MRI techniques are useful to identify the rupture site, including blister aneurysms.

Complications (1)

Complications of diagnostic cerebral angiography include contrast allergy, transient ischemic attack (TIA), stroke (0.5% to 2%), hematoma, and vascular injury/dissection.

Treatment for Ruptured Intracranial Saccular Aneurysm (4,5)

Surgical Aneurysm Treatment: Clipping

1. Intraoperative angiography confirms optimal clip placement and confirms patency of adjacent vessels. Sheaths are placed in the operating room (OR) and sterile access to the sheath established. Rapid recognition and revision of clip placement, when needed, may improve outcome.
2. Proximal control with surgical access to the carotid in the neck may be helpful for temporary reduction of flow in the internal carotid artery at the time of clip placement for the treatment of large paraclinoid or supraclinoid aneurysms.

Endovascular Aneurysm Treatment: Detachable Coils

Indications

1. Anatomical criteria that favor successful coil placement
   a. Consider aneurysm morphology; shape and size; relationship to adjacent branches and other critical structures.
   b. Small neck of the aneurysm compared to the dome; aneurysms with neck to dome ratio >0.5, or neck of 4 mm, will likely require balloon or stent assist or newer endovascular devices such as WEB or flow diverters for endovascular management.
2. Endovascular treatment is favored for posterior circulation aneurysms such as basilar terminus, superior cerebellar and posterior inferior cerebellar artery aneurysms.

Contraindications and Relative Contraindications

1. Severely tortuous and/or atherosclerotic vessels with inadequate access to the aneurysm may require open surgery.
2. Fusiform or dissecting aneurysms: May require stent assist or flow diversion (see below).
3. Vasospasm that inhibits adequate catheterization and deployment of the coils may require endovascular treatment of vasospasm and the aneurysm in the same session.
4. Coagulation disorders, connective tissue disorders and active bacterial infection (mycotic aneurysm) require thoughtful consideration prior to endovascular treatment.

Preprocedural Preparation

1. General anesthesia, arterial line, ventriculostomy, and central venous catheters as needed for patient care.
2. Preparation as per diagnostic angiography, noting that patients may be more unstable and thus require higher levels of care.

Procedure

1. Detachable coil systems for endovascular treatment of aneurysms (available through multiple vendors).
2. Coils are available in a wide variety of diameters, lengths, shapes, and degrees of softness. New technologies include stretch resistance, complex shapes, more precise detachment mechanisms.
3. Platinum microcoils are introduced through a microcatheter placed into the aneurysm using at least a 5-Fr or 6-Fr guiding catheter platform.
4. For balloon-assisted coiling, larger internal diameter (ID) guiding catheters are needed; balloon is inflated across the neck of the aneurysm to protect the parent artery during coil placement. The balloon is deflated just prior to coil detachment in order to identify coil prolapse, although the coil can still be removed. A balloon can also provide some protection in the case of intraprocedural rupture and may be lifesaving.
5. Heparin administration is titrated to an ACT level of approximately 250 to 300 seconds, following 5,000-unit loading dose (70 units per kg).
6. Stent-assisted coiling was initially reserved for unruptured aneurysm patients who could be electively treated with antiplatelet agents prior to treatment.

Currently some aneurysms may be treated with stent assist following acute rupture as needed to secure the aneurysm. The stent is placed crossing the aneurysm neck and the aneurysm accessed through the stent mesh. Alternatively, the aneurysm can be catheterized and the catheter "jailed" by the stent. The aneurysm is coiled, and the microcatheter removed.

Postprocedure Management
1. Intensive care unit (ICU) management, vasospasm monitoring
2. Systemic heparinization (partial thromboplastin time [PTT] 40 to 60 seconds) may be maintained for 12 to 24 hours for large coil masses. Antiplatelet therapy, usually aspirin, may be added after 24 hours
3. Follow-up CTA to assess for vasospasm and vessel patency

Results
1. With endovascular coil techniques, the International Subarachnoid Aneurysm Trial (ISAT) study of treatment for ruptured saccular aneurysms demonstrated an absolute risk reduction for endovascular versus surgery of 7.4%. The metric was death and disability at 1 year. Although there are many criticisms of the study, the basic conclusion remains supported by extended ISAT follow-up and other studies.
2. Aneurysms with smaller sacs will have a higher rate of total occlusion.

Complications
1. Complications of diagnostic cerebral angiography include contrast allergy, TIA, stroke (0.5% to 2%), hematoma, dissection, and death.
2. Risk of aneurysm rupture is low during diagnostic angiography and approximately 1% to 3% during endovascular treatment.
3. Risk of TIA/stroke during endovascular treatment (thromboembolic complications) is 3% to 5% depending on the series. Some authors feel the risk of stroke is reduced by the administration of heparin during the procedure and for 48 hours following endovascular treatment.
4. Compaction of coils within the aneurysm may result in aneurysm recurrence requiring placement of additional coils, stent, flow diversion, or surgical clipping.
5. Perforation or vascular injury with hemorrhage; compromise of adjacent or parent vessel by thrombus or due to compression by the coil mass.

Endovascular Aneurysm Treatment: Parent Vessel Occlusion

Indications
Parent vessel occlusion (deconstructive treatment) remains a viable treatment alternative for selected surgically or endovascularly inaccessible aneurysms.

Preprocedural Preparation
1. Diagnostic arteriography to visualize the aneurysm and the circle of Willis.
2. Balloon occlusion tolerance (BOT) test is performed to determine the patient's ability to tolerate permanent occlusion.
3. The predictive value of BOT may be enhanced by the use of controlled hypotension and clinical assessment during occlusion and cerebral blood flow testing using hexamethylpropyleneamine oxime (HMPAO) single-photon emission computed tomography (SPECT) at the time of occlusion (see "Balloon Occlusion Tolerance Test" for technique).

Procedure
1. Permanent internal carotid or vertebral occlusion via surgical clipping, or endovascular embolization using coils or AMPLATZER plugs. Detachable balloons are no longer available in the United States.
2. Proximal occlusion is sufficient in many cases to induce thrombosis without the need for trapping of the aneurysm.

Contraindications/Relative Contraindications
1. Failure of the BOT precluding parent vessel sacrifice; may require surgical bypass or incomplete treatment strategies.
2. Vascular anatomy precluding device deployment (dissection, stenosis, tortuosity, etc.) favor open surgical options.

Postprocedure Management
1. Optimal ICU management is important to ensure maintenance of cerebral perfusion pressure to reduce the risk of stroke following parent vessel occlusion.
2. Anticoagulation includes heparin infusion following parent vessel occlusion for 48 hours. Antiplatelet therapy, usually aspirin, added after 24 hours.

Complications (1,4,5)
In addition to complications of DSA, stroke, immediate or delayed, is the most worrisome complication of parent vessel occlusion. Tolerance of BOT test is greater than 85% predictive of a good outcome.

Endovascular Aneurysm Treatment: Flow Diverting Stents
1. This novel technology involves deployment of a low-porosity, self-expanding stent, which diverts flow away from the aneurysm and reconstructs the parent vessel lumen, thereby excluding the aneurysm from the circulation. The first one approved for use in the United States was the Pipeline Embolization Device (2011; PED eV3, Irvine, CA) (comprised of braided platinum and nickel-cobalt chromium alloy).
2. Initial indications were for **nonruptured** wide-necked aneurysms of the internal carotid artery from the petrous internal carotid to the superior hypophyseal segment that were not amenable to coiling or clipping.
3. Indications have expanded with successful use of flow diverters for ruptured blister aneurysms not amenable to other treatments.
4. Dual antiplatelet therapy is required to prevent in-stent thrombosis.
5. Complications include delayed thrombosis and/or delayed aneurysm rupture in addition to the risks of DSA.

Treatment of Cerebral Vasospasm (6)
1. Cerebral vasospasm usually results from subarachnoid hemorrhage where blood in the subarachnoid space causes local irritation of the vessels at the level of the circle of Willis and often distally.
2. Loss of autoregulation, narrowing, and flow limitation may result in parenchymal ischemia and clinical deterioration. Angiographic vasospasm occurs in 30% to 70% of patients, but delayed cerebral ischemia (DCI) occurs in 20% to 30% and half of those patients will require endovascular therapy.
3. Vasospasm peaks at 7 to 10 days after subarachnoid hemorrhage. Spasm results in ischemia to the parenchymal territories supplied by the involved vessels.
4. Clinical symptoms vary with the territory of involvement and include depressed consciousness and focal neurologic deficits.
5. Serial transcranial Doppler (TCD) evaluation may be of value in demonstrating early evidence of cerebral vasospasm. CTA and MRA may demonstrate vessel narrowing and diffusion MR can identify associated cerebral ischemia.
6. **Triple-H therapy** to include *hypervolemia, hypertension, and hemodilution* is employed in order to maintain pressure and blood supply through the vessels and is a mainstay of ICU treatment postaneurysmal SAH. Endovascular treatment should commence if there is no response to medical management.

Indications (6)
1. The primary indication for angiography is to confirm diagnosis and for endovascular treatment in the setting of suspected vasospasm (focal or global neurologic deterioration, not responding to medical treatment).

2. Endovascular treatment is initiated early in the course of symptoms that are poorly responsive to initial medical therapy, in order to maximize the opportunity for clinical improvement.
3. Noncontrast CT prior to angiography to identify areas of parenchymal ischemic injury and to exclude nonvasospastic causes of neurologic deterioration, such as hydrocephalus or rebleeding. TCD and CTA may show direct evidence of vasospasm. CTA can reveal both proximal and peripheral vasospasm.

Contraindications
1. Relative contraindications to cerebral angiography include renal failure and uncontrolled hypertension.
2. Relative contraindications to vasospasm treatment include ischemic or hemorrhagic infarction in the involved territory. Revascularization can lead to hemorrhage in severely ischemic and/or infarcted territories.
3. Allergy to medications.

Preprocedural Preparation
1. As per diagnostic angiography.
2. Patient monitoring as in the ICU, including ICP monitoring, arterial and central lines. Anesthesia support with intubation and sedation +/− paralysis are indicated for the majority of patients, especially those undergoing angioplasty.

Cerebral Angiography of Vasospasm
1. Standard heparin bolus may be administered at the time of angiography (2,000 U IV for an average adult). Heparin use is variable and dependent upon the individual situation.
2. Diagnostic angiographic protocol includes both the carotid and vertebral territories with a focus on the vessel supplying the clinically suspected ischemic territory.
3. Angiographic criteria for diagnosis of vasospasm
   a. Narrowing of vessels: Proximal vessel narrowing or sometimes areas of narrowing and dilatation in late stages of vasospasm
   b. Delayed transit time
   c. Parenchymal staining
   d. Comparison with initial CTA and/or initial diagnostic arteriogram may be helpful

Procedure
1. **Endovascular treatment for vasospasm: Vasodilator infusion**
   a. Using a 5-Fr or 6-Fr guide catheter platform, a 4-Fr or 5-Fr catheter can be used for drug infusion into the internal carotid and/or vertebral artery. Alternatively, a microcatheter is placed into the involved territorial branch for more distal infusion. Once vasospasm is confirmed and a stable catheter position achieved, drug infusion is performed.
   b. Calcium channel blockers such as nicardipine and verapamil have replaced papaverine for infusion vasospasm therapy. Nicardipine is given as an infusion at 0.5 to 0.6 mg per vessel and is a more potent vasodilator than verapamil. Verapamil is given as a bolus of 5 mg in 5-mL normal saline administered over 5 minutes for a maximum dose of 15 mg per vessel. Class IIb recommendation, American Heart Association (AHA).
   c. Intermittent control arteriography to document angiographic response. Use the minimum dose needed to provide improvement in cerebral blood flow.
2. **Transluminal balloon angioplasty for vasospasm**
   a. Established vasospasm may not respond to vasodilator therapy and may require angioplasty for treatment; related to the degree of spasm and treatment timing.
   b. Proximal vasospasm, including the internal carotid artery, the M1 segment of the middle cerebral artery, the A1 segment of the anterior cerebral artery, the vertebrobasilar junction, the basilar artery, and the P1 segment of the posterior cerebral artery may be amenable to angioplasty.

c. Angioplasty is most successful in the distal internal carotid artery and the A1 and M1 segments of the anterior and middle cerebral arteries, respectively. The vertebrobasilar system may also respond to angioplasty, but risks are greater in the basilar and the P1 segment of the posterior cerebral artery due to the presence of perforating branches (see below).

d. Angioplasty is performed with a soft, nondetachable silicone microballoon Scepter XC, inflated with gentle intermittent inflation pressures in order to mechanically expand the vessel and improve flow.

e. Angioplasty is reported to be most successful prior to the administration of calcium channel blockers.

Postprocedure Management (After Vasodilator or Angioplasty Treatment)

1. Maintenance of triple-H therapy and close neurologic monitoring for signs of recurrent vasospasm.
2. Daily angiography and vasodilator infusion therapy may be performed in intractable cases of vasospasm.
3. TCD is a useful method to follow the recurrence of vasospasm. CTA is adjunctive.

Results

1. About 66% of patients respond to treatment of vasospasm with vasodilator therapy alone (nicardipine > verapamil).
2. About 54% of the remainder will respond to a combination of vasodilator and angioplasty.
3. The response to therapy is best when initiated within 2 hours of symptom onset. Few patients will demonstrate clinical improvement following endovascular treatment with stable clinical symptoms of greater than 48-hour duration.

Complications of Endovascular Vasospasm Treatment

1. Complications of vasodilator infusion for vasospasm
   a. Increased ICP and retinal hemorrhage were problems seen with papaverine (a phosphodiesterase inhibitor), which is no longer recommended for use.
   b. Hypotension, in response to vasodilator infusion, may lead to decreased cerebral perfusion pressure. Arterial line monitoring is critical during these infusion procedures. Respiratory arrest (vertebral-basilar artery infusion) may lead to heart block in the elderly.
   c. Reperfusion hemorrhage after vasodilator infusion reported in association with vasospasm-induced infarction (hemorrhagic transformation of infarction).
2. Complications of angioplasty for vasospasm
   a. Higher risk than vasodilator infusion
   b. Arterial dissection
   c. Arterial rupture
   d. Arterial thrombosis/occlusion
   e. Secondary embolic sequelae

Nontraumatic Cerebral Parenchymal Hemorrhage (IPH) (7)

Diagnosis

1. Location is often predictive of underlying pathology and helps determine need for cerebral angiography.
2. Noncontrast CT and CTA are the main imaging modalities; MRI is adjunctive.
3. The *spot sign* on CTA imaging is 1 to 2 mm focus (foci) contrast extravasation within the hematoma indicative of active bleeding and is predictive of rapid hematoma expansion. The finding is not associated with any specific pathology.

Etiology

1. Hypertensive hemorrhage: Basal ganglia, pons, cerebellum; thought to be due to microaneurysms (such as Charcot aneurysm from the lenticulostriate vessels), not visible on angiography nor amenable to intervention. If no underlying lesion on CTA, DSA is not indicated.

2. AVMs, DAVF, cavernous malformations, capillary telangiectasia
3. Amyloid angiopathy: Lobar hemorrhages, microbleeds are seen on MRI; rebleeds are common
4. Tumors: metastases; melanoma, thyroid, choriocarcinoma, and primary tumors
5. Cortical vein or dural venous sinus thrombosis causing venous infarction
6. Aneurysmal rupture may also result in intraparenchymal hematoma, usually associated with subarachnoid or intraventricular hemorrhage
   a. Middle cerebral artery and posterior communicating artery aneurysms may rupture into the adjacent temporal lobe
   b. Anterior communicating artery aneurysms may rupture into the medial inferior frontal lobe
7. Mycotic aneurysms may present with IPH alone particularly when distal
8. Hemorrhagic transformation of ischemic infarction
9. Nontraumatic extraaxial hematomas may occasionally result from aneurysm, AVM, or DAVF, often associated with SAH or IPH

Indications
DSA is indicated when the hemorrhage is not associated with hypertension, not confined to the basal ganglia or not typical of amyloid angiography.

Contraindications
Need for emergent decompression due to mass effect; angiography after surgical decompression has added benefit of reducing mass effect, which can compress underlying vascular pathology.

Preprocedural Preparation
1. CT/CTA and/or MRI/MRA obtained in most patients
2. Routine preparation as per diagnostic angiography

Procedure
1. Heparin bolus may be administered at the time of angiography dependent on size and location of the hematoma, coagulation parameters, and the timing of surgical intervention.
2. Angiography (6 vessel) should be performed although it may be tailored to address the clinical problem.
3. Criteria for emergent endovascular intervention for AVM or DAVF
   a. Risk of rebleeding during or immediately following embolization is elevated when intervention is performed shortly after the hemorrhage; due in part to the fragility of the recently ruptured vasculature.
   b. Embolization is usually performed in the nonacute stage; however, if high-risk features are identified, they may be embolized to protect from rebleeding.
   c. Embolic agents include Onyx and *n*-butyl cyanoacrylate; platinum microcoils for associated aneurysms.
4. Criteria for emergent endovascular intervention for ruptured cerebral aneurysm with parenchymal hematoma:
   a. Dependent upon patient condition and the anatomic configuration of the aneurysm, endovascular treatment may be performed prior to or following emergent surgical decompression of the parenchymal hematoma.
   b. Regarding the aneurysms commonly associated with parenchymal hematoma
      (1) Aneurysms at the M1 bifurcation may not be amenable to simple coiling as a primary form of treatment. Balloon or stent assistance, intrasaccular devices and flow diverting stents increase the configurations of aneurysms amenable to endovascular treatment.
      (2) Anterior communicating and pericallosal aneurysms are often successfully treated despite the presence of hematoma.

Postprocedure Management
Routine postprocedural care including high-level neuromonitoring.

Results and Complications
1. Yield of emergent angiography is highly variable and reflects the noninvasive imaging findings regarding location and character of the hematoma.
2. Likelihood of angiographic positivity can be increased with the addition of CTA prior to angiography.
3. Complications include the standard risks of diagnostic cerebral angiography and the relative risks of any intervention previously described.

Otorhinolaryngologic (ENT) Emergencies

Epistaxis (8)

Etiology and Diagnosis
1. **Hereditary vascular dysplasias**
   a. Prototype is hereditary hemorrhagic telangiectasia (HHT), an autosomal dominant disorder with telangiectasias involving the nasal mucosa, skin, and airway. Hepatic and pulmonary AVMs are common.
   b. Clinical and family history help establish the diagnosis.
2. **Tumor**
   a. Primary or metastatic tumors involving the nasal cavity and/or paranasal sinuses.
   b. CT can define the location and extent of the mass and may suggest diagnosis.
3. **Trauma to the nose and face**
   a. Both penetrating and blunt trauma may result in vascular injury, including transection, laceration, occlusion, pseudoaneurysm, and arteriovenous fistula.
   b. CT defines extent of bony injury, proximity of fracture fragments, foreign bodies, and/or projectile path to major vessels of the head and neck. Addition of CTA assists in determining the need for angiography.
4. **Intracranial source for epistaxis**
   a. Ruptured aneurysms of the petrous or cavernous carotid
   b. Traumatic pseudoaneurysms in this location include iatrogenic injury to the internal carotid artery during pituitary or sphenoid surgery
   c. Dural arteriovenous fistula
5. **Idiopathic epistaxis**
   a. May be associated with bleeding diathesis, anticoagulation
   b. Often seen at start of heating season—dry nasal mucosa

Indications
Angiographic indications include intractable epistaxis, not responsive to anterior and posterior packs, often associated with significant blood loss, requiring transfusion.

Contraindications
1. Relative: impaired renal function, advanced atherosclerosis
2. Uncorrectable coagulopathy

Preprocedural Preparation
1. Routine preparation as per diagnostic angiography
2. General anesthesia is recommended for airway control given the risk of uncontrolled hemorrhage.

Procedure
1. Standard heparin bolus administered at the time of angiography (2,000 U IV for an average adult).

2. Angiographic protocol should include examination of the internal and external carotid arteries or, when significant internal carotid occlusive disease precludes safe selective catheterization, both common carotid arteries.
3. Vascular supply to the nasal mucosa must be assessed:
    a. Both the distal internal maxillary and the distal facial arteries supply the nasal mucosa.
    b. The ophthalmic artery may provide a major supply to the nasal mucosa via ethmoidal branches.
4. Other contributions from the internal carotid artery include the inferolateral trunk, the artery of the foramen rotundum, or other petrous or cavernous branches.
5. **Embolization protocol with identifiable source**
    a. Bleeding source should be treated directly.
    b. Proximal occlusions should be avoided to allow for repeat embolization if needed.
    c. Gelfoam pledgets, coils, endovascular plugs, and liquid embolics can be used to occlude shunts, pseudoaneurysms, and pathologic vessels.
6. **Embolization protocol without identifiable source**
    a. Three of the four major external carotid artery branches to the distal nasal mucosa should be embolized, leaving the main trunks intact.
    b. At least one of the four major feeding arteries should be left intact to provide collateral flow and prevent necrosis.
    c. Embolic of choice is polyvinyl alcohol (PVA) particles measuring 150 to 250 or 250 to 355 μm to avoid skin or mucosal necrosis.

Postprocedural Management
1. ICU or step-down unit management for close hemodynamic and neurologic monitoring
2. Nasal packs are removed when the coagulation parameters have normalized after completion of intervention (often the following day)

Complications
1. Local vascular injury
2. Skin or nasal mucosal sloughing when particle size is too small or collateral circulation is inadequate. Consider plastics consult for wound care; O_2 therapy
3. Cranial nerve palsies. Intravenous steroid immediate postop period followed by Medrol dose pack
4. Nontarget embolization; possible ECA-ICA collaterals; post-stroke care

Traumatic Vascular Injuries (9)

Etiology
1. **Blunt trauma**
    a. Typically produces injury at the site of impact ("coup"), although force transmission may result in anatomically remote injury.
    b. CT/CTA is useful for determining the location of hematoma and fracture fragments in relation to vascular structures.
2. **Penetrating trauma**
    a. Often resulting from gunshot or stab wounds or other penetrating foreign-body CT and/or CTA demonstrate the path of the projectile and vessel injury. Vascular injury may manifest as complete or partial transection, occlusion, pseudoaneurysm formation, and/or vasospasm
    b. Clinical presentation
        (1) Patients may present in varying degrees of extremis depending on the severity of the injury.
        (2) Although major injury presents acutely, minor injury may present in a delayed fashion, particularly in those with cognitive limitation.

   c. Diagnosis
     (1) CT should be obtained first, with most major trauma centers having an algorithmic approach to trauma evaluation.
     (2) If vascular injury is known, patients often go directly to the angiography for intervention. If diagnosis uncertain, CTA should be obtained first.

Preprocedural Preparation

The extent of preparation inversely correlates with the urgency of the procedure. It may be necessary to proceed to intervention without preprocedural imaging.

1. As per diagnostic angiography.
2. Standard protocols should include examination of the aortic arch, bilateral common, internal and external carotid arteries, and bilateral vertebral arteries. Adjustments should be made based on the nature of the injury.
3. Heparin bolus is administered unless precluded by the injuries.

Procedure: Selected Angiographic Protocols (Specific Considerations)

1. **Facial fractures with oral or nasal bleeding**
   a. Protocol similar to that for idiopathic epistaxis.
   b. Bleeding usually originates from an external carotid artery branch.
   c. Temporary embolic agents, gelfoam pledgets, or larger PVA (300 to 500 μm or larger) particles may be sufficient for small vessels.
   d. Liquid embolic agents such as *n*-butyl cyanoacrylate or onyx can be used for pseudoaneurysm or fistulas.
   e. When coils are used, care must be taken to ensure sufficiently distal occlusion as the rich collateral network of the face may result in ongoing bleeding distal to the site of occlusion.

2. **Carotid artery injuries**
   a. Evaluation must include both carotid arteries and at least one vertebral artery, both to identify vascular injury and to assess collateral flow through the circle of Willis.
   b. Injury to the cervical carotid most commonly results from direct trauma although acceleration/deceleration injury may occur at fixed points including the level of the skull base where the carotid pierces the dura, at the level of the supraclinoid internal carotid artery, and within the cavernous sinus.
   c. Injury may manifest as laceration, dissection or rupture with resultant occlusion, pseudoaneurysm or carotid cavernous fistula formation.
   d. Treatment for traumatic carotid artery occlusion is expectant. Revascularization by surgical bypass is usually not possible.
   e. Pseudoaneurysm may be treated by parent artery occlusion, if adequate collateral supply can be demonstrated. Endovascular treatment with covered or uncovered stents, with or without detachable coils placed through the stent mesh into the pseudoaneurysm. Surgical repair may be possible depending on the location.
   f. TIAs or hemiparesis which occurs acutely following carotid endarterectomy may result from carotid occlusion, often requiring reoperation. CTA is performed for assessment and DSA may be added depending on whether reexploration or endovascular management is planned. Emergent angiography can establish the etiology of the symptomatology and the nature of the vascular compromise prior to reexploration.

3. **Traumatic carotid cavernous fistula**
   a. May present acutely or in delayed fashion following severe head injury.
   b. Clinical symptoms relate to the pattern of venous drainage.
      (1) Anterior venous drainage into the superior and/or inferior ophthalmic veins leads to ocular symptoms such as chemosis, proptosis, and increased intraocular pressure.

(2) Posterior venous drainage into the superior and/or inferior petrosal sinuses with increased jugular venous drainage and tinnitus.

(3) Cortical venous drainage (cortical venous reflux via the greater sylvian vein or other cortical vein) with venous hypertension and intraparenchymal hemorrhage.

(4) Transcavernous collateral venous egress may result in bilateral symptomatology with a unilateral fistula.

c. Emergency treatment is not necessary unless the vision is threatened or there is IPH secondary to venous hypertension.

d. Closure of the fistula may be performed from an arterial or a venous approach depending on the location of the fistula and pattern of venous drainage.

e. Parent artery occlusion may be needed if the underlying carotid injury is severe.

4. **Vertebral artery injury**

a. Evaluation must include both vertebral arteries and at least one carotid artery, both to evaluate for vascular injury and to assess collateral flow through the circle of Willis.

b. As with the carotid, injury may result from direct trauma. With acceleration/deceleration, injury may occur at points of fixation, such as the entrance into the foramen transversarium at C5–C6, the C1–C2 junction, and between the arch of C1 and the foramen magnum.

c. Cervical spine fractures, particularly those that extend through the foramen transversarium, are commonly associated.

d. Noncontrast CT of the cervical spine without contrast can demonstrate fracture involving the foramen transversarium. CTA is indicated to determine the status of the vertebral artery.

e. Management options include:

(1) Vertebral artery sacrifice, using coils following demonstration of adequate collateral flow.

(2) Recanalization of lacerated or dissected vertebral arteries should be avoided as it may lead to distal embolization and stroke.

5. **Vertebrojugular fistula**

a. More commonly seen following penetrating than blunt trauma.

b. May result in steal phenomenon affecting the brain or the arm. When large, hemodynamic instability may result.

c. Treatment via arterial access with or without sacrifice of the vertebral artery. A venous approach may facilitate preservation of vertebral artery patency. Surgery is uncommonly required.

Complications

These include the routine risks of cerebral arteriography as well as the risk of local vascular injury and stroke. Risks vary according to the therapeutic technique applied.

Postprocedural Management

ICU neurologic and hemodynamic monitoring, particularly when major vessel sacrifice was required for treatment.

Malignant Disease of the Head and Neck (10)

Emergent intervention in malignant disease is usually required when intractable oronasal bleeding develops in a patient with underlying head and neck cancer. Assessment of the distribution of the residual tumor by CT or MRI is useful in planning the endovascular therapy.

Endovascular treatment usually consists of occlusion of tumoral neovascularity derived from the external carotid arterial branches or occlusion of a major branch, common carotid, or internal carotid artery.

Provocative testing using the BOT test is a critical part of the management of these patients in the subacute setting (see the following discussion).

Preprocedural Preparation
1. As per diagnostic angiography.
2. Airway control is paramount in a patient who may hemorrhage while supine on the angiography table. Monitored anesthesia care is preferred, with intubation and sedation when possible, in order to permit clinical testing.

Diagnostic Arteriography
1. In general, angiographic protocols should include examination of both common carotid arteries and the internal and external carotid and vertebral arteries. Intracranial as well as extracranial vessels should be studied.
2. The vertebral artery circulation must be assessed if carotid occlusion is contemplated to evaluate the integrity of the circle of Willis (patency of the anterior and posterior communicating arteries).
3. The vertebral artery muscular branches may provide collateral supply to external carotid branches and contribute to ongoing bleeding.

Balloon Occlusion Tolerance Test
1. A clinical and angiographic test for tolerance of carotid occlusion performed prior to possible surgical or endovascular occlusion of the internal carotid artery.
2. Components include diagnostic arteriography for collateral assessment, clinical testing during occlusion, and HMPAO SPECT evaluation of cerebral blood flow at the time of the temporary occlusion.

Procedure
1. BOT test is performed with placement of a nondetachable balloon catheter into the internal or common carotid artery. A microballoon or a conventional 8.5-mm occlusion balloon may be used for the temporary occlusion.
2. The patient is systemically heparinized during the temporary occlusion (ACT 250 to 300 seconds).
3. Neurologic testing is ongoing during the period of temporary occlusion.
4. Systemic hypotension may be induced with reduction of mean arterial pressure to two-thirds normal using a sodium nitroprusside (Nipride) or other pharmacologic intervention. During this period of pressure reduction, the patient may be injected with HMPAO for a first-pass assessment of cerebral blood flow.
5. The balloon is deflated and withdrawn. The patient is taken to the nuclear medicine department for SPECT imaging, leaving the sheath sutured in place.
6. If the patient tolerates the clinical examination and the SPECT demonstrates no focal abnormalities, the patient returns to angiography for the permanent occlusion (see "Permanent Carotid Sacrifice").

Permanent Carotid Sacrifice
1. **Emergent:** Performed when no option is available to salvage the carotid using stent techniques. Potentially lifesaving.
2. **Elective:**
   a. Patients with local recurrence of head and neck carcinoma in the neck following surgical and/or radiation treatment may be eligible for radical surgical options, often requiring resection of the carotid artery within the surgical block.
   b. Sacrifice of the carotid artery at the time of surgery is associated with a higher risk of perioperative stroke than with elective carotid sacrifice several weeks prior to the definitive surgical procedure.

Preprocedural Preparation
1. As per diagnostic angiography.
2. Prior to endovascular occlusion, the patient undergoes placement of a central line.

Procedure
1. Diagnostic cerebral arteriography is performed with particular attention to the circle of Willis and the patency of the anterior communicating and posterior communicating arteries. The common carotid arteries in the neck are also examined (see earlier discussion).
2. BOT test of the carotid artery is performed, when possible, prior to permanent occlusion. If tolerance is demonstrated, permanent occlusion follows.
3. Endovascular carotid occlusion is performed using detachable platinum coils with or without an AMPLATZER plug or like closure device.

Carotid Blowout Syndrome

Overview
1. Carotid blowout syndrome is a syndrome of acute oral, nasal, or paratracheal bleeding originating from the vasculature of the head and neck secondary to erosion from adjacent malignant tumor.
2. A subset of the carotid blowout patients are those with more chronic or intermittent hemorrhage. Sentinel hemorrhage is not uncommon.

Preprocedural Preparation
1. As per diagnostic angiography.
2. Patient should be intubated for airway control. A central line is important for patient monitoring and hemodynamic management, particularly in the situation where carotid sacrifice may be imminent.

Procedure
1. Angiographic protocol includes bilateral common carotid arteries, both internal carotid arteries, and at least one vertebral artery to localize the lesion and to establish the integrity of the circle of Willis.
2. Rarely is there time for formal BOT prior to treatment.
3. The carotid is occluded using platinum detachable coils.
4. When carotid sacrifice cannot be performed due to incomplete circle of Willis or lack of collateral flow, or a lack of tolerance of temporary balloon occlusion, covered stents have had limited use to stabilize the patient prior to permanent carotid occlusion. Rarely extracranial-to-intracranial bypass may be considered but these have distinct limitations in the setting of the malignant postradiation neck and has no role in acute massive hemorrhage.
5. When carotid blowout manifests as uncontrollable hemorrhage, carotid sacrifice must be performed without BOT in order to be lifesaving. Risk of stroke may be considerably higher in such patients. Perfusion imaging following occlusion may be useful to inform aggressive hypertensive and hypervolemic management.

Postprocedure Management: Major Vessel Sacrifice
1. Neurointensive ICU management, including hypertensive and hypervolemic therapy, is critical to maintain cerebral perfusion and allow the patient to equilibrate and adjust to the changes in cerebral perfusion.
2. Systemic heparinization (PTT 60 to 80 seconds) is maintained for at least 48 hours; antiplatelet therapy, usually aspirin, is added.
3. The femoral access may be maintained for 24 to 48 hours. Alternatively, percutaneous closure devices are utilized to obtain hemostasis in order to allow for the maintenance of systemic heparinization and antiplatelet therapy for several days.

Results and Complications: Major Vessel Sacrifice
1. Carotid and/or vertebral artery sacrifice may be well tolerated in the patient with good collateral circulation and a good clinical +/– HMPAO SPECT response to test occlusion.
2. Aggressive ICU management designed to maximize cerebral perfusion, coupled with anticoagulation.

3. Risks include hypoperfusion stroke and focal infarction during the procedure and during the first week of the postocclusion period.
4. Risks are increased in those patients with poor collateral circulation, poor response to test occlusion, hypoperfusion on HMPAO SPECT, and/or exsanguinating bleeding necessitating emergent carotid sacrifice.

Tumoral Hemorrhage

1. Oral, nasal, or paratracheal bleeding may result from tumoral neovascularity, or erosion through the wall of a small vessel rather than a major vessel erosion.
2. Vascular lacerations or pseudoaneurysms are treated directly with embolization to address the specific site of bleeding.
3. In many patients, subacute assessment of the tolerance for carotid occlusion may be necessary and subsequent carotid sacrifice performed.
4. Preprocedure and angiographic protocols are analogous to those used for epistaxis.
5. Complications include the routine risks of cerebral arteriography as well as the risk of local vascular injury and stroke. Risks vary according to the therapeutic technique applied; in general, the risks are similar to those for epistaxis management.
6. Careful diagnostic angiography and controlled embolization of tumoral bleeding sites are greater than 95% effective in bleeding control.
7. **Postprocedural management**
   a. ICU or step-down management to monitor bleeding, manage hemodynamics.
   b. Packing removal when bleeding parameters stabilize.
   c. Neurologic and hemodynamic monitoring when carotid occlusion has been performed.

References

1. Case D, Kumpe D, Roark C, et al. Neuroangiography: review of anatomy, periprocedural management, technique, and tips. *Semin Interv Radiol*. 2020;37(2):166–174. doi:10.1055/s-0040-1709171
2. Patel J, Huynh TJ, Rao D, et al. Vascular trauma in the head and neck and endovascular neurointerventional management. *J Clin Imaging Sci*. 2020;10(1):44.
3. Connolly ES Jr, Rabinstein AA, Carhuapoma JR, et al. Guidelines for the management of aneurysmal subarachnoid hemorrhage: a guideline for healthcare professionals from the American Heart Association/American Stroke Association. *Stroke*. 2012;43(6):1711–1737.
4. Molyneux AJ, Birks J, Clarke A, et al. The durability of endovascular coiling versus neurosurgical clipping of ruptured cerebral aneurysms: 18 year follow-up of the UK cohort of the International Subarachnoid Aneurysm Trial (ISAT). *Lancet*. 2015;385(9969):691–697.
5. Benomar A, Farzin B, Volders D, et al. Angiographic results of surgical or endovascular treatment of intracranial aneurysms: a systematic review and inter-observer reliability study. *Neuroradiology*. 2021;63(9):1511–1519. doi:http://dx.doi.org/10.1007/s00234-021-02676-0
6. Li K, Barras CD, Chandra RV, et al. A review of the management of cerebral vasospasm after aneurysmal subarachnoid hemorrhage. *World Neurosurgery*. 2019;126:513–527. doi:http://dx.doi.org/10.1016/j.wneu.2019.03.083
7. Cusack TJ, Carhuapoma JR, Ziai WC. Update on the treatment of spontaneous intraparenchymal hemorrhage: medical and interventional management. *Curr Treat Options Neurol*. 2018;20(1):1. doi:10.1007/s11940-018-0486-5
8. Tunkel DE, Anne S, Payne SC, et al. Clinical practice guideline: nosebleed (epistaxis). *Otolaryngol Head Neck Surg*. 2020;162(1_SUPPL):S1–S38. doi:10.1177/0194599819890327
9. Vellimana AK, Lavie J, Chatterjee AR. Endovascular considerations in traumatic injury of the carotid and vertebral arteries. *Semin Interv Radiol*. 2021;38(01):53–63. doi:10.1055/s-0041-1724008
10. Hoffman H, Jalal MS, Masoud HE, et al. Outcomes after endovascular embolization for the treatment of nasal and oropharyngeal hemorrhage: safety, efficacy, and rebleeding. *Neuroradiol J*. 2021. doi:http://dx.doi.org/10.1177/19714009211042893

7 Renovascular Hypertension: Endovascular Management

William F. Browne, MD and David W. Trost, MD

Introduction (1)

Hypertension is the most common modifiable risk factor for cardiovascular morbidity and mortality. Revascularization of renal artery stenosis (RAS) is indicated in the treatment of renovascular hypertension (RVH) and renal insufficiency (RI) due to ischemic nephropathy (IN); RVH and IN frequently coexist but may be present independently of each other. Hemodynamically significant RAS is one of the few potentially reversible causes of RI due to IN and hypertension. Multicenter prospective randomized trials (STAR, ASTRAL, and CORAL) have not shown additional benefit for renal artery stenting in atheromatous disease over optimal medical therapy. The negative results of these trials have been criticized as being based on faulty methodology and statistics. The challenge for physicians is to identify patients with RAS who would benefit from renal revascularization, whether by interventional techniques or open surgery. In order to do so, RAS must first be clinically suspected and anatomically identified, and its hemodynamic significance and causal relationship to hypertension or RI documented. Renal artery denervation (RDN) is emerging as a method of lowering blood pressure (BP) in essential hypertension that is poorly controlled by medication (2). Its place in hypertension management has yet to be defined but potentially could be of benefit to a large number of patients. The risks and benefits of alternative medical and invasive therapies for both procedures must be compared to each other and to the natural history of the disease.

Renovascular Hypertension

RVH accounts for about 5% of all hypertensive patients (3) and is usually due to atherosclerosis (75% of patients with RVH) or fibromuscular dysplasia (FMD) in the renal artery.

Indications for Revascularization (4)

Angiographically documented RAS, greater than 70% diameter, and a history of sustained hypertension (140/95 mm Hg) in the setting of:
1. Failed optimal medical therapy.
2. Multiple antihypertensive agents required for BP control (with an aim toward reducing, if not eliminating, the number of medications needed). Patients treated with greater than four medications or using clonidine may have a higher success rate.
3. A strong clinical suspicion for RVH and a positive radionuclide or medical "Captopril Challenge Test" (plasma renin activity with angiotensin-converting enzyme inhibitor [ACEI])
4. *An arterial pressure gradient greater than 10% of the systemic BP across the stenotic segment of the renal artery* (5). Areas of web-like stenosis that appear noncritical on angiography but have a significant arterial pressure gradient occur more often with FMD than with atherosclerosis. To measure gradients accurately in FMD, especially in the "string of beads" medial form, a pressure wire or a very flexible microcatheter is often necessary—a stiff angiographic catheter may "stent open" the soft fibrotic flaps responsible for the gradient.

Note: Indications 1 through 3 may not be present in every case. Indication 4 must be present in every case.

Ischemic Nephropathy

IN usually results from bilateral atheromatous RAS; FMD virtually never produces IN. Many patients with IN have coexistent RVH. Revascularization may, especially in recent onset IN, reverse the process or prevent further decline of renal function.

Indications for Revascularization (3,4)

Angiographically documented RAS greater than 70% in diameter and recent onset or deteriorating renal function while on optimal medical management and:

1. An arterial pressure gradient greater than 10% of the systemic BP across the stenosis (5).
2. Loss of renal mass demonstrated on serial imaging. A kidney length of >7 cm is considered by some to be the lower limit at which function is likely to be restored (2).

Renovascular Hypertension, Ischemic Nephropathy, or Both, with Any of the Following Conditions

Indications (3–6)

1. **Renal transplant arterial stenosis:** Most transplant RASs are due to neointimal hyperplasia, accelerated atherosclerosis, clamp or other iatrogenic injury, usually at the perianastomotic area. Prior to the procedure be aware if there is an end-to-side external iliac artery or an end-to-end internal iliac artery anastomosis (7).
2. **Renal artery venous, arterial, or synthetic bypass graft stenosis:** These lesions occur most often at or adjacent to anastomoses, and are due to perianastomotic fibrosis or clamp injury. Anastomoses must be examined in multiple projections to identify and quantify stenosis.
3. **Cardiac disturbance syndromes:** Flash pulmonary edema (Pickering syndrome), unstable angina, or acute coronary syndrome (ACS).

Contraindications to Renal Revascularization (3–6)

Absolute

1. Medically unstable patient
2. Hemodynamically nonsignificant stenosis (5)

Relative

1. Long-segment total occlusion
2. Severely diseased aorta predisposing to increased risk of embolization of atheroma

Renal Artery Balloon Angioplasty

Equipment Suggestions

1. **Guidewires:** Initial guidewire introduction should be with a soft atraumatic wire, such as a 0.035 Bentson-type wire. The initial wire should be exchanged for a stiff 0.018 working wire for balloon or stent introduction, such as the Thruway (Lake Region Medical, Chaska, MN). If working through a sheath or guiding catheter, a 0.014-in diameter coronary type guidewire such as the Grand Slam (Asahi Intecc, Aichi, Japan) or Ironman (Abbott Vascular Solutions, Santa Clara, CA) may also be used. Hydrophilic wires, especially the stiff-tipped V-18 (Boston Scientific/Medi-Tech, Natick, MA) should only be used as a last resort because they can easily dissect or perforate; if used, they should be exchanged out as soon

as practical. For 0.035-in systems, suitable wires include the TAD-II and standard Rosen wire (various manufacturers). Embolic protection devices can be considered, but have not been statistically proven to preserve glomerular filtration rate (8).

2. **Angiographic catheters:** Catheters for diagnostic angiography and selective renal artery catheterization are chosen depending on renal artery anatomy. The 4-Fr Sos Omni Selective (AngioDynamics, Queensbury, NY) is often suitable for crossing the RAS.

3. **Guiding catheters/sheaths:** Guiding catheters and sheaths are used for stabilization, angiography, and stent delivery. The frequently used 40-cm Flexor Ansel Sheath (Cook Medical Inc, Bloomington, IN) comes with two dilators: one tapered to a 0.035 in. guidewire and the other tapered to a 0.018 in.

4. **Balloons:** Balloons should be low profile to allow for easy crossing of the lesion, or stent for post dilation. Multiple manufacturers provide balloons for 0.014-in or 0.018-in systems. The Sterling (Boston Scientific, Natick, MA) balloon has both monorail or over the wire configurations.

Preprocedure Preparation

1. Discontinue long-acting antihypertensive medications prior to procedure, if possible; manage BP with short-acting drugs as necessary (in consultation with managing physician).

2. In patients who already have RI or in those at increased risk consider using dilute iodinated contrast or alternative contrast agents such as CO_2. (For an in-depth discussion of periprocedural renal function management, see Chapter 66.)

3. Standard preangiography preparation. Premedicate with ASA and clopidogrel.

4. Review prior imaging studies (computed tomographic angiography [CTA], magnetic resonance angiography [MRA], duplex ultrasound [US], radionuclide studies, and angiograms). CTA and MRA are particularly important for preprocedure planning.

Procedure (Figs. 7.1 and 7.2)

1. **Arterial access**

    a. **Common femoral artery:** Almost all renal interventions can be performed from a right femoral access. Place an arterial sheath (with a side arm for flushing). Patients who have significant iliofemoral atherosclerosis have a higher chance of distal cholesterol embolization. In this case, a 40-cm long Flexor

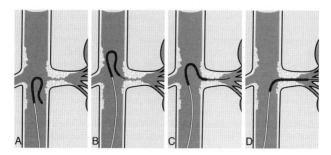

FIGURE 7.1 • Technique of renal angioplasty using a Sos Omni Selective catheter (**A**). After selection of an appropriate renal artery (**B**), a flexible-tipped guidewire is advanced through the lesion under fluoroscopic control (**C**). The catheter is advanced across the stenosis by withdrawing the catheter at the puncture site (**D**). After exchange for a heavy-duty, tight J-tip wire, a sheath is advanced to the renal artery ostium.

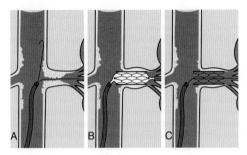

FIGURE 7.2 • Image demonstrating an alternative "no-touch" technique (**A**). An appropriate balloon-expandable stent is deployed across the stenosis (**B**). The balloon is removed and confirmatory angiogram performed via the sheath (**C**).

Ansel Sheath (Cook Medical Inc, Bloomington, IN), is placed initially to minimize disruption of plaque during catheter exchanges and will usually be necessary later for intervention.

b. **Radial artery** (see Ch. 1): is increasingly a matter of physician preference; or can be used for patients with distal aortic occlusion, an unfavorable caudal renal artery angle for a femoral approach, or in obese patients.

2. **Diagnostic angiography:** Begin with a flush aortogram. Review of prior CTA/MRA is critical to determining the optimal obliquity for visualizing the target renal artery ostium, which can be difficult on to visualize on fluoroscopy due to proximal and ostial disease. Classically, the left renal artery is best imaged in 5- to 10-degree left anterior oblique (LAO) and the right renal artery in 20- to 30-degree LAO. If no prior cross-sectional imaging is available and both sides need to be evaluated, a compromise 20-degree LAO projection is preferred. Children or patients with suspected FMD should have selective magnification renal arteriography in at least two oblique views per side. When patients have significant bilateral stenoses, attempt angioplasty on the side with the larger kidney first (usually also technically easier because disease tends to be less severe); if this goes well, and if the patient and operator can tolerate a prolonged procedure, attempt the other side.

3. **Crossing the lesion:** In general, the stenosis should be crossed with a soft, atraumatic guidewire, such as a Bentson, and a recurved catheter such as a 4-Fr Sos Omni Selective or a Simmons (Fig. 7.1). Aggressive/excessive catheter manipulation while finding the renal artery and crossing the stenosis can be the cause of cholesterol or macroparticle embolization. There are several published techniques to minimize this. The "no touch" technique described by Feldman et al. (Fig. 7.2) (9) minimizes the contact between the guiding catheter and the aortic wall, as does the "Sos flick" technique (Fig. 7.1) (10). Once the wire is across the lesion, the Sos Omni Selective catheter can be pulled down across the lesion. After the catheter has crossed, it is often exchanged for a smaller diameter 0.018-in or 0.014-in wire for intervention. Once the catheter is safely across the stenosis, administer an IV heparin bolus of 3,000 to 5,000 U (70 units per kg), followed by an infusion of 750 to 1,000 units per hour. Target activated clotting time (ACT) should be 2.5 times baseline.

4. **Crossing the lesion troubleshooting:** Nitroglycerin (NTG) 100 to 200 µg intraarterial (IA) into the renal artery can be given to prevent or reverse spasm. *If the wire advances with difficulty or the tip curves and is unable to be straightened, stop all wire manipulations.* Assess whether the wire has passed subintimally or perforated. If occlusive dissection is present, prolonged (few minutes) under inflation

with a balloon 1 mm lesser in diameter may restore the lumen. If occlusive dissection persists or perforation has occurred, a stent or covered stent may be necessary to complete the procedure.

5. **Pressure-gradient across stenosis:** A pressure gradient is considered to be significant if it is greater than 10% of the systemic arterial pressure. This is best performed with simultaneous arterial pressure measurements acquired from the distal renal artery and the aorta via the access sheath (i.e., $Pd/Pa \leq 0.90$, where Pd = distal renal artery pressure and Pa = aortic pressure) (5). If there is not a significant gradient, then revascularization should not be continued. Gradients should be measured with the lowest-profile device to avoid inadvertently enhancing the severity of a stenosis. A 0.014-in pressure wire is ideal; a 4-Fr catheter clearly contributes more to an existing stenosis, but it is very useful in excluding unnecessary intervention in those patients who do not meet even this minimal threshold.

6. **Preparation for balloon angioplasty (percutaneous transluminal renal angioplasty [PTRA]) or stent placement (3,4,6)**
   a. For ostial atherosclerotic stenosis, primary stent placement is indicated. If the lesion is nonostial (greater than 1 cm from the origin), whether atherosclerotic or FMD, balloon angioplasty should be primarily performed. Primary stenting of FMD is contraindicated.
   b. Choose a balloon diameter approximately 10% larger than the estimated "normal" diameter of the vessel based on the arteriogram. Take care not to base balloon size on an arterial segment with poststenotic dilatation. If in doubt, use a smaller balloon, at least initially. Balloons utilizing a 0.014-in or 0.018-in guidewire system have almost completely replaced 0.035-in systems.
   c. Guiding catheters or sheaths (5 to 8 Fr) are used to provide support for crossing severe calcific stenosis and better seating within the ostium. They have a soft, blunt distal end, which minimizes arterial trauma but are almost as stiff as guiding catheters.
   d. Place a soft tip, stiff shaft guidewire into a distal branch for the intervention. Exchange the diagnostic catheter for the sheath/guide or directly for the balloon catheter. Prevent motion of the distal wire tip by firmly fixing it; otherwise, spasm may be provoked in the smaller distal vessels. *Perforations can occur if the guidewire is allowed to go too peripherally, especially when using hydrophilic wires.* Place the balloon markers across lesion. Care should be taken not to advance the distal portion of the balloon past a branch point for fear of dissection or rupture.

7. **Dilation (see Figs. 7.1 and 7.2)**
   a. Inflate the balloon slowly until fully inflated or its rated maximum pressure is reached; for angioplasty, inflate for a minute. Discontinue balloon inflation if the patient experiences severe pain.
   b. Deflate the balloon immediately and completely to avoid thrombus formation on the balloon surface and possible vessel occlusion.
   c. It is generally best to avoid recrossing the site of angioplasty after the vessel has been dilated, as this can lead to dissection and subintimal passage of the wire. Do a completion angiogram using a technique that preserves wire position across the lesion. If a guide/sheath is present, the angiogram can be obtained through the sheath. If there is no guide/sheath, the injection can be performed by using a 5-Fr multi–side-hole catheter over the guidewire with the tip just into the renal artery and injecting through a side-arm adapter. A postangioplasty cleft is often seen and usually resolves in about 3 months (4).
   d. If the angiographic result and post-PTRA pressure gradient are acceptable, the procedure is complete. Otherwise, a balloon of 1-mm diameter greater than the one previously used is reintroduced into the stenotic segment over the wire and the angioplasty is repeated until a satisfactory result is obtained.
   e. Make sure the balloon is fully deflated prior to removing it from the artery.

f. Remember, if PTRA/stenting has failed or if the patient is to undergo surgical revascularization without attempted angioplasty, the angiographer must evaluate the donor or source vessels most likely to be used for the reconstruction.

Renal Artery Stenting

Indications (3)

1. Ostial atheromatous RAS (within 1 cm of the aortic lumen). For renal artery less than 4 mm diameter, a coronary drug-eluting stent should be used
2. Restenosis after previous PTRA or stenting. For in-stent restenosis, drug-eluting or covered stents (3) within the stent are used
3. Postoperative stenosis (renal artery bypass and transplant renal arteries)
4. Highly eccentric RAS
5. Acute failure or complication of PTRA due to:
   a. Vessel recoil with threatened closure
   b. Complex dissections which do not respond to prolonged reinflation
   c. Residual stenosis, or residual pressure gradient greater than 10% of mean arterial pressure
   d. Rupture or perforation. These may require use of a covered stent

Contraindications (3)

Relative
1. Branch vessel disease
2. Lesion length exceeding 2 cm
3. Renal artery diameter less than 4 mm (consider coronary size or drug-eluting stent)
4. Unfavorable renal artery anatomy, not permitting sufficient distal vessel length to allow surgical bypass, if needed
5. Diffuse intrarenal vascular disease
6. Noncompliant lesion
7. Kidney size less than 7 cm

Equipment Suggestions
1. Equipment for renal artery stenting is the same as for balloon PTRA described earlier.
2. **Stents:** Balloon expandable metallic stents, such as the Express (Boston Scientific, Natick, MA) and RX Herculink Elite (Abbot Laboratories, Plymouth, MN) are preferred. Drug eluting coronary stents have also been used. Typical stent lengths range from 1 to 2 cm in length and 4 to 8 mm in diameter. They are mounted on 0.014- and 0.018-in monorail/rapid-exchange type and over the wire, and 0.035 in over the wire systems.

Preprocedure Preparation
Preparation for renal artery stenting is the same as for balloon PTRA described earlier.

Procedure
1. Evaluate the stenotic lesion with diagnostic angiography and pressure measurements as described above.
2. There are several techniques for stent deployment; almost all use 0.018 in or lower-profile systems. A long 5- to 6-Fr diameter sheath with a tapered dilator may be initially advanced through the stenosis over the 0.018-in or 0.014-in wire for assured stent delivery, especially if the stenosis is heavily calcified and eccentric. The "bare back" technique utilizes a guide sheath or catheter that never crosses the lesion.
3. Choose a stent and balloon combination that will adequately cover the lesion and expand the stent to the normal vessel diameter. Take care not to size the balloon on an arterial segment with poststenotic dilatation. If there is any doubt, use a smaller balloon and postdilate to a larger diameter, if necessary. If the lesion is

ostial, the stent length should be sized to ensure that it extends approximately 1 to 2 mm into the aortic lumen and past the stenosis.

4. Carefully introduce the stent across the hemostatic system of the delivery sheath. If a standard vascular sheath is used, be careful that the stent is not displaced from the balloon during passage through the hemostatic valve.

5. Keeping the sheath immobile, observe fluoroscopically as the stent is advanced through the sheath to the site of the lesion.

6. After initial stent positioning, hold the stent immobile and retract the sheath to uncover the stent. Once the stent is completely unsheathed, do not try to resheath it because the stent may slide off the balloon. When using the "bare back" technique, the stent system should be carefully advanced through the lesion making sure that the stent does not catch on the stenosis.

7. Angiography must be performed through the sheath prior to stent deployment to confirm positioning. Be sure to image the artery in the oblique view that best shows the lesion. This is most important for optimal positioning of a stent at ostial lesions.

8. Using an inflating device, steadily inflate the balloon under fluoroscopic monitoring until fully expanded. Do not inflate the balloon above its rated burst pressure.

9. Deflate the balloon completely, and aspirate with a 50-mL syringe, if necessary. Retract balloon, keeping the wire fixed, and remove through the sheath. If the stent moves during balloon removal, the sheath can be used to hold it in place or even to begin to enfold the balloon as described earlier to keep the stent from becoming displaced.

10. Perform a repeat angiogram, either through the sheath or through a catheter (advanced over the wire) proximal to the stent. Preserve the wire position across the stent if possible. Angiographically evaluate wall contact and any residual stenosis.

11. If necessary, use a larger balloon and expand the stent further.

12. If more than one stent is necessary, extra care must be used when advancing a wire, a sheath or a new stent *to avoid displacing or deforming the previously deployed stent—a very soft-tipped wire should be used to avoid passing under or through the stent struts. A sheath (with its introducer in place) may be necessary to traverse the first stent.*

13. When stenting in series, approximately 2 mm of stent overlap is advised. Avoid gaps as well as excessive overlap because these may contribute to local formation of intimal hyperplasia.

14. After deployment of stents to their final desirable diameter, perform a repeat arteriogram, measure pressure gradients across the stented segment, and, if necessary, evaluate with intravascular US to assess proper wall apposition and full stent expansion in any region.

Postprocedure Management

Percutaneous Renal Revascularization by PTRA and/or Stent

1. Remove femoral sheath when the ACT is less than 180 seconds. Obtain puncture site hemostasis by groin compression or alternatively with a closure device. Follow standard postangiography management.

2. Monitor renal function (serum creatinine [SCr] and blood urea nitrogen [BUN]) as appropriate for at least the first 24 hours.

3. Monitor BP for 24 hours (4).
   a. If BP drops significantly below normal levels, administer normal saline by IV infusion.
   b. If BP increases during or after procedure, consider ACEI or short-acting medication.

4. Postprocedure, continue aspirin 81 mg by mouth (PO) and an antiplatelet agent (e.g., clopidogrel) for up to 6 months if a drug-eluting stent was used.

5. Follow BP and renal function at frequent intervals for the first few months. Most recurrences of hypertension tend to occur within 8 months.

Results—Percutaneous Revascularization (3–5,11)

1. **Initial** technical success rate: >90% (3)
2. **Immediate** therapeutic success rate
   a. **Hypertension:** Favorable (improved or cured) BP response as percentage of technical successes
      (1) FMD: 90% to 100% improvement (3), 40% to 60% cure rate (11)
      (2) Atherosclerosis: 50% to 90% (3,4)
   b. **Azotemia:** Improvement or stabilization of renal function: 68% to 74% of patients (11)
   c. **Renal transplant:** Clinical improvement: 76% (7)
3. Definitions for evaluating of BP after revascularization
   a. **Cured**—BP of 140/90 mm Hg or less without medication
   b. **Improved**—Decrease in diastolic BP of 15 mm Hg or greater on same or less medicines *OR* decrease in diastolic BP less than 15 mm Hg but normal BP on medicines
   c. **Stable**—Diastolic BP ±15 mm Hg on same or less medicines
   d. **Failure**—Diastolic BP greater than 15 mm Hg on same or less medicines
4. Definitions to grade success with renal dysfunction
   a. **Improved**—Decrease in SCr of 20% or more over baseline
   b. **Stable**—SCr within 20% of baseline
   c. **Failure**—Elevation SCr of 20% or more over baseline
5. **Stent patency**:
   a. Primary patency: 80% at 5 years.
   b. One-year restenosis rates by vessel diameter:
      (1) 36% for vessels <4.5 mm
      (2) 16% for vessels between 4.5 and 6 mm
      (3) 6.5% in vessels >6 mm (2)

Complications

1. **Complication rates have diminished to 1.5% to 2%** as equipment and endovascular expertise has evolved. The *highest* reported overall complication rate in recent years is 9% (3).
2. **Thirty-day mortality:** Less than 1%
3. **Angioplasty-site** complications (1)
   a. Arterial dissection: 2%
   b. Local thrombus: 1%
   c. Arterial rupture: 1%
4. **Angioplasty-related** complications (1)
   a. Wire perforation/hematoma: 1%
   b. Peripheral renal embolism: 1%
   c. Acute renal failure or acute exacerbation of chronic renal failure: 1.5% to 6.0% (3). This may be due to many factors; contrast-induced nephropathy and microcholesterol embolization being the most common.
5. **Access site complications:** Hematoma, pseudoaneurysm, AV fistula, distal emboli to extremities.
6. **Management of complications**
   a. If local thrombus occurs without significant dissection or vessel perforation, a trial of local IA thrombolysis may be useful: 5-mg tissue plasminogen activator (tPA) over 30 minutes, followed by 0.5 mg per hour for up to 24 hours.
   b. If arterial rupture occurs, retroperitoneal hemorrhage may be prevented or slowed by gently reinflating the balloon across the tear. A covering stent may be utilized to seal the leak.
   c. If the balloon ruptures and no arterial damage is present, exchange the balloon catheter for a new one and proceed with angioplasty.
   d. Dissections: Angioplasty is always accompanied by minor dissections that heal within months. Non–flow-limiting dissections may be managed

conservatively even if they are severe in appearance (3). *Flow-limiting dissection should be treated by prolonged reinflation of a 1-mm undersized balloon or a stent.*

e. Chronic steroid therapy: Extra caution is urged when contemplating angioplasty in patients on chronic steroid therapy because they tend to be more prone to vessel rupture.

f. Patients with untreated hyperlipidemia and those who continue to smoke may also have increased risk of complications and restenosis.

Renal Artery Denervation (2)

Interrupting sympathetic nerves located in the adventitia and perivascular fat via a catheter placed in the renal arteries in appropriately selected patients with essential hypertension results in a statistically significant decrease in systolic BP of 5 to 15 mm Hg for at least 3 years with surprisingly minimal morbidity. Catheter-based treatments most frequently use radiofrequency, however focused ultrasound, cryoablation and injected alcohol are also available and appear to be equally efficacious. Preprocedure imaging, technique of renal artery access and postprocedure care are as described earlier in this chapter, except that as the renal arteries are typically normal (RDN is contraindicated in patients with RAS), the procedural component is more straight forward. Each device has unique procedural characteristics; it is essential that the interventionalist become familiar with them. The optimal patient is described as one with high sympathetic tone; the best method of identifying this remains elusive. It is important to understand this is not a cure, however regardless of the patients' baseline blood pressure even these seemingly modest reductions significantly reduce cardiovascular morbidity and mortality.

Acknowledgment

We thank Dr. Thomas Sos for his work on prior versions of this chapter and continued dedication to this field.

References

1. Cooper CJ, Murphy TP, Cutlip DE, et al. Stenting and medical therapy for atherosclerotic renal-artery stenosis. *N Engl J Med*. 2014;370(1):13–22.
2. Kandzari D. Catheter-based renal denervation therapy: evolution of evidence and future directions. *Circ Cardiovasc Interv*. 2021;14(12):e011130.
3. Prince M, Tafur JD, White C. When and how should we revascularize patients with atherosclerotic renal artery stenosis? *JACC: Cardiovasc Interv*. 2019;12(6):505–517.
4. Sos TA, Pickering TG, Sniderman K, et al. Percutaneous transluminal renal angioplasty in renovascular hypertension due to atheroma or fibromuscular dysplasia. *N Engl J Med*. 1983;309(5):274–279.
5. De Bruyne B, Manoharan G, Pijls NH, et al. Assessment of renal artery stenosis severity by pressure gradient measurements. *J Am Coll Cardiol*. 2006;48(9):1851–1855.
6. Touma J, Constanzo A, Boura B, et al. Endovascular management of transplant renal artery stenosis. *J Vasc Surg*. 2014;59(4):1058–1065.
7. Chen W, Kayler L, Zand M, et al. Transplant renal artery stenosis: clinical manifestations, diagnosis and therapy. *Clin Kidney J*. 2015;8(1):71–78.
8. Cooper CJ, Haller S, Coyler W. Embolic protection and platelet inhibition during renal artery stenting. *Circulation*. 2008;117(21):2752–2760.
9. Feldman RL, Wargovich TJ, Bittl JA. No-touch technique for reducing aortic wall trauma during renal artery stenting. *Catheter Cardiovasc Interv*. 1999;46(2):245–248.
10. Sos TA, Trost DW. Renal angioplasty and stenting. In: K. Kandarpa, ed. *Peripheral Vascular Interventions*. Lippincott Williams & Wilkins; 2008:287–314.
11. Martin L, Rundback J, Wallace M, et al. Quality improvement guidelines for angiography, angioplasty, and stent placement for the diagnosis and treatment of renal artery stenosis in adults. *J Vasc Interv Radiol*. 2010;21(4):421–430.

8 Acute Mesenteric Ischemia

Meghan R. Clark, MD, Luke R. Wilkins, MD, Daniel P. Sheeran, MD, and Alan H. Matsumoto, MD, FACR, FSIR, FAHA

Introduction

Acute mesenteric ischemia (AMI) is a medical emergency, necessitating prompt diagnosis and intervention to achieve favorable outcomes (1). Historically, the mortality associated with AMI has been incredibly high, between 60% and 80% (1). Emerging data suggest that mortality due to AMI has improved over the last two decades, and currently falls somewhere between 17% and 40% (2–4). These findings are likely reflective of the increased utilization of primary endovascular revascularization in AMI in addition to concurrent advancements in medical and surgical management of the diseases and comorbidities that commonly occur in this population (3).

Although grouped as a common disease process, AMI reflects a heterogeneous group of entities based on underlying etiology that typically fall into four broad categories—arterial embolism, arterial thrombosis, nonocclusive mesenteric ischemia (NOMI), and venous thrombosis. Less common entities such as trauma, strangulated hernias, adhesions, intestinal obstruction, cholesterol emboli, and aortic dissection can also cause intestinal ischemia.

Risk factors for AMI vary depending on the underlying etiology. Common risk factors for thromboembolic causes of AMI include older age, atherosclerosis, cardiac arrhythmias (most commonly atrial fibrillation), dilated cardiomyopathies, severe cardiac valvular disease, endocarditis, recent myocardial infarction, recent arterial intervention, hypercoagulability, and intraabdominal malignancy (5). Predisposing factors associated with the development of NOMI include critical illness, recent cardiac surgery, prolonged hypotension, older age with cardiovascular disease, hypovolemia, major burns, hemodialysis, mesenteric stenosis, and medications such as vasopressors (5). It is also important to note that many patients presenting with NOMI are found to have an underlying superior mesenteric artery (SMA) stenosis. Risk factors for AMI attributable to venous thrombosis include dehydration, hypotension, portal hypertension, hypercoagulability, oral contraceptives, estrogen use, thrombophilia, history of pulmonary embolism, sickle cell disease, DVT/PE, abdominal infection, abdominal malignancy, pancreatitis, trauma, and splenectomy (5). The critical nature of mesenteric ischemia warrants a high index of clinical suspicion, particularly in elderly patients with cardiovascular disease or embolic or thrombotic risk factors.

NOMI typically results from mesenteric arterial vasoconstriction in the setting of a low-flow state, which is usually precipitated by hypotension and/or use of vasopressors. Despite resolution of the hypotension or discontinuation of the vasopressors, persistent mesenteric arterial vasoconstriction (diffuse vasospasm) persists, causing bowel hypoperfusion and intestinal ischemia. Other causes of NOMI include drugs (i.e., cocaine), vasculitides and abdominal compartment syndrome/intraabdominal hypertension (5). NOMI can also be seen in association with mesenteric venous thrombosis or distal to an SMA embolus.

The clinical presentation of AMI is classically described as acute, severe, periumbilical abdominal pain that is out of proportion to physical examination findings. The presence of peritoneal signs raises concern that the bowel ischemia has progressed to transmural infarction. Anorexia, nausea, vomiting, diarrhea, and hematochezia are common. Unfortunately, the clinical manifestations of AMI overlap with many other, more common clinical entities, such as bowel obstruction, pancreatitis, diverticulitis, and peritonitis, which can often lead to a delay in diagnosis. Therefore, the clinical presentation must be considered in the context of the clinical history and patient-specific risk factors, physical examination, and laboratory and radiographic findings.

In the last two decades there has been a paradigm shift to an "endovascular-first" approach at many institutions, demonstrating improved patient outcomes in comparison to traditional open surgery (2,3,6,7). A study looking at trends in the treatment and mortality for AMI from 2000 to 2012 in the United States found that the incidence of endovascular treatment increased from 0.6 to 1.8/million; during that same period mortality of AMI decreased from 12.9 to 5.3 million deaths per year (3). Another study using the National Inpatient Sample database noted an almost 1.5-fold increase in use of endovascular therapies in the primary management of AMI from 2003 to 2011 (8). The benefits to an endovascular-first approach include decreased morbidity and mortality, potential avoidance of general anesthesia and open surgery, more targeted and limited bowel resections, decreased times for revascularization, a reduced need for parenteral nutrition, shortened lengths of stay, and fewer postoperative complications (2,4,6). Table 8.1 summarizes the differences between the etiologies for AMI and their management. A treatment algorithm employed at our institution is demonstrated in Figure 8.1.

Indications

1. Diagnosis of AMI and determination of etiology
   a. Although angiography remains the gold standard in the diagnosis of AMI because of its ability to resolve both large- and small-vessel disease as well as provide information on flow dynamics, its diagnostic role has largely been replaced by computed tomographic angiography (CTA) and magnetic resonance angiography (MRA). Multiphase CTA is considered the first-line imaging modality for anyone suspected of having AMI as it is widely available, can be performed rapidly, and is the most sensitive and specific modality (5). CTA has the benefit of delineating etiology, excluding other potential causes of abdominal pain, and providing information on the potential viability of the bowel. MRA is less useful in the setting of AMI due to its poorer spatial resolution, lack of widespread availability, and longer acquisition time.

      CTA and MRA generate two- and three-dimensional images of the mesenteric arterial and venous anatomy facilitating accurate diagnosis and treatment planning for occlusive AMI, while also providing suggestive findings of NOMI.
      (1) CTA protocol: Noncontrast, arterial phase (30-second delay), and venous phase (60- to 70-second delay) multidetector CT images should be obtained from the dome of the liver through the pelvis. The use of oral contrast is contraindicated in the setting of suspected AMI as it obscures evaluation of bowel mucosa and causes further delays in diagnosis.
   b. Angiography has diagnostic utility in cases with equivocal findings by CTA or MRA or in patients in whom endovascular intervention is likely.
      (1) Angiography may reduce contrast load and potential renal injury by bypassing the CTA examination in select patients.
      (2) Angiography is usually now performed in anticipation of an endovascular treatment solution.
2. Treatment of AMI
   a. For patients with acute bowel ischemia without evidence of bowel infarction or for patients that are poor surgical candidates, endovascular management alone is an acceptable therapeutic option (4,6,9).

Table 8.1 Summary of the Different Causes of Acute Mesenteric Ischemia and Respective Treatments

(a) SMA Embolus

General	• 40–50% of cases • Frequent association with cardiac disease (e.g., atrial fibrillation) • Abrupt presentation with severe abdominal pain and diarrhea (hematochezia) • 20% with simultaneous peripheral arterial embolus; 33% with history of prior embolic event
Imaging features	• Filling defect outlined by contrast, convex meniscus, and location that is typically at least 3 cm beyond origin of SMA • Lack of collaterals • Poor distal flow • 15% found in proximal SMA, 50% found at middle colic artery bifurcation, 25% at the ileocolic branch, and 10% in the distal small bowel branches of the SMA • Ileus, mucosal edema, bowel infarction
Treatment	• Endovascular therapy (direct intrathrombus infusion) may be considered first line in cases with short occlusion, adequate distal collateral circulation, and no peritoneal signs or elevation of lactic acid • Intraoperative thrombectomy or thrombolytic therapy may be considered in a hybrid OR setting, if available • Exploratory laparoscopy/laparotomy if clinical/imaging evidence of end-organ ischemia • Papaverine administered when arterial vasoconstriction present • Systemic anticoagulation

(b) SMA Thrombosis

General	• 25% of cases • Typically occurs in patients with underlying atherosclerotic lesions, especially of the visceral branches • 50–75% of patients with history of intestinal angina • May have acute on chronic symptoms
Imaging features	• Occlusive lesion commonly located 1–2 cm from the origin of the SMA • Collateral vessels may be present suggesting underlying chronic occlusive disease • Ileus; mucosal edema; bowel infarction
Treatment	• End-organ ischemia/infarction (e.g., elevated lactic acid or peritoneal signs) requires prompt surgical exploration • Consider endovascular thrombolysis/thrombectomy vs. primary surgical bypass and/or thromboendarterectomy • ± preoperative papaverine (may not be feasible because of proximal nature of these lesions) • Second look operation 24–48 h later may be required • Postoperative vasodilators as warranted • Primary endovascular management if no peritoneal signs or lactic acidosis • May perform primary stenting ± filter wire ± lytics • Because lesions often represent acute clot superimposed on underlying chronic lesion, thrombolytics may be administered prior to stenting to reduce the risk of distal embolization

Table 8.1   **Summary of the Different Causes of Acute Mesenteric Ischemia and Respective Treatments (*continued*)**

(c) NOMI

General	• 10–15% of cases
	• Typically occurs in patients with a prior hypotensive event, even if resolved
	• Associated with low cardiac output, hypovolemia, hypotension, and splanchnic vasoconstriction. Also affiliated with vasoactive drugs (e.g., vasopressin, α-agonists, and digoxin)
	• May be an insidious onset
Imaging features	• Diffuse arterial vasospasm with segmental, such as narrowing or diffuse narrowing of vessels commonly identified near branch points
	• Delayed filling of distal arterial and intramural branches
	• Delayed bowel wall enhancement and/or venous filling
	• Improved flow at angiography after administration of 60-mg papaverine into the SMA
	• Ileus, mucosal edema, bowel infarction
Treatment	• Papaverine infusion directly into the SMA at 1 mg/min is the mainstay of therapy and is continued until the symptoms resolve (typically within 12–36 h). If peritoneal signs develop, surgery is indicated to explore for dead bowel while continuing papaverine infusion

(d) SMV Thrombosis

General	• Accounts for less than 5% of all acute mesenteric ischemia
	• Predisposing factors include portal hypertension, abdominal inflammatory disease, oral contraceptives, prior surgery on the portal venous system, trauma, and hypercoagulable states
	• Mesenteric venous thrombosis causes mucosal edema leading to arterial hypoperfusion
Imaging features	• Intraluminal filling defect in the mesenteric veins with venous congestion and mucosal edema
	• Secondary arterial vasospasm and diminished perfusion
	• Prolonged mucosal enhancement
	• Lack of or delay in opacification of the mesenteric veins
	• Prolonged opacification of venules or larger regional veins
	• Ileus, mucosal edema, bowel infarction
Treatment	• Hydrate patient and correct predisposing factors
	• Systemic anticoagulation
	• If bowel infarction, surgery is warranted
	• Pre- and postoperative anticoagulation
	• Intraarterial papaverine if coexistent mesenteric arterial vasoconstriction
	• If no peritoneal signs or lactic acidosis, endovascular options include transarterial, systemic, and direct transhepatic or transjugular access for venous thrombolysis, mechanical thrombectomy, angioplasty, and/or stent placement
	• Most patients can be managed conservatively with supportive care and anticoagulation

(*continued*)

Table 8.1	**Summary of the Different Causes of Acute Mesenteric Ischemia and Respective Treatments (*continued*)**

(e) Aortic Dissection

General	• 5% of all cases of acute mesenteric ischemia • High (90%) operative mortality in this cohort • Mesenteric vasculature can be supplied from the true or false lumen with static and/or dynamic obstruction • Inadequate flow results when blood flow fails to meet the metabolic needs of the bowel
Imaging features	• Identification of true and false lumens with possible visualization of a dissection flap extending into the SMA or compromise of the lumen perfusing the SMA • Ileus, mucosal edema, bowel infarction
Treatment	• Operative mortality is high • Endovascular—Intravascular ultrasound (IVUS) helpful • Endograft therapy to cover primary entry tear • Creation of *de novo* fenestrations to equalize pressures between the true and false lumens • SMA stenting for persistent malperfusion from obstructive intimal flap

b. Catheter-based techniques can provide a potential therapeutic role for AMI, regardless of the underlying etiology. However, the first-line choice of treatment varies depending upon the underlying cause (Table 8.1).
   (1) Treatment options include vasodilator infusion, thrombolysis and mechanical thrombectomy with or without use of a filter wire, angioplasty, and stenting.
c. Because of the high mortality associated with surgery, some authors advocate a broader use of endovascular therapy both alone and in combination with surgery for AMI, including patients with evidence of bowel infarction (peritoneal signs and lactic acidosis) (4,6). Recent evidence suggests that even in patients with intestinal necrosis, endovascular revascularization prior to open surgery can reduce morbidity and mortality, likely due to decreased ischemic times (7).
d. Hybrid operative and endovascular procedures of various forms have gained significant traction in recent years. The broader use of hybrid operating and interventional suites allows endovascular revascularization in the same setting as surgical removal of bowel. In addition, in the case of failed antegrade endovascular revascularization, exposure of the mesenteric root with retrograde open mesenteric stenting, as well as open antegrade and retrograde mesenteric bypass has been described.

Contraindications

1. Renal insufficiency is not a contraindication for contrast administration, as contrast-induced renal failure may be less of a risk for a patient than delaying the diagnosis and treatment of a highly lethal disease (5).
2. Performance of a diagnostic CTA or endovascular intervention in a patient with a severe contrast allergy history is typically contraindicated. In patients in whom the diagnosis of AMI is highly suspected, the use of general anesthesia for CTA and the endovascular intervention may obviate the concerns about the contrast allergy risks. MRA may be an acceptable alternative diagnostic modality.
3. Evidence of bowel infarction mandates emergent surgical exploration and resection of dead bowel. Use of an endovascular solution alone is not appropriate.

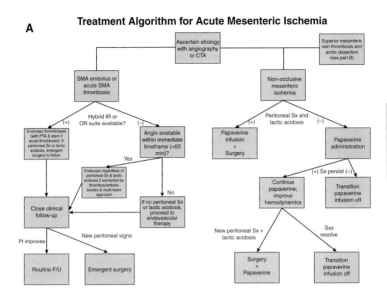

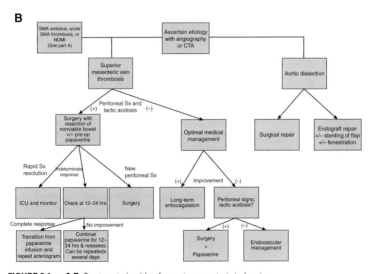

FIGURE 8.1 • A,B: Treatment algorithm for acute mesenteric ischemia.

However, adjunctive endovascular therapy is known to improve surgical out-comes while also helping to minimize the amount of bowel resected (4,6,7). Catheter-based interventions also provide the opportunity to relieve mesenteric vasospasm by pre-, intra-, and/or postoperative catheter-directed intraarterial infusion of vasodilators, such as papaverine, nitroglycerin, glucagon, and pros-taglandin E1.

4. Relative contraindications to angiography and an endovascular intervention include uncontrolled bacteremia and uncorrectable bleeding diatheses.
5. Other contraindications will be guided by the specifics of the intended therapy
   a. Papaverine is contraindicated in patients with complete heart block and papaverine allergies. Other relative contraindications exist as well (Table 8.2).
   b. Thrombolytics are relatively contraindicated in patients with active bleeding or hemorrhagic disorders, recent trauma, uncontrolled hypertension, recent gastrointestinal bleeding, hemoptysis, epistaxis, pregnancy, recent surgery, retinal detachment, a recent cerebrovascular accident, or an acute or recent (less than 3 months) intracranial or intraspinal process.

Preprocedure Preparation and Evaluation

1. Pathophysiology of AMI
   a. AMI manifests a complex pathophysiology, an understanding of which is imperative for successful management. A common pathway with associated severe morbidity and mortality is a systemic inflammatory response syndrome (SIRS), multiorgan dysfunction syndrome (MODS), and acute respiratory distress syndrome (ARDS). The vicious cycles of these clinical entities can be further propagated by reperfusion of infarcted bowel.
   b. The viscera are supplied by three vessels from the aorta—the celiac artery (CA), SMA, and inferior mesenteric artery (IMA). They receive 10% to 25% of the cardiac output in a resting state and up to 35% postprandially (10). The mucosal and submucosal layers receive up to 70% of the splanchnic blood

Table 8.2 **Papaverine Administration**

Indications	• Primary therapy for nonocclusive mesenteric ischemia or adjunctive therapy for acute mesenteric ischemia regardless of the cause • Can also be used pre- and postoperatively in those patients requiring surgical revascularization

Contraindications	• **Absolute**
	   • Complete AV heart block
	 • **Relative**
	   • Simultaneous administration of alkaline substances through the same catheter, including lactated Ringer's, urokinase, heparin, etc. (can cause precipitation)
	   • Narrow-angle glaucoma
	   • Severe cardiac disease (particularly with bradyarrhythmias)
	   • Severe liver dysfunction

Dose	• Intraarterial bolus of 45–60 mg followed by steady infusion of 0.5–1.0 mg/min. Initial treatment period of 12–24 h prior to reevaluation
Optional	• Nifedipine 10–20 mg PO q6h can be given as an adjunct to papaverine and may confer some beneficial vasodilatory effect, but may worsen hypotension • Risk for inducing reflex tachycardia and cardiac ischemia
Common complications	• Systemic vasodilatation/hypotension, but >90% of the drug is metabolized on first pass through the liver • Diarrhea and abdominal pain are common after reestablishing flow to the bowel

flow, due to their high metabolic demands. The muscular and serosal layers rely on the remaining 30% (10). There is extensive collateralization between the CA, SMA, and IMA—so much so that it is possible for the entire gut to be supplied by a single artery if the collateral pathways are mature and patent. Important collaterals between the CA and SMA are pancreaticoduodenal arcade and arc of Bühler. The SMA and IMA are connected among others by the arc of Riolan and the marginal artery of Drummond. There is a complex interplay between neural and humoral influences and locally acting factors that regulate visceral perfusion that are beyond the scope of this chapter (10). Vascular occlusive disease ultimately produces splanchnomesenteric hypoperfusion and mesenteric vascular vasoconstriction (10). Hypoxia, acidosis, and epithelial permeability develop which allows for bacterial transgression of the mucosal barrier and subjects the immune system to massive stimulation from bacterial antigens, stimulating the proinflammatory pathways. Enteric decontamination has been shown to decrease transmural necrosis and improve survival in ICU patients (11).

2. Once the diagnosis of AMI is entertained, a review of the history, serial clinical examinations, laboratory data, and available imaging studies are requisite.

   a. Unfortunately in AMI, most laboratory abnormalities are nonspecific. Serum L-lactate levels remain the most common marker of bowel ischemia and infarction, but it is a nonspecific marker of tissue hypoperfusion and is often elevated in the setting of critical illnesses in the absence of bowel infarction. However, the higher the L-lactate levels, in general the worse the patient prognosis. Perhaps more importantly, a normal serum lactate level does not rule out the presence of AMI (1,5). However, in the ICU setting where the incidence of AMI is much higher (especially NOMI), novel biomarkers may be of potential use to help guide diagnostic and treatment decisions (like whether to go to the CT scanner, the angiography suite, or the OR) in suspected AMI (12). Although not commonly used, a recent meta-analysis of serologic markers in AMI found ischemia-modified albumin has the highest sensitivity and specificity of any biomarker thus far, 94% and 86%, respectively (12). Intestinal fatty acid-binding protein (I-FABP) has also shown some promise, with a sensitivity of 79% and a specificity of 91%.

   b. A multidisciplinary team consisting of vascular surgeons, general surgeons, intensivists/anesthesiologists, diagnostic radiologists, and interventional radiologists is essential for the initial evaluation and treatment planning of each patient with suspected AMI due to the complexity and acuity of their circumstances that requires carefully orchestrated treatment plans.

3. Medical optimization/preparation (1,5):

   a. Blood volume resuscitation to achieve a mean arterial pressure (MAP) > 65 mmHg and urine output > 0.5 mL/Kg/hr.

      (1) Typically requires central venous access and invasive monitoring with an arterial line

      (2) Treat hemodynamic instability with volume. Patients with AMI can require an astounding amount of resuscitative fluid—up to 10 to 20 L within the first 24 hours

   b. Systemic heparinization +/− ASA for embolic or thrombotic events

   c. Broad-spectrum enteric decontamination with PO and IV antibiotics (see specific recommendations in "Postprocedure Management" section)

   d. IV proton pump inhibitors

   e. Supplemental O_2

   f. Bowel rest with nil per os +/− gastric decompression tube if ileus

   g. Nutritional support with TPN as needed

   h. Transfusion as needed

   i. Urgent ECHO or cardiac CT to evaluate for thrombus in the setting of embolic AMI

4. If bowel infarction is present, the patient will require surgery. Depending on the operator and institutional capabilities, endovascular revascularization can be attempted first to allow better definition of the ischemic versus infarcted bowel segments at the time of surgery. After revascularization, a delay for surgery should be minimized to reduce the risk for developing a reperfusion syndrome. Hybrid operating rooms or endovascular suites equipped to do open surgery confer the advantage of allowing operative and endovascular intervention in a single session.

5. Assess the patient for the appropriateness for the intended procedure (e.g., papaverine and/or thrombolytic infusion; or a direct transhepatic or transjugular approach for mesenteric venous thrombosis). If NOMI is present, strongly consider pre- and perioperative intraarterial papaverine infusion as there is usually no fixed obstruction to treat with balloon angioplasty, stenting, or surgical bypass.

6. Consider using general anesthesia for the uncooperative patient or whom a bowel exploration is planned.

7. Correct underlying hypotension, coagulopathy, and electrolyte imbalances as soon as possible, while initiating definitive treatment.

8. Continue physiologic monitoring (pulse oximetry, blood pressure, pulse, and EKG) until treatment is complete.

Procedure

1. Arterial access: Access may be obtained via either the femoral artery, the left brachial or radial artery for arterial interventions. Regardless of the chosen access site, an appropriately sized sheath should be placed and secured.

   a. Although advances in catheter and sheath technology have reduced the need for brachial arterial access, certain clinical situations mandate use of the brachial or radial artery, including inaccessible groin access (i.e., total aortic or iliac artery occlusions, active groin infections, and flexion contractures) and mesenteric anatomic factors (when the mesenteric vessels have a very sharp caudal angle relative to the aorta). In these situations, catheter access and intervention may be more favorable from an antegrade approach.

   b. The brachial artery is a second-line approach since it is associated with a higher rate of complications relative to a femoral access. Use of the radial artery reduces the risk of brachial nerve injury, but there is a defined risk for radial artery thrombosis. Therefore, a Barbeau test should be performed to ensure an intact palmar arch. Having devices of appropriate lengths to perform the necessary interventions may be more challenging with a radial artery approach. In addition, the operator is typically constrained to using devices that can be used through a 6-Fr sheath.

   c. Arterial access should be obtained with ultrasound guidance to ensure atraumatic single-wall entry into the artery, especially if thrombolytics are under consideration.

2. Preliminary imaging

   a. Using a pigtail catheter, obtain a lateral and anterior–posterior (AP) abdominal aortogram, preferably simultaneously (biplane). These images can be eliminated to minimize contrast load and expedite the procedure if a prior CTA or MRA defined the mesenteric vascular anatomy well enough to allow a more targeted approach to treatment.

      (1) The AP aortogram is particularly useful in the assessment of aortic disease, collateral vascularization, and the overall perfusion of the bowel. In addition, while most occlusive pathology involves the proximal main and first-order branch vessels of the mesenteric circulation, the more distal arterial anatomy is better appreciated on the AP projection.

(2) Delayed imaging on the AP projection allows visualization of the superior mesenteric vein (SMV), inferior mesenteric vein (IMV), and portal vein (PV) to assess for mesenteric venous patency.

(3) The lateral aortogram should define the origins and the patency of the proximal CA, SMA, and IMA.

3. Catheterization of the SMA

    a. A variety of commercially available 4-Fr and 5-Fr catheters (AngioDynamics, Queensbury, NY; Boston Scientific, Natick, MA; Cook Medical, Bloomington, IN) will readily engage the SMA. Although the RC1, RC2, and C2 Cobra catheters are commonly used to select the SMA, reverse curve catheters such as the Sos 1 and Sos 2 and the Simmons 1 and Simmons 2 catheters confer better catheter stability for further intervention (e.g., papaverine infusion).

      (1) The RC 1 or 2 and C2 catheters are placed above the vessel of interest and retracted slowly in order to engage the target vessel. A soft-tipped wire can then be advanced through the catheter more distally into the SMA over which the catheter is subsequently maneuvered to obtain a more stable catheter position.

      (2) Once formed, reverse curve catheters (Sos or Simmons) are advanced cranially from an inferior position until the catheter tip selects the target vessel. A soft-tipped wire is then advanced into the target vessel and the catheter is gently retracted over the wire to seat the catheter into the SMA in a more stable position.

    b. Use of a long sheath (e.g., Ansel 2, Cook Medical, Bloomington, IN) advanced over a support wire with the inner dilator or alone over a catheter to the origin of the SMA may be helpful if additional interventions (i.e., stenting, mechanical thrombectomy, and/or suction embolectomy) are intended.

4. SMA angiography

    a. The diagnosis of AMI and the ascertainment of its etiology are often made from a previous CTA or MRA, but can readily be made with a combination of aortography and/or selective SMA angiography as well. The angiographic findings of the various etiologies for AMI are outlined in Table 8.1.

      (1) The selective AP SMA injection of contrast should be at a rate of 4 to 6 mL per second for a 5-second duration (20 to 30 mL total volume). Filming should be carried out for at least 30 to 40 seconds to allow visualization of the mesenteric veins. Selective SMA angiography is specifically helpful in making the diagnosis of NOMI, especially if there is significant improvement in the flow characteristics and visualization of the vasa recta with repeat angiography after intraarterial administration of 60 mg of papaverine directly into the SMA. In addition, mesenteric ischemia due to vasculopathies, volvulus, hernias, distal emboli, and mesenteric venous thrombosis can be detected with selective SMA arteriography.

5. Treatment (see Table 8.1, Fig. 8.1)

    a. Embolic etiology

      (1) Endovascular options

        (a) Depending on the clinical scenario, endovascular treatment may be used in lieu of or as adjunct to open surgery. It is accepted first-line therapy for nonoperative patients or patients with short occlusions, adequate distal collateralization, absent peritoneal signs, minimal lactic acidosis, and less than 12 hours of symptoms. Initial endovascular revascularization followed by pro re nata damage control laparotomy is increasingly being used as a treatment algorithm (13).

        (b) On occasion, an SMA embolus can be managed with exclusion with a covered stent with use of an embolic protection device (EPD). More commonly, catheter-directed mechanical thrombectomy, suction embolectomy with a nontapered guide catheter, or intrathrombus infusion of a thrombolytic agent may be performed (6). Recombinant tissue plasminogen activator (rtPA; Genetech, South San Francisco, CA) is the most commonly used lytic agent in the United States. Its use is an off-U.S. Food and Drug Administration (FDA) label application of an FDA-approved drug. It is administered as a drip infusion of rt-PA through an infusion catheter positioned in direct contact with the clot, at a rate of 1 mg per hour with or without a prior bolus. Short-term (e.g., every 4 to 8 hours) angiographic reassessment, frequent serum lactate levels, and monitoring for the development of peritoneal signs for response to therapy are necessary. Concomitant use of heparin is variable depending upon the institutional preference. However, we prefer to administer heparin systemically to keep the patient fully anticoagulated, if the patient is at risk for further embolization or thrombosis.

(c) Papaverine infusion can also be used to reduce the ischemia from diffuse vasospasm which frequently occurs distal to the embolus. A coaxial infusion system is usually used. Papaverine should not be infused via the same catheter as heparin, as the two agents will precipitate if mixed together.

(d) Underlying occlusive lesions may be treated with angioplasty and/or stenting as necessary.

(2) Surgical options: Multiple "hybrid" techniques are described in the literature. One commonly described hybrid approach is primary endovascular revascularization followed by damage control laparotomy in a hybrid angio suite/OR to reduce ischemic bowel time and time to resection of dead bowel. Open surgery with direct puncture of the SMA and retrograde stenting, followed by resection of necrotic bowel has also been described.

(a) Adjunctive peri- and postoperative papaverine infusion into the SMA can help to enhance perfusion to residual ischemic bowel segments in order to preserve as much bowel as possible.

b. Thrombotic etiology

(1) Endovascular options

(a) When possible, endovascular revascularization with primary stent placement should be attempted first, with or without use of an EPD (to prevent distal clot migration) or thrombolysis of any underlying acute thrombus prior to stent placement (4,6). A balloon-expandable covered stent or self-expanding covered stent may help to trap any acute clot between the stent and vessel wall and prevent herniation and distal embolization of thrombotic material through the cells of a bare-metal stent.

(b) Adjunctive IA vasodilator administration is more difficult in these patients because the occlusion of the SMA is often at its origin and stable positioning of the infusion catheter can be problematic.

(2) Surgical options: Surgical revascularization may be indicated in the setting of ostial occlusion that cannot be crossed or long-segment occlusions. Surgical revascularization strategies include antegrade and retrograde aortomesenteric bypass and/or thromboendarterectomy with patch angioplasty.

c. NOMI: Typically occurs in critically ill patients who are generally hypoperfused, seen most commonly in elderly patients postcardiac surgery or florid sepsis. This is a particularly challenging clinical scenario that requires vigilance to diagnose because these patients typically are noncommunicative (intubated/sedated), critically ill with multiple comorbidities, who slowly develop abdominal distention and increasing vasopressor requirement. DSA is the gold standard to diagnose NOMI.

(1) Endovascular options: Vasodilators administered intraarterially are the mainstay of therapy. Surgery is indicated only if peritoneal signs or bowel infarction develops.

    (a) Papaverine is administered through a 4-Fr or 5-Fr catheter into the SMA as a 45- to 60-mg bolus followed by a continuous infusion at a rate of 30 to 60 mg per hour (0.5 to 1 mg per minute—most often 1 mg per minute). Typically, it is titrated for effect for an initial 12- to 24-hour period. After 12 to 24 hours, if the symptoms of ischemia have resolved, the papaverine is stopped and replaced with heparinized saline. If the patient remains asymptomatic for 6 to 12 hours and is hemodynamically stable (no longer hypotensive or on vasopressors), the catheter is removed. Repeat angiography is only performed if there is a question about the mesenteric vascular anatomy relative to the patient's symptoms.

        i. Papaverine may have an adjunctive role with surgery as described earlier and is administered before and 12 to 24 hours after surgery.

        ii. More information about papaverine is detailed in Table 8.2.

    (b) The use of other IA vasodilators including alprostadil (prostaglandin E1), nitroglycerin, and glucagon has also been described.

    (c) Patients with NOMI found to have underlying SMA stenosis on DSA should be revascularized with angioplasty and stenting.

    (d) As with all types of AMI, surgery is indicated for the resection of infarcted bowel.

    (e) Intraabdominal compartment syndrome/intraabdominal hypertension can contribute to NOMI, and if that case, papaverine infusion and decompressive laparotomy are recommended (14,15).

d. SMV thrombosis

(1) The initial goal is to hydrate the patient, stabilize their cardiovascular status, and correct the precipitating event(s).

(2) Anticoagulation is a critical facet of management, since these patients are highly prone to recurrent thrombosis.

(3) Most of these patients do well with supportive care, hydration, and meticulous anticoagulation. However, in cases when patients do not clinically improve, endovascular therapy is implemented.

    (a) Thrombolytics with or without mechanical thrombectomy are the mainstay of endovascular therapy and are directly administered into the thrombosed SMV or PV via a transhepatic or transjugular access.

    (b) Mechanical thrombectomy, angioplasty, and stent placement are performed as needed. Successful mesenteric venous recanalization has been demonstrated with all methods but appears to be most effective, as with other catheter-directed thrombolysis (CDT), when the catheter is directly positioned within the clot.

(4) As with all cases of AMI, signs of peritoneal irritation or elevated lactic acid indicative of bowel infarction may warrant emergent surgical exploration.

e. Aortic dissection

(1) Mesenteric ischemia secondary to an aortic dissection can be the result of direct extension of the dissection flap into the SMA or due to the false lumen compressing the true lumen, causing diminished perfusion pressures in the SMA. Open surgical repair in a patient with mesenteric ischemia in the setting of an acute aortic dissection is associated with mortality rates approaching 90%. Therefore, endovascular solutions are being used more frequently to address this clinical problem.

(a) The goal of aortic endografting is to exclude the primary entry tear with a stent graft to decrease the perfusion pressure in the false lumen, induce false lumen collapse, and increase perfusion pressure in the true lumen to allow better perfusion of the SMA via the true lumen. In cases in which the dissection flap extends directly into the SMA, use of a self-expanding uncovered stent may result in reapproximation of the dissection flap against the SMA wall to allow better mesenteric perfusion. Intravascular ultrasound (IVUS) is critical in helping to determine the true versus false lumens and to ensure that the stent will be in the true lumen.

(b) When an endograft or stent solution is not feasible, creation of perivisceral de novo fenestrations to facilitate pressure equalization in the true and false lumens can be beneficial. The ability to measure simultaneous pressures in both lumens is very helpful so that the size of the fenestrations can be increased by using larger balloons until the pressure in both lumens has equalized.

f. Surgery remains an important component of therapy, especially in the presence of bowel infarction. Expeditious removal of necrotic bowel is imperative in order to mitigate the effects of reperfusion injury. As previously stated, the first goal of therapy should be to restore visceral perfusion. Ideally damage control surgery is performed immediately following revascularization in patients who are suspected of having transmural necrosis based on preprocedural imaging, severe lactic acidosis, peritoneal signs, or clinical deterioration.

(1) In general, when a patient is too unstable to tolerate definitive surgical repair a "damage control" operation is performed to temporize immediately life-threatening pathology until they are appropriately resuscitated to withstand a reparative operation, usually within 24 to 48 hours. In the setting of AMI, if frankly necrotic bowel is encountered and resected, the bowel is sometimes left in discontinuity with a temporary abdominal closure device. A second look laparotomy is performed at the discretion of the surgeon, typically at 12 to 24 hours, and the bowel is anastomosed. Once the bowel is back in continuity and the patient has started to improve clinically, the abdominal fascia can be closed.

Postprocedure Management

1. All patients treated for AMI should be admitted to the ICU regardless of the underlying etiology. The goals of therapy in the perioperative or periprocedural period are resuscitation, avoidance of reperfusion injury, prevention of clot propagation, prevention of sepsis, and minimizing the extent of bowel injury.

a. Close monitoring of arterial blood pressures and cardiac indices may be necessary. Hypotension may develop with use of vasodilators, although this occurrence is rare since >90% of papaverine administered into the SMA is metabolized on first pass through the liver. In the setting of hypotension, historically vasopressors or cardiotonic agents including dopamine (2 to 5 µg/kg/min) or dobutamine (0.5 to 1.0 µg/kg/min titrated to 2.5 to 20 µg/kg/min), have been recommended, however no studies have ever been done comparing different vasopressive agents in the setting of AMI, so it is hard to give a recommendation. Theoretically vasopressin and α-agonists should be avoided because of the concern for worsening mesenteric vasoconstriction.

b. Correction of acidosis and fluid and electrolyte disturbances is necessary in order to minimize the risk for arrhythmias or further hypotension.

c. Anticoagulation with IV heparin is recommended. The initial heparin bolus should be 70 to 100 U per kg, unless a major intervention (i.e., transhepatic puncture) is planned and then titrated to maintain a partial thromboplastin time (PTT) of 60 to 80 seconds. Use of low–molecular-weight heparin (LMWH) should be discouraged if endovascular therapy is contemplated, as LMWHs have long half-lives and their excretion is affected by changes in renal function. In addition, there is no easy test to monitor their activity (i.e., PTT) without doing factor Xa assays.

d. A recent prospective study at an intestinal stroke center found that oral antibiotics were associated with decreased incidence of transmural necrosis and improved mortality, HR = 0.16, (95% CI 0.03–0.62; p = 0.01) (11). Mesenteric venous thrombosis can lead to edema and/or breakdown of the intestinal mucosa, with secondary seeding of the clot by gastrointestinal bacteria. Therefore, these patients are at risk of developing septic thrombophlebitis from gram-negative and anaerobic organisms, so broad-spectrum antibiotic therapy is recommended for these patients.

(1) Piperacillin/tazobactam (Zosyn): Given intravenously every 6 hours (typical IV dose is 3.375 g).

(2) Metronidazole (Flagyl): Loaded at a dose of 15 mg per kg given over 1 hour and then continued at a dose of 7.5 mg/kg every 6 to 8 hours.

(3) Levofloxacin (Levaquin): Provided in conjunction with Zosyn or Flagyl at a dose of 500 mg every 24 hours.

e. Prevention of reperfusion injury.

(1) Glucagon may be used as an adjunct for patients undergoing papaverine therapy. Glucagon causes intestinal vasodilatation and hypotonicity, reducing the demand for oxygen. The dose is 1 µg/kg/min titrated up to 10 µg/kg/min as tolerated; however, nausea and vomiting are frequent with this medication, so its use in this setting is infrequent.

(2) Other agents such as allopurinol and enalapril that can theoretically act as free-radical scavengers may decrease the risk of reperfusion injury, but there is limited experience with the use of these medications.

2. Patients undergoing papaverine or other vasodilator therapy should be monitored for signs or symptoms indicative of bowel infarction.

a. Worsening lactic acidosis (normal = 0.5 to 2.2 mmol per L) is an indicator of advancing ischemia and possible bowel infarction, and although nonspecific, may be very helpful, in patients with an altered mental status or those on steroids or analgesics, where assessment for peritoneal signs and serosal irritation may not be helpful.

b. Papaverine treatment can be continued for up to 5 days if the patient remains stable, but most often, if NOMI is the etiology and the cause for hypotension has been reversed, papaverine infusions greater than 36 hours are unusual (16).

3. Patients undergoing thrombolysis are reevaluated angiographically at frequent intervals (e.g., ~4 to 8 hours). Plasma fibrinogen levels are concurrently monitored to assess for a systemic lytic effect. The infusion dose may be reduced in order to maintain fibrinogen levels above 100 g per L. Fresh-frozen plasma (FFP) is transfused in select cases in which fibrinogen levels decrease to below 100 g per L.

4. The development of peritoneal signs and worsening lactic acidosis is suggestive of bowel infarction and requires prompt surgical exploration.

a. Patients that have undergone extensive bowel resection are at risk for developing short-gut syndrome, and appropriate diet modifications in consultation with a gastroenterologist and nutrition specialist are necessary.

5. Follow-up CTA can be performed at 1 month if a proximal occlusion has been treated. If stents are placed, a follow-up CTA or duplex ultrasound at 6 to 12 months to evaluate for in-stent restenosis is warranted.

6. Patients with stents should be placed on clopidogrel (Plavix; Bristol Myers Squibb, New York, NY) using a 300-mg loading dose and 75 mg per day thereafter, for 3 to 6 months and ASA at 81 to 325 mg per day for life.

Results

1. Optimal results are attained with early and rapid diagnosis and intervention (9,10,17):
   a. Emerging data suggest that morbidity and mortality associated with AMI have been improving over the last two decades, along with rates of endovascular interventions. A recent meta-analysis of 26,104 patients from 2000 to 2012 showed total revascularizations in AMI has increased over time, but open surgery has remained stable (3). Over that same period, in-hospital mortality rates decreased from 28% to 17% in patients who received endovascular treatment and from 40% to 25% in those who underwent open revascularization (3). Combined in-hospital mortality rates decreased from 37% to 21%. Annual population mortality from AMI decreased from 12.9 to 5.3 deaths per million people/year (3).
   b. Predictors of increased mortality in the setting of AMI include an elevated SVS comorbidity score, the presence of CHF, chronic kidney disease, cerebrovascular disease, bowel resection, peripheral vascular disease, coronary artery disease, lactate > 2.2 mmol per L, advanced age, and the presence of connective tissue disease. Conversely, the presence of chronic mesenteric ischemia appears protective, likely from the development of collateral blood flow (6,9).
   c. Higher rates of survival are attainable with a multimodal, multispecialty strategy. This is achieved by prompt recognition, a specific medical protocol, and rapid revascularization.
2. While surgery remains an essential component in the management of AMI, there is growing evidence for early endovascular intervention and some practitioners advocate for an "endo-first" approach, even in the setting of infarcted bowel (4,6,14).
   a. Benefits of endovascular therapy include a reduced need for anesthesia and an urgent laparotomy, less bowel resection, decreased need for TPN, the potential for more rapid revascularization, lower morbidity, and possibly improved mortality. In a retrospective study, Arthurs et al. reported that 31% of patients with AMI avoided laparotomy altogether, and in comparison with the traditional surgery, patients who underwent endovascular therapy first had a mean of 52 cm of bowel resected compared to 160 cm in the surgery-first group. Mortality for the endovascular group was 36% compared with 50% for the surgical group (6). Other groups have confirmed marked reduction in bowel resection, decreased hospital stays, and decreased mortality using an endovascular first approach (4). However, the nature of these studies remains subject to considerable selection bias and there remains a lack of prospective randomized trials comparing surgical and endovascular outcomes, likely in part because of the logistical and ethical challenges inherent with such a study.
3. The authors advocate a multidisciplinary approach to AMI with a team comprised of vascular and general surgery, interventional and diagnostic radiology, gastroenterology, and intensive care specialists. In the setting of bowel necrosis, endovascular therapy is not a substitute for surgical therapy, but an adjunct which can improve subsequent surgical outcomes (4,6). In the acute setting, the decision between surgery and endovascular as first-line therapy is made on an individual patient basis and should incorporate the specific resources and expertise available to the institution. An endo-first approach should not be embraced if this approach substantially delays surgical resection of necrotic bowel.
4. The results of endovascular therapy are also influenced by the specific etiology of AMI.
   a. Use of vasodilators has a high reported efficacy for AMI due to NOMI.
   b. Thrombolysis for SMA emboli is also effective. The largest reported series (10 patients) found 90% achieved angiographic success, and 70% had resolution of symptoms following IA thrombolysis of the SMA (14). A study found 62.5% of patients with AMI achieved clinical success after thrombolysis (15).

c. In select patients with SMA thrombosis, use of angioplasty and/or stenting with thrombolysis is beneficial. One report showed technical success in 71% of patients with AMI. Of those successfully treated, 80% experienced clinical success with improvement in their symptoms (15). One series reported a good clinical outcome in 81% (17 of 21) of patients presenting with either acute SMA thrombosis or an SMA embolus with aggressive endovascular therapy, sometimes combined with surgery, even in patients presenting with bowel infarction (18).

Complications

1. Access site
   a. Hematoma or pseudoaneurysm formation
      (1) Increased risk with thrombolysis and anticoagulation
2. Papaverine (or other vasodilator) associated hypotension
   a. More commonly occurs if catheter inadvertently disengages SMA and direct infusion into the aorta occurs
3. Contrast-related complications
   a. Renal toxicity: Increased risk with dehydration, renal insufficiency, and associated renal emboli
   b. Allergic reactions
4. Thrombolysis-associated complications
   a. Access site or distant site bleeding, embolization, stroke, and intraperitoneal bleeding with transhepatic approaches for mesenteric venous thrombosis
5. Angioplasty-associated complications
   a. Vessel injury: dissection, rupture
   b. Distal embolization
6. Reperfusion injury manifested as a systemic inflammatory response or ARDS
7. Cardiac arrhythmias

R e f e r e n c e s

1. Clair DG, Beach JM. Mesenteric ischemia. *N Engl J Med*. 2016;374(10):959–968.
2. Salsano G, Salsano A, Sportelli E, et al. What is the best revascularization strategy for acute occlusive arterial mesenteric ischemia: systematic review and meta-analysis. *Cardiovasc Intervent Radiol*. 2018;41(1):27–36.
3. Zettervall SL, Lo RC, Soden PA, et al. Trends in treatment and mortality for mesenteric ischemia in the United States from 2000 to 2012. *Ann Vasc Surg*. 2017;42:111–119.
4. Beaulieu RJ, Arnaoutakis KD, Abularrage CJ, et al. Comparison of open and endovascular treatment of acute mesenteric ischemia. *J Vasc Surg*. 2014;59(1):159–64.
5. Bala M, Kashuk J, Moore EE, et al. Acute mesenteric ischemia: guidelines of the world society of emergency surgery. *World J Emerg Surg*. 2017;12(1):1–11.
6. Arthurs ZM, Titus J, Bannazadeh M, et al. A comparison of endovascular revascularization with traditional therapy for the treatment of acute mesenteric ischemia. *J Vasc Surg*. 2011;53(3):698–705.
7. Hsu A, Bhattacharya KR, Chan HK, et al. Effect of timing on endovascular therapy and exploratory laparotomy outcome in acute mesenteric ischemia. *Ann Gastroenterol*. 2019; 32(6):600.
8. Eslami MH, Rybin D, Doros G, et al. Mortality of acute mesenteric ischemia remains unchanged despite significant increase in utilization of endovascular techniques. *Vascular*. 2016;24(1):44–52.
9. Ryer EJ, Kalra M, Oderich GS, et al. Revascularization for acute mesenteric ischemia. *J Vasc Surg*. 2012;55(6):1682–1689.
10. Oldenburg WA, Lau LL, Rodenberg TJ, et al. Acute mesenteric ischemia: a clinical review. *Arch Intern Med*. 2004;164(10):1054–62.
11. Nuzzo A, Maggiori L, Paugam-Burtz C, et al. Oral antibiotics reduce intestinal necrosis in acute mesenteric ischemia: a prospective cohort study. *Am J Gastroenterol*. 2019; 114(2):348–351.

12. Treskes N, Persoon AM, van Zanten AR. Diagnostic accuracy of novel serological biomark-ers to detect acute mesenteric ischemia: a systematic review and meta-analysis. *Intern Emerg Med.* 2017;12(6):821–836.
13. Liu Y-R, Tong Z, Hou C-B, et al. Aspiration therapy for acute embolic occlusion of the superior mesenteric artery. *World J Gastroenterol.* 2019;25(7):848.
14. Simo G, Echenagusia AJ, Camúñez F, et al. Superior mesenteric arterial embolism: local fibrinolytic treatment with urokinase. *Radiology.* 1997;204(3):775–9.
15. Simonetti G, Lupattelli L, Urigo F, et al. Interventional radiology in the treatment of acute and chronic mesenteric ischemia. *Radiol Med (Torino).* 1992;84(1–2):98–105.
16. Demir IE, Ceyhan GO, Friess H. Beyond lactate: is there a role for serum lactate measure-ment in diagnosing acute mesenteric ischemia? *Dig Surg.* 2012;29(3):226–35.
17. Corcos O, Castier Y, Sibert A, et al. Effects of a multimodal management strategy for acute mesenteric ischemia on survival and intestinal failure. *Clin Gastroenterol Hepatol.* 2013;11(2):158–65.
18. Acosta S, Sonesson B, Resch T. Endovascular therapeutic approaches for acute superior mesenteric artery occlusion. *Cardiovasc Intervent Radiol.* 2009;32(5):896–905.

9 Acute Gastrointestinal Hemorrhage

Michael Darcy, MD and Alexander Ushinsky, MD

Introduction

Angiography and embolization are a critical component of the modern man-agement of gastrointestinal (GI) bleeding, not only providing important di-agnostic information but also potential lifesaving therapy. In general, these procedures can be performed with high level of success and low complication rates.

Indications

1. For upper GI bleeding (UGIB), endoscopy is usually the first approach because a diagnosis can be made in the majority of cases and the bleeding can be treated at the same time by injection, heater probe coagulation, etc. Angiography is usually not used for diagnosis but instead is used to manage ongoing hemorrhage (usually with embolization). Indications include the following:
   a. Bleeding so vigorous that the endoscopist is unable to define the source
   b. Bleeding not controllable by endoscopic therapy
   c. Patient unable to undergo endoscopy for medical or anatomic reasons
   d. Lack of availability of a qualified endoscopist
2. For lower GI bleeding (LGIB), colonoscopy is the preferred initial diagnostic and therapeutic intervention. In practice, colonoscopy for LGIB is technically chal-lenging due to lack of bowel prep or profound bleeding. Often angiography is requested in lieu of endoscopy to localize and stop bleeding (1). Angiography can also be used to identify the source of bleeding in planning for surgery. Situa-tions in which angiography, with planned embolization, is indicated include the following:
   a. Ongoing bleeding documented by computed tomography (CT) or tagged red blood cell (RBC) scan. Because these studies have better sensitivity for detect-ing bleeding, angiography is usually not indicated if these studies are nega-tive. These procedures can detect bleeding at rates of 0.1 mL per minute for tagged RBC scan, 0.3 mL per minute for CT (2), in contrast to 0.5 to 1.0 mL per minute for angiography.

b. For massive LGIB, one may proceed to angiography without waiting for a scan to confirm bleeding.

c. Angiography can be indicated to look for a structural lesion in patients with intermittent chronic LGIB.

Contraindications

Absolute

1. Given that angiography and embolization may be needed as lifesaving procedures, there are no absolute contraindications.
2. History of life-threatening contrast reaction is a serious contraindication, but rapid steroid preparation can be given if angiography is required to stop critical hemorrhage.

Relative

1. There are several relative contraindications that may help guide the decision to defer arteriography, especially if the indications are marginal in the first place.
   a. Renal insufficiency
   b. Contrast allergy
   c. Uncorrectable coagulopathy
   d. If the rate of bleeding is massive, surgery may be preferable to angiography because angiography may not be able to control the bleeding as quickly as surgery

Preprocedure Preparation

1. History and physical examination
   a. Adequate history may provide clues as to the source of bleeding. For example, history of recent polypectomy in a patient with LGIB would point to post polypectomy bleeding; significant recent vomiting in a person with UGIB would suggest a Mallory–Weiss tear.
   b. Other medical conditions (especially cardiac and pulmonary conditions and allergies) that might increase the risk of angiography should be assessed.
2. Ensure adequate monitoring
   a. Frequent blood pressure monitoring is essential because GIB patients can become hypotensive.
   b. Electrocardiogram (ECG), pulse oximetry, capnography—loss of blood and dilution of the blood pool by crystalloid infusion decreases the oxygen-carrying capacity of the blood, increasing the potential for cardiac ischemia, and possibly arrhythmias or infarcts.
   c. Body temperature—hypothermia due to exposure or transfusion of large amounts of fluid can induce coagulopathy by reducing the effectiveness of various clotting factors. Keep patients covered, use blood warmers, and consider use of warming blankets.
3. Resuscitation efforts—although resuscitation is critical, it cannot be performed as an isolated event prior to angiography. Some patients cannot be stabilized until the bleeding is actually stopped. Thus, angiographic therapy needs to be undertaken quickly, and resuscitation should be an ongoing process that continues into the angiography suite.
   a. Ensure adequate intravenous (IV) access for infusion of boluses of crystalloid or transfusion of blood. Typically, two large-gauge (16-gauge) IVs are recommended.
   b. Correct hypotension—in relatively compensated patients, resuscitation with crystalloid can be initiated. In critically ill patients, resuscitation with RBCs, plasma, and platelet transfusion in a ratio of 1:1:1 or whole blood is derived

from the trauma literature (1). A goal hemoglobin of 7 g/dL for most patients and 9 g/dL for cardiac patients is recommended.

c. Correct coagulopathy—embolization is much less effective when done in a coagulopathic patient because many embolic agents only partially occlude vessels and they rely on the clot formation they initiate to complete the vessel occlusion.

4. CT Angiogram (CTA). With rare exception, catheter angiography should not be done without prior CTA, done within the time of the acute bleeding episode (see Appendix 5 for CTA protocols). Catheter angiography is usually not indicated if CTA does not show active bleeding or a focal vascular abnormality. In addition it can provide anatomic information such as vessel tortuosity, or occlusive or aneurysmal disease which may influence route of access or catheter type, or even feasibility of endovascular treatment.

Procedure

1. Diagnostic angiography
   a. A sheath must be placed in the artery to avoid losing access if the angiographic catheter becomes occluded during embolization. A femoral artery approach is used in most cases, barring more proximal occlusions.
   b. Radial artery access has become increasingly utilized for angiographic interventions and may be the preferred approach where there is femoral occlusion or femoral access is considered high risk, for example morbid obesity or bleeding disorder.
   c. Aortograms are usually not performed because visualization of contrast extravasation into the GI tract requires more selective injection.
   d. The vessel selected first should be based on suspicion of the likely source of bleeding according to history, clinical signs, as well as localization provided by tagged RBC or CT scans. If there is no good clue as to the source, some prefer to select the inferior mesenteric artery (IMA) first to study the rectum before the overlying bladder fills with contrast. For suspected UGIB, the celiac and superior mesenteric arteries (SMAs) are the primary targets. For LGIB, the IMA and SMA need to be studied first. However, if these runs are negative, the celiac artery (e.g., gastroduodenal artery [GDA]) should be injected because rapid distal duodenal bleeding can present as LGIB. If extravasation is not seen on injection of the main trunks, more subselective injection may be needed. For duodenal or gastric fundus bleeding, the GDA, or left gastric arteries, respectively, should be studied. Choice of subselective injections can be guided by localization provided by CT, tagged RBC scan, or endoscopic findings.
   e. Contrast injections are at a rate of 5 to 6 mL per second for celiac and SMA, and 2 to 3 mL per second for the IMA. Four- to five-second long injections help maximize visualization of contrast extravasation while avoiding overlap between the arterial injection and the venous phase.
   f. Imaging should be continued until the venous phase has cleared out to help distinguish contrast extravasation from persistent venous opacification. Although digital subtraction angiography (DSA) is the standard technique, viewing the images in nonsubtracted mode is important to distinguish true extravasation from misregistration artifacts caused by respiratory or peristaltic motion. Use of glucagon (1 mg IV) before the angiogram can help reduce artifacts from bowel motion.
   g. Unfortunately, GI bleeding is often intermittent, and an angiogram may be negative even after positive CT or tagged RBC scans. CT is the preferred diagnostic test over tagged RBC scan due to better anatomic resolution and because RBC scan can be overly sensitive for slow bleeds which are undetectable at catheter angiogram.

h. If a bleeding source is not identified at angiogram, some authors advocate using provocative maneuvers such as infusion of vasodilators, heparin, or even thrombolytics such as tissue plasminogen activator (tPA) (3). The goal is to stimulate bleeding to allow the pathology to be localized, which will then allow treatment. In one series, these infusions helped identify the bleeding site in 31% of cases without causing any hemodynamic instability (3).

2. Vasopressin infusion to stop bleeding
   a. Vasopressin works by constricting the mesenteric vessels, thus reducing the blood flow to the site of bleeding potentially allowing stable clot to form at the bleed site.
   b. Compared to embolization, it has several disadvantages so is rarely used except when the patients are not a candidate for embolization, that is, a diffuse bleeding source or bleeding site inaccessible for embolization.
   c. Patient should be on continuous cardiac monitoring because vasopressin can induce coronary vasoconstriction.
   d. The angiographic catheter is positioned in the main trunk of the artery supplying the bleed. It should not be advanced selectively. Infusion is started at 0.1 units per minute.
   e. Repeat angiography is performed after 15 to 20 minutes to ensure that bleeding has stopped and that the vessels are not excessively constricted. If bleeding persists, dose is increased to 0.2 units per minute. Repeat the process and increase up to a maximum of 0.4 units per minute. DSA runs are repeated after each increment to see if the bleeding has stopped and to ensure that the vessels have not been overconstricted. On the DSA runs, contrast should flow through the vessels all the way to the antimesenteric wall of the bowel. If contrast does not flow to the bowel wall, stop, or decrease the infusion and repeat the arteriogram in 10 minutes to assess for excessive vasoconstriction. Excessive vasoconstriction can lead to bowel infarction.

3. Upper GI embolization
   a. The vessel supplying the bleed (usually GDA or left gastric arteries) should be subselectively catheterized. For left gastric bleeds, a common technique is embolization with Gelfoam (Pharmacia and Upjohn Co, Kalamazoo, MI), allowing blood flow to carry the particles to peripheral branches. For GDA bleeding, a microcatheter is usually advanced beyond the site of bleeding and the vessel is occluded there with either coils or Gelfoam to prevent backflow to the bleeding site. The catheter is then withdrawn depositing more emboli until the GDA is occluded back to its origin. Care must be taken when depositing the final embolus to avoid having coils or Gelfoam move in a retrograde manner out of the GDA causing nontarget embolization of the hepatic artery.
   b. In patients with coagulopathy, *n*-butyl cyanoacrylate (NBCA) glue or ethylene vinyl alcohol (EVOH) copolymer (Onyx; ev3 Endovascular Inc. Plymouth Minnesota) can be effectively used because they do not rely on the patient's ability to form stable clot; however, considerable technical expertise is required to use these agents and avoid nontarget embolization (4,5).
   c. Just placing coils at the vessel origin should be avoided because collaterals will rapidly reconstitute flow to the bleeding site beyond the coils.
   d. After GDA embolization, it is essential to do an SMA arteriogram to make sure there is no collateral flow to the bleeding via the pancreaticoduodenal arcade.
   e. Empiric embolization (embolizing a suspected target vessel even though extravasation was not seen on angiography) may be indicated if the site of bleeding is well localized by endoscopy. For example, the GDA may be embolized for a duodenal ulcer or the left gastric artery may be embolized if bleeding is localized to the fundus or gastroesophageal junction region.

4. Lower GI embolization
   a. Avoiding ischemic complications in lower GI embolization requires super-selective catheterization. After engaging the origin of the parent vessel with a 5-Fr angiographic catheter, a microcatheter (3 Fr or smaller) is advanced coaxially through the 5-Fr catheter. The microcatheter should be advanced as close as possible to the point of extravasation. For colonic bleeds, it is often possible to advance all the way into the vasa recta in the bowel wall.
   b. If the catheter can be advanced right up to the site of bleeding, a 0.018-in microcoil can be pushed through the microcatheter. Usually, only one or two microcoils are needed, and they should be short in length to avoid embolizing too large of a vascular territory.
   c. If the bleeding site is more diffuse (as from an angiodysplasia) or if the micro-catheter can be advanced close to but not right next to the bleed, then injec-tion of flow-directed polyvinyl alcohol (PVA) particles can be done. Care must be taken to inject only a very small amount of particles to avoid embolizing an excessively large arterial territory. Particles should be larger than 300 microns because smaller particles may travel too peripherally and are associated with a higher rate of bowel infarction.
   d. NBCA glue has been gaining increasing acceptance as an embolic agent for LGIB. NBCA has advantages of being a fluoroscopically visible, flow-directed agent that is more permanent than flow-directed particles. In addition, because it is occlusive without having to rely on thrombus formation, it works better in coagulopathic patients (5).
   e. EVOH copolymer is an alternative liquid embolic which is highly viscous and conforms to the vessel in a manner which does not depend on vascular flow. Limitations of this agent include its high cost, and 15- to 20-minute prepara-tion time (4).

Postprocedure Management

1. Routine postangiography orders/puncture site management
   a. Vital signs (VS) need to be taken frequently to look for any signs of new bleed-ing, such as a retroperitoneal hematoma that may be caused by an inadver-tent puncture above the inguinal ligament.
   b. The access site should be inspected for a hematoma with each VS check.
   c. Neurovascular checks of the extremity distal to the puncture site should be done to assess for arterial occlusion or distal embolization.
2. Assess if the GI bleeding has stopped.
   a. Follow VS looking for hemodynamic stability. Persistent hypotension or tachycardia could be signs of ongoing hemorrhage.
   b. Check serial hemoglobin and hematocrit levels.
   c. Follow the nature and volume of bloody output from GI tract, either naso-gastric (NG) aspirates for UGIB or degree of hematochezia/melena for LGIB. Realize that the colon is a large reservoir and has the capacity to hold a lot of blood. Thus, passage of blood per rectum may occur for some time after the bleeding has actually been controlled. This clinical finding must be taken in context. Continued active bleeding is unlikely if passage of dark blood occurs in a patient with stable VS and stable hematocrit.
3. Vasopressin infusion
   a. If a vasopressin infusion was started, the patient must be monitored in an intensive care unit (ICU) on continuous cardiac monitoring.
   b. The infusion should be continued in the ICU at the final starting rate for ap-proximately 12 hours. At that point, the infusion rate is decreased by 0.1 units per minute every 12 hours. After being at 0.1 units per minute for 12 hours, the vasopressin infusion is replaced with a saline infusion for several more hours. If there is no further evidence of bleeding, the catheter may be removed.

Results

1. Vasopressin
   a. Although vasopressin effectively stops bleeding in over 85% of cases of diverticular bleeding, the constrictive effect stops after the infusion is terminated. Rebleeding in as many as 50% of cases and the necessity for prolonged catheterization are why vasopressin infusions are rarely used (6).
2. Upper GI embolization
   a. Technical success is defined as the ability to deliver the embolic agent to the desired spot with termination of active bleeding. This is distinguished from clinical success because some patients have continued bleeding despite a technically successful embolization. This can be due to a diffuse source of bleeding (such as angiodysplasia), collateral flow around the therapeutic emboli, or coagulopathy preventing stable clot formation.
   b. Clinical success is considerably lower than technical success because of the multitude of collaterals in the celiac arterial system and because UGIB often arises from more diffuse processes such as gastritis. Control of bleeding may require additional intervention (7). Embolization performs comparably to surgery with regard to durable hemostasis and mortality in UGIB refractory to endoscopic treatment. A systematic review of 711 patients from 9 studies found that patients referred for embolization tended to have worse comorbidities, but although surgery was associated with lower rebleeding rates, there were no differences in mortality between the 2 treatments (8).
   c. Success after empiric embolization has been reported to be as good as embolization done after identification of extravasation. Rebleeding rates are comparable after empiric and targeted embolization, although it is not clear if mortality is similar or higher in those undergoing empiric rather than targeted embolization.
3. Lower GI embolization
   a. Technical success for lower GI embolization is high, greater than 90% (9). This is made possible by the use of microcatheters which can be advanced close to the bleed. Technical failure is most often due to vessel tortuosity or spasm preventing advancing the catheter to the desired point of embolization.
   b. Clinical success is reported as low as 75% with a proportion of patients rebleeding soon after embolization (9). Rebleeding after embolization is more common in the small bowel than in the colon. This is likely because there are more collateral vessels in the small bowel mesentery than in the colonic mesentery. Success also varies with the type of lesion being treated. Rebleeding may be less commonly seen with diverticular bleeds compared to patients with angiodysplasias. This is because diverticular bleeds usually have a simple single vasa recta arterial source, whereas angiodysplasias have multiple feeding arteries.

Complications

1. Standard complications common to all angiograms
   a. Puncture site bleeding or occlusion, and dissection of vessels, can occur but are rare.
   b. Contrast reactions.
2. Vasopressin complications
   a. Bowel infarction can occur but is rare.
   b. Cardiovascular complications including myocardial infarction (MI), arrhythmia, and hypertension (HTN) are most common and occur at a rate of 4.2%.
3. Embolization complications
   a. Nontarget embolization involves embolic material inadvertently passing into a vascular bed that was not the intended target. This may result from excessive pressure when injecting flow-directed particles or from buckling of the delivery catheter out of the target vessel during coil deployment. This complication is rare.

    b. End-organ ischemia as a result of embolization
        (1) This is extremely rare for UGIB embolization due to the rich collateral network around the stomach and duodenum. The potential for ischemia is increased if the patient has had prior upper GI surgery because collateral pathways may be disrupted.
        (2) After superselective embolization for LGIB, minor ischemic complications occur at a rate up to 20% but include self-limited abdominal pain, asymptomatic elevation of serum lactic acid levels, or asymptomatic mucosal changes discovered at follow-up endoscopy, most of which require no therapy. Major ischemic complications such as bowel infarction or ischemic strictures are uncommon occurring at a rate of 0% to 6% (6,10).
    c. Rare complications include coil erosion through the bowel wall.

Management of Complications

1. Puncture site complications (see Chapter 3)
    a. Hematomas are usually self-limited and require no treatment.
    b. Retroperitoneal hematoma with ongoing bleeding can be life threatening and may require surgical or endovascular repair of the puncture site. Surgery consult is indicated.
    c. Pseudoaneurysm of the puncture site can often be closed by ultrasound-guided injection of thrombin compression.
2. Contrast reactions (see Chapter 65).
3. Arterial dissection
    a. If a larger artery (such as an iliac artery) was dissected, it may be possible to place an intravascular stent to restore a patent lumen.
    b. For smaller vessels (<5 mm in diameter) stents may not be a good choice because of limited patency. Balloon angioplasty can be attempted to tack the dissection flap against the vessel wall but may also extend the dissection.
4. Nontarget embolization
    a. The need to treat the nontarget embolization depends on whether the errant emboli are lodged in a critical vessel or one that can be sacrificed. If noncritical (e.g., a distal hepatic arterial branch), the emboli should be left in place.
    b. If the nontarget embolic blocks a critical vessel, removal should be carefully attempted. Suction with a catheter can be used for some particulate emboli, but errant coils need to be retrieved with snares. If NBCA glue or Onyx gets into nontarget vessels, it cannot be removed. Thus, NBCA or Onyx should only be used by those with considerable expertise.
5. Ischemic complications
    a. Temporary changes such as self-limited abdominal pain or asymptomatic serum lactic acid elevation require no therapy.
    b. If true bowel infarction occurs, surgical resection is generally required.
    c. For more chronic ischemic complications such as bowel stricture, balloon dilation may be possible, but resection of the strictured bowel segment may be required if there is symptomatic obstruction.

References

1. Strate LL, Gralnek IM. ACG clinical guideline: management of patients with acute lower gastrointestinal bleeding. *Am J Gastroenterol.* 2016;111(4):459–474.
2. Kuhle WG, Sheiman RG. Detection of active colonic hemorrhage with use of helical CT: findings in a swine model. *Radiology.* 2003;228(3):743–752.
3. Kim CY, Suhocki PV, Miller MJ Jr, et al. Provocative mesenteric angiography for lower gastrointestinal hemorrhage: results from a single-institution study. *J Vasc Interv Radiol.* 2010;21(4):477–783.

4. Kolber MK, Shukla PA, Kumar A, et al. Ethylene vinyl alcohol copolymer (onyx) emboliza-tion for acute hemorrhage: a systematic review of peripheral applications. *J Vasc Interv Radiol.* 2015;26(6):809–815.
5. Kim PH, Tsauo J, Shin JH, et al. Transcatheter arterial embolization of gastrointestinal bleeding with N-butyl cyanoacrylate: a systematic review and meta-analysis of safety and efficacy. *J Vasc Interv Radiol.* 2017;28(4):522–531.e5.
6. Darcy M. Treatment of lower gastrointestinal bleeding: vasopressin infusion versus embo-lization. *J Vasc Interv Radiol.* 2003;14(5):535–543.
7. Padia SA, Geisinger MA, Newman JS, et al. Effectiveness of coil embolization in angiograph-ically detectable versus non-detectable sources of upper gastrointestinal hemorrhage. *J Vasc Interv Radiol.* 2009;20(4):461–466.
8. Beggs AD, Dilworth MP, Powell SL, et al. A systematic review of transarterial embolization versus emergency surgery in treatment of major nonvariceal upper gastrointestinal bleed-ing. *Clin Exp Gastroenterol.* 2014;7:93–104.
9. Hur S, Jae HJ, Lee M, et al. Safety and efficacy of transcatheter arterial embolization for lower gastrointestinal bleeding: a single-center experience with 112 patients. *J Vasc Interv Radiol.* 2014;25(1):10–19.
10. Nykanen T, Peltola E, Kylanpaa L, et al. Transcatheter arterial embolization in lower gas-trointestinal bleeding: ischemia remains a concern even with a superselective approach. *J Gastrointest Surg.* 2018;22(8):1394–1403.

10 Aortoiliac Interventions

Jessica H. Yoon, MD, MBA, Sun Ho Ahn, MD, FSIR, and Timothy P. Murphy, MD

Introduction

Peripheral arterial disease (PAD) is a progressive common medical disease with a presentation that can vary from asymptomatic to extremity gangrene. Since the first percutaneous transluminal revascularization was performed by Dotter and Judkins in 1964, revolutionary changes have occurred in manage-ment of PAD. With advances in angioplasty and stents, endovascular manage-ment has become the mainstay therapy for aortoiliac arterial occlusive disease.

Indications

1. Disabling or lifestyle altering intermittent claudication—often reported using the Rutherford Classification of Chronic Limb Ischemia (Table 10.1)—that is refrac-tory to medical therapy and lifestyle modifications
   a. Rutherford 3: severe intermittent claudication
   b. Rutherford ≥4: critical limb ischemia as evidenced by persistent severe pain +/− tissue loss
2. The TransAtlantic Inter-Society Consensus (TASC) provides a general algorithm for surgical versus endovascular management of aortoiliac disease (TASC II) based on lesion morphology and location (Table 10.2). While TASC II type C and D lesions have traditionally been surgically managed, more and more data support the efficacy of long-term endovascular repair. Thus, first-line endovascular treat-ment is indicated in nearly all cases of aortoiliac disease with surgery indicated for those who fail endovascular treatment.
3. Historically, angioplasty was reserved for concentric, noncalcified, short (<3 cm) lesions and primary stent placement was recommended for complex stenosis and chronic total occlusions (CTOs). Secondary stent placement was indicated

Table 10.1 Rutherford Classification for Chronic Limb Ischemia		
Category	Clinical Presentation	Objective Data
0	Asymptomatic	Normal treadmill test
1	Mild claudication	Completes treadmill test—ankle pressure (AP) <50 mm Hg and >20 mm Hg less than resting AP after test
2	Moderate claudication	Between 1 and 3
3	Severe claudication	Cannot complete treadmill test—AP <50 mm Hg after test
4	Ischemic rest pain	Resting AP <40 mm Hg, flat or barely pulsatile ankle pulse volume recording; toe pressure <30 mm Hg
5	Minor tissue loss—nonhealing ulcer, focal gangrene, diffuse pedal edema	Resting AP <60 mm Hg, flat or barely pulsatile ankle pulse volume recording; toe pressure <40 mm Hg
6	Major tissue loss—extending above transmetatarsal, functional foot no longer salvageable	Same as category 5

Sabri SS, Choudhri A, Orgera G, et al. Outcomes of covered kissing stent placement compared with bare metal stent placement in the treatment of atherosclerotic occlusive disease at the aortic bifurcation. *J Vasc Interv Radiol.* 2010;21(7):995–1003.

for technically unsuccessful angioplasty (mean residual gradient >5 mm Hg or greater than 30% residual stenosis) and complications, including flow-limiting dissection and vessel perforation.

4. Current endovascular practice typically utilizes a primary stenting strategy.

Contraindications

There are no absolute contraindications. Relative contraindications to arteriography apply to aortoiliac endovascular interventions.
1. Uncorrectable coagulopathy
2. History of life-threatening iodinated contrast allergy/reaction
3. Severe non–dialysis-dependent renal insufficiency

Preprocedure Preparation

1. History and physical examination should be performed, with a focus on the vascular system. The operator should perform the peripheral vascular examination and document pulses in the bilateral extremities.
2. Claudicants should demonstrate failure of medical therapy including a supervised exercise program, where possible, and cilostazol for at least 3 months.
3. Pertinent noninvasive imaging (pulse volume recording [PVR], multilevel segmental lower extremity brachial indices, computed tomographic angiography [CTA], or magnetic resonance angiography [MRA]) should be reviewed or obtained if necessary.
4. Preprocedure laboratory evaluations should include platelet count, estimated glomerular filtration rate (eGFR), and coagulation profile.
5. Baseline ankle-brachial index (ABI) should be obtained prior to the procedure.
6. Appropriate evaluation for conscious sedation per American Society of Anesthesiologists (ASA) guidelines should be performed.
7. Patients should be "no oral intake" per institutional protocol.
8. Morning insulin dose should be reduced to half as appropriate.

Table 10.2   TASC II Classification for Aortoiliac Disease (7)

1. Type A—Endovascular treatment is the treatment of choice
   a. Unilateral or bilateral stenosis of common iliac artery (CIA)
   b. Unilateral or bilateral single-short stenosis of external iliac artery (EIA) (≤3 cm)
2. Type B—Endovascular treatment is preferred
   a. Short (≤3 cm) stenosis of infrarenal aorta
   b. Unilateral CIA occlusion
   c. Single or multiple stenoses up to 3–10 cm of EIA not extending into common femoral artery (CFA)
   d. Unilateral EIA occlusion not involving the origins of internal iliac artery (IIA) or CFA
3. Type C
   a. Bilateral CIA occlusions
   b. Bilateral EIA stenosis, 3–10 cm long not extending into CFA
   c. Unilateral EIA stenosis extending into CFA
   d. Unilateral EIA occlusion involving the origins of IIA and/or CFA
   e. Heavily calcified unilateral EIA occlusion with or without involvement of origins of IIA and/or CFA
4. Type D
   a. Infrarenal aortoiliac occlusion
   b. Diffuse disease of aorta and both iliac arteries requiring treatment
   c. Diffuse multiple stenoses involving unilateral CIA, EIA, CFA
   d. Unilateral occlusions of both CIA and EIA
   e. Bilateral occlusions of EIA
   f. Iliac stenosis in patients with abdominal aortic aneurysm (AAA) requiring treatment not amenable to endograft or other lesions requiring open aortic or iliac surgery

Bosch JL, Hunink MG. Meta-analysis of the results of percutaneous transluminal angioplasty and stent placement for aortoiliac occlusive disease. *Radiology.* 1997;204(1):87–96.

9. If a contrast allergy exists—steroid pretreatment should be given (see Chapter 65: Contrast Media Reactions: Treatment and Risk Reduction).
10. Most patients with PAD are likely on a sole antiplatelet or dual antiplatelet regimen of aspirin and/or clopidogrel.
11. Urinary bladder catheter is usually placed prior to the procedure.
12. Sterile preparation, including surgical clipping, of both inguinal regions and/or arm is performed.
13. Procedures are performed under conscious sedation with incremental intravenous aliquots of midazolam and fentanyl with hemodynamic and respiratory monitoring.
14. Prophylactic antibiotics are not routinely administered.

Procedure

Diagnostic Arteriogram

1. CFA access is preferred. Left arm access may be required on occasion. If preprocedure imaging indicates stenoses primarily in the external iliac artery, contralateral CFA access may be preferable. If disease is primarily located in the common iliac artery, ipsilateral CFA access is preferred. A second CFA access may be required, especially in the case of ostial CIA lesions, or inability to traverse a chronic occlusion from the initial approach.
2. Ultrasound-guided CFA access is now routine. Care should be made to avoid inadvertent ultrasound creep and access of the EIA. Fluoroscopically guided puncture of CFA using landmarks and/or vessel calcifications can also be performed. Preprocedure CTA or MRA can assist in determining optimal access.
3. A diagnostic arteriogram of the infrarenal aorta and lower extremity(ies) should be performed. The diagnostic arteriogram may be tailored depending on preoperative CTA or MRA findings and/or in the presence of renal insufficiency to reduce contrast load.

4. Lesion significance can be determined by hemodynamic gradient measurements or diameter reduction measurement. In general, a resting mean transstenotic gradient ≥5 mm Hg or a systolic gradient >10 mm Hg is considered significant. Following augmentation by a vasodilator (e.g., 100-μg nitroglycerin given intraarterially), a mean gradient >10 mm Hg or systolic gradient >20 mm Hg is significant. Diameter reduction >50% is considered significant. Hemodynamic measurements across total occlusions are unnecessary.
5. Pressure gradients are considered the gold standard and can be measured by several methods.
   a. Double access simultaneous measurement above and below the lesion is most accurate.
   b. Coaxial simultaneous measurement requires a 2-Fr-sized difference between the sheath and the catheter.
   c. Pullback pressures may be unreliable and affected by temporal variation in blood pressure.
   d. Pressure wires may be more accurate in smaller-sized arteries due to less flow reduction by the catheter or the sheath but add to the cost and procedure time.

Techniques General to All Interventions
1. Once the determination to intervene has been made, systemic anticoagulation is achieved with intravenous heparin unless contraindicated. Activated clotting time (ACT) during the procedure can be done with a working goal of 250 seconds.
2. Intervention should be performed through an appropriately sized sheath. A 6-Fr sheath can accommodate most stents and balloons used in the iliac system. For contralateral intervention, a long sheath (e.g., Pinnacle Destination, Terumo Medical, Somerset, NJ; or BRITE TIP, Cordis, Bridgewater, NJ) should be advanced over the bifurcation.
3. The lesion must be crossed. Most stenoses can be negotiated with a long taper (LT) straight guidewire and an angled-tip catheter. More complex stenoses may require a steerable hydrophilic guidewire (e.g., Glidewire, Terumo Medical, Somerset, NJ) with a directable catheter (e.g., Kumpe, Cook Medical, Bloomington, IN).
4. CIA lesions, especially ostial, are best treated by an ipsilateral approach, whereas EIA lesions are best treated by a contralateral approach.
5. After lesion traversal, an appropriate-sized sheath should be placed across the lesion over an exchange guidewire. An angioplasty balloon or stent is then positioned at the lesion and the sheath is retracted. Angioplasty or stent placement is then performed.
6. After an intervention, an arteriogram is performed to determine technical success (<30% residual stenosis) and to exclude complications (i.e., arterial rupture, dissection, distal embolization, etc.).
7. Postprocedure pressure gradient may be performed. Less than 5 mm Hg mean gradient after intervention defines technical success.
8. Puncture site hemostasis, with manual compression or a closure device, is achieved after the effects of anticoagulation have expired (1 to 2 hours, partial thromboplastin time [PTT] <1.5 times normal, or ACT <160 seconds).
9. *Pearls*
   a. Always maintain guidewire purchase across the treated lesion until completion angiogram. This will preserve treatment options in case of complication such as dissection or rupture.
   b. Minimize the number of lesion traversals with wires and catheters to avoid potential distal embolization.

Angioplasty Technique
1. Angioplasty balloon is positioned to cover the lesion. Appropriate placement of the balloon usually can be confirmed with contrast injection via the sheath just prior to deployment, but fluoroscopic landmarks or digital road mapping can also be done.

2. Angioplasty balloon is inflated with an inflation device until the waist is resolved. In general, 8 atm is sufficient; however, if greater than 10 atm is required, beware of potential arterial rupture especially if the patient reports significant pain during balloon inflation. Persistent pain after balloon deflation can be indicative of arterial rupture, and if present, an immediate angiogram of the angioplasty site is warranted.

3. Postangioplasty arteriogram is performed to assess technical success, failure, and complications. If a residual stenosis (>30%) or flow-limiting dissection is present, a repeat prolonged dilation or stent placement may be required.

Stent Placement Technique (Fig. 10.1)

1. Stent diameter should be chosen with consideration for intimal hyperplasia, which may narrow the lumen by, on average, a millimeter. Stent length should be sufficient to cover the entire lesion. Care must be taken when using self-expanding (SE) stents, which tend to foreshorten after deployment. Measurements can be obtained from a prior CTA or by using digital angiography software calibrated to an internal standard or marker catheters.

2. Stent positioning can be confirmed with road mapping or contrast injection. The vascular sheath is retracted and stent is deployed. For balloon-mounted stents, care should be given to ensure that stent does not become dislodged when

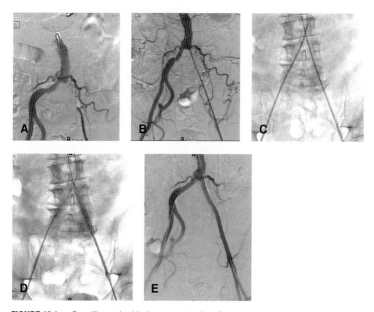

FIGURE 10.1 • Case illustrating kissing stent technique for complete left common iliac artery occlusion and stenotic right common iliac artery. **A:** Digital subtraction angiogram shows complete left common iliac artery occlusion and stenosis of right common iliac artery. Corresponding waveforms taken at right common femoral artery (118/51) and left common femoral artery (60/46). **B:** DSA demonstrating bilateral catheters extending to the distal aorta. It is important to take note of the IMA takeoff and other branching vessels to avoid obstruction if possible. **C:** Positioning of balloon-expandable covered stents. Real-time hand-injection was performed to confirm positioning (not shown). **D:** Simultaneous balloon inflation, taking care to keep balloon pressures equal during deployment. **E:** DSA after stent deployment demonstrating near-equal flow through bilateral common iliac arteries.

traversing the lesion or aortic bifurcation. Minimize this risk by crossing the lesion with a vascular sheath that has an adequate inner diameter to ensure the safe passage of the stent.

3. SE stents can be landed accurately at the distal external iliac artery more easily when placed from a contralateral access. Conversely, they can be placed more accurately for a proximal common iliac artery lesion when placed ipsilaterally.

4. Traversal of the lesion with the sheath and dilator "dotters" the stenosis and thus balloon predilation is rarely required.

5. Balloon-mounted stents are expanded with the provided balloon, using an inflator that has a pressure gauge. For SE stents, withdrawing the outer sleeve covering the collapsed stent on the delivery catheter initiates deployment. When unsheathing the SE stent, the hand holding the inner catheter should be stationary to avoid the tendency to advance the stent during deployment. Some SE stents may have measured incremental retraction systems such as a wheel. Some nitinol stents are known to "lurch" forward if redundancy isn't removed from the introducer catheter prior to unsheathing, so it is recommended with these devices to advance the catheter beyond the desired location and then retract the entire device into position prior to unsheathing.

6. SE stents usually require postdeployment dilation with a balloon.

7. As with angioplasty, a poststent arteriogram is mandatory.

8. Lower extremity run-off or in-suite peripheral vascular clinical examination should be performed to assess for distal thromboembolic complications.

Available Stents

1. There is a myriad of available stents for use in the aortoiliac segment and a detailed analysis is beyond the scope of this chapter. The general categories of stents are SE, balloon-expandable (BE), and stent grafts (SGs).

2. *SE stents* are composed of nitinol and possess shape memory. They are compressed into a delivery catheter and are delivered by unsheathing.
   a. Advantages: SE stents generally possess greater flexibility, conformability, and trackability. Their elasticity allows them to be placed in segments that may experience intermittent external compression.
   b. Disadvantages: SE stents generally have lower hoop strength than BE stents, and due to foreshortening are more difficult to precisely place, for example, at bifurcation or ostial locations.
   c. Examples of SE stents (selective list and not exhaustive): Zilver (Cook, Bloomington, IN) (Fig. 10.2A), Absolute Pro (Abbott Vascular, Santa Clara, CA), Luminexx (C.R. Bard, Covington, GA), SMART (Cordis Endovascular, Miami Lakes, FL)

3. *BE stents* are typically premounted on a balloon. Larger sizes (>14 mm), may need hand mounting, should be placed on an appropriate-sized scratch-resistant balloon using a crimper or by hand.
   a. Advantages: BE stents possess stronger radial force, the ability for precise placement, and superior radiopacity.
   b. Disadvantages: BE stents have the potential for dislodgment from the balloon, are more rigid, and possess plastic deformity. Use of a sheath as suggested earlier should minimize stent dislodgment. Rigidity may be detrimental in tortuous arteries. Finally, BE stents undergo plastic deformation that make them unsuitable in areas subject to external compression.
   c. Examples of BE stents (selective list and not exhaustive): PALMAZ (Cordis Endovascular, Miami Lakes, FL), Express LD (Boston Scientific, Natick, MA), Omnilink Elite (Abbott Vascular, Santa Clara, CA) Assurant (Medtronic, Minneapolis, MN).

4. *Covered stents* are generally composed of synthetic material such as polyethylene terephthalate (e.g., Dacron) or extruded polytetrafluoroethylene (PTFE) covering or lining a stent. They may be SE or BE depending on the properties of the stent scaffold.

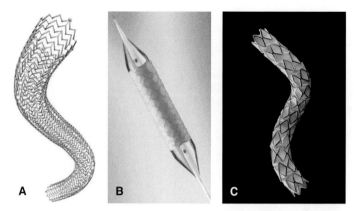

FIGURE 10.2 • Examples of stents commonly used for common iliac stent disease. **A:** Zilver SE stent. **B:** Atrium iCAST stent. **C:** Gore Viabahn VBX.

    a. Advantages: SGs are theorized to limit restenosis by their barrier effect and are essential for the treatment of arterial rupture or aneurysms.
    b. Disadvantages: They require a larger delivery system and increase device cost.
    c. Examples (selective list and not exhaustive): Atrium iCAST (BE) (Getinge, Goteborg, Sweden) (Fig. 10.2B), VIABAHN (SE) (W.L. GORE, Flagstaff, AZ), and VIABAHN VBX (BE) (W.L. GORE, Flagstaff, AZ).

Stent Selection
Choose an appropriate stent based on lesion characteristics (diameter, location, length, calcification, and eccentricity).
1. Diameter—Usually, stent diameters of 10 to 15 mm in the aorta (although in some cases, an 8-mm diameter is satisfactory, e.g., small, elderly person with critical limb ischemia and severe aortic stenosis), 8 to 10 mm in the CIA, and 7 to 9 mm in the EIA are desirable. The lumen diameter achieved after stent placement usually will be reduced by 0.5 to 1 mm by the development of neointimal hyperplasia within the stent, and this must be considered when sizing stents.
2. Location—Data suggest placement of covered BE stents for CIA ostial stenosis. For aortic bifurcation lesions, BE stents may also be preferred for their superior radial strength and precise placement ability.
3. Length—Short, focal lesions are ideal for BE stents. Longer lesions or occlusions are better treated by SE stents. Although multiple BE stents can be overlapped to treat diffuse iliac artery stenoses, their inelasticity prevents motion in the stented artery. Pulsatile wall motion produces strains within the stents, which may result in stent fracture due to metal fatigue. Alternatively, if the stents are not overlapped but are placed contiguously in close proximity, stent motion may result in shearing of the artery and pseudoaneurysm formation in the gaps between stents.
4. Calcification and eccentricity—Calcified and/or eccentric atherosclerotic plaques generally require a stent with higher radial force, that is, BE stents.

Special Situations
1. Chronic total occlusions (Fig. 10.3)
    a. Most CTOs can be successfully treated with endovascular methods. Most occlusions are traversed using an angled-tip hydrophilic guidewire and a directable catheter. Specialty crossing wires and devices can be utilized, but are not typically needed.

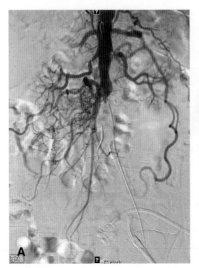
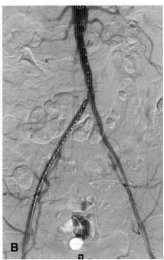

FIGURE 10.3 • A 78-year-old female with left lower extremity rest pain. Preprocedure LLE ABI of 0.2. **A:** DSA of abdominal aorta demonstrating complete occlusion of distal aorta, aortic bifurcation, and bilateral common iliac arteries. *(Not shown: Careful crossing of the occlusion from bilateral CFA access. Balloon-expandable stenting of distal abdominal aorta and bilateral common iliac arteries via kissing stent technique into the distal aortic stent.)* **B:** Poststenting angiogram demonstrating opacification of the distal abdominal aorta and bilateral common iliac arteries. Please note, pre-stent imaging demonstrates significant collateral arterialization, which is no longer seen post-stenting.

b. In long occlusions where guidewire traversal is easily performed, a trial of thrombolysis may reduce the length of occlusion, reveal stenosis, reduce potential for emboli, and improve stent wall apposition. Disadvantages include increased procedure time, prolonged hospitalization, presence of chronic thrombus resistant to thrombolysis, and risks of bleeding. Because of the chronic nature of CTOs, routine prestent thrombolysis has fallen out of favor.

c. Subintimal wire passage may be unavoidable in some cases. This is acceptable as long as reentry into the true lumen is gained. This may require approaching the occlusion simultaneously from both antegrade and retrograde directions.

(1) Modified "wire-loop" technique—If a wire but not a catheter can be passed, the wire can be snared from a contralateral approach and be tightly fixed from both ends to pass a catheter.

(2) Sharp needle recanalization may be required in certain situations when a wire cannot be passed into the true lumen. When attempting sharp needle recanalization, (a) a compliant balloon is inflated as a target, (b) the distance between the target balloon and the sharp needle should be minimized, (c) indentation effect on the balloon should be confirmed and viewed on multiple projections, and (d) contrast should be injected in the tract prior to stent placement to ensure that the location is subintimal and has not perforated the artery.

(3) Reentry devices (e.g., Outback Ltd, Cordis Endovascular, Miami Lakes, FL) or intravascular ultrasound (IVUS) may be useful.

2. Aortic bifurcation lesions

a. These include stenosis and/or occlusion involving the origin(s) of the CIA(s) and a distal abdominal aortic plaque extending to the ostia of the CIA(s). A supporting stent may be required in the contralateral CIA even if there is no hemodynamically significant stenosis. This is so the contralateral stent may protect the nonstenotic ostium from compression by the therapeutic stent and may also minimize turbulent flow. Alternatively, a low compliance angioplasty balloon can be inflated in the nonstenotic CIA to stabilize stent placement and protect the unaffected ostium.

b. Technique—Stent placement in the distal abdominal aorta should be done only after consideration of the origin of the inferior mesenteric artery (IMA) and the status of the superior mesenteric, celiac, and hypogastric arteries. Ideally, the intervention should preserve the IMA origin; however, this is not always possible. An appropriate length vascular sheath should be inserted via each CFA. Digital road mapping or real-time hand injection through one of the sheaths is critical for precise deployment of stents at the aortic bifurcation. Ideal positioning of stents is less than 5 mm cephalad to the aortic bifurcation. Extending the stents into the aorta should be limited as that reduces the durability of the procedural result. Stents should be deployed using a "kissing stent technique," that is, simultaneous balloon inflation while attempting to keep inflation pressures equal during deployment.

3. Coexistent CFA stenosis—In cases with CFA stenosis, in addition to ipsilateral iliac artery disease, CFA endarterectomy should be considered to preserve durability of the iliac intervention. Surgery should ideally be done at the time of, or at the least during the same hospital admission as, the aortoiliac intervention to reduce the risk of stent thrombosis. Alternatively, percutaneous transluminal (balloon) angioplasty (PTA) or atherectomy may be considered for CFA lesions.

Postprocedure Management

1. Most patients with uncomplicated interventions may be safely discharged the same day of the procedure, although some may require overnight observation.
2. Serial vascular examinations and ABI are performed in the recovery area.
3. In the presence of renal insufficiency, the authors perform overnight hydration.
4. Patients are seen in follow-up in the office within 1 to 4 weeks and then longitudinally.
5. Antiplatelet medications and regimen
   a. There are not yet definitive recommendations for the use and duration of single versus dual antiplatelet administration *after* stent placement.
   b. The VOYAGER PAD trial (2020) demonstrated a statistically significant benefit of aspirin and 2.5 mg of rivaroxaban over aspirin alone in reducing incidence of acute limb ischemia, major amputation for vascular causes, myocardial infarction, ischemic stroke, and death from CV causes in patients who had undergone lower extremity revascularization (1).
   c. The authors of this chapter routinely continue 75 mg of clopidogrel for 1 to 3 months and 81 mg or 325 mg of aspirin indefinitely.
6. Smoking cessation, lipid optimization, and blood pressure reduction should be pursued, either by the treating interventionist or in conjunction with the primary care physician.
7. All patients with PAD should be on a statin, regardless of lipid profile, with few exceptions (e.g., chronic liver disease, statin-induced myopathies).
8. If patient was on cilostazol preprocedure, this should be continued.

Results

Intervention, Medical Therapy, and Exercise
1. Stenting technical success and patency
   a. Overall high technical success varying somewhat with lesion type (2,3)
      (1) TASC A to C, 94% to 100%; TASC D, 85% to 95%
   b. Primary patency rates vary between reports but overall are 90%, 75%, 70%, and 50% at 1, 3, 5, and 10 years, respectively. Long-term secondary patency

rates are substantially higher—90%, 80%, and 65% at 3, 5, and 10 years, respectively (3,4).

   c. Recent data demonstrate traditionally complex lesions (TASC C/D) have similar patency rates at up to 95% (3).

   d. Balloon angioplasty alone has lower patency rates compared with stenting with 75%, 60%, and 50% primary patency at 1, 3, and 5 years.

2. Claudication: Exercise versus Endoluminal Revascularization (CLEVER) prospective randomized trial (5)

   a. There were 111 patients randomly assigned to optimal medical care (OMC group), supervised exercise plus optimal medical care (SE group), or stent revascularization plus optimal medical care (ST group).

   b. Change in peak walking time for SE was significantly greater than ST. Both were significantly greater than OMC.

   c. Quality-of-life measurements and validated walking scores are greater for ST than SE.

   d. Supervised exercise programs have been increasing in availability and insurance coverage, mainly Medicare.

3. Meta-analysis has shown improved ABI and treadmill walking times when stenting is added to medical therapy and supervised exercise. However, there was no significant difference between stenting alone and supervised exercise alone.

Stenting versus Angioplasty

1. The Dutch Iliac Stent Trial (DIST) randomized patients to primary angioplasty with secondary stent placement, or primary stent placement for iliac disease (6).

   a. There was no significant difference in short-term or long-term patency.

   b. However, the primary PTA with selective stent group had a high number of secondary stent placement (43%) and higher complication rates (4% vs. 7%).

2. Meta-analysis of 14 series (6 angioplasty and 8 stent) of 2,116 patients showed better results with stent placement compared with angioplasty (7).

   a. Technical success rate was higher for stent group: 96% versus 91%.

   b. Four-year patency rate was higher for stent group: 77% versus 64%.

   c. Complications and mortality rates were not significantly different.

Covered Stent Grafts versus Bare-Metal Stents

1. Prospective, randomized trial comparing covered BE SG versus BMS (Covered vs. Balloon-Expandable Stent Trial [COBEST]) (8)

   a. Freedom from restenosis greater with SG than BMS at 18 months (95.4% vs. 82.2%) to 60 months (74.7% vs. 62.5%).

   b. Subgroup analysis revealed significantly higher patency and survival benefit for TASC C and D lesions treated with SGs (HR 8.639).

   c. Fewer patients in SG group received target limb revascularization (OR 2.32).

   d. There was no statistically significant difference in rates of subsequent amputations.

2. Conversely, a retrospective study compared SG and BE BMS in 162 patients (9).

   a. Three-year primary patency (89% vs. 72%), assisted primary patency (98% vs. 90%), and secondary patency (98% vs. 92%) all significantly better in the BE BMS group.

   b. SG 2.5 times more likely to require repeat intervention.

3. Emerging data suggest SE may be more suitable for iliac artery occlusions than BE.

   a. The randomized ICE trial (Iliac Artery Stents for Common or External Iliac Artery Occlusive Disease, based in Europe) compared BE stents versus SE in 660 patients (10)

     (1) 12-month primary patency were 94.5% for SE versus 87.0% in BE.

     (2) Restenosis rate at 12 months for SE was superior to BE (6.1% vs. 14.9%).

     (3) No statistical difference in rates of target limb amputation, cardiovascular death, or stroke.

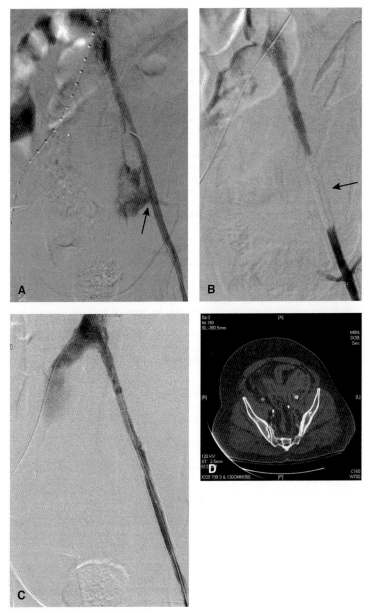

FIGURE 10.4 • Left EIA rupture. **A:** Poststent placement angiogram reveals brisk extravasation of contrast from the EIA (*arrow*). **B:** Balloon was immediately placed for tamponade (*arrow*). Contrast injection from above and below confirming correct placement and adequate tamponade. **C:** No further extravasation after stent-graft placement. **D:** Axial CT demonstrating EIA stent with surrounding hematoma. Patient recovered well and is without claudication at 2 years.

Complications and Management

1. Society of Interventional Radiology (SIR) definition of major complications—those complications requiring therapy or minor hospitalization (<48 hours); require major therapy, unexpected increase in level of care, or prolonged hospitalization; result in permanent sequelae or death.
2. A meta-analysis of 1,300 iliac PTA and 816 iliac stent patients showed all-inclusive 30-day mortality rates of 1% and 0.8%, respectively. The rates of major complications requiring therapy for PTA and stent groups were 4.3% and 5.2% (7).
3. Major complications include arterial rupture, dissection, thromboses, distal embolization, access site hematoma and pseudoaneurysm, and stent infections.
   a. Arterial ruptures (Fig. 10.4)
      (1) Aortoiliac interventions are rarely complicated by arterial ruptures. Rates between 0.8% and 0.9% have been reported.
      (2) Usually diagnosed during the procedure as patients may report persistent pain after intervention, or extravasation of contrast may be seen. Patient resuscitation should begin immediately with intravenous fluids, pressure support medications, reversal of anticoagulation with protamine sulfate, and transfusions as required. A balloon covering the rupture site should be simultaneously inflated to a low pressure (3 to 4 atm), and contrast should be injected above and below to ensure appropriate seal. An SG may be required to exclude the rupture. Emergent surgical management may be needed, if the above fails.
   b. Dissections: may occur during catheterization, PTA, or stenting. If a flow limitation is seen, the flap may be sealed with PTA or a stent.
   c. Distal embolization: Most emboli may be resolved with catheter suction, aspiration devices (e.g., AngioJet [Boston Scientific, Natick, MA] and Indigo System [Penumbra Medical, Alameda, CA]), and thrombolytics. Traditional surgical open thrombectomy may be required in severe rare cases.
   d. Access site pseudoaneurysm and hematoma: See Chapter 4: Management of Vascular Complications.
   e. Stent infections: occur rarely but may have devastating results including limb loss or death. Fever, pain, and positive blood cultures are clues for stent infection. Pseudoaneurysm formation and sepsis may ensue. Aggressive antibiotic administration is imperative, and surgical exploration may be warranted.

References

1. Bonaca MP, Bauersachs RM, Anand SS, et al. Rivaroxaban in peripheral artery disease after revascularization. *N Engl J Med.* 2020;382(21):1994–2004.
2. Ye W, Liu CW, Ricco JB, et al. Early and late outcomes of percutaneous treatment of transatlantic inter-society consensus class C and D aorto-iliac lesions. *J Vasc Surg.* 2011; 53(6):1728–1737.
3. Bracale UM, Giribono AM, Spinelli D, et al. Long-term results of endovascular treatment of TASC C and D aortoiliac occlusive disease with expanded polytetrafluoroethylene stent graft. *Ann Vasc Surg.* 2019;56:254–260. doi:10.1016/j.avsg.2018.07.060
4. Schürmann K, Mahnken A, Meyer J, et al. Long-term results 10 years after iliac arterial stent placement. *Radiology.* 2002;224(3):731–738.
5. Murphy TP, Cutlip DE, Regensteiner JG, et al. Supervised exercise versus primary stenting for claudication resulting from aortoiliac peripheral artery disease: six-month outcomes from the claudication: exercise versus endoluminal revascularization (CLEVER) study. *Circulation.* 2012;125(1):130–139.
6. Tetteroo E, van der Graaf Y, Bosch JL, et al. Randomised comparison of primary stent placement versus primary angioplasty followed by selective stent placement in patients with iliac-artery occlusive disease. Dutch Iliac Stent Trial Study Group. *Lancet.* 1998;351(9110):1153–1159.
7. Bosch JL, Hunink MG. Meta-analysis of the results of percutaneous transluminal angioplasty and stent placement for aortoiliac occlusive disease. *Radiology.* 1997;204(1):87–96.

8. Mwipatayi BP, Sharma S, Daneshmand A, et al. Durability of the balloon-expandable covered versus bare-metal stents in the Covered versus Balloon Expandable Stent Trial (COBEST) for the treatment of aortoiliac occlusive disease. *J Vasc Surg.* 2016;64(1):83–94.e1. doi:10.1016/j.jvs.2016.02.064
9. Humphries MD, Armstrong E, Laird J, et al. Outcomes of covered versus bare-metal balloon-expandable stents for aortoiliac occlusive disease. *J Vasc Surg.* 2014;60(2):337–343.
10. Krankenberg H, Zeller T, Ingwersen M, et al. Self-expe12wanding versus balloon-expandable stents for iliac artery occlusive disease: the randomized ICE trial. *JACC: Cardiovas Interven.* 2017;10(16)1694–1704.

11 Superficial Femoral Artery Interventions

Andrew S. Niekamp, MD, Ripal T. Gandhi, MD, FSVM, and James F. Benenati, MD

Introduction

Technology has rapidly advanced in the last several years, and the endovascular options available to treat superficial femoral artery (SFA) disease have markedly increased. Although percutaneous transluminal angioplasty (PTA) was previously considered the initial therapy for treatment of femoropopliteal disease, this therapy has largely been replaced with a wide variety of treatment options such as bare-metal stents (BMS), covered stents, drug-eluting stents (DES), and drug-coated balloons (DCBs). Atherectomy can be performed as an adjunct and may be valuable in the treatment of in-stent restenosis. As new clinical trials emerge, the precise role of each of these new technologies in the ever-expanding SFA endovascular landscape continues to evolve.

Indications

1. Lifestyle-limiting moderate to severe claudication (Fontaine category IIb, Rutherford stages 2 and 3) in patients who have failed medical management (i.e., cilostazol and/or exercise program)
2. Critical limb ischemia (CLI) characterized by rest pain, nonhealing ulcerations, or gangrene
3. Pre- or postbypass surgery to increase inflow or outflow
4. Salvage of failing bypass graft with significant flow-limiting stenosis of the anastomosis or outflow vessels

Contraindications

There are no absolute contraindications to endovascular therapy for the SFA. Most of the contraindications listed below are relative.

1. Uncorrectable coagulopathy
2. Severe renal insufficiency (glomerular filtration rate [GFR] <30) in the absence of hemodialysis. Patient should be hydrated, contrast use minimized, and carbon dioxide angiography should be considered
3. Active phase of vasculitis
4. Nonambulatory critically ill patients with limited life expectancy and/or dementia
5. Patients who have mild claudication symptoms
6. Unfavorable anatomy
   a. SFA occlusion with involvement of the popliteal artery and trifurcation vessels
   b. Hemodynamically significant common femoral artery (CFA) disease. A combined femoral endarterectomy with endovascular treatment of the SFA or

femoropopliteal bypass is recommended. Common femoral angioplasty and/ or atherectomy may be considered in patients who are not surgical candidates. Stenting of the CFA is not desirable and may preclude future surgical options

c. Significant calcification involving a long SFA segment, especially "coral reef" calcification

d. Absent runoff via at least one vessel to the foot

e. Presence of hemodynamically significant inflow disease, which cannot be corrected by endovascular or surgical means

f. Severe aneurysmal disease at intended access site

Preprocedure Preparation

1. Obtain preprocedure physiologic studies with an arterial noninvasive examination with and without exercise (exercise examination not performed in patients with CLI) including baseline ankle-brachial index (ABI) values, segmental plethysmography with pulse volume recordings, and toe pressures when appropriate.

   a. Preprocedural imaging with computed tomography (CTA) or magnetic resonance angiography (MRA) can be utilized to develop a patient-specific course of treatment. Cross-sectional imaging is valuable in determining access site and planning the procedure, which may ultimately allow for a safer procedure with reduced contrast and radiation exposure.

2. Preangiography preparation: Verify stable renal function relative to baseline. Emergent or nonpostponable procedures in patients with impaired kidney function necessitate the use of preventative measures such as aggressive hydration with or without concomitant acetylcysteine. Ascertain allergy history to contrast mediums and treat as needed.

3. Premedication: All patients should be on antiplatelet therapy with aspirin and/or clopidogrel.

   a. Per the Clopidogrel versus Aspirin in Patients at Risk of Ischemic Events (CAPRIE) trial, there was a profound superiority in patients with peripheral arterial disease (PAD) treated with clopidogrel over aspirin in the prevention of stroke, myocardial infarction, and vascular death (1). As a result of this trial, many advocate that clopidogrel be the antiplatelet medication of choice in the PAD population given that the safety profile of this drug is at least as good as aspirin.

   b. All patients treated with drug-eluting balloons and DES require dual antiplatelet therapy for a short period of time. Per instructions for use (IFU), a minimum duration of dual antiplatelet therapy is 1 month and 2 months for Lutonix drug-eluting balloon (Bard, New Providence, NJ) and Zilver PTX DES (Cook Medical, Bloomington, IN), respectively.

   c. In patients who were not previously on antiplatelet mediations, a loading dose of 81 mg of aspirin and 300 mg of clopidogrel can be given at the time of the procedure.

   d. Whether all patients should be treated with dual antiplatelet therapy remains controversial and continues to evolve; this decision should be patient-specific, and the risks of vascular occlusion must be balanced with risk of hemorrhage.

Procedure

1. Obtain initial arterial access.

   a. A contralateral common femoral approach is the norm for SFA procedures; however, this approach may not be feasible in patients with a steep native aortic bifurcation, prior endovascular aneurysm repair, or aortobifemoral bypass.

b. Ipsilateral antegrade access is advantageous if tibial interventions are also necessary provided the patient's body habitus and CFA anatomy allow it.

c. If the occlusion involves the origin of the SFA or the very proximal SFA, a contralateral approach is generally required.

d. In patients with proximal SFA occlusion and significant disease in the contralateral CFA, a popliteal or distal SFA access may be considered.

e. At the current time, devices are not of sufficient length to perform mid to distal SFA interventions via an upper extremity brachial or radial access.

f. Tibiopedal arterial puncture may be used in conjunction with antegrade or contralateral common femoral access in recanalizing complex occlusions.

2. Perform initial angiography including distal runoff.

a. Multiple views may be required to establish a vascular map exhibiting the exact location and morphology of some lesions.

b. We generally perform both anteroposterior and lateral views of the foot in patients without renal insufficiency prior to intervention to establish a baseline.

3. In general, stenoses of more than 50% are considered hemodynamically significant in symptomatic patients.

a. Orthogonal views and correlation with noninvasive imaging and physiologic studies are of paramount importance.

b. Although pressure wires may be utilized to determine the hemodynamic significance of questionable lesions, this is rarely performed in the femoropopliteal segment.

4. Anticoagulation during interventions

a. Patients are generally anticoagulated with either heparin or bivalirudin when performing endovascular intervention to minimize risk of intraprocedural thrombus. Patients with SFA stenosis are anticoagulated prior to crossing the lesion, whereas patients with chronic occlusions are anticoagulated immediately after successful crossing of lesion.

(1) Typically, a heparin bolus dose of 70 to 100 units per kg is given with approximately 1,000 IU per hour subsequently.

(2) Bivalirudin dosing is as follows: initial bolus of 0.75 mg per kg followed by standard infusion of 1.75 mg/kg/h. Infusion dose is reduced to 1.0 mg/kg/h in patients with renal insufficiency (GFR 10 to 29 mL per minute) and to 0.25 mg/kg/h in patients on dialysis.

b. Activated clotting time (ACT) >250 seconds is recommended prior to SFA interventions.

c. The unpredictability associated with heparin therapy has popularized the use of direct thrombin inhibitors (bivalirudin) in more extensive lower extremity interventions as these drugs circumvent the pitfalls associated with heparin therapy.

(1) Unlike heparin, bivalirudin cannot be reversed with protamine; however, it does have a short half-life of approximately 25 minutes.

(2) Because bivalirudin is excreted in the urine, it is important to note that its half-life is increased in patients with renal insufficiency. In patients with GFR between 10 and 29, half-life is approximately 57 minutes.

5. Technique for crossing an SFA occlusion

a. Before treatment can be initiated, a guidewire must cross the lesion. In 80% to 85% of SFA occlusions, only a catheter and guidewire are necessary to successfully recanalize the lesion.

b. Although there are a multitude of guidewires and catheters on the market and every operator has their respective favorites, the technique described here is that preferred by the authors. A .035 system is recommended to cross the majority of SFA occlusions. A .035 Cerebral Newton LLT Guidewire (Cook Medical, Bloomington, IN) in conjunction with a straight or angled catheter is our initial guidewire of choice in crossing SFA occlusions. If this guidewire is not successful in crossing the lesion, hydrophilic guidewires such as an angled GLIDEWIRE (Terumo, Somerset, NJ) or Roadrunner (Cook Medical, Bloomington, IN) are employed. It is desirable to achieve an intraluminal path across the lesion (Fig. 11.1).

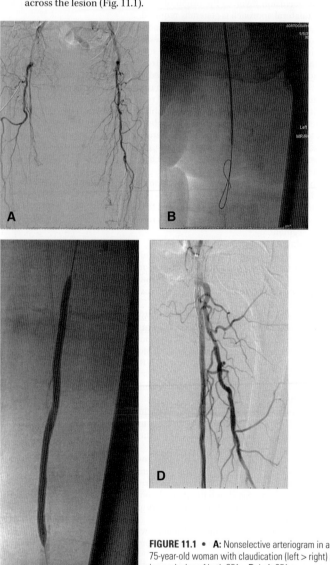

FIGURE 11.1 • **A:** Nonselective arteriogram in a 75-year-old woman with claudication (left > right) showing occlusion of both SFAs. **B:** Left SFA was recanalized advancing a wire loop through the occluded segment. **C, D:** SFA was then balloon dilated and stented with good flow. (Courtesy of Razavi MK, Gilbert M, and Razavi M)

   c. There are a variety of chronic total occlusion (CTO) crossing devices available on the market; however, there are no randomized clinical studies assessing the safety and efficacy of these devices.

   (1) Crossing devices include Viance (Covidien/Medtronic, Mansfield, MA), TruePath (Boston Scientific, Natick, MA), Crosser (Bard, New Providence, NJ), FRONTRUNNER XP (Cordis, East Bridgewater, NJ), Wildcat (Avinger, Redwood City, CA), and Ocelot (Avinger, Redwood City, CA). The latter device utilizes optimal coherence tomography to help direct the device and achieve intraluminal crossing.

   (2) Most of the crossing devices require that an occlusion has not been previously manipulated with a catheter and guidewire as the devices have a tendency to follow the same path created by the guidewire.

   (3) Because the majority of femoropopliteal occlusions can be crossed successfully with a guidewire and catheter and there is an up-front cost to utilizing CTO devices, we generally do not utilize these devices. A study comparing conventional guidewire techniques to CTO devices, focusing on end points including crossing success, cost, time to recanalization, need for re-entry, and complications would be valuable.

   d. If the lesion cannot be crossed intraluminally, a subintimal approach (Bolia technique) will be used.

   (1) A guidewire loop (typically with a hydrophilic .035 guidewire) is formed and advanced subintimally with a catheter providing support. This is extended until the point of target vessel reconstitution. It is important to limit the extension of the subintimal dissection beyond the occlusion because this may result in loss of important collaterals.

   (2) If still subintimal, attempts will be made to re-enter the true lumen with the guidewire and catheter.

   (3) If this is unsuccessful, re-entry devices are extremely helpful in achieving controlled re-entry into the true lumen (Fig. 11.2).

   (a) There are a multitude of re-entry devices available on the market including the OUTBACK (Cordis, East Bridgewater, NJ), Pioneer (Volcano, San Diego, CA), OffRoad (Boston Scientific, Natick, MA), and Enteer (Covidien/Medtronic, Mansfield, MA).

   (b) Advantages of re-entry devices include increased technical success; ability to treat more complex lesions (Trans-Atlantic Inter-Society Consensus [TASC] C and D); and the potential for decreased procedure time, contrast dose, and fluoroscopy time.

   (4) Patency rates after subintimal angioplasty are comparable to intraluminal angioplasty.

   e. If the guidewire very easily crosses an SFA occlusion (known as the "guidewire traversal test"), there is likely acute thrombus, and the patient should generally be treated with thrombolysis or mechanical thrombectomy prior to further endovascular intervention to minimize risk of distal embolization.

   (1) Thrombolysis will generally uncover an underlying lesion, which is typically shorter than the initial occlusion.

   (2) Covered stents may be used in the presence of small amounts of acute thrombus; however, there is a risk of distal embolization, and an embolic protection device should be considered if this strategy is entertained.

6. SFA intervention following crossing lesion/occlusion: Once the wire has been advanced across the stenoses/occlusions, it is critical to perform an angiogram to confirm an intraluminal position.

   a. For lesions <5 cm, PTA using appropriately sized balloons may be performed. For longer and more complex lesions, we generally favor drug-eluting balloons, BMS, DES, or covered stents over PTA.

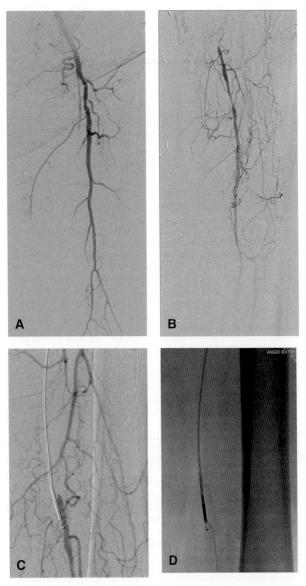

FIGURE 11.2 • A 78-year-old woman with severe left lower extremity claudication. Selective angiogram confirmed occlusion of left SFA (**A**) with reconstitution of popliteal artery (**B**). Re-entry into the true lumen was achieved by using OUTBACK (Cordis, Inc, East Bridgewater, NJ) device. OUTBACK is positioned next to the reconstituted segment (**C**) and actuator applied projecting a nitinol needle into the adjacent flow lumen (**D**) (*continued*).

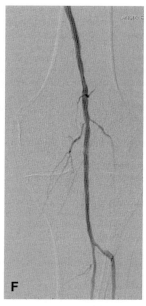

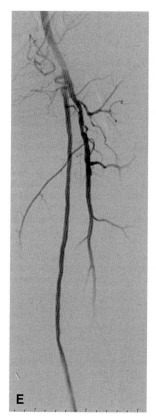

FIGURE 11.2 • (*Continued*) SFA was then balloon dilated and stented (**E** and **F**). (Courtesy of Razavi MK, Gilbert M, and Razavi M)

b. If stenting, angioplasty with a balloon 1 mm in diameter less than the diameter of the target vessel should be performed prior to introduction of the stent. Following placement of stent, postdilatation is performed to the diameter of the native artery.

c. If the plan is to use a drug-eluting balloon, the vessel should initially be predilated with a conventional balloon (PTA) matching the diameter of the artery. If there is a good angiographic result (i.e., no flow-limiting dissection, <30% residual stenosis), the drug-eluting balloon may be subsequently advanced and dilated. The initial angioplasty prevents loss of drug coating during advancement of the balloon.

d. If there is significant residual stenosis or dissection after PTA, the lesion should be stented.

e. For very long lesions (i.e., >20 cm), covered stents (VIABAHN, GORE Medical, Flagstaff, AZ) are favored.

f. If atherectomy is being considered, an embolic protection device is favored.

g. The precise algorithm and choice of device for SFA disease continues to evolve. See "Results" section for review of the data on the various SFA endovascular technologies.

7. Final angiography must be performed after intervention to confirm there is no residual stenosis. It is essential to perform runoff imaging as well to ensure that there has not been distal embolization from the procedure.
8. Vasospasm
   a. Vasospasm is not uncommon when performing endovascular interventions and is more likely to occur when treating small vessels and with poor runoff. Nitroglycerin 100 to 300 µg, intraarterial bolus, is our medication of choice if vasospasm is observed.
   b. Blood pressure should be monitored closely when administering vasodilating medications.

Postprocedure Management

1. If manual compression is used to achieve hemostasis at access site, ACT should be less than 180 seconds to minimize risk of bleeding. We generally do not reverse heparin with protamine unless there is a bleeding complication as there is a risk of anaphylaxis.
2. Closure devices impart a benefit in reducing the time to patient ambulation. See Chapter 2 for more information.
3. Although there is no consensus with regard to dual antiplatelet therapy, lifelong antiplatelet therapy with aspirin (81 mg) or clopidogrel (75 mg) is essential in all patients with PAD. As previously stated, patients who are treated with drug-eluting balloons or stents require dual antiplatelet therapy for a short period of time (1 month for Lutonix drug-eluting balloon, 2 months for Zilver PTX [Cook Medical, Bloomington, IN] per IFU).
4. Recently, the COMPASS trial demonstrated that low-dose rivaroxaban (2.5 mg) twice daily plus aspirin (100 mg) had better cardiovascular outcomes compared to patients who received aspirin alone in patients with stable cardiovascular disease (2). This was further investigated in the VOYAGER PAD trial which demonstrated that patients who underwent lower extremity artery revascularization and received rivaroxaban (2.5 mg) twice daily plus aspirin had a significantly lower incidence of adverse outcomes compared to those who received aspirin alone. These trials may represent a new postinterventional treatment paradigm for patients with PAD (3).
5. Risk factor modification is mandatory with a focus on aggressive management of diabetes, hypertension, hyperlipidemia, and smoking. Unless there is a contraindication or allergic reaction, all patients should be prescribed a statin medication. Statins have been shown to decrease cardiovascular mortality in patients with PAD.
6. Although there are no standard guidelines, surveillance after treatment of femoropopliteal disease is advised. A noninvasive arterial examination with measurement of the ABIs following intervention is recommended to establish a postintervention baseline. Clinic visits with or without duplex follow-up studies should be considered at 1, 3, 6, and 12 months, and yearly thereafter. Patients with CLI may require more frequent follow-ups.

Results

SFA treatment is rapidly evolving. Although some general recommendations are provided, there is clinical equipoise in many areas, and the interventionalist must remain up to date as new clinical data change the treatment approach.
1. Balloon angioplasty (PTA). According to the RESILIENT clinical trial, angioplasty and bare-metal stenting were equivalent for lesions <5 cm in length. PTA alone should be reserved for these short lesions provided that a flow-limiting dissection does not occur.

2. Bare-metal stents
   a. The RESILIENT trial compared PTA to BMS placement in the femoropopliteal segment with mean lesion length of 64 mm and 71 mm, respectively. The 12-month primary was 36.7% in the PTA group and 81.3% in the stent group with freedom from target lesion revascularization (TLR) of 45.1% and 87.3% (2). At 3 years, freedom from TLR (75.5% vs. 41.8%) and clinical success (63.2% vs. 17.9%) were significantly improved in the stent group. A 4.1% stent fracture rate was observed at 18 months.
   b. Supera stent (Abbott Vascular) is a newer-generation BMS made with a flexible and strong interwoven wire technology utilized for the treatment of SFA and proximal popliteal disease. The Comparison of the SUpera PERipheral System in the Superficial Femoral Artery (SUPERB) clinical trial, which evaluated this stent in lesions with a mean length of 7.8 cm, demonstrated 1-year primary patency of 78.9%. Freedom from TLR was 89%, 84%, and 82% at 1, 2, and 3 years, respectively. Patency rates were decreased when stents were inadvertently elongated beyond nominal during deployment. Stent fracture rate was 0.6% at 3 years.
3. DES (Zilver PTX, Cook Medical, Bloomington, IN; Eluvia, Boston Scientific, Marlborough, MA) have been shown to be superior to both balloon angioplasty and provisional BMS placement. In the Zilver PTX randomized clinical trial, 5-year freedom from TLR was 83.1% for the Zilver PTX group compared to 67.6% for the standard group, which included optimal angioplasty and provisional stent placement (4). The IMPERIAL trial compared the Eluvia DES to Zilver PTX DES and demonstrated a statistically significant lower rate of clinically driven TLR of 12.7% for patients treated with Eluvia versus 20.1% for those treated with Zilver PTX (5).
   a. The ZILVERPASS study evaluated the use of Zilver PTX compared to surgical bypass and demonstrated noninferiority results at 12 months with primary patency of the Zilver PTX arm of 74.5% compared to 72.5% in the surgical bypass arm (6).
4. DCBs have better patency than standard angioplasty balloons.
   a. The IN.PACT SFA randomized clinical trial has now demonstrated superiority of the IN.PACT Admiral Paclitaxel-Coated balloon (Medtronic, Fridley, MN) compared to PTA (74.% vs. 65.3%) at 5 years.
   b. U.S. Food and Drug Administration (FDA) approval of the Lutonix DCB in 2014 (as the first approved DCB in the United States) is on the basis of the LEVANT 2 clinical trial, which demonstrated a 29.4% improved primary patency of the Lutonix DCB (Bard) compared to PTA (73.5% vs. 56.8%) at 1 year.
   c. The ILLUMENATE trial evaluated the efficacy and safety of the Stellarex DCB (Philips, Andover, MA) demonstrating 4-year freedom from TLR of 28.2% versus 34.1% in patients undergoing PTA.
5. Controversy continues to surround the use of paclitaxel-coated devices due to a meta-analysis released by Katsanos et al. in 2018. This meta-analysis demonstrated an increased risk of all-cause death up to 5 years of 14.7% in patients receiving paclitaxel-coated devices compared to 8.1% in the control groups (7). This study has launched multiple follow-up evaluations by device companies and clinicians alike. The results continue to show contradictory results and the true mortality risk signal is still largely considered controversial. The FDA released recommendations in 2019 that state "For individual patients judged to be at particularly high risk for restenosis and repeat femoropopliteal interventions, clinicians may determine that the benefits of using paclitaxel-coated device outweigh the risk of late mortality." They also recommend discussing the risk and benefits of paclitaxel-eluting therapy and alternatives with PAD patients (8). The FDA acknowledges the more recent data demonstrating no difference in all-cause mortality between patients treated with paclitaxel-coated devices versus those with non–paclitaxel-coated devices; however, they strongly recommend that these patients must be followed, and long-term outcomes must be

reported. The Society of Interventional Radiology recommends adhering to the recommendations put forth by the FDA.

   a. Furthermore, a Multi-Specialty Paclitaxel Coalition was assembled consisting of representatives from multiple prominent societies and issued the following talking point:

      (1) "There may be other options for the treatment of your symptoms, including medications, exercise, balloons, stents or other devices that do not contain paclitaxel, and surgery. You and your doctor should discuss the possible risks and benefits of all treatments to identify those options that are best for you."

6. Covered stents/stent grafts. Long-segment disease (>20 cm) is best treated with a covered stent (VIABAHN, GORE, Flagstaff, AZ) in the presence of adequate runoff.

   a. According to the VIABAHN endoprosthesis with heparin bioactive surface in the treatment of superficial femoral artery obstructive disease (VIPER) trial, which evaluated lesions with a mean length of 19 cm, there was a 73% primary patency rate of the VIABAHN which was not affected by the diameter or length (<20 cm vs. >20 cm) of the device. If the stent grafts were oversized, greater than 20% in diameter compared to the native vessel diameter, the patency rates were decreased (9).

   b. The multicenter, prospective Viabahn endoprosthesis with PROPATEN bioactive surface versus bare nitinol stent in the treatment of long lesions in superficial femoral artery occlusive disease (VIASTAR) trial randomized patients to the Viabahn versus BMS with mean lesion length of 19 cm in the former and 17.3 cm in the latter. The overall primary patency rate at 1 year was 78% in the Viabahn group versus 54% in the BMS group; for lesion length >20 cm, patency rates were 73% versus 33%, respectively. This study provides level 1 evidence that long SFA lesions are likely best treated with a stent graft.

      (1) For optimal results, predilatation should be performed prior to the deployment of this device and post–stent-graft deployment PTA requires the utilization of balloons matching the diameter of the device used.

      (2) There has been some concern that coverage of collaterals from a covered stent may result in an increased incidence of acute limb ischemia when there is occlusion of the stent. However, the incidence of acute limb ischemia after covered stent occlusion is no higher than that observed after BMS occlusion.

7. Atherectomy

   a. There are several atherectomy devices available on the market. These include SilverHawk and TurboHawk (Covidien/Medtronic, Mansfield, MA), Diamondback (Cardiovascular System Inc, St. Paul, MN), Jetstream (Pathway Medical, Garden Grove, CA), Turbo-Elite and Turbo-Tandem (Spectranetics Inc, Colorado Springs, CO), Phoenix (Volcano, San Diego, CA), Crosser (Bard, New Providence, NJ), Pantheris (Avinger Medical, Redwood City, CA), Rotarex Rotational Excisional Atherectomy Device (BD, Franklin Lakes, NJ), and Auryon (Angiodynamics, Latham, NY).

   b. According to the DEFINITIVE LE study, directional atherectomy with the SilverHawk or TurboHawk device is a safe and effective therapy for patients with claudication and CLI (10). The 12-month primary patency rate was 78% with no difference between patients with diabetes and patients without diabetes. Complications included distal embolization (3.8%), perforation (5.3%), and abrupt closure (2.0%) with a bailout stent rate of 3.2%.

   c. In the authors' institution, atherectomy is generally not used as a primary therapy for SFA disease, although debulking may be helpful for certain clinical scenarios enumerated below:

      (1) Adjunctive treatment of heavily calcified disease, especially "coral reef" and eccentric calcification, which may not be adequately treated with angioplasty or stenting alone.

(2) Treatment of lesions in the CFA, profunda femoral artery, and popliteal artery where stenting is not ideal.

(3) Treatment of in-stent restenosis in conjunction with other modalities. FDA has cleared the Turbo-Tandem and Turbo Elite laser atherectomy devices (Spectranetics Inc, Colorado Springs, CO) to be used in conjunction with PTA. According to the EXCImer Laser Randomized Controlled Study for Treatment of FemoropopliTEal In-Stent Restenosis (EXCITE ISR) multicenter, randomized clinical trial, laser atherectomy with PTA demonstrated improved procedural success compared to PTA alone (93.5% vs. 82.7%). Average lesion length was 20 cm.

d. Vessel perforation is a known complication of atherectomy and is often the result of aggressive cutting of plaque. Care must be taken during debulking, and covered stent may be necessary should a significant perforation be encountered.

e. Distal embolization is not uncommon during atherectomy procedures. An embolic protection device is recommended when performing atherectomy. At the time of this writing, the only FDA-approved embolic protection device in the periphery is the SpiderFX (Covidien/Medtronic, Mansfield, MA). The authors prefer the NAV6 Emboshield embolic protection device (Abbott Vascular, Santa Clara, CA), which must be loaded onto a 315-cm .014 Barewire (Abbott Vascular, Santa Clara, CA) to be utilized in the periphery.

8. Intravascular Lithoplasty is a new technology extrapolated from lithotripsy therapy utilized in treating renal calculi. The Shockwave balloon (Shockwave Medical, Fremont, CA) is a PTA balloon that is inflated to low pressure and emits pulsatile sonic pressure waves that fracture calcium in the intima and media to improve vessel compliance. The DISRUPT PAD trials have demonstrated efficacy and safety of this device.

9. The TACK endovascular System (Philips, Andover, MA) is a small nitinol insert developed to address focal dissections in treatment of PAD. The Tack Optimized Balloon Angioplasty (TOBA) studies have demonstrated strong results of dissection resolution with TOBA III showing 97.7% dissection resolution and 95% vessel patency at 1 year.

Complications

1. Interventions of the femoropopliteal vessels carry a complication rate up to 10%, with 3% to 4% necessitating treatment.

2. Access site complications are common and include hematoma, pseudoaneurysm, arteriovenous fistula (AVF), vascular occlusion, and retroperitoneal hemorrhage. The latter is usually due to inadvertent "high puncture" of the external iliac artery (above the inguinal ligament). Special care must be taken when performing antegrade common femoral puncture to avoid external iliac puncture. Ultrasound-guided arterial access is beneficial.

3. Distal thromboembolism resulting in vascular occlusion. Factors predisposing to thromboembolism include acute limb ischemia with thrombus, inadequate anticoagulation during intervention, treatment of long occlusions, and atherectomy.

4. Flow-limiting dissection is more common after aggressive balloon dilatation.

5. Arterial rupture/perforation. Perforation may be due to guidewire, CTO device, atherectomy device, or aggressive dilatation with balloon or stent. Patients with underlying collagen vascular disease, vasculitis, and on chronic steroids are at increased risk.

6. Infection.

7. Contrast-induced nephropathy (CIN), especially in patients with baseline compromised renal function. See Chapter 66.

Management of Complications

1. Access site including pseudoaneurysm and AVF—see Chapter 3.
   a. Retroperitoneal hemorrhage due to puncture of the external iliac artery may present as a life-threatening complication because the access site cannot be adequately compressed and closure devices typically will not work through the inguinal ligament. Recognition of the problem followed by reversal of anticoagulation and immediate placement of a covered stent or surgery are crucial. Volume expansion, blood transfusion, and vasopressors may be needed if the patient becomes hemodynamically unstable.
2. Distal embolization may be treated with aspiration thrombectomy, thrombolysis, or surgical Fogarty balloon thromboembolectomy.
   a. Aspiration thrombectomy may be performed with a large profile guide catheter, specially designed aspiration catheters, or rheolytic thrombectomy.
   b. Administration of nitroglycerin may help differentiate whether occlusion is due to embolization versus vasospasm.
   c. It is critical to ensure that the patient is adequately anticoagulated by checking the ACT.
3. Flow-limiting dissection
   a. Initially treated with prolonged low-pressure balloon angioplasty in an attempt to tack down the dissection flap.
   b. Flow-limiting dissections which fail to resolve with prolonged angioplasty are treated with a stent.
4. Arterial rupture/perforation should be immediately tamponaded with a balloon, and consideration should be given to reversing anticoagulation if the perforation is large.
   a. If this strategy is not successful in resolving the bleeding, placement of a covered stent is recommended.
   b. Small guidewire perforations during crossing of an occlusion are not uncommon and can be self-limited.
   c. If significant bleeding occurs from a small branch or subintimal tract, coil embolization may be considered if the occlusion has not been crossed.

R e f e r e n c e s

1. CAPRIE Steering Committee. A randomised, blinded, trial of clopidogrel versus aspirin in patients at risk of ischaemic events (CAPRIE). *Lancet.* 1996;348:1329–1339.
2. Eikelboom JW, Connolly SJ, Bosch J, et al. Rivaroxaban with or without aspirin in stable cardiovascular disease. *N Engl J Med.* 2017;377(14):1319–1330.
3. Bonaca MP, Bauersachs RM, Hiatt WR. Rivaroxaban in peripheral artery disease after revascularization. *N Engl J Med.* 2020;382(21):1994–2004.
4. Dake MD, Ansel GM, Jaff MR, et al. Durable clinical effectiveness with paclitaxel-eluting stents in the femoropopliteal artery: 5-year results of the Zilver PTX randomized trial. *Circulation.* 2016;133(15):1472–1483.
5. Gray WA, Keirse K, Soga Y, et al. A polymer-coated, paclitaxel-eluting stent (Eluvia) versus a polymer-free, paclitaxel-coated stent (Zilver PTX) for endovascular femoropopliteal intervention (IMPERIAL): a randomised, non-inferiority trial. *Lancet.* 2018;392(10157):1541–1551.
6. Bosiers M, Setacci C, De Donato G, et al. ZILVERPASS study: ZILVER PTX stent vs bypass surgery in femoropopliteal lesions. *J Endovasc Ther.* 2020;27(2):287–295.
7. Katsanos K, Spiliopoulos S, Kitrou P, et al. Risk of death following application of paclitaxel-coated balloons and stents in the femoropopliteal artery of the leg: a systematic review and meta-analysis of randomized controlled trials. *J Am Heart Assoc.* 2018;7(24):e011245.
8. Farb A, Malone M, Maisel W. Drug-coated devices for peripheral arterial disease. *N Engl J Med.* 2021;384:99–101.

9. Saxon RR, Chervu A, Jones PA, et al. Heparin-bonded, expanded polytetrafluoroethylene-lined stent graft in the treatment of femoropopliteal artery disease: 1-year results of the VIPER (Viabahn Endoprosthesis with Heparin Bioactive Surface in the Treatment of Superficial Femoral Artery Obstructive Disease) trial. *J Vasc Interv Radiol.* 2013;24(2): 165–173.

10. McKinsey JF, Zeller T, Rocha-Singh KJ, et al. Lower extremity revascularization using directional atherectomy: 12-month prospective results of the DEFINITIVE LE study. *JACC Cardiovasc Interv.* 2014;7(8):923–933.

12 Infrapopliteal Arterial Interventions

Crystal Razavi, MD and Mahmood K. Razavi, MD, FSIR, FSVM

Introduction

Below-the-knee (BTK) arterial interventions are almost exclusively performed in the setting of chronic critical limb ischemia (CLI) or the more descriptive term chronic limb threatening ischemia (CLTI). Although peripheral arterial disease (PAD) is a common condition, CLTI occurs in only about 10% of patients with PAD (1). The term CLTI should only be used when symptoms are caused by ischemia (see Differential Diagnosis below).

Diagnosis is established by history and physical examination and confirmed by measurement of ankle-brachial index (ABI), toe pressures (TP)/ toe-brachial index (TBI), and/or transcutaneous oxygen pressure (TcPO$_2$). ABI has high specificity but a variable sensitivity in the diagnosis of CLTI, especially in the presence of medial calcinosis and noncompressible ankle arteries. Hence measurement of TP and TBI is mandatory if CLTI is suspected. Various blood flow and perfusion diagnostic modalities are on the horizon and will likely have an important role in the diagnosis and monitoring of this patient population (2,3).

Although the focus of this chapter is on endovascular revascularization, the reader should be reminded that revascularization in isolation is insufficient for the management of patients with CLTI. Optimal medical management including risk factor modification, lipid lowering therapy, diabetes management, antihypertensive treatment, and intensive wound care including antiinfective therapies are integral to best outcome.

Definition of Critical Limb Ischemia

CLTI refers to chronic rest pain requiring analgesics or opioids (Rutherford-Becker Category 4) and tissue loss resulting from severe ischemia (Rutherford–Becker Categories 5 and 6). In patients with rest pain, the ankle pressure is usually ≤50 mm Hg (TP ≤30 mm Hg). In those with tissue loss, ankle pressure should be ≤70 mm Hg (TP ≤50 mm Hg) to be classified as CLTI. Although the Rutherford–Becker classification is now known to be insufficient to classify patients with CLTI, it is used in this chapter because of its simplicity and wide recognition. Readers are referred to Mills et al. (4) for a review of the WIfI classification.

Differential Diagnosis

Pain

1. Diabetic neuropathy: often described as "burning" which is worse at night with symmetrical distribution in feet or legs. Other signs and symptoms of neuropathy are often present.

2. Complex regional pain syndrome: formerly known as sympathetic dystrophy; patients often have normal arterial flow.
3. Peripheral sensory neuropathy: isolated sensory neuropathy can be caused by various conditions such as vitamin B_{12} deficiency, syringomyelia, alcohol toxicity, and other toxins such as some chemotherapeutic agents.
4. Nerve root compression: various spinal conditions can give rise to continuous leg pain. There is usually no evidence of ischemia.
5. Thromboangiitis obliterans (Buerger disease): usually occurs in younger smokers. The etiology is distal ischemia due to an inflammatory vascular disease involving both arteries and vein.

Foot Ulceration

1. Venous ulcers: usually occur above the forefoot (ankle and calf) with adequate arterial flow.
2. Diabetic foot ulcers: can be divided into three general categories: ischemic, neuropathic, and neuroischemic. Neuropathic is the more common form of diabetic foot ulcers.
3. Mixed arterial and venous: The location is usually malleolar causing mild pain as opposed to purely ischemic ulcers that are usually more distal and cause severe pain.
4. Skin infarcts: usually due to systemic disease or thromboembolism.

Indications

1. Arterial disease in the setting of rest pain or tissue loss
   a. Depending on the availability of expertise, endovascular approach can be and often is the first-line therapy for revascularization in CLTI.
   b. Surgical bypass can be reserved for failures of endotherapy.

Contraindications

Absolute
1. Contraindications to angiography

Relative
1. Cases deemed futile or with low patency of endovascular therapy due to severe advanced disease such as no distal target vessels or occlusion of all three runoff arteries.
2. Nonambulatory patients with advanced disease: these patients should be counseled for amputation. Revascularization should be focused toward healing of amputation site.

Preprocedure Preparation

1. Fundamentals are similar to any other patient undergoing catheter angiography.
2. Ensure adequate hydration unless presence of end-stage renal disease or congestive heart failure prevents aggressive hydration.
3. General anesthesia or use of deep sedation can make the procedure easier on both the patient and the operator. Patients with CLTI often experience severe pain and cannot hold their legs and feet in one position for prolonged periods. Furthermore, patients with degenerative disc disease may experience back pain during prolonged immobility.

4. Preprocedural antiplatelet therapy is mandatory if there are no contraindications to such. Dual antiplatelet therapy with aspirin and a thienopyridine is recommended when patients can tolerate them.

5. Optimal medical therapy for comorbidities such as diabetes, hypertension, infection, heart failure, and pain are mandatory. Management of patients with CLTI is a multispecialty task and consultation with appropriate specialists should be sought.

6. Imaging: Noninvasive duplex examination with hemodynamic measurements is the standard preprocedural imaging. Magnetic resonance angiography (MRA) and computed tomographic angiography (CTA) are useful preprocedural imaging tools to better delineate BTK arterial anatomy in centers where both the technical and diagnostic expertise exists. CTA can be limited in BTK applications due to the presence of dense calcifications in small-caliber vessels or those with poor renal function.

Procedure

The overall strategy is focused on reestablishing direct inline flow into the foot or the area of nonhealing ulcer. In general, we treat all inflow lesions (aortoiliac and femoropopliteal) in the same session as the BTK when possible. In case of three-vessel disease, the initial focus should be to revascularize the artery feeding the most ischemic region of the foot (ischemic angiosome). In our practice, we attempt to treat all treatable hemodynamically significant lesions when possible, including those below the ankle. In general, short lesions with <50% or <60% stenosis should be left alone. Injury to these arterial segments changes the natural history of the lesion in favor of more rapid disease progression in the form of neointimal hyperplasia as opposed to the natural progression of atherosclerotic plaque.

1. Arterial access: Various anatomic sites can be used. Regardless of the approach, the tip of the access sheath/guide catheter should be placed as close to the diseased area as possible to gain maximal torque and forward force advantage.

   a. Contralateral common femoral artery (CFA): Preferred in patients with hostile groins (e.g., scarring from prior surgery), morbid obesity with large pannus, or high occlusion of the superficial femoral artery (SFA), all of which can make an antegrade ipsilateral approach difficult or impractical.

   b. Ipsilateral CFA: This is the preferred approach in most patients with BTK disease excluding the situations described earlier. Antegrade CFA access:

      (1) Allows better manipulation and improved pushability of wires/catheters/ devices.

      (2) Allows a shorter distance to the target lesions.

      (3) Below-the-ankle lesions can be treated with better advantage.

      (4) In case of complications such as thromboembolism, proximity to the target site improves ability to aspirate through shorter catheters, which improve aspiration efficiency.

   c. Tibiopedal access: can be utilized if attempts at antegrade recanalization of chronic total occlusions (CTO) fail (5). Dedicated pedal access needles and sheaths (3 to 5 Fr) make this approach more practical. Ultrasound-guided access is the preferred method, but direct access using fluoroscopic or angiographic images can also be utilized. The authors use pedal access as the sole interventional approach only in case of failure of antegrade approaches. Others use pedal access in patients with severe back pain or respiratory compromise who cannot tolerate flat positions for long (6).

   d. Radial access: with the popularity of radial access for coronary interventions some operators use this for peripheral arterial interventions. The radial-to-peripheral (R2P) approach has many disadvantages, especially for BTK including the long distance to the target disease, loss of pushability and torque control, and lack of optimized instrumentation. It can be utilized in the absence of other arterial access sites.
2. Crossing the lesions: can be time consuming in the BTK territory. This is especially true of long-segment CTO because the vessels are often calcified, small-caliber, and effective reentry devices for these specific arteries do not currently exist. A variety of specialty wires and support catheters have been developed to assist in such lesions. The optimal devices and techniques are in continuous evolution.
   a. *Specialty wires*—have variable performance characteristics suitable for crossing and navigation through CTO caps, plaque, calcification, fibrotic lesions, etc. Some operators prefer 0.018-in wires in combination with compatible crossing catheters. The 0.014-in wires, however, have emerged as the preferred choice in the majority of cases due to compatibility with existing low-profile balloons, stents, reentry devices, etc. Wire tip load, torqueability, support, and flexibility are among the performance characteristics to consider when choosing a wire or matching an appropriate wire to lesion and anatomy. Understanding features and trade-offs of wires is critical in procedural success. A detailed description of what wire to choose when is beyond the scope of this writing and readers are encouraged to educate themselves about BTK wires and try to gain experience with a variety of such. Escalation and deescalation of wires is common in complex BTK lesions.

   Several companies including Abbott Vascular, Asahi, Terumo, Boston Scientific, and Cook make wires that are particularly well suited for BTK interventions. They have different performance characteristics, and their use remains the operator's preference. Interventionists should become familiar with these wires to be able to choose their favorite platform.
   b. *Support catheters*—have improved pushability, trackability, and high longitudinal support characteristics. These devices are sometimes referred to as "microcatheters" without the distinction between small bore catheters used for navigation (microcatheters) versus those used for crossing (support catheters). Similar to wires above, the choice of a support catheter will depend on the lesion and anatomy. While traversing a tortuous segment or using a transcollateral route for recanalization may require more flexibility and trackibility, crossing the straight segment of a posterior tibial artery CTO, for example, will require maximal longitudinal support. On other occasions where a support catheter may not cross, use of rotational support catheters may be helpful. As with wires, many companies make low-profile crossing catheters of varying characteristics.
   c. *Crossing tools*—In majority of cases the use of appropriately selected catheter/wire combination is sufficient to cross BTK lesions. Occasionally passage of wires through long-segment occluded calcified lesions is not possible using specialized support catheters. Hence, some manufacturers have developed BTK crossing tools to assist with recanalization of long-segment CTO. Current examples include Viance (Covidien, Plymouth, MN), Crosser (Bard Peripheral Vascular, Tempe, AZ), TruePath (Boston Scientific, Natick, MA), Turbo-Elite laser catheter (Spectranetics/Philips, Colorado Springs, CO), Wingman (ReFlow Medical, Mission Viejo, CA), KittyKat (Avinger, Redwood City, CA), and PowerWire (Baylis Medical, Montréal, Quebec, Canada). In addition, a variety of rotational catheters with "corkscrew" features are available to improve technical success.
   d. *Alternative techniques:* Failure of standard catheter/wire techniques may require alternative methods and reentry maneuvers such as bidirectional

approach (tibiopedal access), single- or double balloon–assisted reentry, hydrodynamic boost, or rendezvous maneuvers (5,6). Recently methods for better perfusion of the foot have been devised that includes diversion of blood from occluded arteries into the veins. This is referred to as distal venous arterialization (DVA) and has been attempted in patients with no distal arterial target or patients with no revascularization options. Ongoing studies will better elucidate the utility of this approach.

3. Treatment tools: Once the target lesions have been crossed, flow is reestablished through a variety of techniques.

   a. Angioplasty—is the mainstay of therapy in BTK (often referred to as "plain old balloon angioplasty" or POBA). Most manufacturers make high-performance balloons of various diameters and lengths for BTK applications. The longest balloon that best matches the diseased segment should be used. Care should be taken to closely match the diameter of the balloon to that of the nondiseased adjacent segment. *Under-sizing of balloon diameter is a common mistake that can lead to recoil or suboptimal results.*

   b. Debulking—for example, rotational or directional (excisional) atherectomy, or laser. All current debulking systems in the market have dedicated BTK tools. Although the authors prefer "front-cutting" atherectomy devices for BTK, experience and comfort level of the operator should determine which device is used. There is currently no data proving the superiority of one debulking system to another in BTK interventions.

   c. Specialty balloons: A variety of balloons have been devised to overcome the common shortcomings of POBA such as recoil and dissection. Examples include the Flextome Cutting Balloon (Boston Scientific, Natick, MA) or AngioSculpt scoring balloon (Spectranetics/Philips, Colorado Springs, CO). Flextome has the disadvantage of not having longer balloons and being too bulky to cross most BTK lesions. Due to its lower profile, AngioSculpt is more suited for such applications. Another specialty balloon that is designed to theoretically reduce angioplasty trauma is the Chocolate Balloon (Medtronic, Minneapolis, MN). Serranator (Cagent Vascular, Wayne, PA) creates controlled "serrations" into the plaque which may reduce the rate of dissection or recoil. Studies to prove such are pending.

   It should be noted that while the specialty balloons mentioned above may improve technical success, none have been shown to improve long-term outcome beyond POBA alone.

   d. Drug-coated balloons (DCBs): These devices have shown success in the femoropopliteal segments but all randomized, prospective, multicenter trials to date have missed their primary efficacy endpoints in BTK and as such are not the standard of care. Furthermore, presence of drug on the balloon is designed to prevent neointimal hyperplasia and hence does nothing to prevent recoil or dissection, which are the prevailing causes of early failure of BTK angioplasty.

   e. Scaffolds: These have the advantage of treating both recoil and dissection. Currently Tack (Intact Vascular/Philips, Wayne, PA) is the only FDA-approved scaffold for BTK. The device has five short self-expanding nitinol scaffolds and has a relatively low radial force. It is used to spot stent dissections after angioplasty. No other dedicated BTK bare-metal stents (BMSs), drug-eluting stents (DESs), or bioabsorbable drug-eluting vascular scaffolds (BVSs) have approval in the United States. Their use in the EU and rest of the world has also been limited. Coronary BMS and DES are used off-label when stents are needed. Another off-label BMS is the Xpert stent (Abbott Vascular, Santa Clara, CA), which is a 4-Fr compatible self-expanding nitinol stent that is supplied in diameters 3 to 8 mm. The authors' preferred technique in treating recoil and dissection in BTK arteries is to spot stent using coronary DES. Balloon expandable coronary DES have the advantage of having ultra–low profile delivery catheters with a high radial force suitable for calcified BTK lesions as well as limus drugs to reduce restenosis.

  f. Procedural pharmacology: Intraprocedural anticoagulation can be accomplished by heparin with a target-activated clotting time above 250 seconds. An alternative anticoagulant is bivalirudin, which is administered intravenously at standard doses. The more precise and predictable anticoagulation properties of bivalirudin may be preferable when treating patients with infrainguinal long-segment CTO.

Postprocedure Management

1. Management of patients with CLTI is best done in a multispecialty setting. Optimal wound care, management of pain and infection, and active risk factor modification such as smoking cessation are all integral parts of the optimal treatment of patients with CLTI. Diabetes, dyslipidemia, hypertension, and antiplatelet/anticoagulation use should all be optimized.

2. Patients with foot ulceration should be evaluated in wound-care centers and treated accordingly before and after the revascularization procedures.

3. Postprocedure antiplatelet therapy is continued indefinitely. Dual antiplatelet, when used, can be discontinued 3 months after the procedure with continuation of monotherapy. It should be noted that there are no current standards for dual antiplatelet therapy in CLTI patients. Recent studies have indicated that the postprocedural addition of anticoagulant rivaroxaban to aspirin may be preferable in certain patient populations (7).

4. Follow-up imaging using duplex arterial evaluation should be done at regular intervals according to the routine of treating physician and reimbursement policies of the local payers. Evaluation outside of the routine windows must be performed if there is persistence or recurrence of symptoms.

Results

1. *Limb salvage and control of pain and infection*—Various studies have documented 1-year limb salvage rate of 50% to 96% in such patients using different endorevascularization strategies, which is similar to surgical bypass outcomes. Outcome in CLTI patients is highly dependent on the stage of disease and comorbidities such as diabetes, heart failure, renal failure, and nutritional status. Safety data and patient preferences favor an endovascular first approach over open surgical bypass.

  a. A meta-analysis of the results of randomized trials comparing various treatments for BTK vessels showed no significant difference in limb salvage rates and hence recommended treatment with POBA with bailout stenting using BMS when possible (8). It should be noted that limb salvage is a relatively insensitive tool to measure incremental differences between various technologies and techniques. Patency and freedom from target lesion revascularization (TLR) is highest when coronary DESs are used.

2. *Patency, improvements in disease classification, TLR*—there are varying outcomes between the different techniques and devices in BTK intervention. Variables affecting results include lesion length, presence of CTO, diabetes, renal failure, etc.

  a. POBA: Despite a poor patency of 50% to 60% at 1 year in BTK, limb salvage rates are high as mentioned above.

  b. DCB: Prospective, randomized, multicenter trials such as IN.PACT DEEP failed to show any difference between the POBA and DCB (9). Other completed pivotal studies of DCB in BTK have also missed their primary efficacy endpoints and hence not currently approved by the FDA in the United States.

  c. Various atherectomy studies have shown excellent limb salvage rates of >80% at 1 year. Results of orbital atherectomy using Diamondback device (CSI, Minneapolis, MN) have shown >95% limb salvage at 1 year. Superiority of any form of atherectomy over POBA alone in randomized trials has not been established.

d. Scaffolds: BMS have better technical results as compared to POBA but long-term patency has generally not been demonstrated to be better. Results of the TOBA-II BTK showed 74.5% patency at 12 months in patients with CLTI, which is an improvement over POBA.

Use of DES improves 1-year patency, wound healing, and event-free survival as well as reduce restenosis and need for reintervention as compared to POBA in relatively short lesions (10,11). For these reasons, spot stenting using DES is the authors' preferred approach in BTK.

3. Given a lack of standardized treatment for patients with CLTI, local results and individual experiences will likely determine the strategy used. Results of ongoing trials should clarify the role of various devices in the treatment of patients with CLTI.

Complications

1. The most common complications are those related to catheter angiography such as access site complications and contrast nephropathy.

2. Vascular injury such as rupture is rare and can be treated by placement of stent grafts, BMS, or prolonged balloon inflation. Focal contrast extravasation due to false passage of wire is frequently self-limiting and does not require any specific treatment.

3. Embolization into the distal circulation can occur. Risk factors for distal emboli include the use of atherectomy devices, PTA of thrombotic lesions, and recanalization of long CTOs. Loss of distal flow has been correlated with poorer outcome and emboli should be treated by one of a variety of aspiration devices currently available. Authors typically prefer the Jeti-6 (Walk Vascular, Irvine, CA) for more proximal emboli/thrombus (e.g., trifurcation occlusion or proximal one-third of tibial arteries) and CAT-Rx (Penumbra, Alameda, CA) for more distal emboli. Debris into the arteries of the foot can be aspirated by CAT-3 (Penumbra, Alameda, CA) or equivalent devices.

4. Acute failures of intervention can also occur depending on the devices used and the operator experience.

a. Inability to cross an occluded segment occurs in 5% to 10% of cases (12). In this scenario, tibiopedal access can often be successful in achieving recanalization. Technical details of instrumentation and approaches to such are beyond the scope of this writing and can be found elsewhere (5).

b. Other causes of acute failure include recoil, dissection, and uncommonly thrombosis. The former is common in BTK interventions, and use of scaffolds, debulking devices, or specialty balloons may be required (12).

References

1. Hiatt WR. Medical treatment of peripheral arterial disease and claudication. *N Engl J Med.* 2001;344(21):1608–1621.

2. Razavi MK, Flanigan DP, White SM, et al. A novel real-time blood flow measurement device for patients with peripheral artery disease. *J Vasc Interv Radiol.* 2021;32(3):453–458.

3. Rogers RK, Montero-Baker M, Biswas M, et al. Assessment of foot perfusion: overview of modalities, review of evidence, and identification of evidence gaps. *Vasc Med.* 2020;25(3):235–245.

4. Mills JL Sr, Conte MS, Armstrong DG, et al. The Society for vascular surgery lower extremity threatened limb classification system: risk stratification based on wound, ischemia, and foot infection (WIfI). *J Vasc Surg.* 2014;59:220–234.e1-2.

5. Razavi MK, Kafai NM. Re-entry and wire snaring techniques in CLI interventions. In: Mustapha J, ed. Critical Limb Ischemia: CLI Diagnostics and Interventions. HMP Communications, LLC; 2014.

6. Mustapha JA, Saab F, McGoff T, et al. Tibio-pedal arterial minimally invasive retrograde revascularization in patients with advanced peripheral vascular disease: the TAMI technique, original case series. *Catheter Cardiovasc Interv.* 2014;83(6):987–994.

7. Bonaca MP, Bauersachs RM, Anand SS, et al. Rivaroxaban in peripheral artery disease after revascularization. *N Engl J Med.* 2020;382(21):1992–2004.

8. Jens S, Conijn AP, Koelemay MJ, et al. Randomized trials for endovascular treatment of infrainguinal arterial disease: systematic review and meta-analysis (Part 2: Below the knee). *Eur J Vasc Endovasc Surg.* 2014;47(5):536–544.

9. Zeller T, Baumgartner I, Scheinert D, et al. Drug-eluting balloon versus standard balloon angioplasty for infrapopliteal arterial revascularization in critical limb ischemia: 12-month results from the IN.PACT DEEP randomized trial. *J Am Coll Cardiol.* 2014;64(15):1568–1576.

10. Fusaro M, Cassese S, Ndrepepa G, et al. Drug-eluting stents for revascularization of infrapopliteal arteries: updated meta-analysis of randomized trials. *JACC Cardiovasc Interv.* 2013;6(12):1284–1293.

11. Katsanos K, Spiliopoulos S, Diamantopoulos A, et al. Systematic review of infrapopliteal drug-eluting stents: a meta-analysis of randomized controlled trials. *Cardiovasc Intervent Radiol.* 2013;36(3):645–658.

12. Razavi MK, Mustapha JA, Miller LE. Contemporary systematic review and meta-analysis of early outcomes with percutaneous treatment for infrapopliteal atherosclerotic disease. *J Vasc Interv Radiol.* 2014;25(10):1489–1496.

13 Acute Limb Ischemia: Pharmacomechanical and Thrombolytic Therapy

Matthew J. Scheidt, MD

Intraarterial Catheter-Directed Thrombolytic Therapy

Pioneered by Dotter in the 1970s, intraarterial (IA) catheter-directed thrombolysis (CDT) has become routine medical practice in the emergent treatment of an acutely ischemic limb with the goal of rapidly restoring blood flow to the threatened limb (Fig. 13.1), minimizing amputation rate and mortality. Angiography can also help identify the underlying culprit lesion(s) for subsequent surgical and/or endovascular treatment including both CDT and mechanical thrombectomy.

Indications

Thrombotic or embolic occlusion(s) of native arteries or bypass grafts with new-onset claudication or limb-threatening ischemia (Table 13.1) (1–4). Both acute (less than 14 days' duration) and chronic thrombi are amenable to treatment (2,5).

Contraindications (1–4)

Absolute
1. Active clinically significant bleeding
2. Irreversible limb ischemia with major tissue loss or permanent nerve damage (severe sensorimotor loss, paralysis/muscle rigor)

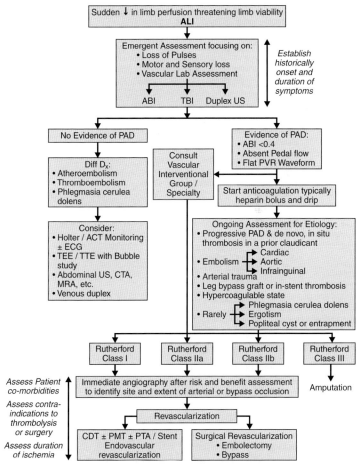

FIGURE 13.1 • Algorithm for the evaluation and management of acute limb ischemia (ALI). Once diagnosed, anticoagulation is initiated with subsequent treatment depending on classification of the ALI. Initial options include catheter-directed thrombolysis (CDT) with or without percutaneous mechanical thrombectomy (PMT) or surgical revascularization. Clinical categories of ALI include limbs that are (a) viable, with no immediate threat of tissue loss, intact muscle power and sensations, and audible arterial/venous Doppler signals; (b) marginally threatened, with a threat of tissue loss, minimal or no sensory loss, intact muscle power weak, and often inaudible arterial Doppler signals but intact venous Doppler signals (treated promptly, these limbs are salvageable; these limbs afford time for vascular imaging); (c) immediately threatened and need prompt attention without delay and manifest as limbs with sensory (more than the toes) and motor loss (mild to moderate) with inaudible arterial Doppler signals but audible venous Doppler signals; these limbs are salvageable; and (d) irreversibly ischemic or nonviable, with major tissue loss, profound sensory and motor loss (paralysis), and inaudible arterial/venous Doppler signals.

Table 13.1 **Classification of Acute Limb Ischemia**

Rutherford Class	Category	Prognosis	Sensory Loss	Muscle Weakness	Arterial Doppler	Venous Doppler
I (Reversible ischemia)	**Viable limb**	Not immediately threatened	None	None	Audible	Audible
IIA (Reversible ischemia)	**Salvageable limb**: threatened marginally	Salvageable if promptly revascularized	Minimal (toes) or none	None	Often inaudible	Audible
IIB (Reversible ischemia)	**Salvageable limb**: threatened immediately	Salvageable if immediately revascularized	More than toes and associated with rest pain	Mild to moderate	Usually inaudible	Audible
III (Irreversible ischemia)	**Nonviable limb**	Limb loss or permanent damage with major tissue loss or permanent nerve damage inevitable	Profound anesthetic loss	Profound paralysis (rigor)	None	None

Reprinted with permission from McNamara TO. Thrombolysis as an alternative initial therapy for the acutely ischemic limb. *Semin Vasc Surg*. 1992;5:89–98.

3. Presence/development of compartment syndrome
4. Intracranial hemorrhage
5. Absolute contraindication to anticoagulation

Relative
Although thrombolysis is not usually considered in the following conditions, clinical decision making revolves around the anticipated benefit and attendant risks. Careful clinical evaluation and sound judgment in patient selection, especially elderly patients, are essential.
1. Bleeding diathesis
2. Disseminated intravascular coagulation
3. Established cerebrovascular accident (within 2 months)
4. Neurosurgery or intracranial trauma (within 3 months)
5. Cardiopulmonary resuscitation (within 10 days)
6. Major surgery or trauma (within 10 days)
7. Eye surgery (within 3 months)
8. Intracranial tumor, vascular malformation, aneurysm, or seizure disorder
9. Uncontrolled hypertension
10. Recent internal hemorrhage or visceral biopsy
11. Recent major gastrointestinal bleeding (within 10 days)
12. Serious allergic reaction to thrombolytic agent, anticoagulant, or contrast which cannot be controlled by premedication
13. Severe thrombocytopenia
14. Pregnancy or immediate postpartum state
15. Severe liver dysfunction with associated coagulopathy
16. Bacterial endocarditis

17. Diabetic hemorrhagic retinopathy
18. Life expectancy <1 year

Preprocedure Preparation

1. **Good-quality noninvasive imaging**. Review of available imaging is mandatory. Vascular ultrasound, computed tomography angiography (CTA) or magnetic resonance angiography (MRA) can define the distribution of disease, determine the etiology of the patient's symptoms, and aid with planning subsequent interventions including access site and equipment needed.
2. **Standard laboratory evaluation**. Generally includes hematocrit (Hct)/hemoglobin (Hgb) (>10 g per dL and 30% by volume), platelet count (>100,000 per μL), baseline blood urea nitrogen (BUN)/creatinine (Cr), estimated GFR (eGFR), prothrombin time (PT) with international normalized ratio (INR), partial thromboplastin time (PTT), and fibrinogen levels (optional).
3. **Access site selection**. Review all available prior imaging. Occlusive disease can be approached from either the contralateral or the ipsilateral side. An ipsilateral antegrade approach may be necessary when up-and-over sheath access cannot be obtained due to iliac artery occlusion, kissing iliac stents, or presence of an aortoiliac/aortobifemoral bypass. Careful, direct puncture of a graft is usually risk-free. Brachial and axillary artery puncture should generally be *avoided* when thrombolytic therapy is anticipated.

Procedure

1. After obtaining the desired IA access and placing the appropriately sized vascular sheath, a baseline arteriogram is performed to document the extent of the thrombus and arterial disease (Fig. 13.2).
2. After identifying the occlusion and deciding on CDT (Fig. 13.3), the 5-Fr short sheath (typically placed at time of access) is replaced with a 6-Fr crossover sheath (when possible, tip of the sheath is placed in the external iliac artery, in case of occlusion of all lower extremity branches).

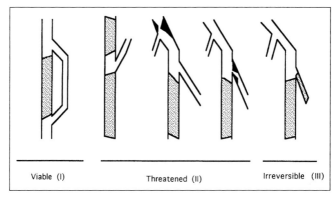

Viable (I)   Threatened (II)   Irreversible (III)

FIGURE 13.2 • Arteriographic patterns typically corresponding to clinical acute ischemia categories: *(I)* Viable limbs often show a single segmental occlusion with patent collaterals and reconstitution of calf runoff vessels; *(II)* threatened limbs can have tandem lesions in series or in parallel with patent collaterals and reconstitution of calf runoff vessels; and *(III)* irreversibly ischemic limbs have extensive parallel thrombotic occlusions, occluded collaterals, and no distal reconstitution of runoff vessels. (Borrowed from McNamara TO. Thrombolysis as an alternative initial therapy for the acutely ischemic limb. *Semin Vasc Surg.* 1992;5:89–98.)

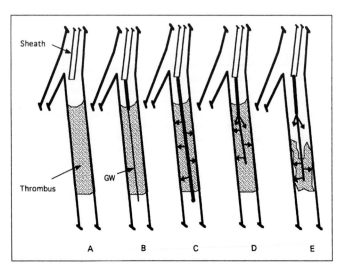

FIGURE 13.3 • Stages of IA thrombolysis. **A:** An occluded segment of vessel is demonstrated arteriographically. **B:** A coaxial catheter is introduced through the IA sheath and advanced into the proximal thrombus, and a guidewire is then advanced to the distal end of the thrombus (GWTT). **C:** A tip-occluded multiside-orifice catheter is advanced into the entire thrombus, which is saturated with a lacing dose of lytic agent deposited by rapid pulse-spray infusion. (Alternatively, an end-hole catheter or a catheter with fewer distal side-holes is advanced distally and then retracted proximally while depositing small doses of lytic agent at each site.) **D:** Continuous infusion is administered with an end-hole catheter with its tip in the proximal thrombus and a smaller side-hole catheter that is advanced much farther into the clot. (A distal untreated segment of thrombus is shown here, but a side-hole catheter, with its tip occluded, may be advanced so as to bathe the thrombus with lytic agent throughout its length.) **E:** As thrombolysis progresses, both catheters may be advanced, but with this configuration, the inner catheter alone may be advanced into the receding thrombus front. The process continued until the entire thrombus is dissolved and an underlying obstructing lesion is uncovered for treatment by angioplasty or surgery.

3. Attempt is next made to traverse the occlusion. This is often done using a combination of 0.035" guidewire (Bentson, angled hydrophilic wire) and a 4- or 5-Fr angled catheter, for example, Bernstein/glidecath/MPA/straight or angled crossing catheter. Progress is monitored by periodic angiography, and catheter position is adjusted appropriately. Oblique views may help find the entry orifice of the thrombus. Once the wire is through the occluded segment, the catheter is advanced over it, and confirmatory angiography is then performed to demonstrate intraluminal positioning. A more sturdy, exchange length working wire is then placed through the catheter across the occlusion.

4. After determining the length of the occlusion, a thrombolytic infusion catheter is placed over the working wire. Typically, the infusion catheter should cover the entire length of the occlusion, extending at least 2 cm from both ends.

   a. A thrombus that is resistant to passage of a standard guidewire (Guidewire Traversal Test or GWTT) is likely more chronic and can be difficult to resolve with CDT alone. However, this should not necessarily discourage a trial of thrombolysis (1).

   b. If the catheter tip cannot be successfully placed across the thrombus, it may be positioned proximal to the occlusion with initiation of (regional) lysis to

Table 13.2	Popular Dosing Schemes for Treatment of Peripheral Arterial Occlusions with Thrombolytic Agents[a]			
Agent	**Plasma Half-life (min)**	**Concentration**	**Dosing Scheme**	**Systemic Heparin**
Streptokinase (SK)	30	1,500 IU/mL	Intrathrombic lace: 20,000–50,000 IU Infusion: 5,000 IU/h (optional)	May be needed early; perhaps unnecessary or optional beyond 12 h
Urokinase (UK)	15	3,000 IU/mL	Intrathrombic lace: 250,000–500,000 IU Infusion: 4,000 IU/h × 2 h; 2,000 IU/h × 2 h then 1,000 IU/h for duration (optional)	Full therapeutic dose
rt-PA	5	0.2 mg/mL	Intrathrombic lace: 5–10 mg Infusion: 0.5–1.0 mg/h (optional)	Subtherapeutic (2,500 U IV bolus + 500 U/h IV infusion); optional
Reteplase	15	0.5 U/mL	Intrathrombic lace: 2–5 U Infusion: 0.5–1.0 U/h (optional)	Subtherapeutic; optional

rt-PA, recombinant tissue plasminogen activator; IV, intravenous.
[a]For a more complete listing and descriptions, please see references (2), (4), and (9).

soften the proximal thrombus for a later attempt at intrathrombic catheter placement.

c. Failure to place the catheter within or across the thrombus will decrease the efficacy of the lytic therapy due to decreased access of the drug to fibrin-bound plasminogen.

5. **Infusion wire or catheter selection:** A variety of 4- and 5-Fr infusion catheters (e.g., Cragg-McNamara Valved Infusion catheter [Medtronic, Minneapolis, MN] and Uni-Fuse Infusion catheter [Angiodynamics, Latham, NY]) and possibly smaller infusion catheters and wires as commercially available devices are constantly changing. The catheter and wire combinations are typically used for slow, continuous infusion of the thrombolytic.

6. **Thrombolytic agents** (see Table 13.2 for dose administration): CDT relies on diffusion of the agent into the thrombus, a slow process that requires a high concentration gradient to drive the reagent into the clot.

a. Several thrombolytic agents have been described in the literature, and currently none has U.S. Food and Drug Administration (FDA) approval for use in peripheral arteries or veins. Prospective randomized trials comparing the agents directly are limited and thus do not yield a meaningful comparison.

(1) UK was the most commonly used agent in the United States until it was temporarily removed from the market in 1999. Alteplase, a second-generation

rt-PA with more fibrin specificity, and Reteplase (rt-PA), a recombinant deletion mutant of rt-PA, are currently the most widely used thrombolytic agents in the United States for peripheral vascular applications.

(2) The general consensus is that UK and rt-PA are equally efficacious and safe (1,2) and that both are superior to SK for treating peripheral arterial occlusions (2,3,8). Tissue-plasminogen activator produces more rapid early lysis than UK (4,5,10). Experience with peripheral thrombolysis using rt-PA has grown, and efficacy and safety profile appears to be acceptable (2,4,9).

b. *Intrathrombic lacing* involves depositing concentrated agent into the thrombus using multiple side-hole catheters and the pulsed-spray technique. High-dose intrathrombic lacing of the agent saturates the thrombus and significantly decreases treatment duration, total dose, and complication rates but slightly increases incidence of major hemorrhage (2). Lacing is performed through a multi-sidehole infusion catheter or an end-hole catheter positioned distally and slowly retracted proximally. Some advocate leaving a distal plug of thrombus in place in order to avoid possible embolization caused by the forced infusion. Others lace the entire thrombus in order to reestablish flow quickly. Small distal emboli of thrombus usually dissolve with continued infusion of the lytic agent.

c. Slow, *continuous, low-dose intrathrombus infusion* represents the current state of practice with follow-up angiography in 6 to 24 hours which can be variable based on each individual case.

7. **Concomitant intravenous anticoagulation:** Heparin is given as an IV bolus dose of 70 U per kg and then as a continuous IV infusion at 500 to 1,200 U per hour (1–4) to prevent thrombus formation around an occlusive catheter. This may be initiated as soon as the thrombus is crossed with a guidewire.

a. Heparin should be adjusted to maintain either the PTT or ACT in the therapeutic range. However, several operators use a lower-rate heparin infusion at a fixed rate of 500 U per hour to maintain PTT in the lower range (40 to 50 seconds).

b. Interactions between heparin and lytic agents can cause precipitate formation (data from Abbott Laboratories, Abbott Park, IL; and Genentech Inc, San Francisco, CA), and so the two drugs should not be mixed together prior to administration (1–4).

8. **Ultrasound-assisted thrombolysis:** It has been demonstrated that energy transmitted by the ultrasound waves separates/loosens the fibrin strands, increasing the surface area of the thrombus and making more thrombus available to the lytic agent. In vitro studies have demonstrated accelerated clot lysis by accelerating the contact of the lytic agent with the thrombus, increasing thrombus permeability, and increasing available plasminogen receptors (2). The EKOS infusion catheter (Boston Scientific, Natick, MA), is based on these principles and FDA approved for use in pulmonary artery thrombolysis. However, there is no current data to support the improved efficacy of this device in peripheral arterial or venous thrombolysis compared to traditional infusion catheters. Therefore, it remains difficult to determine if use of ultrasound-thrombolysis in this clinical scenario justifies the associated extra cost.

Postprocedure Management

1. **Pressure bandage** at site of catheter entry; puncture site is checked every 30 minutes for 2 hours and then every 2 hours during infusion.

2. Patients are usually managed in the intensive care or step-down unit and vital signs monitored frequently per institutional thrombolysis protocol. Extremity pulses (palpation/Doppler) are checked every 4 hours or more frequently as clinically indicated.

3. Laboratory monitoring
   a. Hct, PT and PTT/ACT every 2 hours ×2 and then every 6 hours during infusion

b. Desired PTT is 2.0 to 2.5 times control level (with a control level of 35 seconds, target PTT would be 70 to 90 seconds or lower as per operator preference). The ACT should be >250 seconds during lytic therapy.

4. Fluid input/output are monitored closely.

5. Intramuscular injections are best avoided during this period.

6. Heparin is administered at 500 to 1,000 U per hour through the vascular sheath to avoid peri-sheath thrombosis. However, small series have demonstrated no improvement in efficacy and similar complication rates whether heparin was or was not used during CDT (2,4).

7. In case of fever, acetaminophen is suggested, *not* aspirin.

8. The patient is usually returned to the interventional laboratory for repeat angiogram in 6 to 24 hours to check for dissolution of the thrombus or as deemed necessary clinically.

9. Therapy is terminated on evidence of successful recanalization (angiographic resolution with clinical improvement, return of Doppler signals), complication, or failure.

a. Both the lytic agent and heparin are discontinued. The infusion catheter is removed over a guidewire (maintaining wire access across the site of occlusion). Heparinized saline infusion is continued via the IA sheath. A postlysis angiogram is then performed.

b. Attempts to treat the underlying obstructing lesion(s) promptly by percutaneous endovascular methods or surgery (1–4) should be undertaken as soon as possible.

c. Once definitive endovascular treatment has been undertaken (mechanical thrombectomy, angioplasty, and/or stent), the sheath can be removed, or when ACT is <180 seconds. For earlier removal (1 to 2 hours), if PTT or ACT is elevated, protamine sulfate 25-mg slow IV infusion, may be given, barring contraindications. Alternatively, percutaneous access–site closure devices may be used to obtain hemostasis at the arteriotomy. There is no evidence to suggest these devices increase access site infections post multiday thrombolysis.

d. IV anticoagulation can be restarted in 3 to 6 hours after removal of IA sheath and successful groin compression, or possibly sooner if closure device was used to obtain hemostasis at the access site. Indications for restarting IV anticoagulation include peripheral thromboembolism still present, anticoagulation needing to be continued until surgery, bridge to conversion of oral therapy, or for other indications (e.g., atrial fibrillation).

Results

1. Despite widespread use, evidence for thrombolysis versus open surgery in ALI is limited. A review of current literature found only five studies comparing lysis directly to surgery. In addition to the RCTs, a large database of thrombolysis was maintained in the United Kingdom: the National Audit of Thrombolysis in Acute Leg Ischemia (NATALI).

2. Three randomized trials—ROCHESTER, STILE, and TOPAS—comparing thrombolysis to primary surgery have largely defined the role of CDT in the treatment of ALI. ALI, associated with acutely occluded bypass grafts, was seen to have a better outcome than acute occlusion in native vessels in both the TOPAS and STILE trials. In addition, the studies demonstrated a reduction in the magnitude of interventions required with CDT relative to open thrombectomy. However, use of thrombolytic therapy is associated with hemorrhagic complications and stroke, and there are also reports of recurrent ischemia (5–9). Therefore, CDT is mainly recommended for graft thromboses or in situ thromboses of native vessels of short duration (<14 days).

3. A Cochrane meta-analysis concluded that there is no significant difference in limb salvage, amputation rate, or mortality at 30 days, 6 months, and 1 year between

CDT and open thrombectomy (8). Published series on thrombolysis with urokinase for acutely ischemic lower limbs reveals a positive thrombolytic outcome in 85% to 95% patients with mean duration of infusion approximately 24 hours. A rapid early (<2 hours) response to thrombolysis is associated with improved initial success. Infusion duration is generally reported to be shorter with rt-PA, and much longer with SK. However, duration of treatment may vary with the doses and infusion rates used.

4. Long-term patency is improved if the underlying lesions are treated promptly by percutaneous and/or surgical techniques. Long-term patency is generally better for successfully treated suprainguinal occlusions (vs. infrainguinal occlusions) and vein grafts (vs. synthetic grafts).

5. When thrombolysis fails, simple thrombectomy and/or graft revision also do poorly.

6. Evidence suggests that CDT is associated with an increased risk of hemorrhagic complications and distal embolization versus open surgical intervention. No statistically increased risk of stroke between the two groups (8).

7. Patients with chronic occlusions (duration >14 days) reportedly have a better long-term prognosis with initial surgical intervention, but thrombolysis remains a viable option for them (5).

Complications

1. The probability of a major complication increases dramatically with the duration of thrombolysis. Reported incidences of various complications are shown in Table 13.3.

Table 13.3 Overall Incidence of Complications of Peripheral Arterial Thrombolysis	
Complication	**Incidence (%)**
Major bleeding	6.6
Intracranial hemorrhage	0.5
Retroperitoneal hemorrhage	0.3
Minor bleeding	6.3
Limb-related complications	
Distal embolization	5.2
Amputation	
Due to distal embolization	0.8
Due to preexisting severe ischemia	8.0
Reperfusion syndrome	0.7
Compartment syndrome	2.0
Concurrent rethrombosis	3.0
Local arterial dissection	0.6
Systemic complications	
Acute renal failure	0.3
Acute myocardial infarction	0.2
Other	
Nonhemorrhagic stroke	<1.0
Death	0.8

Compiled from two reviews of the literature on regional thrombolysis for peripheral arterial occlusions by Gardiner GA, Sullivan KL. In: Kadir S, ed. *Current Practice of Interventional Radiology.* CB Decker; 1991:87–91. (*n* = 1,787 cases) and McNamara et al. (McNamara TO, Goodwin SC, Kandarpa K. Complications associated with thrombolysis. *Semin Interv Radiol.* 1994;2:134–144.) (*n* = 1,000 cases).

2. The incidence of a major allergic reaction with SK is under 0.5% but is lower with UK; however these first-generation thrombolytics are no longer used in ALI due to increased hemorrhagic risk and slower thrombus resolution time given the lack of fibrin-bound specificity of these products.

3. Because many of the factors that increase hemorrhagic complications remain uncertain, it is prudent to direct efforts toward early detection and appropriate management of hemorrhage.

4. Avoidance of arterial puncture in noncompressible anatomical areas is advisable (e.g., axillary artery).

5. Other reported incidences of complications of thrombolysis are as follows (2):
   a. Intracranial hemorrhage 0–2.5% (threshold 2)
   b. Major bleeding requiring transfusion or surgery 1–20% (threshold 10)
   c. Compartment syndrome 1–10% (threshold 4)
   d. Distal embolization not corrected with lysis 1–5% (threshold 5)
   e. Mechanical distal embolization 1.8% (threshold 2)
   f. Sepsis or renal failure <1%
   g. Pseudoaneurysm formation at the puncture site, <1%

Management of Complications During Lytic Agent Infusion

1. Severe bleeding
   a. Immediate discontinuation of the thrombolytic agent and IV heparin.
   b. Consider transfusion of fresh whole blood, packed red blood cells, or fresh frozen plasma.
   c. If the fibrinogen is less than 100 mg per dL, give 0.15 units per kg of cryoprecipitate rounded up to the nearest unit.
   d. For severe continuing hemorrhage, consider aminocaproic acid (Amicar 5 g by mouth [PO] or slow IV infusion over 20 minutes and then 1 g per hour for 2 to 4 hours).
   e. Meticulous search for source of internal bleeding to take specific corrective measures (e.g., computed tomography scan for occult retroperitoneal hemorrhage).

2. Distal embolization of thrombus occurs in about 5% to 10% of cases, usually resolving with continued lytic therapy or suction embolectomy. Surgical embolectomy is rarely needed.

3. Allergic reaction
   a. Rare with UK and rt-PA, most frequently associated with SK.
   b. Occasional reports of chills and rigors following large rapid-bolus infusions of UK (e.g., 500,000 IU for treatment of occluded dialysis access grafts) have been reported. Prophylactic treatment consists of acetaminophen 1 g PO and diphenhydramine hydrochloride (Benadryl) 50 mg PO, given 30 to 60 minutes prior to UK infusion. For reactions occurring once UK infusion has started, treat with meperidine hydrochloride (Demerol) 50 mg IV or cimetidine 300 mg IV.

Mechanical Thrombectomy in Acute Limb Ischemia

In addition to CDT, other minimally invasive techniques, such as percutaneous aspiration thrombectomy (PAT) or PMT, are used in the treatment of ALI (2,4). PMT allows rapid debulking of a large thrombus burden, as a stand-alone thrombectomy therapy or as an adjunct to IA thrombolytic therapy to decrease symptomatic ischemia time.

1. **Manual aspiration thrombectomy** catheters are an inexpensive, rapid technique that is often underestimated.
   a. Essential tools involve a sheath with a removable hub, end-hole catheters of appropriate diameter, and/or hydrophilic guidewires.

b. Several, low-profile, rapid exchange aspiration thrombectomy catheters are available. These tend to work well as an adjunct to thrombolysis or attempt removal of distal emboli.
    (1) Pronto extraction catheter (Teleflex, Wayne, PA)
    (2) Export catheter (Medtronic, Minneapolis, MN)
    (3) Xpress-Way catheter
    (4) ASAP catheter (Merit Medical, South Jordan, UT)
    (5) Eliminate aspiration catheter (Terumo, Somerset, NJ)
c. When aspirating the clot, the end of the catheter is brought into contact with the proximal end of the clot and negative suction applied by use of a 20-mL or 50-mL syringe; suction is continued while the catheter is pulled back into the sheath. Suction is stopped when easy aspiration of blood occurs indicating loss of thrombus or successful aspiration. Most of the PAT catheters are low-profile, dual-lumen, rapid-exchange catheters compatible with a 0.014-in wire. Although successfully used in acute myocardial infarction during coronary interventions and for mesenteric arterial interventions, the use of PAT catheters in ALI remains anecdotal.

2. **Mechanical aspiration thrombectomy**
   a. QuickClear Mechanical Thrombectomy (Phillips)
      (1) 6-, 8-, and 10-Fr aspiration catheter sizes.
      (2) Simple design, no capital equipment costs as aspiration pump is disposable.
      (3) Directionality is obtained with 8- and 10-Fr angled guide catheters.
   b. Indigo Aspiration System (Penumbra, Alameda, CA).
      (1) Several catheter sizes are available (3 to 12 Fr) including rapid exchange device. Aspiration device is powered by the Penumbra ENGINE pump which aspirates at near true vacuum.
      (2) Typically, the catheter is advanced to the proximal aspect of the thrombus and attached to the aspiration device. Slowly advance through clot, then can use the separator (sized to each catheter) to agitate the thrombus if needed. Advance from proximal to distal in clot (arterial and pulmonary) and peripheral to central for DVT.
      (3) Lightning technology is a microprocessor on the pump allowing for continuous aspiration in clot and pulsed aspiration in flowing blood to reduce blood loss. Available in 7 and 12 Fr.

3. **Rheolytic thrombectomy (RT)** uses the Venturi principle for thrombus removal. High-speed saline jets are delivered retrograde from the outflow window of the catheter which simultaneously disrupt thrombus from the vessel wall while causing a low-pressure vacuum zone allowing the thrombus to enter the in-flow windows of the catheter and be removed. The AngioJet system (Boston Scientific, Marlborough, MA) is an example of this technology.
   a. Under ideal circumstances, the procedure is isovolumic, avoiding fluid overload in the patient.
   b. The AngioJet Rheolytic Thrombectomy System is extensively used currently and is the only FDA-approved device.
   c. It is a dual-lumen catheter, one lumen of which accommodates either a 0.014-in or a 0.035-in guidewire, depending on model, and the smaller lumen delivers a high-velocity, pulsatile saline flow to the catheter tip via a high-pressure stainless steel hypotube connected to an external piston pump and drive unit. The hypotube forms a closed loop at the catheter tip, which contains multiple jets aimed retrograde into the larger effluent lumen that is used for both guidewire passage and evacuation of thrombus debris. The jets fragment and dislodge the thrombus, creating a localized low-pressure zone (Bernoulli/Venturi effect) that draws the thrombus into the catheter tip and then out of the vessel through the catheter's effluent lumen.

d. The AngioJet catheter also can be used for the power-pulse spray technique that involves thrombolytic drug infusion through the catheter directly into the thrombus while occluding the outflow port. This technique effectively increases interaction of the tPA with the fibrin-bound plasminogen, increasing the efficiency of thrombolysis and/or "softening" of the thrombus for subsequent aspiration after at least 20 to 30 minutes of dwell time.

4. **Rotational thrombectomy** involves fragmenting the thrombus into small pieces that are small enough to pass through the aspiration port of the respective catheters.
   a. The Rotarex Rotational Excisional Atherectomy System (BD, Tempe, AZ)
      (1) Works over 0.018-in wire and rotates at approximately 40,000 rpm.
      (2) The catheter works by utilizing a rotating catheter head that disrupts and fragments thrombus. The internal rotating helix, which is attached to the tip of the catheter, creates a continuous negative pressure at the tip allowing for aspiration of debris into the catheter.
      (3) The internal "Archimedes screw" continues to fragment the thrombus until it is expelled into the collection bag.
   b. Jetstream Atherectomy and Thrombectomy Device (Boston Scientific, Marlborough, MA)
      (1) FDA approved for both atherectomy and thrombectomy.
      (2) Compatible with 0.014-in wire and 7-Fr vascular sheath.
      (3) Front-end cutting tip that rotates at approximately 70,000 rpm and is designed to treat soft, fibrotic, and calcified lesions as well as thrombus.
      (4) Several catheters' sizes available depending on vessel to be treated, some of the catheters also include expandable cutters to allow "blades down" and "blades up" atherectomy/thrombectomy.
      (5) Continuous and dynamic aspiration of debris and thrombus to limit amount of distal emboli.
   c. Rotational thrombectomy devices have certainly demonstrated efficacy in ALI, however, to be safe and effective, the artery needs to be somewhat larger in diameter than the catheter. Arterial spasm and vessel wall damage are inherent risks.

5. **Salvage therapies**
   a. Although mechanical thrombectomy allows for debulking of the thrombus burden and potentially a shorter thrombolytic infusion time, one of the pitfalls of this technique is increased rate of distal embolization. Many reliable methods of percutaneous thromboembolic retrieval exist including:
      (1) Manual aspiration or PAT
      (2) RT
      (3) Rotational thrombectomy
      (4) Stent placement
         (a) May be used to treat soft thrombotic occlusions. Stents are able to displace a clot to the periphery of the vessel wall and can be utilized as a last resort if mechanical clot removal fails.

6. **Conclusion**
   a. Over the past several years, many new endovascular thromboembolectoy devices have become commercially available. However, it is important to note that use of these devices may increase the risk of distal embolization. The clinical presentation of the patient and operator expertise with the device need to be considered when choosing the appropriate initial intervention.
   b. The PEARL Registry has shown that RT, with or without chemical lysis, leads to effective thrombus removal in a short time and reduces major adverse

events in ALI patients. The 12-month amputation free survival is 81% and overall survival of 91%. Half of the procedures were completed without use of CDT. Use of RT decreased overall procedure time while providing rapid perfusion to the leg (11).

c. These devices perform best for treating acute emboli, an application for which thrombolytic therapy is superior to surgery with respect to long-term, amputation-free survival (6).

d. Mechanical thrombectomy is a feasible concept for the acutely ischemic limb and in most instances allows rapid removal of the clot material and rapid revascularization, avoiding lengthy procedures and repeat angiography. A combination of PMT with IA thrombolysis may speed up clot lysis and decrease time to revascularization.

References

1. Valji K. Evolving strategies for thrombolytic therapy of peripheral vascular occlusions. *J Vasc Interv Radiol.* 2000;11(4):411–420.
2. Patel NH, Krishnamurthy VN, Kim S, et al. Quality improvement guidelines for percutaneous management of acute lower-extremity ischemia. *J Vasc Interv Radiol.* 2013;24(1):3–15. doi:10.1016/j.jvir.2012.09.026
3. Gilliland C, Shah J, Martin JG, et al. Acute limb ischemia. *Tech Vasc Interv Radiol.* 2017; 20(04):274–280.
4. Hage AN, McDevitt JL, Chick JFB, et al. Acute limb ischemia therapies: when and how to treat endovascularly. *Semin Intervent Radiol.* 2018;35(5):453–460. doi:10.1055/s-0038-1676321
5. Results of a prospective randomized trial evaluating surgery versus thrombolysis for ischemia of the lower extremity: the STILE trial. *Ann Surg.* 1994;220(3):251–268.
6. Ouriel K, Shortell CK, DeWeese JA, et al. A comparison of thrombolytic therapy with operative revascularization in the initial treatment of acute peripheral arterial ischemia. *J Vasc Surg.* 1994;19(6):1021–1030.
7. Ouriel K, Veith FJ, Sasahara AA. A comparison of recombinant urokinase with vascular surgery as initial treatment for acute arterial occlusion of the legs. Thrombolysis or peripheral arterial surgery (TOPAS) investigators. *N Engl J Med.* 1998;338(16): 1105–1111.
8. Darwood R, Berridge DC, Kessel DO, et al. Surgery versus thrombolysis for initial management of acute limb ischaemia. *Cochrane Database of Syst Rev.* 2018;8(6):CD002784.
9. Theodoridis PG, Davos CH, Dodos I, et al. Thrombolysis in acute lower limb ischemia: review of the current literature. *Ann Vasc Surg.* 2018;52:255–262.
10. Enezate TH, Omran J, Mahmud E et al. Endovascular versus surgical treatment for acute limb ischemia: a systematic review and meta-analysis of clinical trials. *Cardiovasc Diagn Ther.* 2017;7:264–271.
11. Leung DA, Blitz LR, Nelson T et al. Rheolytic pharmacomechanical thrombectomy for the management of acute limb ischemia: results from the PEARL registry. *J Endovasc Ther.* 2015;22(4):546–557. doi:10.1177/1526602815592849

14 Trauma Management

Brian Stainken, MD

Introduction

Worldwide, the leading cause of death in patients younger than the age of 44 years is trauma. In 2013, trauma claimed over 2.1 million years of potential life with direct costs of over $700 billion in the United States alone. These staggering numbers do not take into consideration the additional expense of disability or the lost financial productivity of survivors (1). The cost to society for lost productivity alone is approximately four times the direct medical expenses. Advances in resuscitation, expedited transfer to accredited centers and emergency department–based CT have revolutionized trauma care. CT imaging allows the trauma team to focus on the most critical injury and expedites triage to the relevant experts in either the OR or IR (2). In trauma centers, expert IRs are key members of the trauma team as they are often best equipped to rapidly address exsanguinating hemorrhage (3). Where infrastructure is lacking trauma and IR communities must advocate for appropriate facilities and staff to provide optimal IR care within the institutional trauma system.

The initial steps in intervention for trauma care are similar regardless of the location of injury. General considerations are discussed first. The details involved in treating specific sites including splenic, hepatic, renal, pelvic, paraspinal, and extremity trauma follow.

Trauma Care in the Interventional Radiology Space

Hemorrhagic Shock

Indications

1. Management recommendations have trended away from anatomic classification schemes (laceration length, hematoma size, associated injuries) toward a focus on management based upon the presence or absence of active bleeding on CT. The sequencing of care in the setting of multisystem trauma is driven by the relative morbidity of each diagnosis.

   a. Once bleeding is identified, most treatment algorithms pivot based on the determination of hemodynamic stability. There is no consensus on the actual criteria which define "unstable." One systematic review suggests that systolic blood pressure and heart rate were the most commonly used parameters for blunt trauma patients but notes there is no consensus on threshold values (4). The Advanced Trauma Life Support (ATLS) manual defines "unstable" as BP <90, HR >120, evidence of skin vasoconstriction, altered level of consciousness and/or shortness of breath (5). Others define instability as a failed response to resuscitation, using criteria such as transfusion demand, base deficit, and need for pressors (6).

   b. Anticipated time to hemostasis is driven by many local factors beyond whether bleeding is arrested with a clamp in the OR or a catheter in IR. The role of IR at a given hospital may depend as much on the preparation and layout of the trauma facility and the dedication of the team to best care as it is by the nature of the injury.

2. "Stable" patient with blunt trauma, bleeding confirmed on CT.

Contraindications

Absolute: Unstable patients, if control can be achieved more rapidly in the OR.

Relative (All Situation Specific)

1. Patients with multiple organ involvement.
2. Patients requiring coincidental laparotomy (e.g., perforated viscus).
3. Unable to access care in a sufficiently timely fashion.
4. Pregnancy. A relative risk assessment may demonstrate that the morbidity of surgery exceeds the theoretical risk of radiation exposure especially in late trimester gestation. Most centers wave pregnancy testing rules when timely care is needed. Advanced planning for such scenarios is paramount.
5. Renal insufficiency: In general terms, for the patient in shock, the benefits of accurate diagnosis and expedited care far outweigh the small risk of contrast nephropathy. Do not let waiting for labs delay imaging or intervention when time is of the essence. Acute kidney injury due to ischemia is far more common than contrast nephropathy.
6. Anaphylactoid reactions to nonionic contrast are also rare. When possible, clarification of the specific nature of a prior reaction (mild, moderate, severe) is important. Depending on the presentation and relative risk, it may be reasonable to proceed in a patient with a known reaction history after consultation with anesthesia and other members of the trauma team (see Chapter 65).

Assessment of the Trauma Patient

1. Resuscitation is critical during all aspects of trauma care including endovascular intervention. This entails ensuring an airway and appropriate ventilation as well as adequate intravenous (IV) access with large-bore IV lines for fluid, medication, and transfusions. IR can be a great help in achieving this access especially in hypotensive patients. Warming the patient and replacement of coagulation factors will aid in hemostasis. Other than cervical stabilization, neurologic assessment can wait in hemodynamically labile patients. Although associated with a poorer prognosis, neurologic injury alone is not likely to cause significant hemodynamic shock.
2. Laboratory studies are not a prerequisite for trauma angiography, and the procedure should not be delayed in anticipation of complete blood count (CBC), chemistry panel, pregnancy tests, or coagulation parameters. A worsening base deficit is the most sensitive laboratory indicator of hemodynamic shock and will precede a drop in hematocrit.
3. CT and any other available imaging studies should always be reviewed to identify potential sites of injury and occult sources of bleeding. The trauma CT is the cornerstone of initial diagnosis. A negative CT in children is 99.6% predictive to exclude **any** intraabdominal injury (7). In penetrating abdominal trauma, CT has far greater sensitivity than focused assessment with sonography for trauma (FAST) and its use (during resuscitation) saves lives (2,8). The React-2 trial showed that whole-body CT did not offer a survival benefit over selective scanning, but it did expedite diagnosis. Nearly half of the selective scan group ultimately received the equivalent of a whole-body scan by the time of discharge (9).
4. Resuscitation should be continued throughout the procedure. A lifesaving procedure should not be postponed while waiting for blood products. Safe embolization in unstable patients can be performed if the patient responds, even transiently, to a 2-L rapid resuscitative bolus (6). Transfusions should be administered while the patient is in route to or on the angiography table to prevent delays. Nursing care should move with the patient.

Procedure

Trauma Embolotherapy

1. Arterial access is traditionally obtained via the common femoral artery however radial access can be a useful alternative (see Chapter 1). In severe hemodynamic shock, the femoral pulses may not be palpable, ultrasound guidance is safer when

they are and essential when they aren't. When possible, upsize the sheath 1 to 2 Fr beyond the planned catheter size and use the side arm connected to a manometer to monitor arterial pressures. The same sheath can be used, when warranted for resuscitation. Be sure to sew the sheath in if you expect it to be left in place after your procedure.

2. Treatment should not be delayed for the purpose of angiographic documentation if CT has been diagnostic. If extravasation is seen on hand-injected fluoroscopic imaging, save it and move on to treatment without a formal angiographic/injector run when the situation calls for speed.

3. Angiographic findings for vessel disruption in the setting of trauma may include:
   a. Extravasation
   b. Occlusion
   c. Arteriovenous (AV) fistula
   d. Intimal tear
   e. False aneurysm

4. Extravasation seen on CT and not seen at angiography may be due to:
   a. Vessel spasm
   b. Slow bleeding rate (e.g., venous bleeding)
   c. Changes in blood pressure
   d. Poor cardiac output
   e. Anomalous anatomy

5. Always obtain orthogonal views when the finding is not clear in one projection. A single angiographic projection should not be relied on to clear a vessel of injury. Selective runs may show extravasation not visible on a flush run.

6. If the CT is clear but there is no extravasation on angiography, if the site can be confidently identified, consider embolization on an empiric basis so as to avoid reintervention.

7. Choice of device for achieving hemostasis should be based on experience, vessel caliber, downstream territory, need for control over device positioning, and delivery catheter inner-lumen diameter (see Chapter 95). These include:
   a. Embolic agents.
      (1) Gelfoam is a mainstay for trauma embolization and is used where rapid, temporary vascular occlusion is needed. It can be delivered as a macerated suspension or slurry, or selectively in the form of a compressed dry pledget (torpedo). Gelfoam slurry works well for managing the diffuse small branch intramuscular bleeding often seen in the setting of pelvic fractures.
      (2) Coils are generally reserved for more focused embolization, occlusion of intermediate size conduit vessels, when longer-term occlusion is preferred, or to isolate arterial fistulae or pseudoaneurysms. Detachable coils allow precise control. Hemostatic plugs can achieve precise immediate hemostasis in medium to large vessels, occlusion is less dependent on intrinsic thrombogenesis. All can be delivered through coaxial microcatheters. Note that there is no standardization of tolerances between devices, manufacturers, and delivery catheters. Follow recommendations on packaging. "Stuck" coils in particular can cause unnecessary delays in care.
      (3) Stent grafts can rapidly control exsanguinating bleeding while preserving luminal continuity. This is helpful when larger conduit vessels such as the aorta, carotid, hepatic, renal, iliac, subclavian, and extremity arteries are involved. Depending on the territory, pay attention to branch vessels which will be sacrificed when crossing with a graft. Late reconstitution can be avoided by careful preemptive branch vessel embolization.
      (4) Temporary balloon occlusion is an underutilized and important technique for achieving hemostasis. Inflating an appropriately sized, compliant balloon within the artery proximal to a site of extravasation may provide immediate hemostatic control with a striking hemodynamic

response. The central lumen can then be used to better study the bleeding site and plan care. Microcatheters can be deployed through the central lumen of most over the wire balloon catheters. Downstream pressures can be measured. Temporary balloon occlusion can achieve proximal control prior to surgical exposure and prophylactic balloon placement may be a useful adjunct when there is high potential risk for bleeding. One example is the use of temporary balloon occlusion in penetrating subclavian artery injury for proximal hemostatic control prior to repair via a clavicular resection rather than via midline sternotomy. Resuscitative endovascular balloon occlusion (REBOA) involves placement of a large caliber balloons in the distal thoracic or abdominal aorta. There is significant risk for downstream ischemic complications if definitive control and deflation are not rapidly achieved (10).

8. Once stabilized, completion angiography is important to confirm hemostasis prior to removal of the access sheath. Closure devices should be considered in this population as patients may be heavily sedated, may proceed for additional procedures, and/or be at high risk for transfusion-related coagulopathy.

Longitudinal Management

1. Follow closely for signs of persistent or delayed hemorrhage with serial blood work, physical examination, vital sign checks, and imaging. It is the responsibility of the treating physician to identify complications and ensure that the patient has fully recovered from the intervention.

2. Adequate prophylaxis for infection and deep vein thrombosis (DVT) should be considered.

Splenic Trauma

The spleen is the most commonly injured organ in blunt trauma however most patients can safely avoid splenectomy. Centers with the highest rates of embolization enjoy the highest rates of splenic salvage. The probability of successful preservation of the spleen is increased when embolization is used for all grade 3 and 4 lacerations (11). When a splenectomy is performed without an attempt at salvage, the trauma team should reasonably ask, why?

Indications

1. Blunt trauma
   a. Extravasation of contrast on arterial phase CT or angiography. There is debate about embolization versus observation for stable patients presenting with a grade 1 to 3 laceration and parenchymal contrast extravasation "blush" on CT (12).
   b. Hemodynamic lability or transfusion requirements greater than 4 units packed red blood cells (PRBC) over 24 hours. While some surgical society standards still advise against embolization in the setting of hemodynamic instability, larger published series demonstrate more patients undergoing embolization without a change in the distribution of splenic injury scores (11).
   c. Grade 3 injury on CT; (laceration >3 cm or >5 cm hematoma) or vascular (involvement of segmental or hilar vessel) laceration with or without active extravasation.
   d. Intrasplenic false aneurysm or AV fistula as demonstrated on CT.
   e. Delayed bleeding as evidenced by recurrent hemodynamic lability or transfusion requirements following initial observation or embolization for splenic trauma.

2. Penetrating trauma
   a. There is limited role for endovascular intervention in penetrating splenic trauma. These patients generally require laparotomy because of the risk for coincident visceral injury.

Splenic Embolization

1. Plan your approach based on CT findings. The celiac axis can be catheterized from the femoral route using cobra or Simmons and from the radial artery long cobra ($\geq$100 cm), multipurpose- or vertebral-shaped catheters, all either 4 or 5 Fr. An angiogram is performed through the portal venous phase to visualize the splenic vein. The catheter is then advanced into the splenic artery, and a dedicated splenic arteriogram in a different projection is performed. This can be achieved with any of the above catheters and a hydrophilic guidewire (straightening vessels by deep inspiration or expiration helps!) but in practice most angiographers use a microcatheter, especially if distal embolization is likely. Consider what treatment method you are likely to use when choosing microcatheter diameter.

2. Extravasation may be extremely subtle. If no extravasation or vascular injury is present at angiography, there is a high probability that nonoperative management will be successful. Delayed rupture is rare in these circumstances.

3. If extravasation or vascular injury is seen, intervention may be performed as described below. Splenic artery embolization is typically characterized as proximal or distal (13,14):

   a. Intrasplenic hemorrhage. Proximal coil embolization will temporarily decrease the arterial pulp pressures such that intrasplenic hemorrhage is controlled. Because collateral circulation is preserved, proximal splenic arterial coil embolization is associated with a low risk for splenic infarction. Proximal embolization should be performed with coils sized 20% to 25% larger than the vessel diameter and positioned just distal to the origin of the dorsal pancreatic artery. The coil should be oversized because the artery is often vasoconstricted in hemodynamic shock. Following restoration of normal hemodynamics, the artery may dilate and allow distal coil migration. Alternatively, vascular plugs can be used, but attention to appropriate sizing to avoid distal migration is important.

   b. Focal intrasplenic hemorrhage can also be managed successfully with more selective (distal) embolization when the extent of injury and the patient's presentation allow. Choice of method should be made by the interventional radiologist based on patient stability and pattern of splenic injury, and operator experience.

   c. Extrasplenic hemorrhage. Selective embolization should be performed because of hemodynamic instability and risk of continued hemorrhage. When significant extrasplenic hemorrhage or combined intrasplenic and extracapsular bleeding are noted, a combination of distal selective embolization and proximal splenic artery coil embolization may be used for maximal hemostatic control.

   d. Intraparenchymal false aneurysm or AVF. In the setting of distal false aneurysm or AVF supplied by a discrete vessel, selective micro coil embolization is warranted to minimize splenic infarction.

   e. Pseudoaneurysms or AVFs of the main splenic artery are occasionally seen in association with penetrating trauma. They may be treated by proximal and distal splenic artery coil embolization to isolate the site of injury. A stent graft may also be used to cover the injury and preserve flow to the spleen.

Results (13,14)

Proximal splenic artery coil embolization in the setting of trauma has a technical success rate of 90% to 95% with a similar clinical success rate in terms of avoiding splenectomy. It appears that outcomes for proximal and distal embolization are equivalent. By requiring embolization for all hemodynamically stable patients with grade 3 to 5 injuries, one institution increased the percentage of spleens salvaged from 52% to 67% while reducing the rate of observation failures from 15% to 5%.

Complications

1. Infarct. Particularly with distal embolization, infarction to some degree is to be expected. The significance of asymptomatic peripheral infarcts on postprocedure CT is questionable.
2. Abscess. Approximately 4%. Risk may be minimized by limiting on table handling and exposure of the gel foam prior to administration.

Hepatobiliary Trauma

The liver is a highly vascular organ with a dual blood supply. Clinically significant traumatic hemorrhage from the liver most commonly arises from the hepatic arterial circulation. The most devastating vascular trauma, however, is hepatic venous injury. A potential advantage of nonoperative management of liver trauma may be avoidance of uncontrolled hemorrhage from an occult hepatic venous laceration uncovered during liver mobilization (15).

Indications

1. Blunt trauma
   a. Recurrent hemodynamic lability despite resuscitation or greater than 4 units of PRBC transfusion requirements over 24 hours
   b. CT findings for significant liver injury include:
      (1) Laceration. American Association for the Surgery of Trauma (AAST) grade 3 or higher or extension to involve a major hepatic vein
      (2) Focal contrast material extravasation
      (3) Large subcapsular or perihepatic hematoma
   c. Persistent hemobilia suggesting an arteriobiliary fistula. Biliary colic, jaundice, and melena following trauma are other highly suggestive signs of hemobilia.
   d. Second-stage procedure following open surgical packing of a severe liver injury. The goal is to definitively treat findings temporized by packing.
   e. Repeat hemorrhage or hemodynamic lability following initial surgical management.
2. Penetrating trauma. Most patients will require laparotomy to exclude traumatic enterotomy. CT may be used to exclude bowel wall injury in specific populations.
   a. Focal penetrating wounds isolated to the right upper quadrant may proceed directly to hepatic angiography if there is no CT evidence for bowel injury or clinical suggestion of peritonitis. Proximity of the injury tract to hilar vessels particularly warrants angiographic evaluation.
   b. Repeat hemorrhage or hemodynamic lability following initial surgical management.

Contraindications

Relative
1. Historically, hemodynamic lability not responsive to initial resuscitation was referred for emergent operative management rather than angiography, but this is changing, as previously discussed.
2. Preexisting liver disease. Embolization of multiple liver segments may place the patient at risk for liver insufficiency. When feasible, meticulous technique and subselective embolization are warranted in patients with evidence of cirrhosis to minimize infarction of the liver.
3. Compromised portal vein blood supply. With portal vein thrombosis or hepatofugal portal vein flow, the patient is at greater risk of hepatic infarct following hepatic artery embolization. However, the relative risk of subselective embolization should be weighed against the risks of continued hemorrhage or the relative risk of surgical management.

Procedure

1. The approach to the diagnostic angiogram should be driven by the acuity of the presentation and findings on CT. In the unstable patient, rapid control matters

more than image quality. Once stabilized, a full diagnostic assessment can be completed.

2. Full assessment should include a superior mesenteric artery (SMA) angiogram through the venous phase demonstrating portal vein patency and integrity. Because variant vascular anatomy of the liver is common, the SMA arteriogram is important to exclude accessory or aberrant vessels such as an accessory right hepatic artery.

3. The celiac axis and SMA can be catheterized from the femoral route using cobra or Simmons, and from the radial artery long cobra (≥100 cm), multipurpose- or vertebral-shaped catheters, (all either 4 or 5 Fr).

4. The diagnostic catheter or a microcatheter can be advanced to the common or proper hepatic artery to allow selective hepatic angiography. Multiple oblique views should be obtained to evaluate for arterial injury including selective left and right hepatic arteriograms, if necessary.

5. Embolization can be performed in several ways depending on the distribution of injury and available time:

   a. Multiple points of extravasation. Scatter embolization using gelfoam slurry or large (over 500 micron) particles into the left and/or right hepatic arteries or the proper hepatic artery (with the 5-Fr catheter). Catheterization of the right hepatic distal to the cystic artery is desirable to avoid nontarget embolization of the gallbladder.

   b. Single point of extravasation. Following subselective catheterization of the injured branch via a microcatheter, focal embolization may be performed using gelfoam, particles, or microcoils.

   c. Fistulas between the hepatic artery and portal vein, hepatic vein, or bile ducts. The inflow vessel should be isolated proximal and distal to the fistula with coils or microcoils. For common or proper hepatic artery fistulas, a covered stent is an attractive treatment option.

Results

Technical success rate—88% to 100%. The probability of success is driven by the severity of the injury, coagulopathy, and acuity (16). In children, a 5-year retrospective series reports 100% success in nonoperative management despite that 46% presented with grade 4 lacerations (17). In adults presenting with grade 4 and 5 injuries, embolization in conjunction with surgery is associated with decreased mortality (18).

Complications

Differentiating complications related to the traumatic event itself from procedural complications is important. A single-center review comparing operative management with embolization in 396 patients showed equal liver-related morbidity and a reduction in mortality from 17% for surgically managed to 3% in patients treated with embolotherapy (19). Prospective randomized trials are needed to best determine the roles of surgical- versus image-guided approaches.

1. Gallbladder injury. Rarely encountered in oncologic embolization and less likely with larger embolics used in trauma. Nevertheless, when possible, confirm that the catheter tip is distal to the cystic artery prior to embolization.

2. Liver necrosis or hepatic insufficiency. Review CT to assess portal venous flow prior to hepatic arterial embolization. Avoid powders or liquid agents. Recognize that the extent of underlying parenchymal trauma and perfusion status may influence the extent of necrosis more than the embolization procedure. The highest-risk group for liver necrosis are patients presenting for definitive embolization after high-grade injuries treated initially with damage control laparotomy/liver packing (16).

Renal Trauma

Most blunt renal trauma is minor, self-limiting, and requires no treatment. Patients with solitary kidneys warrant more aggressive kidney-saving procedures. The most common cause of renal vascular injury is iatrogenic following renal biopsy or nephrostomy.

Indications (20)

The 2020 American Urological Association (AUA) Guidelines recommend either surgery or embolization in hemodynamically unstable patients with no or transient response to resuscitation.

1. Blunt trauma
   a. Hemodynamic lability despite resuscitation or greater than 4 units of PRBC over 24 hours, and significant renal injury on CT such as:
      (1) Fractured kidney
      (2) Subcapsular hematoma greater than or equal to 50% of the kidney volume
      (3) Active extravasation
   b. Renovascular injury on CT
      (1) Contrast extravasation
      (2) Central perinephric hematoma between the kidney and aorta or inferior vena cava (IVC) suggesting a full-thickness injury of the renal artery
      (3) Segmental renal infarct suggesting embolic disease from proximal arterial injury or segmental renal artery occlusion
      (4) Complete renal infarct suggesting main renal artery injury or occlusion. This is associated with a poor prognosis for renal preservation
   c. Abdominal bruit or thrill suggesting a renal AV fistula
   d. Unrelenting gross hematuria and/or severe unremitting urinary colic suggesting an arteriocalyceal fistula
2. Penetrating trauma
   a. When penetrating injury results in concomitant intraperitoneal and retroperitoneal involvement, patients typically require laparotomy to exclude enterotomy; however, if the injury is limited to the retroperitoneum, embolization can reduce the risk for nephrectomy. In particular, embolization is the treatment of choice in iatrogenic renal vascular injury such as following renal biopsy or nephrostomy.
   b. Hemodynamic lability despite resuscitation or greater than 4 units of PRBC transfusion requirements over 24 hours and significant kidney injury on CT as listed earlier without intraperitoneal injury.

Procedure

1. If proximal renal artery injury is suspected, perform an aortogram to evaluate the vessel origin.
2. Selective renal artery catheterization is performed (from the femoral route using cobra or Simmons, and from the radial artery long cobra [≥100 cm], multipurpose- or vertebral-shaped catheters, all either 4 or 5 Fr) and angiogram performed.
3. If the selective arteriogram fails to enhance the entire kidney, obtain additional projections and consider a possible accessory renal artery or thrombosed branch vessel. Review CT images.
4. If vascular injury is seen, intervention may be performed as described below:
   a. Renal artery dissection, laceration, or extravasation. A stent or endograft may be used to preserve flow to the kidney if the lesion can be crossed (see Chapter 7).
   b. Intraparenchymal hemorrhage or false aneurysm. Subselective embolization should be performed, either with original catheter and hydrophilic guidewire or microcatheter. In either case control of depth of guidewire penetration is critical as guidewire capsular perforation can easily happen. Because the renal artery is an end artery, unlike the liver or spleen, there is no issue with

rebleeding via collaterals. Therefore there is not an absolute need for embolization distal to the vascular injury unless more than one renal branch is involved. In the kidney, the goal is to minimize segments devascularized so as to maximize preservation of renal tissue.

c. Intraparenchymal AV or arteriocalyceal fistula. Embolization of the conduit vessel proximal to the injury should be performed with microcoils. Note that arteriocalyceal fistulas may be difficult to diagnose angiographically due to extravasation of contrast into the collecting system. Early opacification of a single calyx on angiograms is highly suggestive of arteriocalyceal fistula.

5. If not assessed on CT, delayed imaging 15 to 30 minutes postarterial contrast can be performed to evaluate ureteral injury. The ureters should be visualized to the level of the bladder.

Results

Multiple series of renal trauma patients have demonstrated a greater than 95% success rate of embolotherapy in treating parenchymal renal injury as a means of obtaining hemostasis, maximizing renal function, and avoiding nephrectomy (20). The long-term patency for stents placed in the setting of acute trauma to the main renal artery needs further evaluation and may not offer benefit over nephrectomy (21).

Complications

Infarction of downstream renal parenchyma is a consequence of successful renal embolization. Selective technique is important to minimize the degree of infarction.

Pelvic Fracture

Patients with pelvic fractures presenting in shock have a mortality rate ranging from 30% to 50%. Bleeding associated with such fractures arises from small- to medium-sized intramuscular branches that are unrecognizable intraoperatively. The first course of action in this population is immediate stabilization of the fracture with a pelvic binder and resuscitation. Ongoing blood loss requires aggressive management to stop continued bleeding. CT is the cornerstone of patient assessment. Once the source is isolated to the pelvis, the next step is angiography. There are clear data correlating time to achieving hemostasis with embolization and survival (22). Surgical options in this population are limited, and the acute care focus is on pelvic stabilization/binding. Definitive orthopedic repair can wait.

Indications

1. Blunt trauma
   a. Persistent or recurrent hemorrhagic shock despite resuscitation in a patient with pelvic fractures or a retroperitoneal hematoma and no evidence for hemoperitoneum. Embolization to treat arterial hemorrhage is the accepted treatment of choice in patients with hemorrhage associated with pelvic fractures and should not be delayed for operative external fixation.
   b. Ongoing hemorrhage from pelvic fractures necessitating transfusion greater than 4 units of PRBC in 24 hours or 6 units of PRBC in 48 hours.
   c. Retroperitoneal contrast extravasation on CT in the setting of hemodynamic instability or evidence for ongoing blood loss despite pelvic binding.
   d. Large or expanding retroperitoneal hematoma identified at laparotomy.
2. Penetrating trauma
   a. A penetrating pelvic injury with concern for bowel injury requires laparotomy. However, if there is no concern for bowel injury, pelvic injury in proximity to major vessels or with imaging findings of vascular injury may be evaluated angiographically.

  b. Following laparotomy for penetrating trauma to the pelvis to exclude vascular injury or provide definitive hemostasis

3. Empiric nonselective embolization of the internal iliac arteries (IIAs) in patients without angiographic or CT evidence of vascular injury is not recommended.

Procedure

1. Pelvic stabilization is a priority. By approximating fracture fragments and limiting pelvic volume venous (marrow) bleeding is managed. While wrapping the pelvis in a sheet is a quick means of pelvic stabilization; there are data suggesting that purpose-designed pelvic binders and C clamps are associated with improved survival. Binders are centered at the level of the greater trochanter. Know what is used at your center. Be ready to cut a hole in the device, or use radial access.

2. Assess CT findings and hemodynamic status. If the patient is not stable, don't waste time with full diagnostics; fix the problem.

3. The IIA can be catheterized using a cobra catheter from the femoral route or vertebral-shaped catheters from the radial artery, either 4 or 5 Fr. A lesser used alternative is to use the Roberts Catheter (Cook Inc, Bloomington, IN) via the femoral artery which can make contralateral and ipsilateral IIA cannulation easier.

4. Select the IIA on the side with the most extravasation on CT or the more displaced fracture and scatter embolize the posterior division with gelfoam. Remember that gelfoam is readily colonized when handled or left exposed on a procedure table. Isolate the gelfoam from any contamination on your gloves or the table and minimize maceration. Excessive plunging in the three-way stopcock can create microparticulate emboli within the slurry (23). When delivering gelfoam in a slurry, image in the ipsilateral oblique to open the IIA bifurcation. Use frequent contrast injections or dilute contrast in the slurry to assess stasis and control administration of emboli. Avoid high-pressure or pulsed injections. It does not take very much gelfoam in the right place to stop bleeding.

5. If necessary, use a proximal occluding balloon to arrest bleeding, then allow the team to catch up with resuscitation. You can still use a microcatheter to select or embolize directly through the balloon lumen depending on positioning. Remember that ultimately, the extent to which your intervention is useful to the patient is driven by the speed with which you achieve initial hemostasis (24).

6. Initial embolization or occlusion will often produce dramatic and rapid stabilization, allowing for an opportunity to assess and complete treatment and confirm adequate and stable hemostasis has been achieved.

7. Second-side IIA cannulation is easily achieved using the same vertebral-shaped catheter from a radial approach. If femoral access was used ipsilateral access can be achieved by:

  a. *Waltman loop.* If a cobra catheter was used:

   (1) With the tip of the catheter at least 5 cm, preferably more, over the aortic bifurcation into the contralateral external iliac artery, a guidewire (e.g., angle-tipped hydrophilic wire) is advanced inside the catheter only as far as the apex of the aortic bifurcation.

   (2) While vigorously rotating the catheter (try counterclockwise first), advance catheter and guidewire as a unit so that the body of the catheter forms a loop in the aorta.

   (3) Advance catheter and guidewire as a unit until tip of catheter is above the aortic bifurcation.

   (4) Rotate the catheter tip so it is pointed toward the origin of the ipsilateral common iliac artery and pull the catheter until tip engages it. This can be done with or without the guidewire protruding from the catheter.

(5) Rotate the catheter and/or protruding guide and withdraw catheter further at groin so it engages the ipsilateral IIA. A stable position is usually best achieved by advancing the guidewire/catheter well into the anterior division.

b. Roberts catheter as described above.

c. Especially in tortuous anatomy, the cobra or a RIM catheter can just be pulled back until its tip engages the origin of the ipsilateral IIA and a coaxial microcatheter used to cannulate the anterior division.

8. External iliac artery or major trunk injuries are uncommon. The external pudendal and external obturator branches are two sites of injury, which may be missed on selective internal iliac arteriography. While end branches of the external iliac may be embolized with gelfoam, plugs or coils, external iliac artery injury typically requires placement of a covered stent.

Results

Technical success rates approaching 100% and clinical success rates of 95% are reported (22,24). In a series of 78 patients who underwent embolization for pelvic trauma, only four demonstrated recurrent hemorrhage, the majority of which responded to a second embolization (25). As noted previously, there is a correlation between time to embolization and survival (22).

Complications

1. Impotence (2%). No studies have shown a causative role of IIA embolization in the setting of trauma. It is unclear whether most posttraumatic impotence is due to the underlying pelvic fracture or the embolization procedure.

2. Gluteal necrosis (6%). One should avoid the use of small particles and recognize that more than one factor (e.g., hypotension, underlying muscular injury, and surgical packing) correlates with this complication.

Paraspinal/Lumbar Artery Injury

Lumbar artery injuries can lead to significant bleeding and are associated with lumbar vertebral body and transverse process fractures. When imaging demonstrates lumbar vertebral body injury, lumbar artery injury should be suspected. In addition, lumbar artery injuries may be seen in association with pelvic trauma.

Indications

1. Blunt trauma

   a. Hemodynamic lability despite resuscitation or greater than 4 units of PRBC transfusion requirements over 24 hours and lumbar vertebral body or transverse process fractures with or without pelvic trauma.

   b. CT findings suggestive of lumbar artery injury such as large retroperitoneal hematoma or active extravasation.

2. Penetrating trauma

   a. Penetrating injuries of the retroperitoneum that traverse the peritoneum generally require surgical exploration. However, CT may exclude intraperitoneal extension in focal penetrating wounds isolated to the retroperitoneum. Endovascular management may then be considered in the setting of recurrent hemodynamic lability or greater than 4 units of PRBC transfusion requirement in 24 hours and CT findings of active extravasation or large posterior pararenal hematoma.

Procedure

1. Usually, an aortogram is performed for initial evaluation. Correlate findings with CT. Typically, active extravasation will not be seen; often, the only finding of

lumbar artery injury on aortography is nonopacification of a vasoconstricted or occluded vessel.

2. Selective lumbar artery angiography is performed at the level of interest as well as levels one vertebral body above and below to exclude collateral filling of the injured vessel. If from femoral access, lumbar artery ostia can be engaged using Mickelson, or less frequently Simmons or cobra catheters, and from the radial artery Mickelson, long cobra (≥100 cm), or multipurpose-shaped catheters, all either 4 or 5 Fr. If injury (occlusion/extravasation or spasm) is found, embolization should be performed as follows:

   a. In general, microcatheters and coils are used, and if the injured vessel can be crossed, they should be deployed distal to proximal across the site.

   b. Usually, the artery of Adamkiewicz (aberrant radiculomedullary artery communicating with the anterior spinal artery) arises from the left lower thoracic intercostal arteries (75%). It can rarely arise from the lumbar arteries. If this is seen, proceed carefully; advance the microcatheter past the anastomosis and avoid use of small particle or liquid embolics.

Results

Angiography for retroperitoneal hemorrhage is hampered by a low sensitivity in identifying the source of bleeding. Retroperitoneal hemorrhage will often be self-limiting. When a vascular injury is found, however, embolization achieves a high technical success rate in control of hemorrhage. As noted, lumbar artery injury can be difficult to access and manage operatively.

Extremity Trauma

Most vascular injury occurs in the extremities and acute loss of limb perfusion can be associated with devastating consequences including exsanguination and acute limb ischemia. Although most vascular injuries involving the extremities are a result of penetrating trauma, blunt trauma, especially crush injury, can cause significant morbidity.

Predictive findings for significant vascular injury can be classified as either hard or soft (26).

The presence of hard signs is associated with a 95% positive predictive value for vascular injury. The hard signs include:

1. Pulsatile or expanding hematoma
2. Active hemorrhage
3. Diminished or absent pulses
4. Bruit or thrill
5. Critical limb ischemia

The presence of soft signs has a 30% positive predictive value for vascular injury. The soft signs include:

1. Nonexpanding hematoma
2. History of pulsatile bleeding
3. Neurologic deficit
4. Unexplained hypotension
5. Proximity to vascular structures

The ankle-brachial index is also a useful tool to exclude significant arterial injury. An index of 0.9 in the absence of symptoms excludes arterial involvement.

Indications (27,28)

1. Blunt trauma

   a. If a pulse deficit persists following reduction of the fracture, CT angiography is warranted.

   b. Associated traumatic injuries
      (1) Knee dislocation or comminuted, displaced fracture of the proximal tibia
      (2) Elbow dislocation
      (3) Shoulder dislocation in the elderly
      (4) Scapulothoracic dissociation
2. Penetrating trauma
   a. Penetrating extremity trauma with hard signs of vascular injury warrants immediate intervention.
   b. Penetration by high-velocity missiles (e.g., assault rifles) in proximity to a major vessel warrants angiography even in the absence of hard signs of injury. The energy of the entering missile can cause cavitation and shock wave injury many centimeters from the bullet tract. Possible resulting injuries include vasospasm, thrombosis, intimal flap, perforation, AVF, and intramural hematoma.

Contraindications

Procedure

1. Opaque markers may be placed at the entrance and exit wounds to identify the injury tract.
2. Initial evaluation should begin with an angiogram in multiple obliquities centered on the site of injury. Contrast injection should be from a sufficiently proximal location to identify potential collateral sources of perfusion.
3. Treatment options are dependent on the location and type of injury as described below:
   a. In large arteries such as the superficial femoral, popliteal, subclavian, and brachial, stent grafts have been reported to be effective in treating false aneurysms, AVFs, dissection, and active extravasation.
   b. In small arteries such as the radial, ulnar, peroneal, and tibial, coil occlusion is advised if proximal and distal control can be accomplished. Prior to embolization, confirmation of adequate distal circulation and patency of collaterals is required. Occlusion may be due to spasm or dissection and should be managed with embolization if proximal and distal access can be achieved. The techniques used in such situations are identical to those used for crossing nontraumatic occlusions. In one series, isolated anterior tibial injuries had a higher incidence of limb loss than posterior tibial or peroneal (29).
   c. Muscular arteries arising from conduit vessels such as the profunda femoral, superficial femoral, and popliteal arteries should be treated by subselective coil or particulate embolization as close as possible to the site of injury.
   d. Management of posttraumatic AVF may be deceptively complicated. All arterial inflow to the fistula must be occluded at the time of initial embolization to permanently seal the fistula. In larger arteries, a covered stent may be used to isolate the vessel wall injury, but if the site of fistulation is a branch vessel, crossing the ostium with a stent graft will be insufficient as the fistula will recruit collateral inflow. Careful angiographic assessment of the actual site of vessel wall injury is required. In smaller vessels, coiling distally and proximally to isolate the fistula is generally effective. Care must be exercised to prevent coil migration into the venous system. Short fistulae may require paired venous and arterial grafts. A follow-up arteriogram is advised to confirm adequate isolation for treated AVFs.
   e. Endografts have been employed to reperfuse acutely devascularized limb in the setting of popliteal trauma or fractures at other sites, even prior to orthopedic stabilization. Endografts play a clear role in the management of penetrating trauma as well.

R e f e r e n c e s

1. Centers for Disease Control and Prevention. Years of potential life lost before age 65 years. http://webappa.cdc.gov/cgi-bin/broker.exe. Accessed October 30, 2015.
2. Sutphin PD, Baliyan V. Postprocessing imaging techniques of the computed tomography angiography in trauma patients for preprocedural planning. *Semin Intervent Radiol.* 2021;38(1):9–17.
3. Padia SA, Ingraham CR, Moriarty JM, et al. Society of interventional radiology position statement on endovascular intervention for trauma. *J Vasc Interv Radiol.* 2020;31(3): 363–369.e2.
4. Loggers S, Koedam T, Giannakopoulos G, et al. Definition of hemodynamic stability in blunt trauma patients: a systematic review and assessment amongst Dutch trauma team members. *Eur J Trauma Emerg Surg.* 2017;43(6):823–833.
5. Committee of trauma of ACS. Advanced Trauma Life Support (ATLS) Student Manual. 10th ed. American College of Surgeons; 2018.
6. Zsolt B, Caldwell E, Heetveld M, et al. Institutional practice guidelines on management of pelvic fracture-related hemodynamic instability: do they make a difference? *J Trauma.* 2005;58(4):778–782.
7. Kerrey BT, Rogers AJ, Lee LK, et al. A multicenter study of the risk of intra-abdominal injury in children after normal abdominal computed tomography scan results in the emergency department. *Ann Emerg Med.* 2013;62(4):319–326.
8. Smith IM, Naumann DN, Marsden ME, et al. Scanning and war: utility of FAST and CT in the assessment of battlefield abdominal trauma. *Ann Surg.* 2015;262(2):389–396.
9. Sierink J, Treskes K, Edwards M, et al. Immediate total-body CT scanning versus conventional imaging and selective CT scanning in patients with severe trauma (REACT-2): a randomised controlled trial. *Lancet.* 2016;388:673–683
10. Bulger E, Perina D, Qasim Z, et al. Clinical use of resuscitative endovascular balloon occlusion of the aorta (REBOA) in civilian trauma systems in the USA, 2019: a joint statement from the American College of Surgeons Committee on Trauma, the American College of Emergency Physicians, the National Association of Emergency Medical Services Physicians and the National Association of Emergency Medical Technicians. *Trauma Surg Acute Care Open.* 2019;4(1):e000376.
11. Miller PR, Chang MC, Hoth JJ, et al. Prospective trial of angiography and embolization for all grade III to V blunt splenic injuries: nonoperative management success rate is significantly improved. *J Am Coll Surg.* 2014;218(4):644–648.
12. Post R, Engel D, Pham J, et al. Computed tomography blush and splenic injury: does it always require angioembolization? *Am Surg.* 2013;79(10):1089–1092.
13. Quencer K, Smith T. Review of proximal splenic artery embolization in blunt abdominal trauma. *CVIR Endovasc.* 2019;2(1):11. doi:10.1186/s42155-019-0055-3
14. Patil MS, Goodin SZ, Findeiss LK. Update: Splenic artery embolization in blunt abdominal trauma. *Semin Intervent Radiol.* 2020;37(1):97–102.
15. Kozar R, Feliciano D, Moore E. Western Trauma Association/critical decisions in trauma: operative management of adult blunt hepatic trauma. *J Trauma.* 2011;71(1):1–5.
16. Lee YH, Wu CH, Wang LJ, et al. Predictive factors for early failure of transarterial embolization in blunt hepatic injury patients. *Clin Radiol.* 2014;69(5):e505–e511.
17. Inchingolo R, Ljutikov A, Deganello A, et al. Outcomes and indications for intervention in non-operative management of paediatric liver trauma: a 5 year retrospective study. *Clin Radiol.* 2014;69(2):157–162.
18. Padia SA, Ingraham CR, Moriarty JM, et al. Society of Interventional Radiology Position Statement on endovascular intervention for trauma. *J Vasc Interv Radiol.* 2020;31(3): 363–369.
19. Bertens KA, Vogt KN, Hernandez-Alejandro R, et al. Non-operative management of blunt hepatic trauma: does angioembolization have a major impact? *Eur J Trauma Emerg Surg.* 2015;41(1):81–86.
20. Lopez-Gonzalez DB, Zurkiya O. Interventional radiology in renal trauma. *Semin Intervent Radiol.* 2021;38(1):113–122.
21. Lopera JE, Suri R, Kroma G, et al. Traumatic occlusion and dissection of the main renal artery: endovascular treatment. *J Vasc Interv Radiol.* 2011;22(11):1570–1574.
22. Wijffels DJ, Verbeek DO, Ponsen KJ, et al. Imaging and endovascular treatment of bleeding pelvic fractures: review article. *Cardiovasc Intervent Radiol.* 2019;42(1): 10–18.

23. Katsumori T, Kasahara T. The size of gelatin sponge particles: differences with preparation method. *Cardiovasc Intervent Radiol.* 2006;29:1077–1083. https://doi.org/10.1007/s00270-006-0059-y

24. Sandhu J, Abrahams R, Miller Z, et al. Pelvic trauma: factors predicting arterial hemorrhage and the role of angiography and preperitoneal pelvic packing. *Eur Radiol.* 2020;30(11): 6376–6383.

25. Velmahos GC, Toutouzas KG, Vassiliu P, et al. A prospective study on the safety and efficacy of angiographic embolization for pelvic and visceral injuries. *J Trauma.* 2002;53(2):303–308.

26. Modrall JG, Weaver FA, Yellin AE. Diagnosis and management of penetrating vascular trauma and the injured extremity. *Emerg Med Clin North Am.* 1998;16(1):129–144.

27. Kuwahara JT, Kord A, Ray CE Jr. Penetrating extremity trauma endovascular versus open repair? *Semin Intervent Radiol.* 2020;37(1):55–61.

28. Padia SA, Ingraham CR, Moriarty JM. Society of Interventional Radiology Position Statement on endovascular intervention for trauma. *J Vasc Interv Radiol.* 2020;31(3):363–369.e2.

29. Scalea JR, Crawford R, Scurci S, et al. Below-the-knee arterial injury: the type of vessel may be more important than the number of vessels injured. *J Trauma Acute Care Surg.* 2014;77(6):920–925.

15 Thoracic Aortic Aneurysms and Dissections

David S. Wang, MD and Michael D. Dake, MD

Introduction

Thoracic Aortic Aneurysm (1–4)

1. Localized dilatation of the thoracic aorta greater than 50% of normal. The upper limit of normal caliber for the descending thoracic aorta is 3 to 3.5 cm.
2. Incidence—5.9 to 10.4 cases per 100,000 person-years
3. Male-to-female ratio—1.5 to 1: 1
4. Classification
   a. Anatomic site: 30% to 40% involve the descending thoracic aorta
   b. Morphology: fusiform (80%) or saccular (20%)
   c. Risk factors—Most are "degenerative," a late stage of atherosclerosis. Other risk factors include dissection, infection, inflammatory antitides (e.g., Takayasu disease), connective tissue diseases (e.g., Marfan syndrome), trauma, and iatrogenesis
5. The natural history is progressive expansion. Risk of rupture, usually fatal, markedly increases when the diameter exceeds 6 cm.
6. Conventional treatment is open surgical repair (OSR). With modern techniques, short-term death rates range from 3% to 15% for elective cases and up to 50% for emergent operations. The risk of spinal cord ischemia is 3% to 8%.

Aortic Dissection (2–4)

1. Begins with a tear of the aortic intima and inner layer of the media, allowing blood to cleave a longitudinal plane within the media. The resulting dissection flap separates the aorta into true and false lumina. The false lumen may compress the true lumen or obstruct aortic branch vessel flow, causing end-organ ischemia. The majority of primary entry tears originate just distal to the left subclavian artery (LSCA) origin or within a few centimeters of the aortic valve. Additional communications between true and false lumina may form.
2. Incidence—2 to 3.5 and 0.5 to 2.1 cases per 100,000 person-years for all dissections and those limited to the descending thoracic aorta, respectively

3. Male-to-female ratio—5 to 2: 1
4. Classifications
   a. Anatomic site
      (1) Stanford system
         (a) Type A—involves the ascending aorta (60% to 70%)
         (b) Type B—confined to the descending thoracic aorta (30% to 40%)
      (2) DeBakey system
         (a) Type I—involves the ascending and descending aorta
         (b) Type II—confined to the ascending aorta
         (c) Type III—confined to the descending aorta without (IIIa) or with (IIIb) extension into the abdominal aorta
      (3) Society for Vascular Surgery and Society of Thoracic Surgery Reporting Guidelines for Type B Aortic Dissections
         (a) Location of entry tear; type A or B location
         (b) Proximal and distal extent of dissection; designated by predetermined zones within the thoracoabdominal aorta
   b. Time from symptom onset
      (1) Acute—1–14 days
      (2) Subacute—15–90 days
      (3) Chronic—>90 days
   c. Clinical course: At initial presentation, 30% to 42% are classified as "complicated" due to aortic rupture or impending rupture, malperfusion of visceral or peripheral arteries, rapid false lumen aneurysmal growth, refractory hypertension, or intractable pain.
5. Risk factors—70% to 90% of patients have hypertension. Other risk factors include existing aneurysm, connective tissue diseases (e.g., Marfan syndrome), bicuspid aortic valve, pregnancy, trauma, and iatrogenesis.
6. The natural history is highly variable. The primary late complication is false lumen dilatation and eventual rupture. Aneurysmal degeneration of the false lumen occurs in 20% to 50% within 4 years despite optimal medical therapy (OMT). Predictors of degeneration include a primary entry tear ≥10 mm, total aortic diameter ≥40 mm, false lumen diameter ≥22 mm, and partial false lumen thrombosis.
7. Conventional treatment
   a. Uncomplicated type B aortic dissection (TBAD): OMT with control of blood pressure (goal systolic blood pressure 100 to 120 mm Hg), heart rate (goal <60 beats per minute), and pain. Lifelong close surveillance is required to monitor for signs of disease progression, false lumen aneurysmal dilatation, and/or malperfusion.
   b. Complicated TBAD: OSR, usually performed emergently, is associated with a mortality rate of 25% to 50% with paraplegia occurring in 7% to 36%. Concomitant OMT is required. Prior to the advent of thoracic endovascular aortic repair (TEVAR), fenestration of the dissection flap to equalize pressures in the true and false lumina or stent placement to open obstructed branch vessels were the primary endovascular treatments for malperfusion.

Stent-Grafts

After the first thoracic aortic stent-graft was implanted in a patient in 1992, a commercial device was first approved by the U.S. Food and Drug Administration (FDA) in 2005. Table 15.1 lists the thoracic aortic stent-grafts which are FDA approved and commercially available as of this writing. Additional devices are available outside of the United States.

Goals of Thoracic Endovascular Aortic Repair

1. **Aneurysms**—To provide a durable conduit for aortic blood flow across the entire longitudinal extent of the aneurysm, resulting in aneurysm sac

Table 15.1 FDA-Approved Thoracic Aortic Stent-Grafts and Stents

Device (Manufacturer)	Stent Material	Graft Material	Diameters (cm)	Lengths (cm)
Gore TAG Conformable (Gore)	Nitinol	ePTFE	21–45[a]	10, 15, 20
Gore TAG Conformable with Active Control (Gore)	Nitinol	ePTFE	21–45[a]	10, 15, 20
RelayPlus (Terumo Aortic)	Nitinol	Woven polyester	22–46[a]	10, 15, 20, 25
Valiant Navion (Medtronic)	Nitinol	Woven polyester	20–46[a]	5.2–22.3
Valiant with Captivia Delivery System (Medtronic)	Nitinol	Woven polyester	22–46[a]	10, 15, 20
Zenith Alpha Thoracic (Cook Medical)[b]	Nitinol	Woven polyester	24–46 proximal,[a] 28–46 distal, 26–46 distal extension	10.5–23.3 proximal, 14.2–21.1 distal, 9.1–11.2 distal extension
Zenith TX2 Dissection Graft (Cook Medical)[b]	Stainless steel	Woven polyester	22–42[a]	7.9–21.8
Zenith TX2 Dissection Stent (Cook Medical)[c]	Nitinol	None	36, 46	8, 12, 18, 18.5

ePTFE, expanded polytetrafluoroethylene.
[a]Straight and tapered versions available.
[b]Modular with proximal and distal components.
[c]Intended use as a bare-stent distal component.

depressurization, thrombosis formation, and eventual stabilization or regression in size.

2. **Aortic dissections**—Complete coverage of the primary intimal entry tear to redirect blood flow into the true lumen while depressurizing the false lumen to promote thrombosis. Reapposition of the aortic wall layers restores true lumen caliber and relieves certain branch vessel obstructions. This may prevent late aneurysmal degeneration of the aorta.

Indications (1–4)

Table 15.2 lists the FDA-approved indications for specific devices.

1. Descending thoracic aortic aneurysms (TAAs)
   a. Asymptomatic with minimum orthogonal diameter of >5.5 cm or more than two times the diameter of adjacent nonaneurysmal aorta
   b. Asymptomatic with growth rate of >1 cm over 1 year
   c. Symptomatic, regardless of aneurysm size

Table 15.2 **FDA-Approved On-Label Indications for Thoracic Aortic Stent-Grafts and Stents**

Indication	Devices
Descending thoracic aortic aneurysm	Gore TAG, RelayPlus, Valiant, Zenith Alpha Thoracic
Penetrating atherosclerotic ulcer	Gore TAG, RelayPlus, Valiant, Zenith Alpha Thoracic
Blunt thoracic aortic injury	Gore TAG, Valiant
Type B aortic dissection	Gore TAG, Valiant, Zenith TX2 Dissection Graft and Stent

2. Type B aortic dissections
   a. Complicated acute TBAD: TEVAR is the treatment of choice for acute TBADs complicated by rupture or impending rupture, malperfusion, early aortic expansion, refractory hypertension, or intractable pain.
   b. Uncomplicated acute TBAD: Proactive endovascular treatment of uncomplicated patients determined to be at high risk for delayed complications is currently under active investigation. Several anatomic and clinical features are being considered as high-risk criteria.
   c. Complicated subacute/chronic TBAD: For patients who were initially uncomplicated and develop delayed complications (i.e., aortic diameter growth >1 cm per year, false lumen aneurysm with total aortic diameter >60 mm, malperfusion syndrome, or recurrent pain) in the subacute or early chronic phase, prompt intervention, whether TEVAR or OSR, is required; however, the optimal approach is unclear.
3. Other thoracic aortic pathologies: penetrating atherosclerotic ulcers, intramural hematomas, blunt traumatic thoracic aortic injuries, and ruptures.
4. Less common investigational applications include pseudoaneurysms, aortic fistulas, and mycotic aneurysms. TEVAR is also used in hybrid surgical procedures, such as the "elephant trunk" technique.

Contraindications (1–4)

Absolute
1. Allergies to device materials
2. Conditions that may increase the risk of endovascular graft infection

Relative
Exclusionary criteria from FDA clinical trials may be bypassed at the discretion of the operator, bearing in mind that outcomes may vary.
1. Inadequate anatomy for TEVAR
   a. Anatomic obstacles may be overcome with adjunctive surgical procedures (see "Special Considerations" section)
2. Allergies to contrast material or renal insufficiency
3. Severe comorbidities with short life expectancy
4. TEVAR is not recommended in patients with underlying connective tissue disease, except as a bailout procedure or adjunct to surgical therapy

Preprocedure Imaging

Imaging should be performed within 3 months of the procedure.
1. Computed tomography (CT) should be performed from the thoracic inlet to the femoral artery bifurcations.

a. Noncontrast images are helpful for evaluation of vascular calcifications, intramural hematoma, and other high-density lesions.

b. Computed tomographic angiography (CTA) performed during the first-pass arterial phase is the most critical component of preprocedural imaging. Cardiac gating should be performed for lesions that may involve the ascending aorta.

c. Reformatting in multiple planes is essential for accurate measurements.

d. For TBAD, delayed imaging should be performed to evaluate branch vessel ischemia and other potential complications.

2. Magnetic resonance angiography (MRA) can be used in patients with impaired renal function or intolerance to iodinated contrast media. Evaluation of calcifications is however limited.

3. Intraprocedural intravascular ultrasound (IVUS) or transesophageal echo (TEE) may be useful for more detailed evaluation of landing zones and localization of side branches and intimal tears.

4. If the target lesion is located near the LSCA origin, CTA or MRA of the head and neck should be considered.

Measurement Techniques and Imaging Assessment

Measurements are made on the arterial phase images. Figure 15.1 illustrates the recommended parameters for case selection and planning.

1. Descending TAA

a. Available proximal landing zone length is the distance from the LSCA (or left common carotid artery [LCCA]) to the proximal extent of the TAA.

b. Available distal landing zone length is the distance from the distal extent of the TAA to the celiac trunk.

c. Total treatment length is the sum of the length of the aneurysm and selected lengths of the proximal and distal landing zones.

d. Landing zone diameter is generally measured from inner wall to inner wall, excluding wall calcifications but including intraluminal thrombi and plaque.

e. Evaluation of landing zone morphology includes assessment of angulation, tortuosity, and presence of intraluminal thrombi and calcifications.

f. Quantitative and qualitative evaluation of potential vascular access pathways are performed as done for the landing zones. This should include the bilateral common femoral, external iliac, and common iliac arteries and the distal infrarenal aorta.

g. The overall morphology and degree of atherosclerotic disease of the aorta should also be assessed.

2. Complicated acute TBAD

a. The primary intimal entry tear must be clearly identified by careful tracing of the dissecting septum. Downstream reentry fenestrations should also be identified.

b. The proximal and distal extents of the dissection and possible involvement of aortic branch vessels should be ascertained.

c. In the presence of branch vessel ischemia, it is important to determine if the ischemic organ is supplied by the true or false lumen.

Selection Criteria for Endograft Repair

Patient selection is based on (1–4):

1. Anatomic considerations—inappropriate anatomy is one of the most common reasons for treatment failure.

2. Clinical considerations—the risk of TEVAR is weighed relative to that of OSR and medical management in the context of overall life expectancy and quality of life.

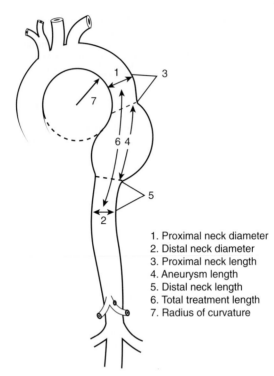

1. Proximal neck diameter
2. Distal neck diameter
3. Proximal neck length
4. Aneurysm length
5. Distal neck length
6. Total treatment length
7. Radius of curvature

FIGURE 15.1 • Recommended aortic dimensions to be measured in evaluation of a descending thoracic aortic aneurysm for stent-graft management.

Anatomic Criteria
1. Proximal and distal landing zones
    a. Descending TAAs: Normal aortic segments ≥20 mm in length are required distal to either the LSCA or LCCA and proximal to the celiac trunk.
    b. Complicated acute TBADs: No strict anatomic criteria. A proximal landing zone of ≥10 mm distal to the LSCA is generally sufficient.
    c. Absence of significant thrombus or calcification
    d. Aortic diameters that can be accommodated by available devices, generally 16 to 42 mm.
    e. A radius of curvature of >35 mm or aortic angulation of <60 degrees is generally preferred.
2. Iliofemoral vascular access
    a. Adequate caliber to accommodate delivery systems or anatomy suitable for a surgical conduit
    b. Absence of significant tortuosity, thrombus, or calcification

Preprocedure Preparation (1–4)

Device Selection for Descending Thoracic Aortic Aneurysms
1. Device diameter: Device diameters are generally oversized 10% to 20% relative to the luminal diameter of the native landing zones.

a. If the distal landing zone diameter is significantly smaller than the proximal, consider a tapered endograft or a combination of devices of different diameters.
2. Device length: Longer landing zones are generally preferred when possible.
   a. If multiple endografts are to be used, the devices should overlap a minimum of 5 cm.
   b. If the landing zone is angulated, the treatment length may need to be elongated. Particularly important for proximal landing zones, the leading edge of the device should not be placed near the apex of an acute angle. Doing so may result in malapposition of the stent-graft along a tight inner curve, increasing the risk of a type I endoleak or endograft collapse.
   c. For a large TAA, redundancy in device length may be needed to account for potential bowing of the endograft into the aneurysm sac.

Device Selection for Complicated Acute Type B Aortic Dissections

1. Device diameter: Endografts are oversized in the lower range of 5% to 10% over the luminal diameter of the nondissected aorta just proximal to the primary entry tear.
2. Device length: The appropriate length remains controversial with strategies ranging from focal coverage of the proximal tear to the less common coverage of the entire dissection. Exclusion of the mesenteric aortic branches is not recommended. If the dissection is complicated by rupture, multiple devices are typically needed to prevent retrograde flow into the false lumen through distal tears. The preferred sequence of multiple device implantation is proximal to distal.

Special Considerations

1. LSCA and celiac trunk
   a. For lesions that extend close to but not proximal to the LSCA, landing zone limitations are increasingly being challenged. Intentional coverage of the LSCA is often needed to effectively extend the proximal landing zone.
   b. Routine preprocedural revascularization of the LSCA (e.g., left carotid to subclavian bypass) in patients with planned LSCA exclusion is recommended, unless TEVAR is performed emergently (9).
   c. Thoracic aortic pathologies that extend proximal to the LSCA require hybrid surgical and endovascular treatments, such as the elephant trunk technique.
   d. Intentional coverage of the celiac trunk without prior revascularization is not recommended. Hybrid surgical and endovascular approaches for treatment of thoracoabdominal aneurysms are being explored.
   e. Other approaches to overcome landing zone anatomic challenges include the development of branched and fenestrated thoracic aortic endografts and percutaneous revascularization techniques (e.g., "chimney" graft).
2. Cerebrospinal fluid (CSF) drainage
   a. CSF drainage can prevent and reverse spinal cord ischemia.
   b. Prophylactic CSF drainage should be considered for patients with perioperative hypotension (mean arterial pressure <70 mm Hg), aortic treatment length >20 cm, endograft coverage between the levels of T8 and L2, and prior history of AAA repair.

Procedure

Deployment procedures are highly specific to each device. The steps described here provide a general outline for thoracic stent-graft deployment.

Vascular Access

1. Arterial access is preferably through the common femoral artery but may be via the external iliac or common iliac arteries or the distal infrarenal aorta. A temporary access conduit may be placed surgically to facilitate device delivery.
2. Vascular access may be achieved by surgical cutdown or using percutaneous approaches.
3. For aortic dissections, select an access site that allows entrance into the true lumen.

Descending Thoracic Aortic Aneurysms

1. Continuous monitoring of vital signs, particularly arterial pressure, is mandatory.
   a. If the LSCA is to be covered, the arterial line should be placed in the right radial artery.
   b. Use of intraoperative somatosensory-evoked potentials and electroencephalography to detect neurologic complications, TEE, or other invasive monitoring techniques is left to the discretion of the operator.
   c. To decrease the risk of spinal cord ischemia, hypotension should be avoided.
2. The procedure is typically performed with the patient under general or regional anesthesia.
3. With the patient supine, sterile access sites are prepared.
4. To allow for lateral angiography, patient's arms should be raised or, if brachial artery access is needed, positioned at 90 degrees.
5. For imaging purposes, cannulate the common femoral artery contralateral to the previously determined site for stent-graft delivery per routine techniques. The brachial artery may also be used.
6. After placement of a sheath, advance a marker pigtail catheter to the proximal aortic arch.
   a. To decrease the risk of atheroembolization, manipulation of guidewires, catheters, and other devices in the aortic arch should be minimized.
7. Perform an initial aortogram with the fluoroscope angled in the left anterior oblique projection, perpendicular to the aortic arch (typically between 45 degrees and 75 degrees) as calculated from the preprocedure CT or MR.
8. Obtain arterial access at the planned endograft insertion site.
9. Once access is obtained, anticoagulate the patient for the duration of the procedure to achieve an activated clotting time of 250 to 300 seconds.
10. Prepare the stent-graft delivery system according to manufacturer instructions.
11. With continuous fluoroscopic guidance angled perpendicular to the proximal landing zone, advance the endograft delivery system to the target site over a stiff 0.035-in guidewire. Use the device's radiopaque markers to confirm positioning.
12. After reconfirming positioning, deploy the device under continuous fluoroscopic visualization per manufacturer instructions.
    a. For intubated patients, transient apnea may aid in deployment accuracy.
    b. Other measures to prevent device malpositioning, such as transient hypotension or adenosine-induced cardiac asystole, are no longer necessary.
13. Carefully withdraw the delivery catheter under fluoroscopic observation.
14. Perform molding balloon angioplasty as needed.
15. Deployment of additional devices is performed in identical fashion. The order of device deployment is dependent on the system used.
16. Completion angiogram is performed with the angiographic catheter placed proximal to the endovascular graft.
17. As needed, deploy additional devices and/or repeat balloon dilatation to ensure adequate coverage, device expansion, and wall apposition.

Complicated Acute Type B Aortic Dissections

The procedure for TEVAR in complicated acute TBAD is performed in similar fashion to that of TAA with the following key differences:

1. Blood pressure should be strictly maintained within a narrow range of normal to minimize progression of the dissection.
2. Exclusive true lumen passage of the principal guidewire is essential as deployment of a stent-graft in the false lumen leads to catastrophic consequences.
3. Intraprocedural TEE or IVUS may be useful for identifying the location of the primary entry tear and other intimal tears, confirming wire passage through the true lumen, and documenting exclusion of the proximal false lumen during deployment.
4. Once the device is deployed, balloon molding is usually not performed and further manipulation is kept to a minimum because the dissection flap is vulnerable to additional perforations or retrograde extension into the proximal aortic arch. Devices with proximal rigid or bare-metal segments are less preferred.
5. If there is persistent malperfusion after the primary entry tear is covered, deployment of bare stent(s) or fenestration of the dissection flap may be performed in the distal aspect of the dissection and/or stents may be placed in each obstructed aortic branch if the false lumen supplies blood to an end organ.

Postprocedure Management

Immediate
1. Patients are monitored in the intensive care unit for a minimum of 24 hours.
   a. Mean arterial pressure should be maintained over 100 mm Hg immediately after device deployment.
   b. Monitor hemodynamic function and for signs and symptoms of paraplegia or paraparesis, stroke, mesenteric or lower extremity ischemia, and other potential immediate complications.
   c. No postprocedural anticoagulation is necessary.

Follow-up Imaging Surveillance (1–4)
1. Follow-up imaging and clinical evaluation are performed at 1, 6, and 12 months and then annually. More frequent imaging is needed if an endoleak is identified.
2. CTA is the default modality for postprocedural imaging.
3. MRA remains an alternative to CT. Although all current FDA-approved devices are MR compatible, evaluation may be limited by compromised image quality in regions immediately adjacent to the device.
4. Chest radiograph: Frontal, lateral, and 45-degree bilateral posterior oblique views are performed for evaluation of device integrity.

Results

Descending Thoracic Aortic Aneurysms
1. Clinical trial outcomes of FDA-approved devices (3,4):
   a. 98% to 99.5% technical success rate
   b. At 1 year
      (1) 91% to 92.9% of TAAs remained stable or decreased (>5 mm) in size
      (2) ≤0.7% aneurysm rupture, ≤0.7% open conversion, and 0.7% to 3.9% stent-graft migration
   c. At 5 years
      (1) Aneurysm-related mortality of 2.8% to 5.9% with TEVAR compared with 11.7% to 12% for OSR
      (2) 81% to 94.1% of TAAs remained stable or decreased in size
2. Medicare study comparing TEVAR (2,470 patients) versus OSR (1,235 patients) of intact descending TAAs (5):
   a. 180-day mortality: 10.2% for TEVAR versus 23.8% for OSR
   b. At 9 years: restricted mean survival time with OSR was 6.9 months less compared to TEVAR

3. Single-center study comparing TEVAR (79 patients) versus OSR (39 patients) of descending thoracic aortic *rupture* from nontraumatic pathologies (6):
   a. 30-day mortality: 16.5% for TEVAR versus 38.5% for OSR
   b. 5-year mortality: 30.4% for TEVAR versus 56.4% for OSR
   c. Aortic reintervention was required more frequently after TEVAR (15.2% vs. 2.6%)

Complicated Acute Type B Aortic Dissections (2)

1. Meta-analysis of 2,531 patients who underwent TEVAR and 1,276 who underwent OSR:
   a. Pooled 30-day/in-hospital mortality rate: 7.3% for TEVAR versus 19% for OSR
   b. Pooled cerebrovascular events and spinal cord ischemia rates: 3.9% and 3.1% for TEVAR versus 6.8% and 3.3% for OSR, respectively
2. Meta-analysis of 942 patients who underwent TEVAR:
   a. Technical success: 95%
   b. Complete false lumen thrombosis: 85%
   c. Stroke and paraplegia: 3.1% and 1.9%
   d. 30-day mortality: 9%
   e. Late mortality (mean 20 months): 3.6%

Uncomplicated Type B Aortic Dissections

Two RCTs compared TEVAR with OMT versus OMT alone

1. Investigation of Stent-Grafts in Patients with Type B Aortic Dissection (INSTEAD) trial (7,8): Subacute/chronic uncomplicated TBAD.
   a. Two-year follow-up: Aortic remodeling in 91.3% of TEVAR with OMT patients versus 19.4% in OMT only patients. However, there was no survival benefit (88.9% vs. 95.6%, respectively).
   b. Five-year follow-up: Reduced aorta-related mortality (6.9% vs. 19.3%, respectively) and disease progression (27% vs. 46.1%, respectively) for TEVAR with OMT patients compared with OMT alone. In the OMT-only group, 21.2% required crossover to TEVAR during follow-up due to evolving complications. After TEVAR, complete false lumen thrombosis was found in 90.6% at 5 years.
2. Acute Dissection: Stent-Graft OR Best Medical Therapy (ADSORB) trial (9): Acute uncomplicated TBAD.
   a. One-year follow-up: Complete false lumen thrombosis in 63.3% of TEVAR with OMT patients versus 6.5% in the OMT-only group with a corresponding significantly larger true lumen diameter in the combined treatment group.

Complications (1–4,10)

Early

1. Postimplantation syndrome: Low-grade fever, mild leukocytosis, elevated C-reactive protein, and possible reactive pleural effusion. This is self-limited and should resolve within a week.
2. Spinal cord ischemia (0.8% to 3%): Paraparesis and paraplegia are less common compared with OSR.
   a. If detected early, may be reversed with prompt CSF drainage and maintaining a mean blood pressure of 80 to 90 mm Hg.
   b. To avoid intracranial hypotension, drainage should be performed over the first 24 to 72 hours and limited to <15 mL per hour or <350 mL per day.
3. Cerebrovascular stroke (2.1% to 3.6%): Associated with longer procedure times and extensive device manipulation within the aortic arch.
4. Aortic perforation, de novo dissection, or extension of an existing dissection. Retrograde dissection into the ascending aorta is reported in 0.7% to 2.5% of TBAD TEVAR cases.

5. Endoleaks (10% to 20%): Endoleaks and their treatment are discussed in Chapter 18.
6. Device malposition, incomplete expansion, migration, and collapse.
7. Vascular access complications include thrombosis, dissection, rupture, and avulsion.

Late
1. Endoleaks (see Chapter 18).
2. Spinal cord ischemia may present as late as 30 days following device implantation.
3. Device migration, collapse, component separation, or fabric tears.
4. Stent fracture: Isolated fractures are often of little clinical consequence.
5. Residual or recurrent disease and progression toward eventual rupture.

References

1. Upchurch GR Jr, Escobar GC, Azizzdeh A, et al. Society for Vascular Surgery clinical practice guidelines for thoracic endovascular aneurysm repair (TEVAR). *J Vasc Surg.* 2020;73(1S):55S–83S.
2. Riambau V, Bockler D, Brunkwall J, et al. Management of descending thoracic aorta diseases: clinical practice guidelines of the European Society for Vascular Surgery (ESVS). *Eur J Vasc Endovasc Surg.* 2017;53(1):4–52.
3. Erbel R, Aboyans V, Boileau C, et al. 2014 ESC guidelines on the diagnosis and treatment of aortic diseases: document covering acute and chronic aortic diseases of the thoracic and abdominal aorta of the adult. The task force for the diagnosis and treatment of aortic diseases of the European Society of Cardiology (ESC). *Eur Heart J.* 2014;35(41):2873–2926.
4. Hiratzka LF, Bakris GL, Beckman JA, et al. ACCF/AHA/AATS/ACR/ASA/SCA/SCAI/SIR/STS/SVM guidelines for the diagnosis and management of patients with thoracic aortic disease. *Circulation.* 2010;121(13):e266–e369.
5. Chiu P, Goldstone AB, Schaffer JM, et al. Endovascular versus open repair of intact descending thoracic aortic aneurysms. *J Am Coll Cardiol.* 2019;73(6):643–651.
6. Ogawa Y, Watkins AC, Lingala B, et al. Improved midterm outcomes after endovascular repair of nontraumatic descending thoracic aortic rupture compared with open surgery. *J Thorac Cardiovasc Surg.* 2019;161(6):2004–2012.
7. Nienaber CA, Rousseau H, Eggebrecht H, et al. Randomized comparison of strategies for type B aortic dissection: the investigation of stent grafts in aortic dissection (INSTEAD) trial. *Circulation.* 2009;120(25):2519–2528.
8. Nienaber CA, Kische S, Rousseau H, et al. Endovascular repair of type B aortic dissection: long-term results of the randomized investigation of stent grafts in aortic dissection trial. *Circ Cardiovasc Interv.* 2013;6(4):407–416.
9. Brunkwall J, Kasprzak P, Verhoeven E, et al. Endovascular repair of acute uncomplicated aortic type B dissection promotes aortic remodelling: 1 year results of the ADSORB trial. *Eur J Vasc Endovasc Surg.* 2014;48(3):285–291.
10. Lee WA. Failure modes of thoracic endografts: prevention and management. *J Vasc Surg.* 2009;49(3):792–799.

16 Pulmonary Vascular Malformations

Todd Schlachter, MD, Katharine J. Henderson, MS, and Jeffrey S. Pollak, MD

Introduction

Pulmonary vascular malformations may involve abnormalities of the arteries, veins, communications between these two, lymphatics, and associated lung abnormalities. This chapter will concentrate on pulmonary arteriovenous malformation as well as acquired fistula, which are often amenable to interventional radiologic management. Conditions having abnormal systemic arterial supply into abnormal or normal lung tissue such as bronchopleural sequestration and scimitar syndrome artery are typically managed surgically or expectantly, although embolization of arterial supply may occasionally be appropriate (1). Conditions with abnormal venous drainage are usually also managed conservatively.

Indications

1. *Pulmonary arteriovenous malformations (PAVMs)* consist of a congenital connection between a pulmonary artery and vein, without a normal capillary bed. These are the most common type of pulmonary arteriovenous connections. Their prevalence may be as high as 1 in 2,600 and they are associated with hereditary hemorrhagic telangiectasia (HHT) (Osler–Weber–Rendu syndrome) in 56% to 97% of patients (2–4), in which setting they are more commonly multiple. Therefore, patients with PAVM must be evaluated for the possibility of HHT.
2. *Acquired pulmonary arteriovenous fistulas* are less commonly clinically significant and can occur in a variety of conditions (5):
   a. Idiopathic. This is the most common etiology for incidentally found macroscopic solitary fistula in an adult without HHT, and it is often unclear whether it is congenital or acquired.
   b. Cirrhosis (hepatopulmonary syndrome). These are rarely large enough to warrant embolization.
   c. Glenn or Fontan shunts for congenital heart disease, with no or minimal hepatic venous return to the lung.
   d. Infections: Schistosomiasis and Actinomycosis.
   e. Hypervascular metastatic cancer such as thyroid carcinoma and choriocarcinoma.
   f. Amyloidosis.
   g. Fanconi syndrome.
   h. Erosion of an aneurysm into a vein.
   i. Trauma, including prior thoracic surgery.

Contraindications

There are no absolute contraindications to pulmonary artery embolization; however, certain situations indicate caution (3,4).
1. Severe pulmonary hypertension. PAVM occlusion in this setting may risk further elevation of pulmonary artery pressure and cor pulmonale, although the precise effect is difficult to predict given the concomitant reduction in flow.
2. Diffuse and innumerable multifocal PAVM. These generally cannot be eradicated and especially when involving extensive regions of the lung, embolization results

in little or no respiratory improvement and should be directed toward only focally larger lesions, if present.
3. Renal insufficiency.
4. Radiation exposure in pregnant women and in children, the latter potentially also having a higher proclivity for reperfusion.
5. Individuals with a history of serious contrast reaction can still be treated using premedication and possibly general anesthesia.

Association of PAVM with Hereditary Hemorrhagic Telangiectasia (3,6)

1. HHT results in scattered arteriovenous malformations (AVMs), manifested primarily as mucocutaneous telangiectases and less frequently as larger visceral AVMs. Its prevalence is estimated at 1 in 5,000 to 10,000.
2. Several different genes have been found to cause HHT, with the three identified ones coding for proteins involved with transforming growth factor-β signal transduction. The two most common are HHT1, which results from a defect in endoglin, and HHT2, resulting in a defect in activin receptor-like kinase 1. The third is a combined syndrome of HHT with juvenile polyposis.
3. A definite clinical diagnosis of the heterozygous, autosomal dominant disorder depends on the presence of at least three of the following four features. The diagnosis is possible if only two are present and doubted with just one:
   a. Multiple telangiectases of the skin and mucous membranes
   b. Repeated episodes of spontaneous epistaxis, occurring in over 90% of patients
   c. An autosomal dominant pattern of inheritance
   d. Typical visceral malformations
      (1) PAVM in approximately 20% to 70%, more common in HHT1 than HHT2.
      (2) Central nervous system in approximately 10%, more common in HHT1 than HHT2. Still, the most common neurologic events in patients with HHT are due to paradoxical embolization through PAVMs.
      (3) Gastrointestinal tract telangiectases and less commonly larger AVMs occur in 55% to 70% and can produce bleeding in approximately 25%.
      (4) Liver AVM occurs in 41% to 74%, but are symptomatic in less than 10%, and these patients generally have HHT2.
4. Genetic testing can identify approximately 85% of patients with HHT.

Pathology of PAVM (4)

1. Types
   a. Simple PAVMs are fed by an artery contained within one pulmonary segment and account for 80% to 90% of PAVMs. The artery may have more than one distal branch supplying the malformation.
   b. Complex PAVMs are fed by arteries from more than one pulmonary segment and account for 10% to 20%.
   c. Diffuse involvement of one or more segments or lobes, typically basilar, accounts for 5%.
   d. The nidus connecting the artery(ies) and vein(s) may be a single aneurysmal sac or a plexiform, septated, multichannelled connection, with complex PAVMs more commonly having the latter type of nidus.
   e. A systemic artery will rarely be found to supply a PAVM.
2. Location
   a. Lower lobes in approximately 65%
   b. Upper lobes, right middle lobe, and lingula in 35%

3. Multiplicity
   a. Multiple PAVMs in over 50%
   b. Bilateral PAVMs in over 40%

Clinical Manifestations of PAVM and Fistula (2,3)

1. Right-to-left shunting can result in:
   a. Arterial hypoxemia. Clinical manifestations include dyspnea, fatigue, cyanosis, clubbing, and rarely polycythemia; however, patients are also often asymptomatic.
   b. Paradoxical embolization. This most commonly manifests in the brain but can affect other organs. Thromboembolic embolization can result in stroke and transient ischemic attack (TIA) in 11% to 55% of patients while bacterial embolization has been reported to result in brain abscess in 5% to 25%, prompting the recommendation for prophylactic antibiotics prior to dental and other procedures that may cause bacteremia.
   c. High-output heart failure. This is uncommon but has been reported in neonates.
2. Rupture of thin-walled PAVMs can result in hemoptysis and hemothorax in 3% to 18%.
3. Migraine headaches are more common in patients with PAVM.
4. Conditions in which the risk of PAVM complications appears greater:
   a. Pregnancy may cause PAVM enlargement from increased blood volume and hormonal effects. Increased mortality has been described (3).
   b. Pulmonary hypertension may accelerate enlargement of PAVM.
5. Conditions in which the risk of PAVM complications appears lower:
   a. Preadolescent children, particularly with smaller lesions.
6. Symptoms can be related to associated disorders, such as other manifestations of HHT.

Embolotherapy for Pulmonary Arteriovenous Malformation and Fistula

Preprocedure Evaluation: Diagnostic Evaluation for PAVM
1. Goals:
   a. Detect PAVM with high sensitivity but also high specificity.
   b. Characterize size, number, and location of PAVMs. This will determine whether the PAVM(s) need specific treatment. For any one PAVM, the presence of a feeding artery of 2 mm or greater is an indication to consider invasive treatment. As smaller lesions can still permit paradoxical bacterial embolization, lifelong antibiotic prophylaxis is essential before procedures prone to result in bacteremia, such as dental work.
2. Who to evaluate?
   a. Patients with symptoms or signs suggestive of PAVM by history, physical examination, or incidentally found on imaging.
   b. Screen all patients with HHT.
3. Diagnostic tests for PAVM (3,4).
   a. Detection of right-to-left shunting. A disadvantage of these studies is the lack of morphologic detail with regard to location, number, and size of PAVMs.
      (1) Pulse oximetry may show oxygen saturation less than 97%, especially in an erect position due to the predilection of PAVMs for the lower lobes. The sensitivity and specificity of pulse oximetry are too low for it to be the sole diagnostic study but due to its completely noninvasive nature, it may be acceptable in young children since they appear to be less prone to develop complications from smaller PAVMs.

(2) Agitated saline bubble contrast echocardiography is considered the most sensitive study for detecting PAVMs, with a delay in the appearance of left atrial echoes by 3 to 10 heartbeats enhancing specificity for intrapulmonary shunts. Stratifying positive studies into three or four grades by the number of bubbles appearing in left cardiac chambers is of value since those having a grade 1 study consisting of only a small number of bubbles (e.g., less than 30 on one static image) will have no PAVMs of sufficient size to embolize. It is even possible that this group may not have PAVM since a percentage of the normal population can have such a low-grade positive study.

(3) Other studies that are now rarely used for specific PAVM evaluation are arterial blood gas measurements on room air plus additionally on 100% inspired oxygen to permit shunt fraction determination and radionuclide shunt studies.

b. Morphologic studies can provide information on the location, size, and number of lesions.

(1) Chest radiographs can show a lobular soft tissue mass with enlarged vascular structures coursing to and from it; however, sensitivity is limited and a normal chest radiograph does not exclude PAVM.

(2) Computed tomography is highly sensitive in diagnosing and characterizing PAVM both without and with IV contrast; although, false positives can occur. The usual appearance is a well-defined lobular soft tissue nodule or serpiginous mass with enlarged connecting vessels that enhance if contrast is administered. Given its noninvasive nature, it has become the gold standard study. It is also very useful for follow-up of the treated patient.

(3) Magnetic resonance imaging holds potential for PAVM detection without ionizing radiation exposure, but its current resolution is generally considered insufficient compared to CT.

(4) Pulmonary angiography is only performed for equivocal findings on noninvasive studies and immediately before embolization. It can miss tiny PAVMs compared to CT. Various projections may be needed to find the optimal one for catheterization of the supplying artery.

4. How to evaluate patients?

a. Patients with symptoms or signs indicative of PAVM by history and/or physical examination may benefit by proceeding directly to CT.

b. Asymptomatic patients at risk for PAVM should undergo screening (see below). This basically means all patients with HHT.

5. Screening for PAVMs Most HHT centers currently rely on contrast echocardiography for screening asymptomatic patients with this condition at least once they reach adolescence. If negative, no further evaluation is necessary. If grade 1, then microscopic or tiny PAVMs may be present and repeat echocardiography is performed every 5 years to assess for possible growth. The need for antibiotic prophylaxis in this group is uncertain. Higher grades of positivity prompt CT scanning to evaluate for PAVMs of a size requiring invasive treatment. If that is negative, currently, repeat CT scanning at 5-year intervals, and probably before pregnancy, is recommended to look for PAVM growth. The management of asymptomatic children is more controversial. Since our center's data indicates that asymptomatic children have a very low rate of complications from PAVM unless they have an oxygen saturation several percentages below normal, our regimen is yearly pulse oximetry (possibly with assessment of changes with differences in posture), waiting to perform contrast echocardiography once they reach mid adolescence.

Periprocedural Considerations

1. Light sedation—the patient should be able to hold their breath. General anesthesia is rarely needed, mainly for children.

2. No air bubbles or clots in the intravenous line or the catheters as these can result in paradoxical embolization.
3. Phlebotomy if markedly polycythemic, to reduce the risk of puncture site and pericatheter thrombosis. Polycythemia is rare given the presence of HHT-related epistaxis in the majority of patients with PAVM.
4. Heparin 3,000 to 6,000 units to prevent pericatheter thrombosis that could result in paradoxical embolization.
5. Antibiotic prophylaxis—typically weight-based cefazolin.
6. Continuous electrocardiographic monitoring, particularly to assess for catheter-induced arrhythmias.
7. Elective procedures are generally performed as an outpatient.
8. If many bilateral PAVMs are present, consider treating over more than one session and embolizing in only one lung at a time to avoid the possibility of bilateral pleurisy.
9. Pregnant women can be treated in the second trimester.

Procedure (2)

1. Catheterization:
   a. Femoral vein approach with placement of a 7- to 8-Fr sheath. Alternate sides should be used if more than one catheterization is needed in a short time interval.
   b. A 5-Fr pigtail is used to obtain pulmonary pressures and perform pulmonary angiography. The angiogram can be restricted to the regions of abnormality based on a prior CT scan. Pulmonary hypertension should raise concern for hepatic AVM, primary pulmonary hypertension (which can be linked to HHT2), or other common etiologies. When severe, embolotherapy should be performed cautiously, especially if the PAVM is large.
   c. The pigtail catheter is exchanged for a coaxial guide catheter-inner selective catheter system, currently typically an 80-cm 8-Fr multipurpose and 100-cm 6-Fr–angled catheters (White LuMax guiding catheter system, Cook Medical, Bloomington, IN). The use of a guiding catheter provides greater support, and permits the coaxial use of a variety of differently shaped inner catheters. The pulmonary artery feeding the PAVM is then selected with the catheter(s), occasionally aided by the use of steerable and hydrophilic wires. Coaxial microcatheters are sometimes necessary. Selective angiography is performed to confirm proper positioning and determine the proper site for occlusion.
   d. Strict attention is needed to avoid air entering any catheters. Guidewires should be removed while a catheter's hub is in a basin of saline.
2. Site of occlusion: Feeding artery embolization is most commonly performed and should be as distal as possible, beyond any significant supply to normal lung and as close as feasible to the arteriovenous connection, preferably within 1 cm (Fig. 16.1). While traditionally it has not been felt to be necessary to embolize the nidus (or aneurysmal sac) itself, some controversy does exist over this.
3. Embolic agents (4): An appropriately sized mechanical agent is used, which can be placed within the distal feeding artery without risk of migrating through the right-to-left shunt.
   a. *Embolization coils* can be used for basically any PAVM. Forming a dense cross-sectional network of metal is important for achieving long-term occlusion; one should not just rely on the promotion of thrombosis by a looser network of coils, fibered or otherwise.
      (1) *Pushable coils.* The first coil should be either 20% or 2 mm larger than the vessel diameter and additional, smaller coils are typically placed within this in all but the smallest lesions. Pushable soft platinum coils such as Nesters (Cook, Bloomington, IN) and Tornados (Cook) are most useful for small- and medium-sized PAVMs and these can be nested into themselves. Higher radial force coils (e.g., MReye coils [Cook]) are used

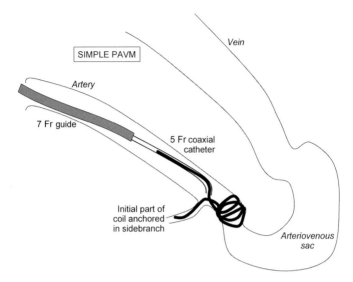

FIGURE 16.1 • Embolization of simple PAVM in the distal feeding artery. In this figure, a push-able coil is used with its initial part anchored in a distal sidebranch, after which additional coil emboli would be placed within and proximal to the first one to achieve a dense network of metal occluding the vessel. Alternatively, a plug could be placed in the feeding artery at this distal location.

for larger, high-flow fistula. Smaller, ~0.018-in gauge microcoils are rarely needed—only if a microcatheter was required to reach the lesion.

(2) *Detachable coils.* These are particularly useful for the first coil in situations where there is concern over distal, transnidal migration, such as with short feeding arteries and intraaneurysmal embolization, and for the final coil when there is concern over proximal prolapse and nontarget embolization of normal pulmonary vasculature. They are generally microcoil in size, but 0.035-in gauge detachable coils are also available, and may be nonfibered, fibered, or have hydrophilic polymer coating.

(3) Techniques to enhance safe use of coils, particularly pushable ones.

(a) *Anchor technique:* The initial 1 to 2 cm of a long coil is placed within a small distal sidebranch, after which the catheter is retracted to deploy the rest of the coil within the actual feeding artery (Fig. 16.1).

(b) *Scaffold technique:* A long, high radial force coil is first placed in a large, high-flow feeding artery (preferably after anchoring its initial 1 to 2 cm in a sidebranch), after which additional high and then soft platinum coils can be placed within this.

(c) An *occlusion balloon* is occasionally useful for high-flow arteries having significant drag or to provide secure positioning in short feeding arteries.

(4) *Intraaneurysmal coil embolization* is needed when embolization of a short feeding artery is not feasible. Microcatheter and microcoil embolization are typically used.

b. *Amplatzer Vascular Plugs* (AVPs) (Abbott, Lake County, Illinois). While more expensive than pushable coils, AVPs have the advantages of detachability, the ability to treat a wide variety of vessel sizes, and the need for fewer devices—typically just one with the AVP II and AVP IV devices, which can offset the cost. Adjunctive use of coils appears desired with the AVP I to reduce the risk of recanalization. Disadvantages are the need for a guide catheter or sheath to be placed at the site of occlusion to deliver AVP I and AVP II devices, but not for the AVP IV, which can be placed through specific 4- to 6-Fr catheters, and the lack of any device compatible with microcatheter delivery. The recanalization rate for these devices appears lower than for coils.

c. *Microvascular Plugs* (Medtronic, Minneapolis, MN). These detachable devices are available in four sizes to treat vessels up to 1.5 to 3, 3 to 5, 5 to 7, and 7 to 9 mm, respectively. The first two have the advantage of delivery through standard and high-flow microcatheters while latter two require at least 4- and 5-Fr catheters. The recanalization rate for these devices also appears lower than for coils.

4. Regional embolization: Diffuse segmental or multisegmental involvement may occasionally be treated by distal embolization of a region of the lung.
5. Postembolization angiography should be done to confirm occlusion and to look for accessory feeding arteries from other nearby regions of the lung.

Posttreatment Care

1. Remove intravenous lines to prevent iatrogenic paradoxical embolization of air or thrombus through residual PAVMs.
2. Incentive spirometry may be used to try and ameliorate atelectasis and pleurisy after embolization of larger PAVMs.
3. Long-term follow-up after PAVM embolization:
   a. Follow-up is indicated to assess for the persistence or recurrence of a treated lesion and for the growth or enlargement of other PAVMs.
   b. Regimen. The following should be done at 6 to 12 months and then every 3 to 5 years:
      (1) Clinical evaluation.
      (2) Physiologic evaluation with pulse oximetry is simple to perform.
      (3) CT scan. This is the most definitive study. The aneurysm and/or draining vein of a treated lesion should shrink by typically 70% or more, although the accuracy of this has been questioned and the lack of enhancement if intravenous contrast was administered for at least the first follow-up study may be more precise (7). Artifact from dense embolization material can interfere with interpretation, particularly with platinum coils.
      (4) Quantitative contrast echocardiography. Early experience suggests that a grade 0 or 1 late right-to-left shunting on follow-up would correlate to the lack of any residual significant PAVM, and so offer an opportunity to avoid ionizing radiation from CT (8).
      (5) MRI and MRA. Experience remains limited for follow-up evaluation.
   c. An abnormality of sufficient size should prompt pulmonary angiography.
   d. Antibiotic prophylaxis remains recommended prior to dental and other "dirty" procedures due to the likely presence of residual tiny or microscopic PAVMs.
   e. Management of other issues related to HHT. In particular, iron deficiency should be corrected given data showing an increased risk of thrombosis in this population (3).

Results (2–4)

1. Technical success with initial complete occlusion is accomplished in 90% to 100%.
2. Subjective improvement may be seen in respiratory symptoms and performance, particularly in patients with initially larger right-to-left shunts.
3. The risks of stroke-TIA and brain abscess are significantly reduced to no more than approximately 3% each, and even lower if all PAVMs of any size are eliminated.

4. Migraines may improve.
5. Persistence or recurrence can occur through recanalization, pulmonary artery collaterals resupplying the lesion beyond the site of embolization, previously missed accessory feeder(s), or systemic collateral supply. The first three result in right-to-left shunting, with the risk of macroscopic paradoxical embolization of course depending on the size of any unimpeded channel(s). Repeat embolization is often more challenging and less successful, particularly with pulmonary artery collaterals, which are of greater concern for developing in younger children. The last method results in a small left-to-left shunt that is of no physiologic significance but rarely may cause hemoptysis due to the higher systemic pressure and fragile collaterals.
6. Persistence or recurrence rates vary by embolization devices, with plugs typically performing better, although no clear advantage yet shown between types of plugs.
   a. Coils. Rates vary greatly, with the average 15% to 25% but range of 0% to 58%. No significant difference has been found between pushable and detachable fibered coils. Hydrogel-coated coils may have a lower rate. Recanalization is the most common method with coils.
   b. Amplatzer vascular plugs. Rates are usually no greater than 10%, and often as low as 0%.
   c. Microvascular plugs. Rates have varied from 0% to 10%.
7. Patient factors may increase persistence, such as smoking and antithrombotic therapy.
8. Growth of previously tiny PAVMs to a size requiring treatment occurs in 14% to 19% and can, of course, cause recurrent symptoms.

Complications and Side Effects
In experienced centers, major and minor complications are quite rare and usually less than 1% to 2%, especially in more recent series.
1. Paradoxical embolization of air, thrombus, or an occluding device.
   a. Clinically, this may result in:
      (1) Angina and/or bradycardia, presumably due to air flowing into the anteriorly positioned right coronary artery in the supine patient. It can be treated with nitroglycerine and atropine. No adverse consequences of this have occurred.
      (2) Cerebral ischemia. Transient ischemic attack and stroke have been reported in less than 1% to 2%, and less common in recent studies.
   b. Paradoxical embolization of an occluding device has occurred in less than 1% to 4%, also less common in recent series, and serious sequelae are rare. The device may need to be retrieved if it has migrated to a critical arterial bed.
2. Rupture of the PAVM with hemorrhage is rare and managed by completion of the embolization.
3. Local venous thrombosis and pulmonary embolism are rare.
4. Pleurisy is the most common side effect after PAVM embolization and is self-limited. It can be treated with nonsteroidal antiinflammatory agents and/or acetaminophen.
   a. Chest pain with possibly fever several days after the procedure is seen in 0% to 36%.
   b. Delayed pleurisy and possibly pulmonary infiltrate after several weeks rarely occurs.
5. Late hemoptysis from systemic collateral supply into a persistent or reperfused PAVM is a rare phenomenon. If systemic embolization is performed, it must be done cautiously given the risk that any particulate agents migrating through systemic supply could then pass through the PAVM and result in paradoxical systemic embolization.
6. Late migration of coil emboli into the bronchial tree is quite rare.

7. Effects of radiation exposure from multiple studies. This underscores the need for follow-up studies that avoid ionizing radiation.

Alternative Treatments for Pulmonary Arteriovenous Malformation

1. Surgical resection such as wedge resection, lobectomy, or even pneumonectomy may be considered in the following situations:
   a. Regional involvement with diffuse or innumerable PAVM.
   b. Previously embolized PAVM with repeated later complications such as episodes of hemoptysis from systemic arterial reperfusion nonresponsive to cautious systemic embolization.
2. Lung transplantation for bilateral diffuse PAVM involvement is almost never indicated given documentation of better longevity than transplant recipients (3).

References

1. Liechty KW, Flake AW. Pulmonary vascular malformations. *Semin Pediatr Surg*. 2008;17(1): 9–16.
2. Pollak JS, White RI Jr. Distal cross-sectional occlusion is the "key" to treating pulmonary arteriovenous malformations. *J Vasc Interv Radiol*. 2012;23(12):1578–1580.
3. Shovlin CL, Condliffe R, Donaldson JW, et al. British Thoracic Society Clinical Statement on Pulmonary Arteriovenous Malformations. *Thorax*. 2017;72(12):1154–1163.
4. Majumdar S, McWilliams JP. Approach to pulmonary arteriovenous malformations: a comprehensive update. *J Clin Med*. 2020;9(6):1927–1951.
5. Albitar HAH, Segraves JM, Almodallal Y, et al. Pulmonary arteriovenous malformations in non-hereditary hemorrhagic telangiectasia patients: an 18-year retrospective study. *Lung*. 2020;198(4):679–686.
6. McDonald J, Bayrak-Toydemir P, Pyeritz RE. Hereditary hemorrhagic telangiectasia: an overview of diagnosis, management, and pathogenesis. *Genet Med*. 2011;13(7):607–616.
7. Belanger C, Chartrand-Lefebvre C, Soulez G, et al. Pulmonary arteriovenous malformation (PAVM) reperfusion after percutaneous embolization: sensitivity and specificity of non-enhanced CT. *Eur J Radiol*. 2016;85(1):150–157.
8. DePietro DM, Curnes NR, Chittams J, et al. Postembolotherapy pulmonary arteriovenous malformation follow-up: a role for graded transthoracic contrast echocardiography prior to high-resolution chest CT scan. *Chest*. 2020;157(5):1278–1286.

17 Stent-Grafts for Abdominal Aortic Aneurysms

Matthew J. Scheidt, MD, Shantanu Warhadpande, MD, and Parag J. Patel, MD, MS

Introduction

1. Abdominal aortic aneurysm (AAA)—Definition:
   a. An increase in diameter of 50% compared to the adjacent normal aortic segment, or
   b. Sac diameter greater than 3 cm.
2. Aneurysms are classified:
   a. Morphologically: fusiform—affecting the entire arterial circumference or saccular—affecting only part of the arterial circumference.
   b. By their relationship to the renal arteries: suprarenal, pararenal, juxtarenal, or infrarenal.

3. Associations include increasing age, male sex, smoking, coronary artery disease, hypercholesterolemia, peripheral vascular disease, hypertension, and family history (higher incidence in first-degree relatives). The reported prevalence ranges from 2% to 8% in adults over the age of 65 (1,2).

4. The natural history of AAA is continuous expansion resulting in increased risk of rupture or distal embolization. Risk factors for AAA rupture include aneurysm size, rate of expansion, poorly controlled hypertension, chronic opstructive pulmonary disease, smoking, and family history (3). Most small aneurysms increase in size by 2.2 mm/y; 4 mm/y is maximum normal growth (3). With progressive enlargement of an AAA, there are also changes in the aorta above and below the aneurysm. The lengths of the proximal neck and distal cuff shorten, the entire aorta lengthens and becomes more tortuous, iliac tortuosity increases, and iliac aneurysms may form.

5. Ruptured AAA is the 10th leading cause of death in men. The annual risk of rupture for AAA (a) less than 5.5 cm: ≤1.0%, (b) 5.5 to 5.9 cm: 9.4%, (c) 6.0 to 6.9 cm: 10.2%, (d) ≥7.0 cm: 32.5%. AAAs >5.5 cm have an annual risk of rupture exceeding the elective 30-day operative mortality, hence, this has been the size criterion for elective repair in men (3,4).

6. The ratio of men to women with AAA is up to 4:1 (5,6). Women have smaller aortic diameters compared to men and a 5.5-cm AAA represents a much larger relative dilatation and has an increased risk of rupture. Thus, some experts have recommended elective repair at 5 cm in women (3).

7. Treatment of AAAs include endovascular aneurysm repair (EVAR) and open surgical repair. The perioperative 30-day mortality rate for EVAR is significantly lower than for open repair. However, the 1-year mortality rates are similar between the two treatments. At present, more than 70% of AAAs are treated via EVAR (3–5). There are currently eight FDA-approved EVAR devices (see Table 17.1).

Goals of Stent-Graft Therapy

1. To provide a less invasive alternative for low-risk patients, lower procedural morbidity and mortality, decreased postprocedure pain and complications, and shortened convalescence.

2. To provide treatment to high-risk patients who are not surgical candidates and would otherwise have no therapeutic option for AAA repair.

Indications

1. Emergent
   a. Known or suspected rupture.
   b. Symptomatic aneurysm (tenderness, abdominal or back pain) regardless of aneurysm diameter.
   c. Rapidly expanding aneurysm: >1-cm growth in 12 months (4).
2. Elective
   a. Asymptomatic fusiform aneurysm: >5.5 cm in diameter for men; >5.0 cm for women (3–5).
   b. Atypical aneurysms such as mycotic, those with penetrating atherosclerotic ulcer, enlarging intramural hematoma, or saccular morphology.
   c. Smaller AAAs with either concomitant common iliac aneurysms requiring repair (>3.0 cm in diameter) or associated thrombotic/embolic complications.
   d. Inflammatory AAAs.

Contraindications

1. Patent inferior mesenteric artery (IMA) in the setting of significant superior mesenteric artery narrowing where the IMA is the predominant blood supply to the bowel.

Table 17.1 FDA-Approved Devices for EVAR

Device	Manufacturer	Fda Approval	Stent Material	Graft Material	Fixation Location	Neck Min. Length (mm)/Max. Diameter (mm)/Max. Angulation (°)	Iliac Seal Zone Diameter/min. Length (mm)	Delivery System	Sheath OD (Fr) for 24-mm Proximal Neck Diameter
AFX2	Endologix	2011	Cobalt chromium alloy	ePTFE	Anatomic at aortic bifurcation	15/32/60	10–23/15	Separate sheath	19
Endurant II	Medtronic	2010	Nitinol	Pressed polyester	Suprarenal with hooks	10/32/60	8–25/15	Integrated sheath	18
Excluder C3	Gore	2011	Nitinol	ePTFE	Infrarenal with hooks	15/32/60	8–25/10	Separate sheath	20
InCraft	Cordis	2018[a]	Nitinol	Woven polyester	Suprarenl with hooks	10/31/60	7–22/15	Integrated sheath	14
Alto	Endologix	2011	Nitinol	ePTFE	Suprarenal with hooks and infrarenal polymer-filled seal rings	7/30/60	8–20/10	Integrated sheath	15
Zenith Flex	Cook	2003	Stainless steel	Woven polyester	Suprarenal with hooks	15/32/60	7.5–20/10[b]	Integrated sheath	21
Zenith Fenestrated	Cook	2012	Stainless steel	Woven polyester	Suprarenal with hooks	4/31/45	Ipsilateral 9–21/30[b], Contralateral 7–21/30[b]	Integrated sheath	23

[a]Not commercially available in the United States.
[b]Iliac diameter measurements for the Cook Zenith devices are from outer wall to outer wall.
FDA, US Food and Drug Administration; EVAR, endovascular aneurysm repair; OD, outer diameter; PTFE, polytetrafluoroethylene.

2. Patients must meet anatomic criteria for successful endograft placement, including appropriate proximal and distal landing zones as well as suitable access vessels (see Fig. 17.1).
3. Relative contraindications include severe concomitant disease with short life expectancy, renal insufficiency, and severe contrast reactions. Endografts have been successfully implanted in patients with renal insufficiency or severe reactions to contrast using reduced amounts of diluted contrast, alternative contrast media such as carbon dioxide, and intravascular ultrasound.

Preprocedure Imaging

As opposed to open surgical repair, EVAR of AAA is entirely dependent upon radiologic imaging for pre-, intra-, and postprocedure management.

Careful imaging to obtain accurate diameter and length measurements is essential to maximize the technical success of the stent-graft deployment. CT angiography (CTA) with three-dimensional (3D) reconstruction is the preferred imaging modality for preprocedural planning and follow-up of EVAR.

1. **CT angiography**
   a. Advantages
      (1) Noninvasive.
      (2) High resolution; able to reveal anatomic details such as calcium and small amounts of mural thrombus.
      (3) Allows for postprocessing at a 3D workstation that provides multiplanar reformatted images and centerline measurements for more accurate and precise length and diameter determination.
   b. Disadvantages
      (1) Radiation exposure.
      (2) Nephrotoxic contrast.
   c. For CTA protocols, see Chapter 72.
2. **Angiography.** Angiography has largely been replaced by CTA or MRA for the preprocedure assessment of anatomy and suitability for EVAR, so is rarely done as a standalone procedure.
   a. Advantages
      (1) Accurate estimation of length and size.
      (2) Defines aortic branch vessels, including renal arteries (main and accessory), mesenteric arteries, hypogastric arteries, and lumbar and visceral artery collaterals.
      (3) Carbon dioxide (CO_2) can be used to decrease contrast medium nephrotoxicity.
   b. Disadvantages
      (1) Invasive.
      (2) Thrombus effect: angiography = lumenography. Only shows flow lumen; therefore, is unreliable to measure diameters; single projection may not show true maximum cross-sectional diameter.
      (3) Unable to demonstrate wall pathology such as thrombus and minimal calcifications.
      (4) Magnification error: Focal point-to-film distance is standard, but patient body habitus may influence magnification error. Calibrated catheters are used to avoid magnification-related measurement errors.
      (5) Foreshortening creating errors in length measurements.
      (6) Parallax error.
      (7) Contrast medium nephrotoxicity.
3. **Magnetic resonance imaging**
   a. Advantages
      (1) Avoids the use of iodinated contrast agents.
      (2) Noninvasive.

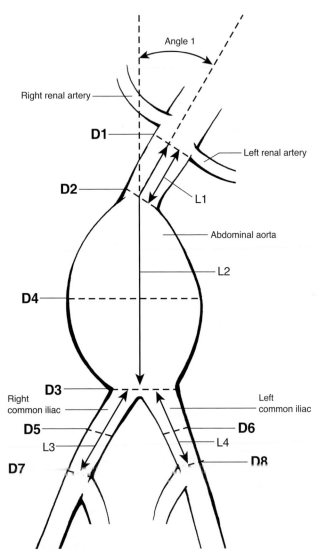

FIGURE 17.1 • Aortic dimensions to be measured in evaluation of an aneurysm for endograft placement. Diameters (D) are measured from transverse images from a CTA that are reconstructed at right angles to the long axis of the vessel being measured. $D1$ = lowest renal artery, $D2$ = 4 to 15 mm distal to the lowest renal artery (distance depending on type of endograft chosen, see Table 17.1), $D3$ = aortic bifurcation, $D4$ = largest aneurysm sac dimension, $D5$ and $D6$ = right and left common iliac arteries, respectively, and $D7$ and $D8$ = right and left distal landing zones, respectively. Lengths (L) are measured from digital subtraction angiography (DSA) obtained with a calibrated catheter or from 3D reconstructions of the vessel on a CTA. $L1$ = neck, $L2$ = lowest renal artery to the aortic bifurcation, and $L3$ and $L4$ = aortic bifurcation to the right and left common iliac artery bifurcations. $Angle\ 1$ = angulation of the proximal neck obtained from DSA or CTA multiplanar reformations.

(3) No radiation exposure.

(4) Excellent soft tissue visualization.

b. Disadvantages

(1) Inferior spatial resolution and may miss collateral vessels less than 2 mm in diameter.

(2) Susceptible to motion artifacts.

(3) Inability to assess the degree of intimal calcification. If MRA is used, then unenhanced CT should be considered in conjunction.

4. **Ultrasound**

a. Advantages

(1) Readily available.

(2) Noninvasive.

(3) No radiation exposure.

b. Disadvantages

(1) Diameter and length measurements are less reliable than other modalities.

(2) Operator and patient body habitus dependent.

5. **Intravascular ultrasound**

a. Advantages

(1) Provides real-time 360-degree cross-sectional view of the vessel being evaluated.

(2) Used in conjunction with contrast sparing angiography or CO_2 angiography to evaluate aortoiliac pathology, confirm branch vessel position, and perform graft sizing.

b. Disadvantages

(1) Operator dependent. The catheter may not lie in a coaxial plane, which distorts the anatomy and may result in inaccurate measurements.

Selection Criteria for Endograft Repair

1. Successful EVAR of AAA depends upon anatomic considerations and patient selection.

2. Anatomic considerations include the morphology of the aorta and access arteries. Correct measurements of the diameter and length are essential to maximize the success of the endograft procedure.

3. Measurements required for the evaluation of an aneurysm for endograft placement are depicted in Figure 17.1. Each EVAR device has a specific protocol for proper sizing, the majority of which are common across all devices. However, there are nuances particular to each device and familiarity with the device is critical for correct sizing. Please refer to each device's instructions for use (IFU) for the sizing protocol.

4. Patient selection is based on elective operative risk, aneurysm rupture risk, concomitant disease, life expectancy, and patient preference.

Anatomic Criteria

1. **Proximal neck**

a. *Definition:* The segment of aorta between the origin of the lowest renal artery and superior aspect of the aneurysm.

b. *Morphology* is of critical importance in aneurysm evaluation and is the most common factor to exclude EVAR.

c. *Length:* Most endografts require at least 15 mm to ensuring adequate proximal seal. Some devices allow for transrenal fixation of the proximal cuff, which enables EVAR in patients with as short as a 4-mm neck.

d. *Diameter:* Requirements depend upon which device is to be deployed. To correctly measure for most devices, the outer wall limits should be used. This measures the outer media and adventitia, the layers that will support and anchor the endograft. Most proximal necks diverge caudally having a conical shape; as a general rule diameter should increase no more than 10% from the proximal to the distal end of the proximal neck. The endograft should be oversized 10% to 20% larger than the neck diameter.

e. *Thrombus:* Thrombus greater than 2 mm in depth involving more than 25% of the proximal neck circumference is considered unfavorable and EVAR is contraindicated by most manufacturers' IFU (4). If EVAR is pursued in cases with appropriate neck length but significant mural thrombus, an endograft with suprarenal active fixation could be considered. Mural thrombus may impair proximal seal and fixation. During EVAR placement, thrombus may be displaced into or across the renal artery ostia.

f. *Angulation:* Angulation between the suprarenal aorta and superior portion of the aneurysm neck is common and can be measured as shown in Figure 17.1. Each endograft has a different threshold of neck angulation in the IFU. However, if it exceeds 60 degrees, the placement of the majority of stent-grafts is contraindicated. Severe angulation may result in kinking or downward migration of the endograft during or after placement.

g. *Advanced Techniques:* 20% to 30% of patients will have aortic neck anatomy considered unfavorable for stent-graft placement (7). A proximal seal is difficult (or impossible) to achieve in short infrarenal necks, highly angulated infrarenal necks, or with suprarenal/juxtarenal aneurysms. Involvement of the visceral arteries by the aneurysm sac can also further complicate the issue. Several advanced techniques are available to treat AAAs with unsuitable proximal aortic neck anatomy: Fenestrated EVAR (FEVAR), Chimney-EVAR (CEVAR), Snorkel and Sandwich techniques.

(1) Fenestrated EVAR (FEVAR)

   (a) Approved for neck lengths >4 mm.

   (b) Custom-made device with suprarenal fixation and specifically sized/aligned fenestrations and/or scallops to allow for cannulation of the involved visceral arteries through the proximal body graft. Once catheterized through the proximal body, covered stents can be deployed through the fenestrations to provide an adequate seal, allow for visceral artery patency, and prevent stent-graft migration. Two devices are currently available for FEVARs and allow for customization: Zenith (Cook Medical, Bloomington, IN) and Anaconda (Terumo, Sunrise, FL); the latter of which is not currently available in the United States.

(2) Chimney-EVAR (ChEVAR)

   (a) Technique used to ensure side-branch artery patency when a FEVAR is not possible (such as during an emergency EVAR when customized stent-grafts are not available). This is achieved by cannulating the side-branch artery *outside* the main body of the stent-graft and deploying a covered stent in parallel to the main-body stent-graft (Fig. 17.2).

   (b) There is one complication unique to ChEVAR that makes the technique controversial. A "gutter" forms in the aorta in between the main-body stent-graft and the chimney stent-graft, as they run in parallel to each other. This can lead to a "gutter endoleak."

   (c) The PERICLES registry from 2015 demonstrated that the ChEVAR technique resulted in favorable outcomes, similar to those seen with FEVARs (8).

2. **Distal aorta**

   a. If an aortic tube graft is being considered, the length of the distal attachment site must be greater than 20 mm and free of significant thrombus. Infrarenal aortic tube grafts are used infrequently due to the aneurysm most commonly extending to the aortic bifurcation.

   b. If a bifurcated device is to be deployed, the diameter of the distal aorta should be evaluated. Distal aortic diameter of 18 mm will accommodate a bifurcated aortic endograft. Distal aortic diameter less than 18 mm may complicate device delivery or result in a hemodynamically significant iliac limb stenosis.

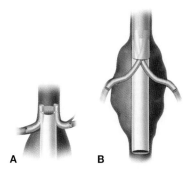

A   **B**

FIGURE 17.2 • Multiple advanced techniques are employed when side-branch patency needs to be preserved and a fenestrated EVAR is not possible. Perigraft leaks are a concern with all these techniques. **A:** A schematic through the aorta with chimney stent-grafts demonstrates the relationship between two chimney grafts along the aortic stent-graft. Chimney/"Snorkel" stent-graft techniques are used in Chimney EVAR (Ch-EVAR) whereby stent-grafts are deployed within the visceral arteries coursing outside and parallel to the aortic stent-graft. The cranially directed side-branch stent is referred to as a chimney/"snorkel" while the caudally directed side-branch stent with retrograde perfusion is referred to as the "periscope" (not shown). **B:** Schematic of the Sandwich technique demonstrates a side-branch stent coursing between the stent-graft material of a proximal stent-graft and a second distal stent-graft. Generally, the proximal stent-graft is deployed first, followed by side-branch cannulation and stenting. The distal stent-graft is then deployed with an overlap with the proximal side-branch stent-graft. The sandwiched chimney graft is within the proximal stent-graft but outside the distal stent-graft coursing in the overlap zone. (Reprinted with permission from Clement Darling R, Ozaki CK. *Master Techniques in Surgery: Vascular Surgery: Arterial Procedures.* Wolters Kluwer; 2016.)

    Significant stenoses at the native aortic bifurcation may require angioplasty both before and after endograft deployment. In these situations, consideration should also be given for the use of an EVAR device that preserves the native aortic bifurcation (Endologix AFX) or placement of an aorto-uni-iliac device plus a femorofemoral bypass.

  c. Evaluate the distal aorta for important branch vessels such as accessory renal arteries and the IMA.

    (1) Small accessory renal arteries can be covered by an endograft. However, this increases the risk of postprocedural renal insufficiency and is a possible source for type II endoleak.

    (2) Patients with a chronically occluded SMA and secondary IMA hypertrophy have an unfavorable anatomy for EVAR and would be at significant clinical risk of bowel ischemia if EVAR were attempted.

3. Iliac arteries

  a. The length and diameter of the common iliac arteries (CIAs) must be carefully assessed, as these are the target sites for distal attachment of a bifurcated endograft. The CIA diameter should be <25 mm and >10 mm of length is required for adequate seal.

  b. Up to 20% to 30% of patients with an AAA have a concomitant iliac artery aneurysm (3).

  c. *Single CIA aneurysm:* If a single common iliac aneurysm extends to the iliac bifurcation, then often the ipsilateral external iliac artery becomes the target site for distal attachment. This may require coil or plug embolization of the ipsilateral hypogastric artery to prevent a type II endoleak from retrograde filling. Assessment of contralateral hypogastric artery patency is important to prevent debilitating buttock claudication, and less commonly erectile dysfunction, spinal ischemia, gluteal necrosis, or colonic ischemia (9).

d. *Bilateral CIA aneurysms:* Endovascular treatment of bilateral CIA aneurysms extending to the level of the iliac bifurcation can be handled in several different ways including staged bilateral hypogastric artery embolization, unilateral iliac branch device, or bilateral iliac branch device placement.

   (1) Bilateral hypogastric artery embolization.

      (a) Although pelvic or bowel ischemia may occur, several studies suggest that the risks associated with bilateral hypogastric artery occlusion are generally limited to buttock claudication and erectile dysfunction (9,10). The risks of bilateral hypogastric artery occlusion can be mitigated by performing a staged occlusion of each hypogastric artery (procedures performed 4 to 6 weeks apart) and embolization limited to the main trunk so as to preserve pelvic collateral vessels. This may be the best option in patients who are otherwise high risk for operative repair.

      (b) Alternatively, the "sandwich" technique, which involves the placement of two parallel endografts within an iliac limb to create an "off-the-shelf" bifurctated iliac component, can be considered to preserve flow to the hypogastric artery.

   (2) Iliac branch endoprosthesis

      (a) The Gore Excluder Iliac Branch Endoprosthesis (IBE) is the only commercially available iliac branch device in the United States. Use of this device, if anatomically feasible, allows for continued perfusion of the internal iliac artery (IIA) distribution.

      (b) The device is deployed prior to the main-body component of the bifurcated abdominal aortic endograft. It is advanced and positioned from an ipsilateral approach and requires a CIA diameter ≥17 mm and length of 55 mm. The IIA gate is precanulated and a through-and-through access to the contralateral common femoral artery is obtained. The ipsilateral iliac branch component is deployed through a 16-Fr sheath. A 12-Fr sheath is then advanced from the contralateral CFA up and over the aortoiliac bifurcation and used to cannulate the ipsilateral IIA limb. The IIA component is then deployed, ensuring that the ipsilateral IIA has a diameter of 6.5 to 13.5 mm and a landing zone of at least 10 mm (10).

      (c) Bilateral IBE placement is technically feasible without significantly increased morbidity, but is beyond the scope of this chapter.

4. Vascular access

a. Common femoral and iliac arteries are the conduits for device introduction. Significant atherosclerotic changes with heavy calcification and plaque formation, diminutive diameter, and marked tortuosity are factors that may complicate device delivery and contraindicate EVAR. The most common causes of technical failure are the inability to deliver the device through the iliac arteries or rupture of the iliac arteries during device withdrawal.

b. Women tend to have smaller caliber iliac arteries than men.

c. In the absence of heavy calcification, tortuosity can often be reduced with the introduction of a rigid guidewire such as the Amplatz Super Stiff or Lunderquist guidewire.

d. Focal stenoses can often be pretreated with simple angioplasty. Heavily calcified lesions may need to be pretreated with simply angioplasty, lithoplasty, or possibly stenting.

e. *Percutaneous versus surgical cutdown*: Compared to open femoral exposure, percutaneous endovascular aneurysm repair (PEVAR) using a suture-mediated closure device (SMCD) "preclose" technique with the Perclose ProGlide (Abbott Vascular, Inc. Redwood City, CA) is less invasive and associated with decreased operative time and major access-related complications compared to surgical cutdown with experienced operators (3,9). Use of SMCD "preclose" technique has been FDA approved for use with up to 21-Fr delivery sheaths. Percutaneous technique is not recommended in patients with small common femoral arteries (<5 mm in diameter), and careful consideration should be taken in patients with extensive anterior wall or circumferential calcification. Ultrasound access within the CFA, 1 cm proximal to the femoral bifurcation and at the 12 o'clock position is strongly recommended.

Procedure

1. Specific detailed procedural steps are unique to each device used. However, in general, some basic steps employed by all devices are discussed.
2. Bilateral common femoral artery access is obtained either percutaneously or via a surgical cutdown and systemic anticoagulation achieved with intravenous heparin.
3. A pigtail marker catheter is advanced via the contralateral access to the level of the renal arteries. An abdominal aortogram can be performed to confirm preprocedural length measurements.
4. The ipsilateral floppy guidewire access is exchanged through a diagnostic catheter for a superstiff guidewire that is positioned in the descending thoracic aorta.
5. The main body of the device and the introducer sheath are advanced over the superstiff guidewire so that the superior end of the endograft is at the level of the lowest renal artery.
6. Under magnification, the superior end of the covered portion of the endograft and lowest renal artery are centered on the field so as to reduce errors caused by parallax. Additionally, the image intensifier is angulated and/or rotated so as to best profile the lowest renal artery.
7. Intermittent angiography at this location is performed with adjustments made to position the endograft immediately distal to the lowest renal artery. Once appropriate position is confirmed, the trunk and contralateral limb are deployed under fluoroscopic guidance.
8. At this time, the contralateral gate is cannulated with a guidewire. Once cannulated, a pigtail catheter is advanced over the guidewire and spun within the main body of endograft to confirm appropriate location within the endograft rather than alongside the graft in the aneurysm sac.
9. A superstiff guidewire is advanced through the pigtail marker catheter, which is then positioned with a marker at the bottom of the contralateral gate. A retrograde contralateral sheath angiogram is performed in the appropriate obliquity so as to profile the hypogastric artery origin. This will allow correct length determination and positioning of the contralateral iliac limb so as to preserve hypogastric artery flow.
10. The pigtail catheter is exchanged over the superstiff guidewire for the contralateral limb, which is positioned appropriately and then deployed. If an ipsilateral iliac extension is needed, a similar technique can be used to determine length and position.
11. At this time, proximal, distal, and overlapping attachment sites are balloon dilated to achieve a maximum profile ("ironing").
12. A pigtail catheter is reintroduced to the level of the renal arteries and a final aortogram is performed. Particular attention is made to renal and hypogastric arterial flow as well as the presence of endoleaks. If necessary, secondary interventions can be performed as needed.

Postprocedure Management

1. Immediate and in-hospital postprocedure management entails the evaluation of bilateral groin access sites for infection or hematoma, assessment of distal perfusion and renal function, and early ambulation. Hospital stay is typically 1 to 3 days.
2. Following recovery from the initial procedure, indefinite long-term imaging surveillance is required. Particular attention is made to AAA diameter, detection and classification of endoleaks, and evaluation of the endograft morphology.

3. Specific imaging modalities and their advantages/disadvantages were discussed previously. CTA remains the most widely used modality for follow-up after EVAR. In patients with renal insufficiency, a noncontrast CT or color Duplex ultrasound and plain radiography are performed.
4. Physical examination and imaging follow-up are recommended at 1 to 3 months and 6 months after the procedure. If no endoleak is identified, then patients are followed at yearly intervals. If an endoleak is present, the patients are followed every 6 months for the first 2 years and yearly thereafter unless treatment is mandated (discussed below).

Results

1. EVAR is associated with significantly less blood loss, fewer days in intensive care, fewer hospital days, fewer systemic complications, and decreased in-hospital and 30-day mortality versus open repair of AAAs. Furthermore, aneurysm-related mortality is significantly lower with EVAR compared with open repair (3).
2. The major disadvantages to EVAR versus open repair are the necessity for lifelong imaging follow-up and need for secondary interventions, especially the treatment of endoleaks.
3. Results of long-term studies are still forthcoming and will help to better define EVAR's clinical efficacy, durability, and cost effectiveness.

Complications

1. EVAR is less invasive than open surgery and has low annual rates of late AAA rupture. Complications include endoleak, aneurysm sac expansion, endograft migration, stent fracture, graft stenosis, graft thrombosis, graft infection, and groin and retroperitoneal hematoma (4).
2. Approximately 30% of patients with AAA treated with EVAR may require secondary interventions, significantly higher than for open repair (2).

Management of Complications

1. Stenosis within or immediately distal to iliac limb. This frequently is related to severely calcified arteries or orientation of the distal orifice of the limb into the vessel wall due to vascular tortuosity or change of stent-graft position with aneurysmal remodeling. Balloon angioplasty may work, but more often a bare metal stent or limb extension is required.
2. Limb occlusion. Options include:
   a. Reopening the limb by balloon thrombectomy or thrombolysis. Once the clot is cleared, search for an underlying mechanical problem by angiography, and if necessary, intra-arterial pressure assessment, is mandatory.
   b. Leaving the limb occluded and performing a femorofemoral bypass graft.
3. Endoleaks and their treatment are discussed in Chapter 18.

References

1. Dua A, Kuy S, Lee CJ, et al. Epidemiology of aortic aneurysm repair in the United States from 2000 to 2010. *J Vasc Surg.* 2014;59(6):1512–1517. doi:10.1016/J.JVS.2014.01.007
2. Kent KC. Clinical practice. Abdominal aortic aneurysms. *N Engl J Med.* 2014;371(22):2101–2108. doi:10.1056/NEJMCP1401430
3. Chaikof EL, Dalman RL, Eskandari MK, et al. The Society for Vascular Surgery practice guidelines on the care of patients with an abdominal aortic aneurysm. *J Vasc Surg.* 2018;67(1):2–77.e2. doi:10.1016/J.JVS.2017.10.044
4. Walker TG, Kalva SP, Yeddula K, et al. Clinical practice guidelines for endovascular abdominal aortic aneurysm repair: written by the Standards of Practice Committee for the Society of Interventional Radiology and Endorsed by the Cardiovascular and Interventional Radiological Society of Europe and the Canadian Interventional

Radiology Association. *J Vasc Interv Radiol.* 2010;21(11):1632–1655. doi:10.1016/J.JVIR.2010.07.008

5. Wanhainen A, Verzini F, van Herzeele I, et al. Editor's Choice – European Society for Vascular Surgery (ESVS) 2019 Clinical Practice Guidelines on the Management of Abdominal Aorto-iliac Artery Aneurysms. *Eur J Vasc Endovasc Surg.* 2019;57(1):8–93. doi:10.1016/J.EJVS.2018.09.020

6. Carino D, Sarac TP, Ziganshin BA, et al. Abdominal aortic aneurysm: evolving controversies and uncertainties. *Int J Angiol.* 2018;27(2):58. doi:10.1055/S-0038-1657771

7. Antoniou GA, Georgiadis GS, Antoniou SA, et al. A meta-analysis of outcomes of endovascular abdominal aortic aneurysm repair in patients with hostile and friendly neck anatomy. *J Vasc Surg.* 2013;57(2):527–538. doi:10.1016/J.JVS.2012.09.050

8. Donas KP, Lee JT, Lachat M, et al. Collected world experience about the performance of the snorkel/chimney endovascular technique in the treatment of complex aortic pathologies: the PERICLES registry. *Ann Surg.* 2015;262(3):546–552. doi:10.1097/SLA.0000000000001405

9. Smeds MR, Charlton-Ouw KM. Infrarenal endovascular aneurysm repair: New developments and decision making in 2016. *Semin Vasc Surg.* 2016;29(1–2):27–34. doi:10.1053/J.SEMVASCSURG.2016.06.001

10. DeRoo E, Harris D, Olson S, et al. Conformability of the GORE EXCLUDER iliac branch endoprosthesis is associated with freedom from adverse iliac events. *J Vasc Surg.* 2021; 74(5):1558–1564.e1. doi:10.1016/J.JVS.2021.05.026

18 Management of Stent-Graft Endoleaks

*David R. Bamshad, MD and
Robert Lookstein, MD, MHCDL, FSIR, FAHA, FSVM*

Endovascular Aortic Aneurysm Repair and Endoleaks

1. As discussed in the previous chapter, endovascular aortic aneurysm repair (EVAR) represents a significant evolution in treating aortic aneurysms and offers reduced morbidity and mortality compared to open aortic repair. However, EVAR requires lifelong surveillance to evaluate for possible complications.

2. Endoleaks are the most common complication of EVAR (25% to 35% of patients). An endoleak is defined as persistent perfusion of the excluded aneurysm sac after stent-graft treatment. This can potentially progress to aneurysm expansion and rupture (1). But with proper surveillance and intervention, recent long-term studies suggest no association between the occurrence of endoleaks and increased mortality.

3. Certain anatomic considerations that predispose to endoleak complications include proximal/distal attachment sites, angulation and tortuosity of the aorta, and the presence of calcification or occlusive disease in the access arteries (2).

4. There are five types of endoleaks, which are defined by the etiology of blood flow into the aneurysm sac (3).

Endoleak Classification (see Table 18.1)

1. Type I endoleak

   a. Blood flows from a stent-graft attachment site (either proximal attachment site [IA], distal attachment site [IB], or from an incompletely occluded, contralateral common iliac artery in aortouniiliac stent-grafts [IC]) (2,3).

   b. Type I endoleaks occur more commonly in the thoracic aorta and in aortas where the attachment sites are complicated by thrombus, short and/or angulated necks, and dilated, irregular iliac arteries (2,3).

   c. Type I endoleaks can be seen immediately after deployment as a result of incomplete expansion of the stent-graft, aortic tortuosity, or steep aortic angulation.

   d. Late development of type I endoleaks can be related to anatomical changes in the configuration of the aorta as the aneurysm sac shrinks (3).

Table 18.1 Classification of Endoleaks

Endoleak Type	Etiology	Incidence[a]	Clinical Significance	Treatment/Management
I	Blood flows from a stent-graft attachment site (either proximal [IA], distal [IB], or from contralateral common iliac artery in aortouniliac stent-grafts [IC])	10%	Immediate treatment is necessary because of direct communication with high-pressure systemic arterial blood flow which increases risk of rupture	Secure suboptimal or compromised attachment site with angioplasty balloons, stents, or stent-graft extensions; alternatively, open repair
II	Blood flows retrograde from aortic branch vessels (most commonly IMA, lumbar artery) into the aneurysm sac (single vessel involved [IIA], or two or more vessels involved [IIB])	25%	Often seals spontaneously and does not require immediate intervention. Monitor with imaging for sac expansion	Embolization of feeding vessel; alternatively, open repair
III	Blood flows through a stent-graft structural defect (either between junctional separations of overlapping modular devices [IIIA], or through stent-graft fractures or fabric holes [IIIB])	2%	Immediate treatment is necessary due to higher risk associated with communicating high-pressure arterial flow	Stent-graft extension to cover the separated modular component or defect within the original graft
IV	Blood flows through the porosity of the stent-graft material itself and manifests as a "blush" in the immediate postimplantation angiogram in patients who are fully anticoagulated	<1%	Rarely seen; resolves spontaneously once the patient's coagulation status is normalized	Monitor for resolution on follow up imaging
V	Continued aneurysm expansion without an obvious cause; also referred to as "endotension"	2%	All diagnostic modalities must be considered to exclude other types of endoleak	Close surveillance imaging for sac expansion; typically treated with open repair

[a]Incidence of endoleaks after EVAR (4).

2. Type II endoleak
   a. Blood flows retrograde from aortic branch vessels into the aneurysm sac (single vessel involved [IIA], or two or more vessels involved [IIB]) (3).
   b. The inferior mesenteric artery and lumbar arteries are most commonly involved. Other less common sources include the hypogastric, median sacral, accessory renal, or gonadal arteries.
   c. Type II endoleaks are the most common (40%) type of endoleak.
3. Type III endoleak
   a. Blood flows through a stent-graft structural defect (either between junctional separations of overlapping modular devices [IIIA], or through stent-graft fractures or fabric holes [IIIB]) (2).
   b. Type III endoleaks may be related to stresses resulting from aneurysm sac shrinkage or stresses caused by arterial pulsations.
4. Type IV endoleak
   a. Blood flows through the porosity of the stent-graft material itself. This may manifest as a "blush" in the immediate postimplantation angiogram in patients who are fully anticoagulated (2). They are typically self-limited and resolve spontaneously with normalization of coagulation status.
   b. Type IV endoleaks are now rare due to improved stent-graft construction. They are a diagnosis of exclusion as other types of endoleaks can mimic type IV endoleaks.
5. Type V endoleak
   a. Continued aneurysm expansion without an obvious cause, also referred to as "endotension."
   b. The exact etiology is unknown, but type V endoleaks may represent occult instances of types I, II, or III endoleak, ultrafiltration of blood across the stent-graft, or a thrombus/atheroma at an attachment site resulting in an ineffective barrier to pressure transmission (3).

Post-EVAR Imaging Modalities

Postoperative imaging surveillance is necessary after EVAR for early detection and characterization of endoleaks (5). Complications such as endoleak, graft migration, limb stenosis, and sac growth can occur months to years after EVAR. Early detection of these events with surveillance imaging may help to prevent associated morbidity and mortality from aneurysm rupture or limb occlusion. Lifelong imaging surveillance is necessary after EVAR.

1. Radiography
   a. Useful to monitor for stent migration, detect kinks in abdominal stent-grafts, and evaluate conformation of thoracic stent-grafts.
   b. Typical projections include anteroposterior (AP) and lateral (for migration and component separation) and oblique (to improve sensitivity for detecting stent-graft wire fractures).
2. Computed tomography (CT)
   a. Most common modality used for surveillance imaging after EVAR.
   b. Highly accurate in determining aneurysm size and volume and can detect endoleaks with a higher sensitivity than conventional angiography.
   c. Because endoleaks have variable flow rates and are detected at variable times after contrast administration, multiphase CT angiography (CTA) is essential. Typical protocol includes three phases: precontrast, arterial phase, and delayed venous phase.
   d. Precontrast imaging is useful for differentiating true endoleaks from high-density mimics such as calcium or metal.
   e. Arterial phase imaging is useful for detecting endoleaks and for planning translumbar embolization of endoleaks.

    f. Venous phase imaging is more sensitive than arterial phase imaging for detection of endoleaks (especially distal type I leaks).

    g. To reduce radiation exposure, precontrast scanning can be obtained for the first post-EVAR examination, with all subsequent examinations acquiring only postcontrast images, using the initial precontrast scan for comparison.

3. Magnetic resonance (MR)

    a. Gadolinium-enhanced MR has been shown in many studies to be comparably as accurate as CTA in determining aneurysm size and stent-graft position as well as being useful in detection of endoleaks in nitinol-based stents.

    b. Gadolinium-enhanced studies are useful for detection of small endoleaks and demonstrate superior sensitivity for slow-flow type II leaks as compared with CT (6).

    c. Time-resolved MR angiography correctly reclassified multiple type 1 endoleaks that were initially labeled type II via CTA (7).

    d. Patients with a long life expectancy, for whom cumulative radiation exposure is of greater concern, and those allergic to iodinated contrast are more suitable for surveillance with MR than CT.

    e. Stainless steel stents can cause extensive susceptibility artifact and elgiloy stents can obscure the lumen of the stent-grafts; therefore, these stents cannot be evaluated with MR (2).

    f. MR imaging is more time consuming and expensive than CT.

4. Ultrasound (US)

    a. Recent studies suggest a high degree of correlation between CT imaging and color duplex US in the detection of clinically significant endoleaks (4). Some centers recommend annual post-EVAR surveillance with color duplex US alone if the first annual contrast-enhanced CT fails to demonstrate an endoleak or enlargement of the residual abdominal aortic aneurysm (AAA) sac.

    b. Some investigators have reported using contrast-enhanced US with microbubble contrast agents as an accurate way to screen for and further characterize endoleaks (6).

    c. Although portable, safe, and inexpensive, US is limited due to its dependence on operator skills, technique, and poor image quality in evaluating obese patients.

5. Digital subtraction angiography (DSA)

    a. The gold standard for endoleak categorization because of its ability to demonstrate flow direction as well as its high spatial and temporal resolution.

    b. Long acquisitions can be used for detection of slow-flow endoleaks that may have been otherwise missed during the delayed phase of CT.

    c. Nearly all endoleaks cause contrast material to appear in the inferior mesenteric or lumbar arteries on CTA which may represent outflow contrast from a type I or type III endoleak or inflow contrast supplying a type II endoleak. Therefore, DSA is the gold standard for classification of endoleaks. Assessment with DSA is usually performed prior to intervention (2).

Surveillance and Management Strategies

Official guidelines regarding surveillance frequency have not been well established and are debated. Many observational studies have reported high rates of noncompliance (30% to 40%) with follow-up imaging. Although there is data demonstrating a lack of association between noncompliance and worse outcomes, many studies suggest higher overall mortality with failure of surveillance (8).

1. Typical initial modalities include radiography and CT unless the patient is severely allergic to iodinated contrast or has poor renal function. US, MRI, and DSA may be performed to further evaluate endotension or endoleak not detected by CT.

    a. One month, 6 months, 1 year, and then annual follow-up with radiography and CT may be performed after EVAR (2).

2. If the size of the aneurysm sac is increasing (more than 5 mm in diameter), suggesting higher pressure, there is a relatively higher long-term risk of rupture. More urgent treatment is required regardless of the type of endoleak.
   a. High-pressure endoleaks (types I and III) are treated immediately.
   b. Low-pressure endoleaks (types II and IV) are considered less urgent.
3. Evaluation by angiography or direct sac puncture is warranted if there is continued growth of the aneurysm sac.
4. Delayed endoleak up to 7 years after EVAR has been reported (2).

Endoleak Treatment

Treatment depends on the type of endoleak. Type I and type III endoleaks are high-pressure endoleaks and usually require some sort of intervention in all cases. Endoleak type II is considered a "low-pressure" endoleak and usually only requires treatment in cases of aneurysm enlargement (9). In cases of a persistent type IV, other endoleak types need to be excluded because in the majority of cases, this type of endoleak is self-limited. Type V endoleak is very rare; therefore, other types of endoleak need to be ruled out first with an additional diagnostic modality and technique.

1. Type I endoleak
   a. Immediate treatment is necessary because of the direct communication with high-pressure systemic arterial blood flow and the risk of aneurysm rupture (2).
   b. These endoleaks are treated with endovascular techniques by securing the attachment site with angioplasty balloons, stents, or stent-graft extensions (2).
   c. Embolization with glue or microcoils is another option that has been reported.
   d. If endovascular approaches are unsuccessful, open surgery remains an option to remove or adjust the stent-graft or in some cases to reinforce the aorta with an external aortic band.

2. Type II endoleak
   a. Selective intervention of type II endoleaks is a safe approach. Most patients with type II endoleaks who are not exhibiting aneurysm sac expansion do well without intervention, as these endoleaks often spontaneously thrombose (2). One study showed approximately 80% of patients with type II endoleaks remained free of sac enlargement greater than 5 mm during a 4-year period and that approximately 75% of type II endoleaks sealed spontaneously within 5 years when observed without intervention (10). Despite the very low rupture risk, type II endoleaks are usually treated in cases of AAA enlargement >5 mm. Feeding vessels can be embolized via transarterial, trans-graft, or trans-lumbar access sites as described below in detail (2).
   b. Transarterial treatment
      (1) Retrograde embolization of feeding arteries
         (a) Possible in the majority of cases, particularly if the feeding vessel is of large caliber, however technically challenging and time consuming.
         (b) Perform an aortogram to identify the vessels supplying and draining the endoleak nidus.
         (c) With a 4-Fr or 5-Fr catheter, engage the major vessel from which the feeding vessel arises. Internal iliac, median sacral, and superior mesenteric artery (SMA) are the most frequent sources.
            i. If the vessel arises from the contralateral internal iliac artery to the side of initial vascular access, it is easier to puncture the ipsilateral groin than to cross the flow divider of the stent-graft.

(d) Insert a coaxial microcatheter and advance as far as possible. Advancement through the nidus of the endoleak and into the draining artery is ideal.

(e) Selectively occlude the feeding and draining arteries and the nidus, if possible.

(f) No embolic agent has been shown to be superior. The most commonly used agents are stainless steel or platinum coils, but cyanoacrylate glue, thrombin, and Onyx (ev3/Covidien/Medtronic, Dublin, Ireland) have also been used.

(f) Following embolization, inflow can shift to another artery and recanalize the endoleak. This may explain a recurrence rate of 36% for type II endoleaks treated with transarterial embolization versus 19% for type II endoleaks treated using a translumbar approach (1).

(2) Transarterial perigraft access to the endoleak

(a) After femoral access, an angle-tipped catheter (e.g., Kumpe or Cobra, Cook Medical, Bloomington, IN) and hydrophilic guidewire (e.g., 0.035-in angled Glidewire, Terumo Medical, Tokyo, Japan) are manipulated under fluoroscopic guidance between the inferior aspect of an iliac limb and an arterial wall.

(b) It is helpful to insert a stiff guidewire and manipulate a sheath with a tapered central stylet into the perigraft space.

(c) The diagnostic catheter is then advanced into the nidus of the endoleak, enabling embolization of feeding and draining arteries, as well as the nidus.

(3) Translumbar approach

(a) Using preprocedural cross-sectional imaging, estimate the location of the endoleak. Determine the most accessible area and assess its position in relation to the stent-graft flow divider.

(b) With the patient in prone position, a fluoroscopically guided puncture of the aneurysm sac is performed with a 21-gauge or 22-gauge needle. The skin puncture site should be at least one handbreadth from the midline.

(c) Once the endoleak sac is accessed, a 6-Fr sheathed needle is inserted using the parallel needle puncture technique. Alternatively, a long micropuncture set can be used.

(d) The needle/sheath combination is advanced just beyond the estimated endoleak site, the needle removed, and the sheath slowly withdrawn until pulsatile blood flows from the sheath.

(e) A left-sided approach is used most commonly; however, if necessary, a transcaval right-sided puncture can be performed.

(f) Angiography is performed through the translumbar sheath or coaxial catheter and pressures are recorded.

(g) Depending on the anatomy of the endoleak sac, position of the puncture, and choice of embolic agent, embolization may be performed directly through the sheath. Alternatively, a coaxial microcatheter may be advanced through the sac into the origins of feeding and draining vessels and selective embolization performed.

(h) Limited data from a 2013 systematic review suggests an overall higher success rate with a lower risk of complications via translumbar embolizations when compared to transarterial approaches (1).

(4) Open or laparoscopic surgical ligation of the inflow and outflow vessels has also been performed.

3. Type III endoleak

a. Like type I endoleaks, these endoleaks are treated immediately at diagnosis because of the direct communication between the high-pressure systemic arterial blood and the aneurysm sac.

    b. A stent-graft extension is typically used to cover the separated modular component or defect within the original graft.
4. Type IV endoleak
    a. These leaks are self-limited and now very rare. They usually self-resolve once the patient's coagulation status is normalized.
5. Type V endoleak
    a. Endotension is very rare and typically treated with open aneurysm repair. Therefore, all diagnostic modalities (CT, MRI, and US) should be performed before a definitive diagnosis of endotension is made (3).

Special Considerations

1. The number of patent aortic branches and amount of thrombus on the aneurysm sac preoperatively correlate with the risk of endoleak development (2).
2. Contrast located in the periphery of the aneurysm sac without contact with the stent may represent a type II endoleak. A tubular configuration abutting the aortic wall also suggests a type II endoleak. If located anteriorly, the most likely vessel is the IMA. If located posterolaterally, the most likely vessel is a lumbar artery.
3. Contrast located centrally around the graft but not peripherally within the aneurysm sac likely represents a type I or III endoleak and must be treated immediately.

R e f e r e n c e s

1. Sidloff DA, Stather PW, Choke E, et al. Type II endoleak after endovascular aneurysm repair. *Br J Surg.* 2013;100(10):1262–1270.
2. Stavropoulos SW, Charagundla SR. Imaging techniques for detection and management of endoleaks after endovascular aortic aneurysm repair. *Radiology.* 2007;243(3):641–655.
3. Veith FJ, Baum RA, Ohki T, et al. Nature and significance of endoleaks and endotension: summary of opinions expressed at an international conference. *J Vasc Surg.* 2002; 35(5):1029–1035.
4. Dooley C, Medani M, O'Hare M, et al. Color duplex ultrasound as suitable alternative for CTA in post EVAR surveillance. *Eur J Vasc Endovasc Surg.* 2018;56(5):e21–e21. doi:10.1016/j. ejvs.2018.06.013
5. Walker TG, Kalva SP, Yeddula K, et al. Clinical practice guidelines for endovascular abdominal aortic aneurysm repair: written by the Standards of Practice Committee for the Society of Interventional Radiology and endorsed by the Cardiovascular and Interventional Radiological Society of Europe and the Canadian Interventional Radiology Association. *J Vasc Interv Radiol.* 2010;21(11):1632–1655. doi:10.1016/j.jvir.2010.07.008
6. Zaiem F, Almasri J, Tello M, et al. A systematic review of surveillance after endovascular aortic repair. *J Vasc Surg.* 2018;67(1):320–331.e37. doi: 10.1016/j.jvs.2017.04.058.
7. Lookstein RA, Goldman J, Pukin L, et al. Time-resolved magnetic resonance angiography as a noninvasive method to characterize endoleaks: initial results compared with conventional angiography. *J Vasc Surg.* 2004;39(1):27–33.
8. Grima MJ, Karthikesalingam A, Holt PJ, EVAR-SCREEN Collaborators. Multicentre Post-EVAR Surveillance Evaluation Study (EVAR-SCREEN). *Eur J Vasc Endovasc Surg.* 2019;57(4):521–526. doi: 10.1016/j.ejvs.2018.10.032. Epub 2019 Feb 6.
9. Chaikof EL, Dalman RL, Eskandri MK, et al. The Society for Vascular Surgery practice guidelines on the care of patients with an abdominal aortic aneurysm. *J Vasc Surg.* 2018;67(1):2–77.e2
10. Silverberg D, Baril DT, Ellozy SH, et al. An 8-year experience with type II endoleaks: natural history suggests selective intervention is a safe approach. *J Vasc Surg.* 2006;44(3):453–459.

19 Visceral Aneurysms

Sebastian Kos, EBIR, FCIRSE and David M. Hovsepian, MD

Introduction

Visceral arterial aneurysms (VAAs) are rare entities, occurring in approximately 2% of the population, based on autopsy series. Most commonly, VAAs are discovered in asymptomatic patients during cross-sectional imaging, suggesting that their prevalence may actually be higher than previously estimated. More importantly, 22% of patients with VAA present with leak or rupture—true emergencies that have a mortality rate of 8.5% (1).

Criteria for intervention are based on whether all three layers of the arterial wall are involved (true aneurysms) or not (pseudoaneurysms). True aneurysms are treated based on their size, location, and symptoms, whereas all pseudoaneurysms require treatment due to significantly higher rates of rupture (~25%) and mortality (~50%) (2).

Etiology (3)

1. Idiopathic
2. Atherosclerosis
3. Hereditary disorders complicated by cystic medial necrosis (e.g., Ehlers–Danlos type IV, Marfan syndrome) or arteriopathy (neurofibromatosis type 1 [NF-1])
4. Segmental arterial mediolysis (SAM)
5. Fibromuscular dysplasia
6. Blunt or penetrating trauma—includes iatrogenic injuries
7. Inflammatory
   a. Proteolytic degradation, for example, pancreatitis
8. Infection
   a. Direct invasion
   b. Septic emboli from intravenous (IV) drug abuse, endocarditis
9. Vasculitis
   a. Polyarteritis nodosa (PAN)
   b. IV amphetamine use
10. Neoplasia

Indications

Calcification of an aneurysm wall does not reduce the risk of rupture.
1. VAAs
   a. Asymptomatic: size >2.0 to 2.5 cm in nonpregnant females of childbearing age or for patients about to undergo liver transplantation. Note: The American College of Cardiology and the American Heart Association guidelines indicate a treatment threshold of 2.0 cm, whereas some authors have suggested a threshold of 2.5 cm (4,5).
   b. Increasing size
   c. Symptomatic (e.g., pain, hemorrhage, renovascular hypertension)
2. Visceral artery pseudoaneurysms
   a. All, including asymptomatic patients, regardless of size

Contraindications

Absolute
None

Relative
1. Contraindications to angiography
   a. Anaphylactoid reactions to iodinated contrast agents (consider carbon dioxide [CO_2] angiography or gadolinium as alternatives)
   b. Uncorrectable coagulopathy
   c. Renal insufficiency
2. Pregnancy
3. Acute or chronic infection in target area
4. Acute hyperthyroidism
5. Thyroid carcinoma and planned radioiodine administration
6. Solitary kidney affected by renal artery aneurysm (RAA)/pseudoaneurysm

Preprocedure Preparation

1. Imaging assessment
   a. Computed tomographic angiography (CTA) or magnetic resonance angiography (MRA) should be obtained to depict the vascular relationships, identify important congenital or postoperative variations, and define the branching anatomy.
   b. Recent laboratory data should include a complete blood count (CBC), platelet count, international normalized ratio (INR), serum creatinine, and estimated glomerular filtration rate (eGFR). For patients on heparin, a partial thromboplastin time (PTT) may be indicated. For suspected vasculitis or inflammatory conditions, a C-reactive protein (CRP) should be obtained.
2. Patient preparation
   a. Obtain informed consent.
   b. Oral intake restrictions according to institutional guidelines (e.g., NPO for 6 to 8 hours for solids, 3 to 4 hours for fat-containing liquids, 1 to 2 hours for water and clear liquids). Typically, oral medications are permitted with sips of water.
   c. Secure IV access.
   d. Periprocedural antibiotic guidelines have not been established.
   e. Attach equipment to monitor vital signs (blood pressure, heart rate, and oxygen saturation).

Procedure

1. Standard sterile skin cleansing and draping.
2. Obtain arterial access. Often a guiding sheath or obturator promotes more stable selective access to the visceral trunks, especially if the origins are acutely angled. Alternative routes of access, such as via the upper extremity, may also provide more favorable orientation in cases of severe downward angulation of the aortic branches.
3. Perform an aortogram if a CTA or MRA has not been obtained or is inadequate or confusing. Some authors advocate the use of IV agents to decrease peristalsis, such as glucagon (1 mg) or hyoscine butylbromide (20 to 40 mg).
4. Select the parent vessel using a 4-Fr or 5-Fr catheter. Useful shapes include the Cobra 2 (Cook Medical Inc, Bloomington, IN) and Sos Omni Selective (AngioDynamics, Latham, NY) catheters. Perform selective angiography.
5. If available, cone-beam computed tomography (CT) can be a helpful tool to better define the three-dimensional anatomy, especially when there are overlapping branches. General guidelines include the following:
   a. 48-cm field-of-view, position isocenter at catheter tip
   b. Inject 3 mL of a 50:50 dilution of contrast and saline for 8 seconds.
   c. Set a 2-second x-ray delay and a rotation rate of 30 degrees per second over the standard 200-degree arc, imaging at 3 degrees per frame.

d. Image reconstruction is performed at a dedicated workstation and should include maximum intensity projections (MIPs) to best plan the approach.

e. Access the branch containing the abnormality. As a rule, if it is less than twice the size of the selective catheter being used, advance a microcatheter coaxially through it to the target. Microcatheter choice is based on the embolic strategy, and care should be taken to size the inner lumen to embolic agent being used. For instance, a 0.028-in inner lumen may allow 0.018-in detachable microcoils to jam and not deploy properly.

f. Options for embolic agents include stainless steel coils, glue, covered and uncovered stents, AMPLATZER Plugs (AGA Medical Corp, Plymouth, MN), or a combination of these.

Embolization Strategies

1. **"Front and back door"** closure involves placement of occlusion devices to block both the arterial inflow and all outflow vessels, trapping the VAA. The outflow is addressed first. Before occluding the inflow, care should be taken to ensure no significant branches are missed because occluding the inflow may render them no longer accessible.

2. **Covered stents** may be deployed across the neck of the VAA, thereby preserving flow to the parent vessel while excluding flow into the aneurysm sac. Thrombosis of the aneurysm should occur without having to embolize the sac itself. The delivery systems for larger devices may be too stiff to track safely to the target area, requiring a different strategy to treat the aneurysm. If the parent artery is small, commercially available stent grafts used for neurologic or cardiovascular applications might be needed.

3. **Coil packing of the aneurysm sac** is a useful strategy for true aneurysms with narrow necks and preserves flow in the parent artery. It is rarely used for pseudoaneurysms because of the risk of perforation or rupture of the sac.

4. **Coil packing through a bare stent** is a good option for true aneurysms that have wide necks. After deployment of a self-expanding stent in the parent vessel, a microcatheter is advanced through the interstices and microcoils are deposited in the aneurysm sac. The stent prevents prolapse of the coils into the parent vessel.

5. **Liquid embolic agents**, such as n-butyl cyanoacrylate (NBCA) glue or Onyx (ethylene vinyl-alcohol copolymer; ev3, Plymouth, MN), generally require greater operator experience than mechanical devices to avoid nontarget embolization but offer some advantages for challenging anatomy. They are often used in conjunction with flow arrest by balloon occlusion or adjunctive deposit of permanent devices.

6. **Thrombin injection** can be performed via catheter or by direct percutaneous injection into the sac of a pseudoaneurysm. For the direct approach, fluoroscopy, ultrasound, or CT can be used to guide advancement of a 22-gauge needle into the sac (6). Placement should be away from the neck of the aneurysm if possible. Confirmation of needle position by injection of contrast during fluoroscopy is ideal. Thrombin injection of 100-unit aliquots (0.1 mL of a 1,000:1 dilution of thrombin in saline) is performed until flow ceases. Color duplex ultrasound of a pseudoaneurysm characteristically reveals a "yin-yang" or "to-and-fro" pattern. Ultrasound easily confirms cessation of flow and decreases the possibility of displacement of thrombus into the parent vessel during contrast injection.

Organ-Specific Comments

1. **Splenic artery aneurysms (SAAs)** are the most common VAA and account for nearly 60% of cases (7). They are four times more common in females. Overall risk of rupture for SAA is 3%.

   a. A 6-Fr renal double curve (RDC) sheath (Destination, Terumo Medical Corporation, Somerset, NJ) is recommended to stabilize access to the celiac trunk when advancing mechanical plugs or other devices into the splenic artery.

b. Most SAAs occur near the splenic hilum. Some degree of splenic infarction can occur following distal embolization. Use of trivalent vaccine remains controversial.

c. Proximal SAA can be treated by stent-graft placement to preserve flow, or by total occlusion with coils. Splenic infarcts are less likely in this setting but can still occur.

2. **Hepatic artery aneurysms (HAAs)** comprise 20% of all VAAs (6). The male-to-female ratio is 2:1. Eighty percent occur in an extrahepatic location.

a. Anatomic variation is common. For example, "replaced" right hepatic arteries from the superior mesenteric artery (SMA) are present in up to 15% of the population and "replaced" left hepatic arteries from the left gastric artery in up to 10%.

b. Intrahepatic rupture may result in hemobilia, whereas extrahepatic rupture may lead to rapid onset of shock and possible exsanguination.

c. The dual blood supply to the liver allows occlusion of hepatic artery branches with minimal risk of organ ischemia. However, portal venous patency should be confirmed prior to arterial embolization.

d. Solitary HAA and hepatic artery pseudoaneurysms can be targeted individually. When multiple (e.g., traumatic), "field" embolization with gelatin sponge slurry is the most effective way to quickly and safely resolve hemorrhage.

3. **RAAs** (7) may cause hypertension or painless hematuria. The male-to-female ratio is 2:3. Most (60%) occur at the main renal artery division. Aneurysms in patients with NF-1 most commonly involve the renal arteries.

a. Renal arteries are "end arteries," and embolization often results in downstream ischemia or infarction. However, this lack of collateralization can be advantageous when the aneurysm is peripherally located, by allowing safer use of liquid embolic agents, including ethanol.

b. When accessing from a femoral approach, a 6-Fr guiding sheath or catheter that has an RDC-type shape is well suited to the angles involved.

c. Frequent variation in renal orientation requires careful technique to obtain an optimal view (true coronal) of the arterial vasculature. Cone-beam CT and/or additional orthogonal views can improve the delineation of anatomic relationships.

d. If RAA or pseudoaneurysm occurs in the setting of angiomyolipoma or other tumor, it should be occluded prior to embolizing the tumor with particulate agents.

4. **Mesenteric artery aneurysms** account for 6% of all VAAs (6,8). They frequently involve the gastroduodenal artery (GDA) or pancreaticoduodenal arcade due to erosion from pancreatitis or a duodenal ulcer. They can occur in any visceral territory in the setting of SAM.

a. For aneurysms occurring in the GDA or its branches, patency of the celiac axis and SMA should be confirmed before embolization. If no stenosis is present in those collaterals, the GDA can be safely occluded.

Postprocedure Management

1. Standard postangiogram observation and management
2. Analgesics as needed
3. For symptoms of postembolization syndrome, antipyretics and antiemetics (e.g., ondansetron) can be added.
4. CTA or MRA within 1 month to assess aneurysm sac and distal organ perfusion, looking for signs of ischemia or infarction

Results

1. No large prospective or comparative series exist—technical success for transcatheter treatment is greater than 90% (7).
2. Overall mortality from ruptured SAA is 10% to 25%. When rupture occurs during pregnancy, there is a 70% risk of maternal death and a 90% risk of fetal demise (9).

Complications and Their Management

1. Angiographic (overall <3%)
2. Embolization related
   a. End-organ ischemia or infarction
      (1) Consider pain management consultation if pain is severe
   b. Abscess formation (overall a rare occurrence, most common after splenic embolization)
      (1) IV and/or oral antibiotic therapy, rarely percutaneous drainage is needed (large abscesses)
   c. Nontarget embolization
      (1) Follow-up cross-sectional imaging (CTA, MRA) if suspected; management in accordance with clinical and imaging findings
   d. Postembolization syndrome (10)
      (1) Fever, malaise, nausea and vomiting, leukocytosis, typically 1 to 3 days postprocedure, self-limited to several days
      (2) IV analgesics, antiemetics, and pain control, as needed; continued observation

R e f e r e n c e s

1. Huang YK, Hsieh HC, Tsai FC, et al. Visceral artery aneurysm: risk factor analysis and therapeutic opinion. *Eur J Vasc Endovasc Surg.* 2007;33(3):293–301.
2. Lookstein RA, Guller J. Embolization of complex vascular lesions. *Mt Sinai J Med.* 2004; 71(1):17–28.
3. Kos S, Liu DM, Jacob AI. Mesenteric aneurysms. In: Geschwind JH, Dake MD, eds. *Abrams' Angiography.* 3rd ed. Lippincott Williams & Wilkins; 2014:712–723
4. Hirsch AT, Haskal ZJ, Hertzer NR, et al. ACC/AHA 2005 guidelines for the management of patients with peripheral arterial disease (lower extremity, renal, mesenteric, and abdominal aortic). *J Am Coll Cardiol.* 2006;47:1239–1312.
5. Sousa J, Costa D, Mansilha A. Visceral artery aneurysms: review on indications and current treatment strategies. *Int Angiol.* 2019;38(5):381–394.
6. Laganà D, Carrafiello G, Mangini M, et al. Multimodal approach to endovascular treatment of visceral artery aneurysms and pseudoaneurysms. *Eur J Radiol.* 2006;59(1):104–111.
7. Vallina-Victorero Vazquez MJ, Vaquero Lorenzo F, Salgado AA, et al. Endovascular treatment of splenic and renal aneurysms. *Ann Vasc Surg.* 2009;23(2):258.e13–258.e17.
8. Nosher JL, Chung J, Brevetti LS, et al. Visceral and renal artery aneurysms: a pictorial essay on endovascular therapy. *Radiographics.* 2006;26(6):1687–1704.
9. Sadat U, Dar O, Walsh S, et al. Splenic artery aneurysms in pregnancy—a systematic review. *Int J Surg.* 2008;6(3):261–265.
10. Barrionuevo P, Malas MB, Nejim B, et al. A systematic review and meta-analysis of the management of visceral artery aneurysms. *J Vasc Surg.* 2019;70(5):1694–1699.

20 The Management of Extracranial Vascular Malformations

Gilles Soulez, MD, MSc, FRCPC, FSIR, Patrick Gilbert, MD, Marie France Giroux, MD, and Josée Dubois, MD, MSc, FRCPC

Introduction

According to the 2018 classification of the International Society for the Study of Vascular Anomalies (ISSVA), vascular anomalies can be classified as (1) vascular tumors that can be divided into benign (infantile and congenital hemangiomas being the most frequent), borderline and malignant and (2) nonproliferative vascular malformations, which can be further subclassified based on vascular channel(s) involved (1).

We will focus in this chapter on the interventional management of vascular malformations. These vascular malformations used to be subdivided into simple malformations based on the type of vessel(s) involved (capillary, venous, and lymphatic) with the exception of arteriovenous malformations (AVMs) which are high-flow malformations containing arteries and veins with arteriovenous shunting. Venous, lymphatic, and capillary malformations (CMs) are low-flow malformations, therefore less at risk of spontaneous bleeding.

Combined vascular malformations involve more than one vessel, typically CM with AVM, venous malformation (VM) or lymphatic malformation (LM) or the combination of VM and LM (1). Finally, these malformations can be associated with nonvascular anomalies in specific syndromes. These syndromes will typically combine vascular malformations with overgrowth of soft tissue and/or bone, the most frequent being the Klippel–Trenaunay syndrome combining a CM, VM ± LM with a limb overgrowth and the Parkes–Weber syndrome combining a CM, AVM, and limb overgrowth.

Significant advances have been made in discovering intracellular signaling pathways often activated by germinal and/or somatic mutations, causing endothelial cell dysfunction. Two major intracellular signaling pathways (RAS/MAPK and PI3K/AKT/mTOR) were identified that may be controlled by inhibitors developed for cancer treatment. This opens the door to potential pharmacologic targeting treatments that can be combined with interventional treatment to improve patient outcome (2).

Vascular malformation patients should be evaluated by a multidisciplinary team involving interventional radiologists, plastic and ENT surgeons, dermatologists, geneticists, and internal medicine specialists.

The goal of interventional treatment is to combine the occlusion of the vascular malformation and the destruction of the endothelial lining to prevent recanalization and recurrence. This often requires the injection of a sclerosing agent. For high-flow malformations such as AVMs, sclerosis is often combined with occlusive agents. Usually, interventional treatment is the first-line of therapy. Surgery can additionally be performed for localized lesions with incomplete response after intervention. Systemic drug therapy is currently reserved for patients with severe forms or failure of interventional treatment. It can be also associated with interventional treatment or surgery in severe presentations to decrease vascular neoangiogenesis and increase therapeutic response (3).

High-Flow Malformation: AVM

Indications

Embolization is now the first line of treatment of AVM. It can be combined with surgery for localized forms (4). The Schobinger classification is useful to evaluate in a standardized fashion the clinical impact of AVMs. In this classification, four stages are described (Table 20.1). Stage I is quiescent and no treatment is warranted. Depending

Table 20.1	Clinical Classification of Schobinger
Stage I	Quiescence: May or may not have vascular skin stain, warmth of the affected tissues, and arteriovenous shunts can be detected by Doppler US. The arteriovenous malformation is present but causes no clinical symptoms
Stage II	Expansion of arteriovenous malformation lesion: Stage I plus enlargement, pulsations, palpable thrill, audible bruit and enlarged arterialized tortuous/tense veins
Stage III	Destructive tissue changes: Stage II plus dystrophic skin changes, skin ulcerations that can be nonhealing, bleeding from ulcerated skin or mucosal surfaces, overt tissue necrosis, and lytic lesions of bone may occur
Stage IV	Decompensation: Stage III plus congestive cardiac failure with increased cardiac output, abnormally lowered peripheral vascular resistance, and venous hypertension secondary tissue and skin changes

Reprinted with permission from Soulez G, Gilbert Md Frcpc P, Giroux Md Frcpc MF, Racicot Md Frcpc JN, Dubois J. Interventional management of arteriovenous malformations. *Tech Vasc Interv Radiol.* 2019;22(4):100633.

on symptomatology and after weighing risks and benefits, treatment could start at stage II (evidence of progression) especially if the angioarchitecture is favorable for embolization. Treatment is definitely indicated for Schobinger stages III (bleeding, ulceration) and IV (cardiac failure). Typically, the symptoms requiring intervention are:

1. Evidence of progression
2. Bleeding
3. Ulceration
4. Pain
5. Cardiac failure
6. Aesthetic concern

For severe lesions, genetic testing to search for a germinal or somatic mutation affecting the RAS/MAPK pathway is recommended. To detect somatic mutation, a biopsy of the affected area should be performed. These forms can benefit from a combined systemic therapy using embolization with an antiangiogenic drug such as thalidomide or trametinib (3).

Contraindications

Absolute
1. Lesion that cannot be accessed and embolized safely by endovascular (arterial or venous) or percutaneous route.

Relative
1. Minimal likelihood of clinical improvement. It is important to weigh potential clinical benefits versus the risk of complications
2. Pregnancy
3. Severe anaphylactic reaction to iodinated contrast
4. Acute renal failure
5. Uncorrectable coagulopathy
6. Infection within the target vasculature

Preprocedure Imaging and Preparation

Preprocedural Imaging
1. Doppler ultrasound is the first examination to perform. It will confirm a high-flow malformation with evidence of arteriovenous fistula(e) (high diastolic flow on the arterial side and arterialization of the flow on the venous side).

2. MRA is usually performed to evaluate extension of the malformation into soft tissues with T1- and T2-weighted sequences showing flow voids. MR angiography with a time-resolved sequence is necessary to evaluate the flow pattern followed by a high-resolution steady-state acquisition to evaluate the angioarchitecture.

3. CTA can also be performed and is particularly useful if there is a bone involvement (5).

4. DSA is the best examination to evaluate the angioarchitecture; it is usually performed in the same session as the embolization.

Preprocedural Preparation

1. Communication with the patient's primary physician is essential, and formal consultations with appropriate specialists within the multidisciplinary group may be required depending on the type and complexity of the malformation.

2. Routine preprocedural laboratory studies should include complete blood count (CBC), electrolytes, creatinine, and coagulation studies. Goals for preoperative testing include an international normalized ratio (INR) <1.5 and platelet count >50,000 per µL.

3. In preparation for sedation or general anesthesia, patients are made nil per os (NPO) for 8 hours or according to hospital guidelines. The authors perform almost all AVM embolization procedures under general anesthesia for patient comfort, close physiologic monitoring, and control of respiration and movement during angiography. General anesthesia is mandatory if ethanol is used as it is extremely painful. Alternatively spinal anesthesia or peripheral nerve block can be used.

4. A preprocedural dose of antibiotics (typically cefazoline) will be used if there is a direct puncture through a contaminated area (oral cavity). Steroids (dexamethasone) to decrease postintervention edema can be administered.

Procedure

Embolization can be performed through an arterial or venous endovascular approach or direct puncture of the nidus. In most cases these approaches will be combined in a single or several embolization sessions. The anatomical classification based on the angioarchitecture is important to select the best approach. Two classifications have been proposed, the Cho classification and the Yakes classification (Fig. 20.1). An algorithm is provided (Fig. 20.2) to guide the reader on the approach based on the Yakes classification.

General Principles of AVM Embolization

1. Always do a comprehensive DSA evaluation with supra selective injection to delineate the main feeders and draining veins, then classify the malformation to confirm your final approach.

2. The goal is to occlude the nidus and if possible, the draining veins.

3. Never do a proximal embolization without occluding the nidus as this will promote recruitment of side branches and worsen patient condition.

4. Liquid agents (Ethanol, Onyx, Glue) are preferred to ensure penetration of the nidus and the draining vein(s). Coils or plugs can be used only (A) on the venous side or (B) on the arterial side for Yakes type I AVMs (direct arteriovenous fistulae).

5. Use pneumatic cuffs and tourniquets to control the flow if needed. Tourniquets can also be used to protect distal vascularization (fingers, toes) for upper or lower limb AVMs. Use negative roadmap technique to evaluate the progression of the embolic agent and prevent proximal reflux or distal migration.

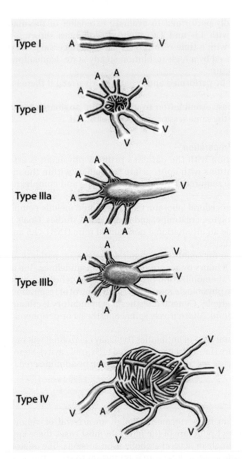

FIGURE 20.1 • Angiographic classification according to Yakes et al. (6) Type I: Direct AV fistula; Type II: Typical AVM nidus with multiple inflow arteries leading to nidus and vein outflow; Type IIIa: Multiple in-flow arterioles shunting into an aneurysmal vein that has a single-vein out-flow. Fistulae are in the vein wall; Type IIIb: Aneurysmal vein with multiple out-flow veins. The fistulae (nidus) are in the vein wall; Type IV: Multiple arteries/arterioles forming innumerable microfistulae that diffusely infiltrate the affected tissue. The innumerable micro-AVF drains into multiple veins. (Reprinted with permission from Yakes W, Baumgartner I. Interventional treatment of arteriovenous malformations. *Gefasschirurgie*. 2014;19(04):325–30.)

6. After completion of your session, image the entire malformation with contrast to identify residual feeders and draining veins. This will help plan the next session, if needed.
7. Stage the sessions to minimize complications.

Arterial Endovascular Approach
1. It is typically used for type I, II, IIIb Yakes AVMs. It is usually the first step to decrease the arterial inflow before proceeding to direct puncture or venous approach.

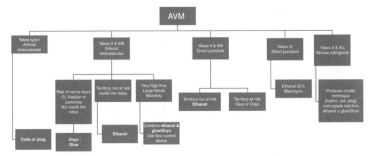

FIGURE 20.2 • Treatment algorithm for AVM based on the Yakes classification.

2. A femoral approach is preferred, with the exception of very distal upper extremity AVMs, which sometimes cannot be reached because of catheter length constraints with very tortuous vessels. Following a comprehensive DSA examination, we usually first target the largest feeder. We use a triaxial approach with a 5-Fr guiding sheath, a 4-Fr glide catheter, and a highly steerable microcatheter. Neurointerventional microcatheters and guidewires are often preferred to reach the nidus as feeding arteries are usually very tortuous.

3. The guiding sheath, which is 1Fr oversized, allows performance of proximal contrast injection if needed during the embolization.

4. Inject close or inside the nidus. Do not inject ethanol if you see normal branches.

5. Flow can be controlled using a pneumatic cuff or a balloon catheter on the arterial or venous side if needed. Pay attention when deflating the cuff or balloon to not allow fast release of ethanol or migration of glue or Onyx.

6. Always obtain a DSA acquisition after each embolization to evaluate carefully flow change, appearance of normal branches, and eventual nontarget embolization. This should be repeated immediately before embolization if there was significant delay since the previous acquisition as hemodynamics might have seriously changed, especially when using ethanol.

Nidus Direct Puncture

1. It is indicated for Yakes type II, IIIb, and IV.

2. Direct puncture is always performed after completing a comprehensive DSA examination to localize the nidus.

3. If the lesion is accessible by ultrasound, direct puncture is targeted using color Doppler ultrasound (CDUS) to detect an aliasing area which is the area of AV fistulization. If not accessible, the use of cone-beam CT with needle guidance software can be useful.

4. We usually use a 22- or 21-gauge needle connected to a flexible tubing. Once you get blood return in your tubing, carefully inject contrast to opacify the nidus and draining veins under DSA.

5. For Yakes type IV AVM with multiple small AV fistulae intravascular injection of ethanol diluted at 50% is recommended. Interstitial injection of bleomycin has also been proposed.

6. For upper- or lower-limb AVM embolization, the use of pneumatic cuffs or tourniquets can be helpful to reflux into the nidus as the puncture is commonly on the venular aspect of the nidus.

Retrograde Venous Approach

1. It is indicated for Yakes type II and IIIa.

2. The vein can be approached endovascularly following selective retrograde catheterization of the draining vein or by direct puncture using a coaxial needle or a micropuncture set.

3. The main draining vein is usually occluded with coils or plugs. It is also possible to occlude the nidus using a retrograde venous approach using the pressure cooker technique. The latter consists of occluding the vein with a microcatheter positioned alongside the plug or coil mass close to the nidus to reflux sclerosant and/ or a liquid embolic into the nidus (Fig. 20.3).

4. Reflux of a sclerosing agent can also be done using an occlusion balloon. However, this approach carries the risk of fast ethanol release or glue/onyx migration when deflating the balloon.

How to Choose and Manipulate the Embolic Agent

Coils and Plugs

1. Usually used for venous retrograde approach, they are often used in combination with a sclerosant and/or a liquid agent.

2. Coils can also be injected in venous cavities accessed by direct puncture. It is particularly important to slightly oversize more than described on the instructions for use, because the pressure on the venous side is high from the arteriovenous fistulae, and the draining vein(s) can expand during its closure and/or Valsalva maneuvers.

3. Complete closure of the vein should be obtained at the end of the procedure to prevent material migration. It is recommended to use detachable coils for the first and last coils. In between, pushable coils can be used to continue packing the coils if deemed safe.

4. On the venous side, 0.035" coils can be used for large-diameter veins. When using a plug, it is recommended to detach the plug only when the flow is completely occluded.

5. On the arterial side, coils or plugs are only recommended for Yakes type I AVMs (which are essentially AVFs), using the usual oversizing.

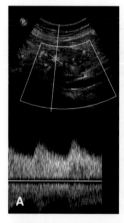
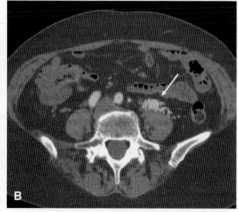

FIGURE 20.3 • A 72-year-old woman with hematuria due to a retroperitoneal AVM in front of the psoas muscle. **A:** Doppler ultrasound showing multiple vascular channels with a high flow and high diastolic component indicating the presence of AV shunting. **B, C:** CT angiography in the arterial phase showing the AVM draining in the left ovarian vein (*white arrows*). (*continued*)

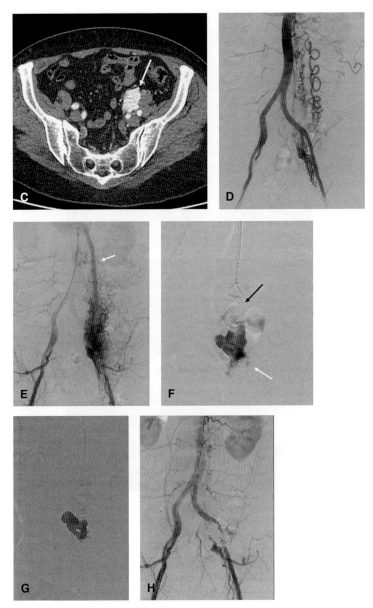

FIGURE 20.3 • (*Continued*) **D, E:** Aortography showing multiple arterial feeders coming from the ureteral, ovarian, inferior mesenteric and internal iliac arteries with single drainage through the left ovarian vein (*white arrow*). **F, G:** Transvenous approach through the left ovarian vein. Pressure cook technique with deployment of an amplatzer plug (*black arrow*) close to the nidus and injection of ethanol to promote sclerosis of the nidus followed by glue injection to occlude the nidus. The injection is performed through a microcatheter positioned distal to the plug with careful injection into the venous side of the nidus (*white arrow*). **H:** Control DSA showing complete closure of the AVM. (*continued*)

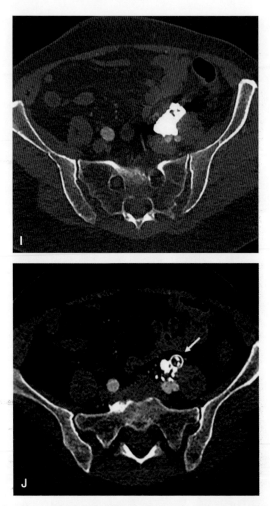

FIGURE 20.3 • (*Continued*) **I, J:** Control CT angiography confirming cure of the AVM with glue filling the AVM and occlusion of the left ovarian vein and around the Amplatzer (*white arrow*).

Ethanol

1. It is the most efficient agent as it will penetrate and destroy the endothelial lining in the nidus. However, there is higher risk of skin necrosis and nerve injury.
2. It should never be injected if there are normal vessels downstream and/or in the vicinity of nerve, bowel or bladder.
3. Monitor pulmonary arterial pressure if you plan injecting more than 20 mL of ethanol. Since ethanol is not radiopaque, evaluate the volume and speed of injection based on an immediately prior DSA injection as well as by the aspect of the contrast column inside the catheter while it is being pushed by the ethanol bolus under negative roadmap fluoroscopy.

4. Never inject more than 5 mL at once, wait 5 minutes between each injection. Do not inject more than 0.5 mL/kg per session.
5. Ethanol diluted at 50% with contrast can be injected in Yakes type IV AVMs with numerous small AV fistulae.
6. Stop injecting ethanol if the pulmonary systolic arterial pressure increases by more than 50% of baseline values. Inject pulmonary vasodilator until return to values close to baseline before resuming injection if necessary.
7. When using flow control devices (balloon, tourniquet, pneumatic cuff), release the occlusion slowly to prevent bolus release of ethanol particularly when using a venous approach.

Cyanoacrylate

1. Adhesive (glue) rapidly polymerizes on contact with any ionic medium and is usually mixed with ethiodol (Lipiodol, Guerbet, Paris). The oil is used to slow glue polymerization time, increase its viscosity, and provide radiopacity.
2. Glue requires experience to find the right dilution and minimize the risk of non-target embolization, catheter gluing, or venous migration. Usually, a ratio ranging between 1:1 and 1:4 is used depending on flow velocity, size of fistulae and draining veins.
3. Glue should be injected through a microcatheter following generous flushing with dextrose 5% water (D5%). It can be injected either as a series of small aliquots (0.2 to 0.8 mL) pushed by D5% in a small vessel nidus or as a "continuous column" when dealing with larger vessels or faster flow.
4. Flow control using balloon catheters on the arterial or venous side is sometimes employed if the flow is too fast, but in most situations, it is preferable to use forward blood flow to carry the agent deep into the nidus.
5. Glue can also be injected by direct puncture or through a venous retrograde approach combined with mechanical vein occlusion using coils and/or plugs as mentioned above (Fig. 20.3).

Ethylene Vinyl Alcohol Copolymer

1. This a nonadhesive polymer that is used in combination with the solvent dimethyl sulfoxide (DMSO). Three products are available on the market (Onyx, ev3, Plymouth, MN; Squid, Emboflu, Switzerland; Phil, Microvention, USA).
2. The agents should be injected through DMSO compatible microcatheters.
3. For AVMs, to have a better nidus penetration, lower or intermediate viscosity formulations are HAVfl (OIIyX 18, Squid 12 or 10, Phil 25 == 20%)
4. Formulations with lower radio opacity are also available; they induce less CT artifacts. The radiopaque component of Onyx and Squid is a tantalum powder which is permanent and can induce skin tattooing whereas Phil uses a chemically bound iodine contrast which leads to less artifacts on CT.
5. Onyx, Squid and Phil have primarily been used in neurointerventions where their safety profiles have been well established. They are used increasingly for peripheral AVMs. Each of these products is injected slowly and continuously forming a lava-like cast of the vessels over a period of minutes.
6. Onyx, Squid, or Phil deposition does not rely on forward flow, which glue does. Therefore, they must be injected directly or close to the nidus.
7. Onyx or Squid can be injected using the plug and push technique to be sure they will progress into the nidus. If there is reflux, wait up to 2 minutes before resuming the injection to form a plug at the tip of the catheter.
8. If necessary, a balloon microcatheter can be used to push the agent more distally. Coils can also be deployed on the venous side to prevent central migration.
9. Avoid Onyx and Squid in superficial lesions close to the skin especially in the face as they can permanently stain the skin.

10. Advantages of Onyx, Squid, Phil include little risk for catheter gluing/fracture, ability to conform to tortuous vessels, and ease of injection control.
11. Disadvantages include ischemic complications if the cast reaches very small vessels and the fact that the marked radiopacity of the agent can obscure anatomic details in subsequent embolization procedures and scans.
12. In addition, Onyx and Squid embolization can be quite time consuming and costly, especially because multiple vials are usually required. Phil embolization seems to be faster.

Combining Ethanol with Glue or Onyx

Glue or Onyx has no or minimal sclerosant effect, thus leading to potential recanalization. On the other hand ethanol alone without mechanical occlusion can also lead to recanalization especially in the presence of large fistulae. The authors often start with ethanol injection into the nidus to promote endothelial ablation in the nidus and draining vein(s) followed by completion with glue or Onyx, Squid to prevent recanalization.

Anatomic Consideration

Pulmonary AVM

Pulmonary AVMs are a distinct type of lesion and are discussed in Chapter 16.

Head and Neck

1. If the AVM involves recruitment of intracranial arteries or involves branches at risk of intracranial anastomoses (internal maxillary, meningeal, temporal, occipital, and facial arteries), working jointly with a neurointerventionalist is recommended.
2. Ethanol should be used cautiously and injected only inside the nidus; avoid it in the vicinity of the facial nerve or in areas at risk of anastomoses with the intracranial vessels and/or the ophthalmic artery.
3. Onyx should be avoided for superficial skin lesions due to the risk of tattooing.

Renal AVM

Type I Yakes AVF can be treated with coils or plugs. For other Yakes classifications, the algorithm presented in Figure 20.2 is valid. In complex AVMs, a dual arterial and venous approach is often necessary.

GI Tract and Pancreas

1. These lesions are more at risk of bleeding, bowel necrosis, or portal thrombosis.
2. High-flow lesions can induce portal hypertension.
3. Ethanol should be avoided. Superselective injection of glue and/or Onyx from an arterial approach is the preferred approach.
4. A staged approach is recommended to minimize the risk of bowel necrosis and portal thrombosis.
5. If reflux in the portal system can be prevented (pressure cooker technique), a venous transportal approach can be performed. In case of failure, surgery with preoperative embolization should be contemplated.

Pelvic AVM

1. The pelvis is a relatively common site for high-flow AVMs. The most common pattern is a multivessel supply from the internal iliac artery, inferior mesenteric artery (IMA), middle sacral, and common femoral branches with drainage into the internal iliac or gonadal veins.
2. If possible, the venous approach should be used, especially if there are numerous feeders with risks of colorectal and/or bladder necrosis.

3. When a single draining vein (Yakes type IIIa) is present, patient cure is usually obtained. In Yakes type II, a first step arterial embolization of the larger feeders can be done before closing the veins.
4. Absolute ethanol should not be used if there is a risk of reflux in vesical or inferior mesenteric arteries.

Uterine AVM

1. AVMs confined to the uterus generally present with menorrhagia and are almost always preceded by an obstetric event (postpartum, postabortion, dilation and curettage, or the presence of trophoblastic disease).
2. There is some controversy whether these are congenital or acquired lesions. In the context of postpartum bleeding, the presence of retained products of conception should first be eliminated.
3. The lesions are fed by one or both uterine arteries and are often amenable to embolization. Lesions are best treated with liquid casting agents.
4. Not only can hysterectomy be avoided, but successful pregnancies have been reported in several patients following embolization.

Extremities AVM

1. These AVMs are usually complex with often Yakes type II, IIIb, or IV classification. Preservation of the distal circulation to prevent amputation is important, especially for AVMs involving the hand or foot.
2. The use of distal tourniquets is recommended to protect fingers or toes from non-target embolization.
3. If an endovascular approach is taken, it is important to inject inside the nidus. Direct punctures are often necessary whereas the venous approach is often limited by the presence of multiple draining veins. The use of pneumatic cuffs is useful to improve the reflux in the nidus if a direct puncture and/or venous approach is privileged.
4. For stage IV AVMs, interstitial injection of bleomycin or endovascular injection of diluted ethanol (50%) or bleomycin has been proposed.
5. Stepwise approach is recommended to decrease the risk of complications.

Postprocedure Management

1. Most patients can be treated on an ambulatory basis with a 6-hour postoperative surveillance. An overnight hospitalization is preferred if there is a risk of airway compromise (AVM involving the oropharyngeal area), an AVM with risk of nerve compression (orbit, forearm, hand), embolization involving the digestive tract or an AVM actively bleeding or at high risk of bleeding
2. Usually, intravenous steroids are administered during the general anesthesia. Postoperative edema can be controlled by NSAIDs. Steroids can be continued for 24 to 48 hours for patients at risk of airway or nerve compression.
3. Pain control often requires parenteral morphine or a morphine analog.
4. If there is no medical contraindication, aggressive intravenous hydration should be prescribed if a significant amount of ethanol (more than 20 mL) was injected. In this setting, urine output should be monitored.

Results

1. The rate of partial or complete response ranges between 68% and 90% (5).
2. Better results are observed with ethanol but at the cost of higher complications.
3. Yakes type IIIa has a higher chance of cure if the draining vein is completely occluded.
4. Embolization followed by complete surgical resection could provide better results and less recurrences (4).
5. Recurrence is always possible therefore, AVM patients need lifelong surveillance.

Patient Follow-Up

Usually, patients are followed at the IR clinic 4 to 6 weeks after each embolization procedure with a clinical and color Doppler ultrasound evaluation. If a residual AVM and/or symptoms are present, another session will be scheduled. In large AVMs requiring multiple sessions, further embolizations will be scheduled systematically 4 to 8 weeks after the first session.

Complications

1. The range of major complications is estimated at 0% to 20% and minor complications range between 6% and 45% (5).
2. Ethanol seems to be more at risk to induce blisters/skin necrosis (15.5%) and transient nerve injury (4.8%) (5).
3. Hemoglobinuria is frequently observed when large volume of ethanol is injected.
4. Cardiac arrest secondary to acute pulmonary hypertension has been reported with ethanol use. It is prevented by rigorously following a protocol of a maximal bolus volume (5 mL), timing between injections (5 to 10 minutes), slow release of temporary occlusion (with balloon, cuff, or tourniquet) and monitoring of pulmonary arterial pressure when large volumes are injected.
5. Nerve injury will recover with time in most cases but can be permanent.
6. Stroke, muscular, gastrointestinal (GI), and bladder necrosis have also been reported.
7. Glue extrusion in superficial AVMs.
8. The arterial endovascular approach carries a higher risk of complications if the injection is proximal to the nidus and involves normal arterial branches, especially when using ethanol.

Management of Complications

1. Skin necrosis and glue extrusion are usually managed conservatively with wound therapy. Sometimes, skin necrosis may require a flap surgery.
2. In case of nerve injury or airway compression, high-dose steroids can improve the recovery.
3. In case of acute pulmonary hypertension, intravenous injection of milrinone, which is a pulmonary vasodilator decreases the pulmonary arterial pressure.
4. In case of hemoglobinuria, hydration is recommended to decrease the risk of acute tubular necrosis.

Low-Flow Malformations: Venous (VMs) and Lymphatic Malformations (LMs)

Introduction

Usually these lesions are less aggressive compared to AVMs but can cause significant symptoms, impairing the quality of life of patients. Mixed VMs and LMs are quite frequent. Both VMs and LMs can be associated with PIK3CA-related overgrowth spectrum (PROS) syndromes. If they are large and compress vital structures, they can be life threatening. If totally asymptomatic, these lesions should be managed conservatively (compressive stocking for VM involving extremities if minor symptoms) and followed.

For severe lesions, genetic testing with a biopsy to search for a germinal and/or somatic mutation in the PIK3CA mTOR pathway is recommended. Combination of systemic therapy using sirolimus (mTOR inhibitor) or alpelisib (PIK3CA inhibitor) can be given (3). Close collaboration with the hemato-oncology or immunology team is recommended.

Indications
Venous Malformation
1. Bleeding is rare in VMs but can occur especially when involving the oral cavity or the GI tract
2. Ulceration can be observed especially in large VMs of the lower limb with venous insufficiency, observed in the context of the Klippel–Trenaunay syndrome
3. Compression of a vital structure or nerve (airway, orbit, forearm)
4. Recurrent phlebitis
5. Localized intravascular coagulation (LIC), which can result in a pre-DIC state, due to recurrent thrombosis-dethrombosis in a large VM, leading to coagulation factor depletion
6. For lower extremity VMs pain and discomfort especially during exercise or standing for long periods
7. Swelling
8. Aesthetic concern

Lymphatic Malformation
1. Lymphatic leakage
2. Recurrent lymphangitis
3. Compression of a vital structure or nerve (airway, orbit)
4. Pain and discomfort
5. Aesthetic concern

Preprocedure Preparation and Imaging

Preprocedural Imaging
1. Doppler ultrasound is the first examination to perform. In VMs a low-flow malformation with compressible vascular lakes and no or minimal flow on Duplex is seen. For LMs, it will demonstrate noncompressible cystic cavities with septa. The latter may contain normal arterial or venous flow. Macrocystic LMs have single or multiple cysts of more than $1~cm^3$. Microcystic LMs usually are more infiltrative and are seen as hyperechoic soft tissue infiltration whereas mixed macro- and microcystic LMs will display both features.
2. MRI is usually performed to evaluate the extension of the malformation in the soft tissue with T1- and T2-weighted sequences followed by T1-weighted fat-saturation postcontrast acquisitions (Fig. 20.4).
3. CT is usually less sensitive and MRI, if possible, is preferred. It will show phleboliths for VMs and the cystic component(s) for macrocystic LMs.
4. DSA does not contribute useful information and should not be performed unless the diagnosis of vascular tumor cannot be excluded.

Preoperative Preparation

1. Communication with the patient's primary physician is essential, and formal consultations with appropriate specialists within the multidisciplinary group may be required depending on the type and complexity of the malformation.
2. Routine preprocedural laboratory studies should include CBC, electrolytes, creatinine, and coagulation studies. Goals for preoperative testing include an INR <2.0 and platelet count >50,000 per µL. For large VMs, routine D-dimer and fibrinogen levels are necessary to exclude local intravascular coagulopathy (LIC).
3. Usually, embolization/sclerotherapy procedures are performed under conscious sedation. For VMs or LMs involving the pharynx, posterior portion of the tongue/nasopharynx or the orbit, general anesthesia is recommended. For malformations

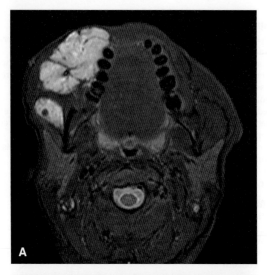

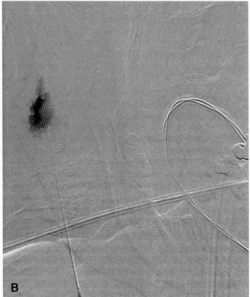

FIGURE 20.4 • A 41-year-old woman with a large venous malformation of the right masticator space and cheek causing significant swelling, pain, and interfering with mastication. **A:** MR STIR acquisition showing two components of the venous malformation (hyperintense) and the presence of phlebolitis (*low signal intensity foci*). **B:** US-guided puncture and percutaneous phlebography confirming a cavitary venous malformation. (*continued*)

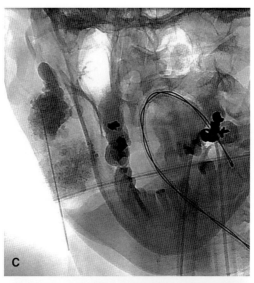

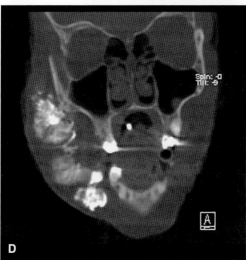

FIGURE 20.4 • (*Continued*) **C:** Single shot acquisition after sclerosis of the malformation with STS foam mixed with lipiodol showing good diffusion of the foam. **D:** Cone-beam CT acquisition showing thorough treatment of the lesion. (*continued*)

involving the hand or foot, locoregional anesthesia or peripheral nerve block can be helpful. In preparation for sedation or general anesthesia, patients are made NPO for 8 hours or according to hospital guidelines.

4. A preprocedural dose of antibiotics (typically cefazolin) is given if there is a direct puncture through a contaminated area (oral cavity). NSAIDs to decrease postintervention edema are also administered. Steroids (dexamethasone) can be considered as well.

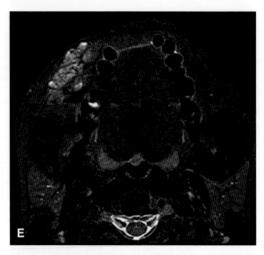

FIGURE 20.4 • (*Continued*) **E:** Control MRI after three sclerotherapy sessions showing significant shrinkage of the malformation. The patient is now asymptomatic.

5. If LIC occurs, preventive treatment with LMWH or oral direct factor Xa inhibitor is required 2 weeks before the procedure (7). Consultation with hematology is recommended as well.

Procedure

Venous Malformation
1. If the lesion is visible on ultrasound, ultrasound-guided puncture is performed using a 21- or 22-gauge needle (Fig. 20.4). If not visible, CBCT with needle guidance can be used (Fig. 20.4). Preliminary image fusion between CBCT and MRI can be useful as well.
2. For VMs involving the posterior oral cavity or the GI tract, combined endoscopic and fluoroscopic guidance can be performed with the ENT or gastroenterology team.
3. Once blood return is obtained, a percutaneous phlebogram is obtained to evaluate the size of the VM and its venous drainage.
4. Central venous drainage can be prevented using local compression with forceps or with a tourniquet. Coil or plug embolization may be required if the risk of deep venous phlebitis is significant.
5. Some authors recommend a vent technique with insertion of a second needle to drain the blood until the foam completely fills the VM.
6. Different sclerosing agents used are detailed below. The authors routinely use sodium sotradecyl sulfate (STS) (Thromboject, Angiodynamics, Latham, NY) as a foam using the Tessari method (8). For deep lesions, the 3% STS formulation is recommended. For very superficial lesions, the 1% STS formulation carries less risk of skin necrosis. The authors are mixing the STS with ethiodol in the following manner: 2 mL STS 3%, 1.5 mL of lipiodol and 3 to 5 mL of air to improve its stability and visibility under fluoroscopy. They use a negative roadmap technique to visualize foam progression. Other authors, just use the negative contrast of the foam displacing the contrast injected during the percutaneous phlebography (8).
7. Following each foam injection, it is recommended to repeat the ultrasound examination to evaluate if there are residual cavities unfilled by the foam therefore requiring additional puncture(s).

8. It is also recommended to inject the deeper aspect of the VM first as the foam will create a superficial screen leading to nonvisualization of the deep portions under ultrasound.

9. When there are dysplastic veins with reflux and venous insufficiency, as may be seen in the marginal vein of a VM in Klippel–Trenaunay syndrome, a combination of mechanical occlusion of the central portion of the vein with coils or plugs and peripheral sclerotherapy with foam can give good results (9). It is important to evaluate if the deep venous system is patent before occluding superficial veins. Attention should be given to avoid deploying coils or plugs in superficial veins (vein less than 1 cm underneath the skin).

10. Alternatively, mechanical occlusion with an adhesive formulation of cyanocrylate purpose designed for saphenous ablation (Venaseal, Medtronic, Santa Rosa, CA), combined with injection of foam in peripheral varicosities can be a good alternative.

11. If sclerotherapy fails, cryotherapy can be considered if the lesion is not too superficial or close to a nerve. It is particularly useful for intramuscular VMs or a specific form of VM involving fat infiltration (fibroadipose vascular anomaly [FAVA]) (10). The technique and precautions are the same as cryotherapy for malignant tumors (see Chapter 59).

Lymphatic Malformation

1. The puncture is usually performed under ultrasound if the lesion is accessible. If not, CBCT with needle guidance can be used. Again, image fusion with a preoperative MRI can be useful.

2. For large macrocystic LMs, we usually insert a pigtail to empty the cavity before injecting the sclerosing agent (Fig. 20.5).

3. If there are residual cavities following drainage, other pigtails or needles should be inserted to completely empty the LM.

4. The different agents used are detailed below. Usually, the authors use doxycycline or bleomycin diluted with 25% iodine contrast.

5. For microcystic LMs, interstitial injection of the sclerosant is usually performed while slowly pulling back the needle. If an acinar pattern with diffusion of the sclerosing agent is observed, the injection can be done while keeping the needle in place.

6. For large LMs with high output, a catheter can be left in place for several days and serial sclerosant injections can be performed on a daily basis until there is no output from the drain.

Sclerosant Agents

Detergents

Detergents are nonionic surfactants promoting endothelial ablation. Sodium tetradecyl sulfate (Thromboject, Angiodynamics, Latham, NY) and polidocanol (Asclera [Merz, Raleigh, NC], Varithena [Boston Scientific, Natick, MA]) are the most commonly used detergents. They are not painful during injection. To improve contact with the endothelium, they are injected as a foam. They are the agents of first intent for VMs. They have been used less frequently for LMs. Thromboject 1% and 3% may contain visible particles that are not soluble therefore use of a filter is recommended for aspiration from the delivery bottle. The maximum per session dose is 10 mL for STS 3%, and 10 mL for polidocanol 3%.

Ethanol

Ethanol is the most powerful sclerosant. It denatures cellular proteins, induces endothelial ablation and medial disruption. It is painful when injected in VMs thus general anesthesia is required. It results in more complications than detergents. Bolus release of ethanol when treating VMs, especially when using a central tourniquet, can lead to acute pulmonary hypertension and death. Thus, the authors are

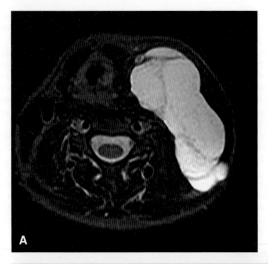

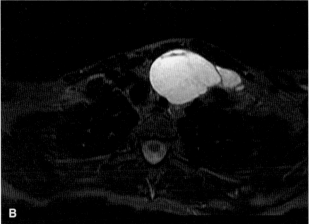

FIGURE 20.5 • A 36-year-old woman with a large macrocystic lymphatic malformation involving the left cervical and cervicothoracic region causing discomfort and aesthetic concern. **A, B:** MR STIR acquisition showing a multiloculated hyperintense cystic lesion with septa involving the left cervical and cervicothoracic regions. (*continued*)

no longer using ethanol for VMs. It occasionally can be used for macrocystic LMs when other agents have failed.

Bleomycin

It is an antitumor agent inhibiting DNA synthesis with a sclerosing effect on endothelial cells and causing a nonspecific inflammatory reaction (11). It induces less edema than detergents and ethanol. It is used primarily for LMs but can be used for VMs after failure of detergents, or for VMs at higher risk for airway or nerve compression due to their location (oropharynx, orbit, and forearm). Not exceeding 15 IU per session is recommended. We usually dilute it in 15-mL NaCl and 5-mL

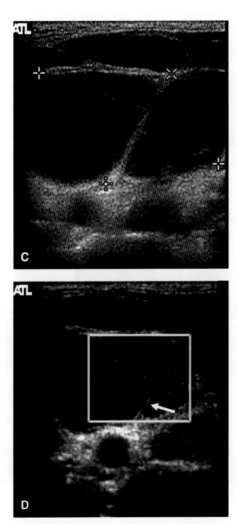

FIGURE 20.5 • (*Continued*) **C, D:** Doppler ultrasound examination confirming the liquid content and little vascularization in the septa (*white arrow*).

iodinated contrast. Chronic lung toxicity has been reported at cumulative doses of 400 IU in oncology. We recommend not exceeding 100 IU. Acute lung hypersensitivity has also been reported; this rare event does not appear to be dose-dependent. Avoidance of hyperoxygenation during the procedure and for subsequent surgeries (SaO$_2$ <92%). Flagellate cutaneous erythema has been reported. Adhesive patches on the skin (EKG electrodes, diachylon adhesive plasters) should be avoided. Pulmonary functional tests are recommended at the end of the sclerotherapy sessions and before further surgeries.

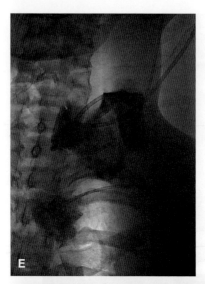

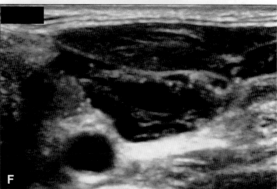

FIGURE 20.5 • (*Continued*) **E:** Sclerosis of the malformation with bleomycin after inserting three drains in the different components of the malformation to empty it before injecting the sclerosant. **F:** Control Doppler ultrasound after three sessions of sclerotherapy showing a small residual cystic component with multiple septations and fibrous organization. The patient is now asymptomatic.

Doxycycline

Doxycycline is an antibiotic inhibiting matrix metalloproteinases, vascular endothelial growth factor induced during angiogenesis, and lymphangiogenesis. It also has a fibrosing and sclerosing effect (11). It is used for LMs. It comes in 100 mg vials. We solubilize it in 5-mL NaCl and 5-mL iodinated contrast. Do not exceed 1,000 mg per session or 20 mg per kg.

Complications

1. Skin ulceration or blistering at the injection site.
2. Glue, coil, and plug extrusion in superficial VMs.

3. DVT due to inadequate outflow control during sclerosant injection.
4. Compartment syndrome (especially calf, forearm).
5. Cardiopulmonary complications (arrhythmia, pulmonary edema, sudden death).
6. Following foam injection, stroke has been reported related to patent foramen ovale. However, these events are very rare and we do not screen for a patent foramen ovale.

Management of Complications

1. Skin ulceration and glue extrusion are usually treated by local wound therapy. Healing generally occurs over a period of weeks with minimal sequelae. Flap surgery is rarely necessary. Coil and/or plug extrusion may need local surgical retrieval of the foreign body.
2. Airway and/or oropharyngeal compression are treated with high-dose corticosteroids. Sometimes, tracheal intubation with mechanical ventilation, tracheostomy or enteral tube feeding can be required.
3. Nerve compression and compartment syndrome require high-dose steroids. Fasciotomy is recommended if it can be performed without cutting into the malformation.
4. DVT should be treated by anticoagulation.
5. Acute lung toxicity related to bleomycin is treated by high-dose steroids and supportive care.

References

1. Wassef M, Blei F, Adams D, et al. Vascular anomalies classification: recommendations from the international society for the study of vascular anomalies. *Pediatrics*. 2015;136(1): e203–e214.
2. Nguyen HL, Boon LM, Vikkula M. Vascular anomalies caused by abnormal signaling within endothelial cells: targets for novel therapies. *Semin Intervent Radiol*. 2017;34(3):233–238.
3. Adams DM, Ricci KW. Vascular anomalies: diagnosis of complicated anomalies and new medical treatment options. *Hematol Oncol Clin North Am*. 2019;33(3):455–470.
4. Goldenberg DC, Hiraki PY, Caldas JG, et al. Surgical treatment of extracranial arteriovenous malformations after multiple embolizations: outcomes in a series of 31 patients. *Plast Reconstr Surg*. 2015;135(2):543–552.
5. Soulez G, Gilbert Md Frcpc P, Giroux Md Frcpc MF, et al. Interventional management of arteriovenous malformations. *Tech Vasc Interv Radiol*. 2019;22(4):100633.
6. Yakes W, Baumgartner I. Interventional treatment of arteriovenous malformations. *Gefasschirurgie*. 2014;19(04):325–330.
7. Han YY, Sun LM, Yuan SM. Localized intravascular coagulation in venous malformations: a system review. *Phlebology*. 2021;36(1):38–42.
8. Legiehn GM, Heran MK. Venous malformations: classification, development, diagnosis, and interventional radiologic management. *Radiol Clin North Am*. 2008;46(3):545–597.
9. Fereydooni A, Nassiri N. Evaluation and management of the lateral marginal vein in Klippel-Trenaunay and other PIK3CA-related overgrowth syndromes. *J Vasc Surg Venous Lymphat Disord*. 2020;8(3):482–493.
10. Cornelis F, Neuville A, Labreze C, et al. Percutaneous cryotherapy of vascular malformation: initial experience. *Cardiovasc Intervent Radiol*. 2013;36(3):853–856.
11. Horbach SE, Lokhorst MM, Saeed P, et al. Sclerotherapy for low-flow vascular malformations of the head and neck: a systematic review of sclerosing agents. *J Plast, Reconstr Aesthet Surg*. 2016;69(3):295–304.

21 Hepatic Metastases: Chemoembolization

Michael C. Soulen, MD, FSIR, FCIRSE

Indications

1. Liver-dominant hepatic metastases. Patients with minimal or indolent extrahepatic disease may be candidates if the liver disease is considered to be the dominant source of morbidity and mortality for that individual. Patients should be evaluated for surgical resection as an alternative.
2. In addition to primary hepatic malignancies such as hepatocellular carcinoma and cholangiocarcinoma, tumors that typically meet these criteria include metastases from colorectal cancer, neuroendocrine tumors (NETs), ocular melanoma, and sarcomas. Atypically, other GI primaries, breast, lung, GU, or other cancers will have liver-only or liver-dominant metastases.

Contraindications

1. Contraindications to angiography
   a. Severe anaphylactoid reactions to radiographic contrast media
   b. Uncorrectable coagulopathy
   c. Severe peripheral arterial disease precluding arterial access
2. Contraindications to administration of chemotherapy
   a. Severe thrombocytopenia (<50,000 per μL) or leucopenia (absolute neutrophil count [ANC] <1,000 per μL)
   b. Cardiac (American Heart Association [AHA] class III to IV failure) or renal insufficiency (creatinine >2.0 mg per dL)
3. Contraindications to hepatic artery embolization
   a. The presence of hepatic encephalopathy or jaundice is an absolute contraindication to embolization.
   b. Tolerance of hepatic artery occlusion is dependent on the presence of portal vein inflow. The portal vein must be carefully assessed at the time of angiography. Compromise in portal venous blood flow is only a relative contraindication to hepatic embolization. Chemoembolization can be performed safely despite portal vein occlusion if hepatopetal collateral flow is present. In this setting, a smaller volume of the liver should be embolized at any one time.
   c. When the parenchyma is diseased, the liver becomes more dependent on the hepatic artery and less on the portal vein. A subgroup of patients has been identified who are at high risk of acute hepatic failure following hepatic artery embolization. They have a constellation of more than 50% of the liver volume replaced by tumor, lactate dehydrogenase (LDH) greater than 425 IU per liter, aspartate transaminase greater than 100 IU per liter, and total bilirubin of 2 mg per dL or greater (1).
   d. Presence of a bilioenteric anastomosis, biliary stent, or prior sphincterotomy allows for colonization of the bile ducts with enteric bacteria. Hepatic artery embolization causes microscopic bile duct injury, leading to liver abscess formation, which can be fatal (2). Aggressive prophylactic regimens decrease the incidence of liver abscess to around 20% (3). Oral moxifloxacin 400 mg daily beginning 3 days before through 2 weeks after TACE is an established and well-tolerated regimen.
   e. Biliary obstruction is a relative contraindication. Even with a normal serum bilirubin, the presence of dilated intrahepatic bile ducts places the patient at high risk for bile duct necrosis and biloma formation in the obstructed segment(s) of the liver.

f. Inability to position the catheter tip selectively, so as to avoid nontarget embolization of the gut, skin, or other vulnerable extrahepatic structures, places the patient at risk for serious injury. Coil blockade of the nontarget vessel can be performed to allow chemoembolization to be performed safely. The cystic artery can be chemoembolized safely, although doing so will increase the intensity and duration of postembolization syndrome (4).

Preprocedure Preparation

Pretreatment Assessment

1. Tissue diagnosis or convincing clinical diagnosis (e.g., liver mass with characteristic features and elevated tumor markers).
2. Cross-sectional imaging of the abdomen and pelvis (computed tomography [CT] or magnetic resonance imaging [MRI]) to identify segmental tumor location, venous and biliary patency, and arterial variants.
3. Exclusion of substantial extrahepatic disease (chest x-ray or CT, positron emission tomography [PET]-CT).
4. Laboratory studies including complete blood count (CBC), international normalized ratio (INR), creatinine, liver function tests, and tumor markers.

Patient Education

Before embarking on this fairly arduous palliative regimen, patients should be carefully assessed and informed of the side effects and risks (5).

Most patients undergoing TACE develop *postembolization syndrome*, which consists of

1. Common (>20% incidence each): variable amounts of pain, fever, nausea, constipation, fatigue, loss of appetite, and elevated blood pressure. These are rarely severe.
2. Less common (10% to 20%): vomiting, diarrhea, accumulation of fluid in the abdomen or chest, limb swelling, and bruising around the catheterization site. These are rarely severe.
3. Uncommon side effects (<10%) include hiccups, confusion, chest pain, infection, liver or gallbladder injury. These can be severe, even life-threatening.
4. The severity of postembolization syndrome is variable and can last from a few hours to a few weeks. Other significant toxicities are rare. Serious complications occur after 5% to 7% of procedures. Given the significant discomforts, hazards, and expense of this treatment, its palliative role should be clearly understood.

Patient Preparation

1. Patients fast overnight.
2. Vigorous hydration is instituted (normal saline [NS] solution at 200 mL per hour).
3. Prophylactic antibiotics (e.g., cefazolin [Ancef] 1 g, metronidazole [Flagyl] 500 mg) and antiemetics (e.g., ondansetron [Zofran] 24 mg, dexamethasone [Decadron] 10 mg, diphenhydramine [Benadryl] 50 mg) are administered intravenously (IV). Patients with well-differentiated NETs get subcutaneous octreotide (Sandostatin) 500 μg. Use of a steroid-based antiemetic regimen is evidence-based. Routine use of prophylactic antibiotics and octreotide is common practice but not evidence-based, with the exception of aggressive antibiotic prophylaxis in the setting of prior biliary instrumentation.

Procedure

1. Diagnostic visceral arteriography (including celiac and superior mesenteric arteriography) is performed under conscious sedation to determine the arterial supply to the liver and confirm patency of the portal vein. Variant hepatic artery anatomy is present in almost half of the population. The origins of vessels supplying the gut (gastroduodenal, right gastric, supraduodenal) are carefully noted

in order to avoid embolization of the stomach or small bowel. The cystic artery should be identified. Chemoembolization of the right hepatic artery proximal to the cystic artery is safe; however, chemoembolization of the gallbladder should be avoided if possible in order to reduce the severity of postembolization syndrome.

2. Once the arterial anatomy is clearly understood, a catheter is advanced superselectively into the right or left hepatic artery, depending on which lobe holds the most tumors. A power-injected superselective angiogram with prolonged imaging should be performed to confirm catheter position and exclude nontarget vessels prior to injecting any chemotherapeutic drugs. Cone-beam CT should be performed routinely because this has been shown to improve outcomes.

3. Catheters: Review of sagittal images from an abdominal CT or MRI is useful to guide base catheter choice. Median arcuate ligament compression of the celiac artery or severe downward angulation often makes selective hepatic catheterization with a Cobra-style catheter difficult, in which case a reverse-curve catheter (e.g., Simmons, Sos) with a coaxial microcatheter works well. Many chemoembolization procedures can be done with a 4-F. hydrophilic-coated Cobra catheter and a long-taper hydrophilic wire. Such catheters should not be advanced into a vessel less than twice the catheter diameter because this will cause iatrogenic stasis. When small vessels or tortuous anatomy is present, a high-flow microcatheter can be advanced through a reverse-curve catheter into the target vessel.

4. A variety of chemoembolic protocols exist, historically 100- to 150-mg cisplatin, 50-mg doxorubicin, and/or 10- to 30-mg mitomycin C dissolved in 10 mL of radiographic contrast and emulsified with 10 to 20 mL of iodized oil. Alternatively, drug-eluting microspheres allow use of doxorubicin or irinotecan in solution. The oil:chemoemulsion ratio is adjusted by the operator based on the size and vascularity of the tumor and but should not be less than 2:1. Dividing the dose into 3 to 4 aliquots allows the interventional oncologist to adjust the emulsion ratio during the embolization to maximize drug delivery at the endpoint of near stasis. Embolization is completed with 100- to 300-micron spherical particles mixed into the final aliquot of the chemoembolic emulsion. All chemotherapy and associated syringes are kept on a separate tray or Mayo stand and must be disposed of according to hospital regulations. Glass or polycarbonate syringes should be used, along with metal or polycarbonate stopcocks. Conventional plastic syringes, stopcocks, and flow switches will disintegrate rapidly after contact with the chemoembolic emulsion. All personnel in the room must have eye protection and a mask on, and anyone handling the chemotherapeutic material must be fully gowned and double-gloved.

5. The patient receives intraarterial lidocaine (30-mg boluses prior to and between aliquots of the chemotherapeutic emulsion, up to 200 mg total) and IV fentanyl and midazolam to alleviate pain during the embolization.

6. For lipiodol chemoembolization (6), the chemotherapeutic drugs should be dissolved in contrast in the pharmacy and delivered in a sterile sealed bottle. The chemotherapy/contrast solution is drawn up in a 20-mL glass or polycarbonate syringe. Lipiodol is drawn up in a separate 20-mL syringe. These serve as reservoirs during the procedure. A 10-mL syringe and a metal or polycarbonate stopcock can then be used to draw off aliquots of chemotherapy/contrast solution and Lipiodol. A second 10-mL syringe is then used to emulsify the two by pumping vigorously back and forth through the stopcock 20 to 25 times. An example would be a 2:1 emulsion of 4-mL lipiodol and 2-mL chemosolution. The chemosolution should always be added to the oil syringe to create a water-in-oil emulsion. This initial aliquot of emulsion is injected slowly through the catheter, followed by a lidocaine flush. If a microcatheter is used, the viscous emulsion will need to be injected using 1- to 3-mL polycarbonate Luer-Lok syringes. Additional aliquots of emulsion are administered, with the addition of one syringe of 100- to 300-micron spherical embolic to the final aliquot. The chemoembolic mixture is injected until nearly complete stasis of blood flow is achieved. The goal is to achieve a "tree-in-winter" appearance, with embolization of the terminal tumor-feeding branches

but preservation of flow in the major arterial trunks. By repeatedly mixing small aliquots of the emulsion, the thickness of the mix can be adjusted to try to deliver as much of the total drug dose as possible before achieving the endpoint of 90% stasis. Large, hypervascular tumors may require a thicker mix by adding more embolic particles or increasing the oil:contrast ratio. Conversely, less vascular tumors may require thinning of the emulsion by using less oil or particles.

7. For drug-eluting microspheres, specific protocols exist for loading of each type of chemotherapeutic drug (e.g., doxorubicin, irinotecan) onto each brand and size of microsphere. Consult the manufacturer's instructions for use. Currently, none of these products are approved in the United States for drug delivery. Typically, 50 to 100 mg of drug in solution is added to a vial of microspheres a few hours before the procedure to allow time for drug uptake. The effluent is then removed, and the drug-loaded microspheres suspended in 10 to 20 mL of dilute nonionic contrast, which is slowly instilled into the target vessel. Because the microspheres are not visible, extra caution is required to avoid nontarget embolization. The endpoint is drug delivery and additional bland embolics are not required. Intra-arterial irinotecan can be painful and additional analgesia may be necessary.

Postprocedure Management

1. Most insurers cover a 23-hour observation period rather than a full inpatient admission. With careful assessment, some patients will be able to be discharged the same day if oral intake is adequate and pain controlled. A protocol should be in place to triage between same-day and observation status incorporating routine post-discharge assessments (7).

2. Vigorous hydration (NS 3 L per 24 hours) and then 5% dextrose, half-normal saline solution (D5½NS) at 80 mL per hour until oral intake is adequate.

3. IV antibiotics until discharge (e.g., cefazolin 500 mg q8h, metronidazole 500 mg q12h)

4. IV antiemetic therapy (ondansetron and Decadron, 8 mg IV q8h)

5. Narcotics, prochlorperazine, ketorolac, and acetaminophen are liberally supplied for control of pain, nausea, and fever. A patient-controlled analgesia (PCA) pump is occasionally required if pain is severe. Typical PCA doses are morphine sulfate 1 to 2 mg per hour, 1 to 2 mg demand, with a 10- to 15-minute lockout. Alternatively, hydromorphone (Dilaudid) can be used at a dose of 0.2 mg per hour and 0.2 mg demand.

6. The patient is discharged as soon as oral intake is adequate and parenteral narcotics are not required for pain control. Most patients are discharged in 1 day. Antiemetics (prochlorperazine [Compazine] 10 mg by mouth [PO] q6h, or granisetron [Kytril] 1 mg PO bid, or ondansetron [Zofran] 8 mg PO bid) and oral narcotics (acetaminophen/codeine [Tylenol with Codeine No. 3], oxycodone/acetaminophen [Percocet], or hydromorphone [Dilaudid] 2 mg), 1 to 2 tablets q4h as needed. Patients taking narcotics should be warned about constipation and given instructions for a concurrent laxative regimen.

7. Laboratory studies are repeated in 3 weeks. Routine liver imaging between procedures is not necessary unless the patient develops signs or symptoms suggesting a complication.

8. At 4 to 8 weeks, the patient returns for a second procedure directed at the other lobe of the liver. Depending on the arterial anatomy, two to four procedures may be required to treat the entire tumor burden, after which response is assessed by repeat imaging studies and tumor markers. Residual viable tumor may indicate the need for additional procedures.

Results

1. Hepatoma (8): 60% to 80% of patients will have disease control and 40% to 60% an objective response of their hepatoma and a decrease in α-fetoprotein level, if elevated, following lipiodol TACE. Median duration of response ranges from 3 to

15 months. Median overall survival is around 19 months, with 70% alive at 1 year, 40% at 3 years, and 32% at 5 years. Important prognostic factors include tumor. Three RCTs have shown no oncologic benefit from doxorubicin-loaded microspheres versus bland embolics.

2. Colon cancer (9): Disease control is achieved in 45% to 65%. No Phase III trials of lipiodol chemoembolization exist to assess survival advantage. For drug-eluting embolics with irinotecan, a review of 10 prospective single-arm trials encompassing 638 subjects noted an ORR of 40% to 78%, PFS of 11 months, and OS of 19 to 33 months among studies with >50 subjects. Randomized trials against standard chemotherapy in the first- and second-line both showed improvement in PFS.

3. NETs (10) have a 50% to 60% response rate to either bland embolization or chemoembolization. The duration of response is mostly driven by the underlying tumor grade. Three prospective trials reported an unacceptable rate of major adverse events following doxorubicin-loaded microspheres among metastatic NET patients; this platform should not be used in this disease.

4. There are limited data for metastases from ocular melanoma, sarcomas, and breast cancer.

Complications

Major complications of hepatic embolization include hepatic insufficiency or infarction (2%), hepatic abscess (2%), biliary necrosis or stricture, tumor rupture, surgical cholecystitis, and nontarget embolization to the gut. With careful patient selection and scrupulous technique, the incidence of these serious events collectively is 5% to 7%. Other complications include cardiac events, renal insufficiency, and anemia requiring transfusion, with incidences of less than 1% each. Thirty-day mortality is <1%.

R e f e r e n c e s

1. Charnsangavej C. Chemoembolization of liver tumors. *Semin Interv Radiol.* 1993;10:150–160.
2. Kim W, Clark TWI, Baum RA, et al. Risk factors for liver abscess formation after hepatic chemoembolization. *J Vasc Interv Radiol.* 2001;12(8):965–968.
3. Parikh RS, Abousoud O, Hunt S, et al. Infection rates following hepatic embolotherapy in patients with prior biliary interventions: comparison of single-drug moxifloxacin and multidrug antibiotic prophylaxis. *J Vasc Interv Radiol.* 2021;32(5):739–744. doi:10.1016/j.jvir.2021.01.273.
4. Leung DA, Goin JE, Sickles C, et al. Determinants of postembolization syndrome after hepatic chemoembolization. *J Vasc Interv Radiol.* 2001;12(3):321–326.
5. Tuite CM, Sun W, Soulen MC. General assessment of the patient with cancer for the interventional oncologist. *J Vasc Interv Radiol.* 2006;17(5):753–758.
6. de Baere T, Arai Y, Lencioni R, et al. Treatment of liver tumors with lipiodol TACE: technical recommendations from experts opinion. *Cardiovasc Intervent Radiol.* 2016;39(3):334–343.
7. Fritsche MR, Watchmaker JM, Lipnick AJ, et al. Outpatient transarterial chemoembolization of hepatocellular carcinoma: review of a same-day discharge strategy. *J Vasc Interv Radiol.* 2018;29:550–555.
8. Lencioni R, de Baere T, Soulen MC, et al. Lipiodol transarterial chemoembolization for hepatocellular carcinoma: a systematic review of efficacy and safety data. *Hepatology.* 2016;44(1):106–116.
9. Fiorentini G, Sarti D, Nani R, et al. Updates of colorectal cancer liver metastases therapy: review on DEBIRI. *Hepat Oncol.* 2020;7(1):HEP16.
10. Chen JX, Rose S, White SB, et al. Embolotherapy for neuroendocrine tumor liver metastases: prognostic factors for hepatic progression-free survival and overall survival. *Cardiovasc Intervent Radiol.* 2017;40(1):69–80.

22 Hepatocellular Carcinoma: Chemoembolization

Andrew R. Kolarich, MD,
Iakovos Theodoulou, BSc (Hons), MBBS, FHEA and
Christos S. Georgiades, MD, PhD, FSIR, FCIRSE

Introduction

Transarterial chemoembolization (TACE) has been established as the standard of care for intermediate-stage (Barcelona Clinic Liver Cancer—BCLC-B) hepatocellular carcinoma (HCC) for nearly two decades with two landmark randomized control trials (1,2) and a subsequent meta-analysis (3) demonstrating improved overall survival compared to best supportive care (BSC). See Chapter 75 for HCC staging. This level 1A evidence has resulted in TACE inclusion in all major HCC treatment guidelines including the American Association for the Study of Liver Diseases (AASLD) and the European Association for the Study of the Liver (EASL). While resection or transplantation in patients with decompensated cirrhosis remains the gold standard for curative treatment of HCC the presence of multifocal disease, limited hepatic function, and liver transplant shortages make these options unavailable to a majority of patients. The rational for chemotherapy administration and selective hepatic artery embolization is based on the fact that HCC tumors derive blood supply almost exclusively through the hepatic artery while liver parenchyma is mainly reliant on the portal vein. In conventional TACE (c-TACE), a cocktail of chemotherapy and lipiodol (an oily contrast medium), (Fig. 22.1) followed by an embolic agent are injected into the tumor vascular bed via selection of branches of the hepatic artery. This allows for fluoroscopic visualization during administration of high levels of local chemotherapy followed by ischemia, extending contact of the agent with the tumor and causing further ischemia of the tumor itself. The most commonly used chemotherapeutic agents are epirubicin, idarubicin, mitomycin C, doxorubicin, and cisplatin used as single agents or in a two or three drug combinations. Drug-eluting beads (DEB) consist of polyvinyl acetate beads that release chemotherapy at a slow rate with advantages of selectivity, better embolic effect, and sustained drug release which results in fewer side effects and prolonged dwell time (4). However, it has not been shown to improve safety or survival over c-TACE (4,5).

Indications

1. The primary indication for TACE is intermediate-stage HCC (BCLC stage B).
2. Secondary indications:
    a. Bridge to transplant, as local control for patients where transplant wait time is predicted to be greater than 4 months regardless of tumor size (6). Almost all HCC transplant candidates fall into this category.
    b. Downstage to resection or transplantation size criteria.
    c. Aid surgery by shrinking a tumor adjacent to a major intrahepatic vascular bundle (e.g., the right or left portal vein).
    d. Palliation of carefully selected patients with advanced HCC (BCLC stage C).

Contraindications

Absolute

1. Advanced liver disease (Child–Pugh C) unless TACE can be performed selectively.
2. Medically refractory hepatic encephalopathy unless TACE can be performed selectively.

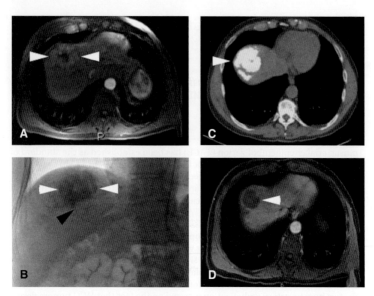

FIGURE 22.1 • Conventional transarterial chemoembolization (cTACE). Axial, T1-weighted, contrast-enhanced MRI (**A**) prior to treatment shows a 4-cm hypervascular lesion (*white arrowheads*) in the dome of the liver. Fluoroscopic image during cTACE (**B**) shows the superselective microcatheter tip (*black arrowhead*) through which lipiodol-chemotherapy cocktail is injected to saturate the target lesion (*white arrowheads*). Post-cTACE non–contrast-enhanced CT (**C**), shows dense lipiodol deposition (*white arrowhead*) within the tumor. Three-month follow-up, axial, T1-weighted, contrast-enhanced MRI (**D**) shows complete necrosis of the dome lesion (*white arrowhead*).

3. Poor performance status. Patients with Eastern Cooperative Oncology Group (ECOG) >2 or Karnofsky Index (<70) do not benefit from TACE.
4. Uncorrectable bleeding diathesis.
5. Large burden of extrahepatic metastatic disease.
6. Active infection.

Relative

1. Total bilirubin >4. TACE can be considered if hyperbilirubinemia is secondary to biliary obstruction and can be reversed with drainage. Drainage should be performed percutaneously and external to avoid crossing the sphincter of Oddi, which can result in bacterial colonization of the intrahepatic bile ducts. This can lead to post-TACE intrahepatic abscess formation and/or cholangitis to the peribiliary plexus which experiences profound ischemia after TACE. An internal–external biliary drain can be advanced after TACE.
2. Anaphylactic reaction to contrast.
3. Anaphylactic reaction to chemotherapy drug.
4. Portal vein occlusion. Portal vein occlusion is a predictor of poor response to treatment with EASL and AASLD against the use of TACE in these patients; studies have shown segmental or subsegmental portal vein occlusion does not increase the risk of complications as long as liver reserve is within criteria and/or collateral flow to the liver exists (7).

Preprocedure Preparation

1. Multidisciplinary review of the patient's disease and functional status to ensure no curative options are overlooked.
2. Clinic visit in which the patient and family are fully informed of the risks, benefits, and reasonable expectations of therapy.
3. Cross-sectional imaging review, with contrast-enhanced magnetic resonance imaging (MRI) preferred over computed tomography (CT).
4. Nil per os (NPO) status except for allowed medications for at least 8 hours prior to sedation or anesthesia.
5. Intravenous (IV) hydration. Dehydration from NPO status, contrast load, chemotherapy nephrotoxicity, and possibility of tumor lysis syndrome increase the risk of acute renal injury. If no contraindication such as heart failure exists, a normal saline bolus (i.e., 500 mL) followed by continuous IV hydration (100 mL per hour) is recommended.
6. Premedication
   a. Dexamethasone 10 mg IV, diphenhydramine 50 mg IV.
   b. Nephroprotectants, if necessary. Most important is hydration.
   c. Antiemetics. Ondansetron 8 mg IV (review of preoperative electrocardiogram to evaluate for QTc prolongation).

Procedure

1. Moderate sedation is adequate for most patients.
2. Sterile preparation of femoral access.
3. Arteriography
   a. Abdominal aortogram may reveal collateral tumor supply. This is important in repeated treatments as phrenic, adrenal, or intercostal arteries may develop tumor supply (Fig. 22.2). Rarely extraabdominal collateral supply may be identified (Fig. 22.3).
   b. Superior mesenteric arteriogram to identify accessory hepatic arteries and assess patency of portal vein
   c. Celiac and hepatic arteriogram for treatment planning
   d. Cone-beam CT imaging could be performed before treatment to ensure proper targeting of the tumor in selected cases.
4. Placement of catheter (or coaxial microcatheter, if necessary) as distal as possible to minimize collateral liver injury but proximal enough to treat the entire targeted lesion.
5. Delivery of chemotherapy/lipiodol/embolization mixture or chemotherapy-loaded DEB under continuous fluoroscopic visualization to avoid the inadvertent delivery of drugs and/or embolic agents into nontarget vessels.
   a. For conventional TACE, a lipiodol (oil): chemotherapy (aqueous) emulsion must be created. Start at a 1:1 ratio and increase for larger, vascular tumors or decrease for tumors with slower arterial flow. The maximum amount of lipiodol should not exceed 20 mL. The amount of lipiodol emulsion to be injected depends on the tumor size. If a visible shunt is identified between the hepatic artery and hepatic vein or more commonly between the hepatic artery and portal vein, complete embolization of the shunt using gelfoam pledgets must be performed prior to the TACE procedure. Additional lidocaine can be given intraarterially after the lipiodol-chemotherapy emulsion has been administered to enhanced cytotoxicity, but before the embolization component of the procedure. Calibrated microspheres in the 100 to 300 μm size should be used to complete the embolization. The angiographic end point should be 2 to 5 heartbeats to clear the contrast column (stasis or near-stasis).

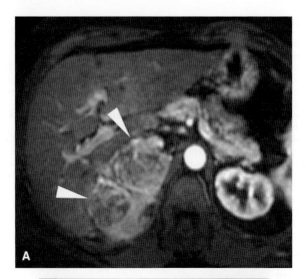

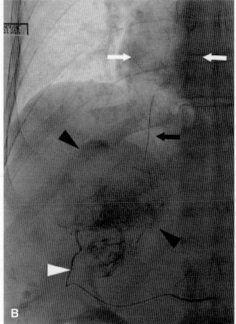

FIGURE 22.2 • Collateral supply to hepatocellular carcinoma (HCC). Pretreatment, axial, T1-weighted, contrast-enhanced MRI (**A**) shows a large infiltrative lesion in segments VI and VII (*white arrowheads*) extending beyond the liver capsule. Fluoroscopic image during angiography (**B**) shows collateral supply to the large HCC (*black arrowheads*) via the right adrenal artery. The superselective microcatheter tip is indicated by the *white arrowhead*. Arterial supply via the right hepatic artery (*black arrow*) is noted supplying a pedunculated mass in the right atrium (*white arrows*). (*continued*)

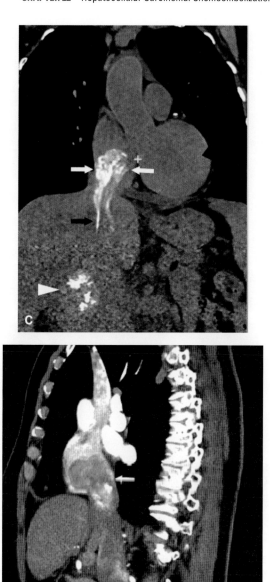

FIGURE 22.2 • (*Continued*) Post-cTACE, coronal, noncontrast CT (**C**), shows lipiodol deposition within the liver mass (*white arrow head*), and its extension to the right atrial component (*white arrows*) via hepatic artery invasion (*black arrow*). Sagittal, contrast-enhanced CT before (**D**) and 3 months after (*continued*)

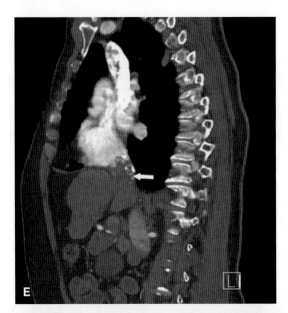

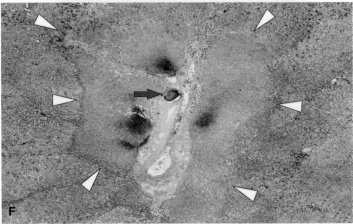

FIGURE 22.2 • (*Continued*) (**E**) cTACE show near complete response of the right atrial tumor (*white arrow*). After this remarkable result the patient went on to resection. H&E histopathology slide (**F**) shows a bead (*red arrow*) embolized in the arteriolar supply of the tumor. The eluted chemotherapy agent (doxorubicin) and ischemia resulted in a well-delineated zone of necrosis (*white arrowheads*) within the targeted HCC.

    b. For DEB-TACE (Fig. 22.4), the use of 100- to 300-μm size DEB is recommended in order to achieve deeper penetration within the tumor(s). Iodinated contrast should be mixed with the DEB in a 3 to 4:1 ratio. Appropriate doxorubicin doses to be used in DEB-TACE range from 50 to 150 mg.

  6. Cone-beam CT imaging (Fig. 22.5) should be performed after treatment in order to confirm appropriate tumor targeting and assess technical success. Additional

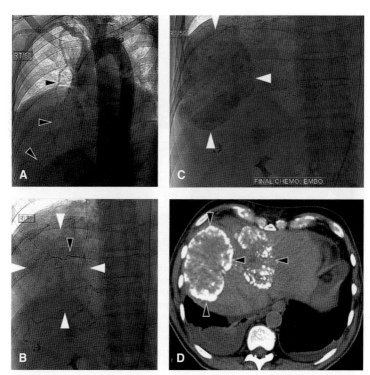

FIGURE 22.3 • Extrahepatic collateral supply to HCC. Left oblique, ascending aortic arch arteriogram (**A**) shows a right internal mammary artery (*black arrowheads*) supplying a tumor artery in the liver. Delayed phase of same arteriogram (**B**) shows collateralization with intercostal artery (*black arrowhead*) and large tumor blush (*white arrowheads*). Frontal single fluoroscopic exposure after cTACE from both the internal mammary and intercostal arteries (**C**) shows excellent coverage of the tumor by lipiodol (*white arrowheads*). Post-cTACE dry CT (**D**) confirms excellent coverage of the targeted tumor by lipiodol (*black arrowheads*).

targeting tools that are available such as automated feeder detection (AFD), 3D overlay, and image-fusion (Figs. 22.6 and 22.7) can further improve response and mitigate nontarget embolization.

7. Access hemostasis.

Follow-Up

Though protocols may vary slightly, standard follow-up consists of a posttreatment contrast-enhanced MRI, laboratory evaluation and clinical examination 4 to 6 weeks after treatment. Response is documented by either EASL criteria or Modified Response Evaluation Criteria in Solid Tumors (mRECIST).

Results

Survival benefit in Child–Pugh A and B patients has been proven compared to best supportive care (BSC) alone.

1. Landmark-randomized control trial by Llovet et al. in 2002 reported mean survival was significantly longer with c-TACE (28.6 months) than BSC (17.9 months;

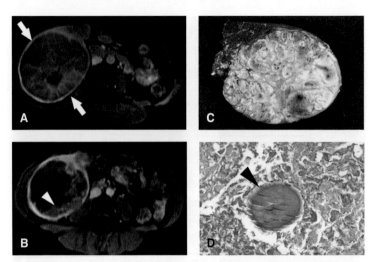

FIGURE 22.4 • Histopathologic correlation after DEB-TACE of a large right lobe HCC. Axial, contrast-enhanced, T1-weighted, fat-suppressed MR image prior to treatment (**A**) shows a 16-cm solidly enhancing HCC (*white arrows*). Three-month post–DEB-TACE image (**B**) shows a shrinking HCC which is mostly necrotic. Small peripheral viable tumor tissue is noted (*white arrowhead*). After this response the patient underwent HCC resection (**C**). Histopathologic examination (**D**) showed more than 90% tumor necrosis centered around DEB embolized in arterioles (*black arrowhead*).

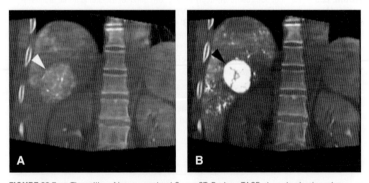

FIGURE 22.5 • The utility of intraprocedural C-arm CT. During cTACE, the subselective micro-catheter was placed in the desired location and contrast was injected at a rate of 1.5 cc per second for a total injection duration of 7 seconds. Arterial and venous phase C-arm CTs were obtained. The first image (**A**) is a coronal reconstruction of a preembolization C-arm CT in this patient with HCC. This shows complete coverage of the targeted HCC (*white arrowhead*) with minimal nontarget enhancement. Coronal reconstruction of a post-cTACE dry CT (**B**) shows complete and dense uptake of lipiodol by the HCC (*black arrowhead*), predictive of excellent response.

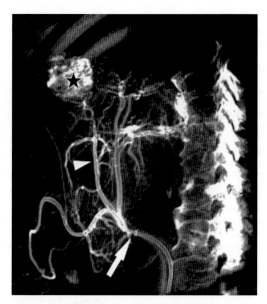

FIGURE 22.6 • Example of embolization planning. Computer-generated arterial vascular pathway connecting the selective catheter (*white arrow*) and the target HCC (*black star*) by selecting the correct branch of the hepatic artery (*white arrowhead*). Knowing this anatomy makes it easier for the operator to subselect the proper arteries for a more selective delivery of treatment.

$p = 0.009$) (1). A similar landmark trial by Lo in 2002 reported benefit in terms of survival rate over BSC (57% vs. 32% at 1 year, 31% vs. 11% at 2 years, 26% vs. 3% at 3 years, $p = 0.002$) (2).

2. Subsequent meta-analyses, including a large systematic review including over 10,000 HCC patients demonstrated overall survival of 19.4 months and a 5-year survival rate of 32.4% (8).

3. No randomized control trials exist to evaluate TACE as neoadjuvant therapy compared to BSC prior to liver transplant. Retrospective comparative studies (level

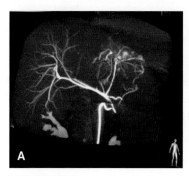
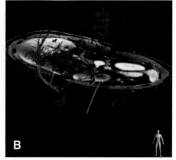

FIGURE 22.7 • Example of image fusion. 3D reconstruction after C-arm CT (**A**) shows the arterial vascular anatomy of the liver. Image fusion with baseline MRI (**B**), confirms the arterial pathway to the target HCC.

3b and 4) have mixed results in terms of comparative waitlist dropout rates and reduction of HCC recurrence with no evidence of increased overall survival after transplant (9).

Complications

The most serious TACE-related complications are liver failure, nontarget embolization, and liver abscess. The expected complications related to TACE are summarized in Table 22.1. The most common side effect of TACE is postchemoembolization syndrome seen in up to 60% to 80% of patients. It is composed of a triad of abdominal pain, nausea, and fever is self-limiting and not indicative of a true complication.

1. Liver failure can be avoided with proper patient selection. Advanced liver disease is indicated by Child–Pugh C, high bilirubin, low albumin, poor performance status, and/or encephalopathy, which are significant predictors of liver failure after TACE. TACE in such patients should be avoided unless a very specific goal exists, such as superselective TACE to improve transplantation candidacy.

2. Liver abscess is a rare complication unless there is bile duct colonization by gastrointestinal (GI) flora as a result of compromised sphincter of Oddi (biliary tube, hepaticojejunostomy). In the latter case, the risk for liver abscess is 60%

Table 22.1 **Complications Related to TACE**

Complication	Risk Factor	% Risk Baseline	After Risk Mitigation	Risk Mitigation Action
Liver failure/ death	Child-Pugh C T. Bilirubin ≥4 mg/dL Albumin ≤2 mg/dL Poor performance status	5–10%	1%	Superselective embolization
Encephalopathy	History of encephalopathy, poor liver function reserve	20–40%	5–10%	Superselective embolization, medication
Liver abscess	Compromised sphincter of Oddi	30–80	0–20%	Broad-spectrum antibiotics Bowel preparation
Nontarget embolization	Aberrant anatomy, difficult vascular anatomy	<10%	<1%	Coil embolization of nontarget vessel, C-arm CT
Pulmonary embolism	Hepatic artery to hepatic vein shunting	<1%	<1%	Gelfoam embolization of shunt
Variceal bleeding	Gastroesophageal varices	1–5%	Unknown but lower	Pre-TACE endoscopic banding
Acute renal failure	Renal insufficiency, diabetes, hypertension	5–10%	<2%	Hydration, renoprotection, minimize contrast

to 80% and only moderately reduced by broad-spectrum antibiotics and colonic preparation prior to TACE. TACE may result in biliary ischemia and cause a local abscess.
3. Nontarget embolization can be catastrophic and can be avoided with intimate knowledge of vascular anatomy, experience, and fastidious technique. High dilution of the DEB with contrast and magnified, continuous visualization limits the chances of reflux. If a nontarget vessel is necessarily close to the target vessel, coil embolization may prevent this complication.

Management of Complications

1. Liver failure, encephalopathy, and death. These complications are related to poor liver function reserve prior to TACE, and the only intervention possible is symptomatic support. IV hydration, pressure support, and metronidazole/lactulose or rifaximin for hepatic encephalopathy may help stabilize the patient until the liver recovers.
2. Liver abscess. Ensuing liver abscess must be drained percutaneously. Such abscesses are notoriously difficult to treat and may require prolonged drainage, repeat drainage, and long-term antibiotics.
3. Nontarget embolization:
   a. Gastric: Symptomatic support, including NPO, IV hydration, proton pump inhibitors, and gastric surface protection. If perforation, surgery may be required.
   b. Gallbladder: Mostly a self-limiting situation. Pain, nausea control, NPO, and IV hydration are adequate in most cases. Gallbladder eventually scars down and symptoms resolve.
4. Pulmonary embolism: Supportive measures to resolution including anticoagulation.
5. Renal failure. Dehydration, contrast nephrotoxicity, chemotherapy nephrotoxicity, and tumor lysis increase the risk for renal injury. Aggressive IV hydration prior to TACE is the single most important maneuver to protect the kidney. Limiting contrast load and using nephroprotectants prior to TACE may help reduce the risk of renal failure.
6. GI bleeding. Two distinct complications:
   a. Arterial bleeding. Nontarget embolization may result in duodenal or gastric ulceration/perforation, which can result in arterial bleeding.
   b. Variceal bleeding. Patients with portal hypertension, gastric varices, and history of variceal bleed have a higher risk of variceal bleeding. This is thought to be due to a transient increase in portal hypertension. Treatment is symptomatic, and if unsuccessful, endoscopic banding/sclerosis is required.

Summary

TACE is the recommended treatment for intermediate-stage (BCLC-B) HCC and it has been shown to offer a substantial survival benefit by multiple level-1 evidence studies. The use of TACE has also been shown to maintain patients on the liver transplant waiting list and downstage patients to within transplantation criteria. These expanding indications are dependent on continued clinical competence of the operator, proper patient selection, multidisciplinary collaborations, and reassertion of these benefits by high-quality studies.

R e f e r e n c e s

1. Llovet JM, Real MI, Montana X, et al. Arterial embolisation or chemoembolisation versus symptomatic treatment in patients with unresectable hepatocellular carcinoma: a randomised controlled trial. *Lancet.* 2002;359(9319):1734–1739.

2. Lo CM, Ngan H, Tso WK, et al. Randomized controlled trial of transarterial lipiodol chemo-embolization for unresectable hepatocellular carcinoma. *Hepatology.* 2002;35(5):1164–1171.
3. Llovet JM, Bruix J. Systematic review of randomized trials for unresectable hepatocellular carcinoma: chemoembolization improves survival. *Hepatology.* 2003;37(2):429–442.
4. Lammer J, Malagari K, Vogl T, et al. Prospective randomized study of doxorubicin-eluting-bead embolization in the treatment of hepatocellular carcinoma: results of the PRECISION V study. *Cardiovasc Intervent Radiol.* 2010;33(1):41–52.
5. Golfieri R, Giampalma E, Renzulli M, et al. Randomised controlled trial of doxorubicin-eluting beads vs conventional chemoembolisation for hepatocellular carcinoma. *Br J Cancer.* 2014;111(2):255–264.
6. Frangakis C, Geschwind JF, Kim D, et al. Chemoembolization decreases drop-off risk of hepatocellular carcinoma patients on the liver transplant list. *Cardiovasc Intervent Radiol,* 2011;34(6):1254–1261.
7. Georgiades, CS, Hong K, D'Angelo, M, et al. Safety and efficacy of transarterial chemoembolization in patients with unresectable hepatocellular carcinoma and portal vein thrombosis. *J Vasc Interv Radiol,* 2005;16(12):1653–1659.
8. Lencioni R, de Baere T, Soulen MC, et al. Lipiodol transarterial chemoembolization for hepatocellular carcinoma: a systematic review of efficacy and safety data. *Hepatology.* 2016;64(1):106–116.
9. Wallace D, Cowling TE, Walker K, et al. Liver transplantation outcomes after transarterial chemotherapy for hepatocellular carcinoma. *Br J Surg.* 2020;107(9):1183–1191.

23 Hepatic Malignancies: Radioembolization

Ahmed Gabr, MD, Riad Salem, MD, MBA, and Robert J. Lewandowski, MD

Introduction

Radioembolization, a form of intraarterial brachytherapy, is a technique where particles of glass or resin, impregnated with the isotope yttrium-90 (90Y), are infused through a catheter directly into the hepatic arteries. 90Y is a pure beta emitter that decays to stable zirconium-90 with a physical half-life of 64.1 hours. The average energy of the beta particles is 0.9367 MeV, with a mean tissue penetration of 2.5 mm, and maximum penetration of 10 mm. Once the particles are infused through the catheter into the hepatic artery, they travel to the distal arterioles within the tumors, where the beta emissions from the isotope irradiate the tumor.

Indications

1. Glass microspheres:
   a. TheraSphere (Boston Scientific, Natick, MA) was approved by the U.S. Food and Drug Administration (FDA) in 1999 under a humanitarian device exemption, defined as safe and probably beneficial for the treatment of unresectable hepatocellular carcinoma (HCC) with or without portal vein thrombosis (PVT), or as a bridge to transplantation in patients who could have appropriately positioned catheters. This device is also approved for the treatment of liver neoplasia in Europe and Canada.
2. Resin microspheres
   a. SIR-Spheres (Sirtex Medical, Lane Cove, Australia) were granted premarket approval by the FDA in 2002, defined as safe and effective for the treatment of metastatic colorectal cancer to the liver with concomitant use of floxuridine.

This device is also approved in Europe, Australia, and various Asian countries for the treatment of liver neoplasia.

Contraindications

Absolute
1. Contraindications to angiography
   a. Uncorrectable coagulopathy
   b. Severe renal insufficiency
   c. Severe anaphylactoid reaction to iodinated contrast agents
   d. Severe peripheral vascular disease precluding arterial access
2. Immediate life-threatening extrahepatic disease
3. Inability to prevent 90Y delivery to the gastrointestinal (GI) tract
4. Hepatopulmonary lung shunting
   a. For TheraSphere, the upper limit of what can be administered to the lungs is based on the lung dose, not lung shunt fraction (LSF) (30 Gy per infusion, 50 Gy cumulative).
   b. For SIR-Spheres, infusion is limited by the LSF (20%).

Relative
1. PVT
   a. Patients with main PVT have poor prognosis; Child–Pugh A patients with main PVT may be safely treated
   b. Radioembolization is not contraindicated in lobar or segmental PVT
2. Poor hepatic reserve
   a. Total bilirubin >2 mg per dL
   b. Risks may be mitigated by selective radioembolization
3. Poor performance status
   a. Eastern Cooperative Oncology Group (ECOG) >2
4. Biliary obstruction
   a. Risks of infectious complications significantly higher in the setting of a compromised sphincter of Oddi

Preprocedure Preparation

1. Patient selection
   a. History, physical examination, and assessment of performance status
   b. Clinical lab workup: complete blood count with differential, blood urea nitrogen, serum creatinine, serum electrolytes, liver function, albumin, lac tate dehydrogenase [LDH], prothrombin time [PT], tumor marker assay: carcinoembryonic antigen [CEA], a-fetoprotein [AFP])
   c. Chest computed tomography (CT) for assessment of lung metastases
   d. CT/magnetic resonance imaging (MRI) scan of the abdomen and pelvis for staging with assessment of portal vein patency
   e. Arteriography/macroaggregated albumin (MAA) lung shunting study
2. Patient preparation
   a. Patients are nil per os (NPO) 6 hours prior to the procedure
      (1) Medications are allowed with sips of water
   b. Peripheral intravenous line placed prior to the procedure
      (1) Hydration of patients with renal insufficiency

Procedure

1. Pretreatment angiography: To define hepatic arterial anatomy, allow embolization of communicating vessels that may lead to aberrant microsphere deposition, and facilitate radiation dosimetry.

a. SMA (3 mL per second for 30 mL)
   (1) Allows for the identification of a replaced right hepatic, replaced proper hepatic, replaced common hepatic, accessory right hepatic, and patency of the portal vein as well as the rare parasitizing of blood flow from the SMA to the liver.
   (2) Retrograde flow (from tumor sumping or celiac occlusion/stenosis) into the gastroduodenal artery (GDA) is also assessed.
b. Celiac artery (3 to 4 mL per second for 12 to 15 mL)
   (1) Allows for the assessment of celiac anatomy and identifies the presence of any possible variants, including a replaced left hepatic artery arising off the left gastric (gastrohepatic trunk), as well as the right and left inferior phrenic arteries. The dorsal pancreatic artery may arise off the celiac.
c. Common hepatic artery (microcatheter; 3 mL per second for 10 to 12 mL)
   (1) Complex variants include:
      (a) A replaced right hepatic artery off the SMA with trifurcation from the CHA into a GDA, left hepatic, and middle hepatic arteries. In such cases, a right gastric is often seen and unless segmental infusions of radioembolization are planned, the GDA/right gastric should be embolized. This functionally converts the CHA into a left hepatic artery.
      (b) Trifurcation of the CHA into a GDA, right, and left hepatic arteries. Given the low margin of error if reflux occurs from a lobar or segmental infusion, the GDA should be embolized in this case, particularly if the more embolic resin microspheres are being administered.
      (c) "Double hepatic" artery: a very early takeoff of the right hepatic artery. Unless sufficient contrast is injected and refluxed to the origin of the celiac, this vessel may be missed.
d. Left hepatic angiogram (microcatheter; 2 mL per second for 8 mL)
   (1) Vessels of interest include the left inferior phrenic artery, accessory left gastric artery, inferior esophageal artery, right gastric artery, and falciform artery. Prophylactic embolization of these vessels may decrease adverse events following radioembolization, such as abdominal pain, gastritis, and ulceration. Furthermore, delayed imaging of the left hepatic angiogram is recommended in order to confirm the lack of opacification of the coronary vein. Finally, injection of the left hepatic artery should outline where there is flow to segment 4 via the medial branch. If the medial branch is absent, a separate middle hepatic artery should be sought, usually off the right hepatic artery.
   (2) If a gastrohepatic trunk is identified, a few vascular observations should be made. Once all of the gastric vessels have branched off, the trunk travels in a horizontal direction. All vessels arising from the horizontal portion of the gastrohepatic trunk are extrahepatic and provide flow to the esophagus and stomach. When delivering glass microspheres, injection should be distal to these vessels. With resin microspheres, these extrahepatic arteries should be embolized; otherwise, vascular redistribution could be considered.
e. Right hepatic angiogram (microcatheter; 2 to 3 mL per second for 10 to 12 mL)
   (1) Vessels of interest include the middle hepatic artery, supraduodenal, and cystic artery.
f. Phrenic arteries (microcatheter; 1 to 2 mL per second for 4 to 6 mL)
   (1) If a portion of the liver tumor (especially HCC) is not opacified by hepatic arteriography, interrogating these vessels may identify the remainder of the blood supply to the tumors.

2. MAA administration
   a. The LSF fraction of Tc-99m MAA observed in the lungs relative to the total Tc-99m MAA activity observed can be determined by infusing 4 to 5 mCi of Tc-99m-labeled MAA particles through the catheter into the desired liver distribution and obtaining planar imaging.

b. The Tc-99m MAA scan can also demonstrate the presence of any stomach or bowel perfusion, especially if single-photon emission computed tomography (SPECT) imaging is performed. Thus, it is recommended that MAA injection be performed once all vessels of concern have been embolized. The shunt evaluation allows the physician to plan for radioembolization therapy and minimize any uncertainty in microspheres distribution at the time of treatment.

3. Dosimetry
   a. Glass microspheres
      (1) As described in the product insert, TheraSphere consists of insoluble glass microspheres where 90Y is an integral constituent of the glass. The mean sphere diameter ranges from 20 to 30 μm. Each milligram contains between 22,000 microspheres and 73,000 microspheres. TheraSphere is supplied in 0.05 mL of sterile, pyrogen-free water contained in a 0.3-mL vee-bottom vial secured within a 12-mm clear acrylic vial shield. TheraSphere are dispensed weekly by the manufacturer (BTG, London, UK) on Wednesdays and are calibrated for noon, Eastern Standard Time of the following Sunday and are available in the activity sizes from 3 GBq (81 mCi) to 20 GBq (540 mCi). The activity per microsphere at calibration is approximately 2,500 Bq.

      (2) The recommended activity of TheraSphere that should be delivered to a lobe of the liver containing tumor is between 80 Gy and 150 Gy. This wide range exists to give the treating physician clinical flexibility.

      (3) Patients with significant cirrhosis should be treated more conservatively (80 to 100 Gy), whereas patients without cirrhosis may be treated more aggressively (100 to 150 Gy).

      (4) Assuming TheraSphere 90Y microspheres distribute in a uniform manner throughout the liver and 90Y undergoes complete decay in situ, radioactivity required to deliver the desired dose to the liver can be calculated using the following formula:

$$A\ (GBq) = [D\ (Gy) \times M\ (kg)] / 50.$$

Given that a fraction of the microspheres will flow into the pulmonary circulation without lodging in the arterioles, when LSF is taken into account, the actual dose delivered to the target volume becomes

$$D\ (Gy) = [A\ (GBq) \times 50 \times (1\text{-}LSF)] / M\ (kg).$$

A is the activity delivered to the liver, D is the absorbed/delivered dose to the target liver mass, and M is the target liver mass. Liver volume (mL) is estimated with CT, and then converted to mass using a conversion factor of 1.03 mg per mL. Note that the dosimetry for TheraSphere is independent of tumor burden.

   b. Resin microspheres
      (1) As described in the product insert, SIR-Spheres consist of biocompatible resin-based microspheres containing 90Y with a size between 20 μm and 60 μm in diameter. SIR-Spheres are a permanent implant and are provided in a vial with water for injection. Each vial contains 3 GBq of 90Y (at the time of calibration) in a total of 5 mL water for injection. Each vial contains 40 to 80 million microspheres. Consequently, the activity per microsphere at calibration for SIR-Spheres is much lower than that of TheraSphere (50 Bq vs. 2,500 Bq, respectively). SIR-Spheres are dispensed three times per week by the manufacturer (Sirtex, Lane Cove, Australia) and are calibrated for 6 pm Eastern Standard Time on the date of treatment. The shelf life is 24 hours following the calibration date and time. Just as with TheraSphere, assuming SIR-Spheres 90Y microspheres distribute in a uniform manner throughout the liver and undergo complete decay in

situ, radioactivity delivered to the liver can be calculated by incorporating the body surface area and the estimate of tumor burden as follows:

$$A\ (GBq) = BSA\ (m^2) - 0.2 + (\%\ tumor\ involvement\ /\ 100),$$
$$where\ BSA\ is\ body\ surface\ area.$$

4. Radioembolization
   a. The selected catheter is advanced into the treatment vessel of choice as determined by pretreatment angiography and either the TheraSphere or SIR-Spheres administration device is utilized for microsphere infusion.
   b. A treatment paradigm that parallels transarterial chemoembolization is recommended, that is, lobar or sub/segmental infusions.
      (1) If a treating physician insists on treatment to the entire liver at once, then a "bilobar lobar" infusion is recommended. This involves placement of the catheter in the one followed by the other hepatic artery where infusion is performed.

Postprocedure Management

1. Outpatient management
   a. Patients are discharged home following the appropriate management of femoral arteriotomy.
   b. Patients are placed on a proton pump inhibitor for 7 to 10 days following treatment.
2. Follow-up
   a. Clinical assessment: Patients are assessed for treatment-related side effects (e.g., fatigue, nausea, fevers, abdominal pain) and potential complications (e.g., radiation cholecystitis, GI ulcer).
   b. Laboratory: Tumor markers (AFP, CEA, CA-19-9, chromogranin A, CA-125), complete blood count, liver function tests, and general chemistries are obtained 4 to 6 weeks postprocedure.
   c. Imaging: Cross-sectional imaging (triphasic CT, dynamic gadolinium-enhanced MRI, perfusion imaging) and functional imaging positron emission tomography (PET) when appropriate are obtained at that time to assess the results of therapy. If bilobar disease, the contralateral lobe is usually treated shortly following the assessment of response. Completion evaluation and assessment of response (CT/PET/MR/tumor markers) are usually complete once both lobes have been treated and 30 to 60 days have elapsed from the last treatment.

Results

1. HCC
   a. Early-stage HCC
      (1) Curative intent: Radiation segmentectomy in solitary tumors ≤5 cm and preserved liver function have high response rate (85% to 90%) and 75% 5-year overall survival rates, which is comparable to survival outcomes of surgical resection and ablation (1).
      (2) Bridging to liver transplantation: Patients with tumors within Milan Criteria benefit of Y90 bridging therapy by achieving tumor response and delaying progression. Time-to-progression of radiation segmentectomy is often >26 months which benefits patients on transplant list (2). A recent single-center intention-to-treat analysis showed that drop-out rate due to disease progression in Y90 treated patients awaiting liver transplant can be as low as 5.2%.
      (3) Downstaging/Bridging to resection: Unresectable solitary HCC with preserved liver function and no signs of portal hypertension can be treated with radiation lobectomy (Lobar Y90) or modified radiation lobectomy (Lobar Y90 + Radiation segmentectomy Y90) to achieve tumor necrosis and stimulate hypertrophy of contralateral hepatic lobe, and subsequently allowing for future surgical candidacy.

b. Intermediate-stage HCC
   (1) Overall survival: Recent studies have shown that intermediate-stage (BCLC B) patients can have a median overall survival of 25 months in Child–Pugh A patients and 15 months in Child–Pugh B patients.
   (2) Time to progression in BCLC B patients is 13 months (median), ranging from 8 to 26 months (3).
c. Advanced-stage HCC
   (1) Treatment in patients with PVT is safe, with a median survival of 8 to 14 months.
   (2) Favorable prognostic factors include baseline bilirubin ≤1.2 mg per dL, tumor burden <50%, and PVTT limited to segmental (third order) of portal vein. In such patients, median overall survival is 14.1 (CI: 6.9 to 21.3) months (4).
   (3) In two major phase III randomized controlled trials comparing radioembolization versus sorafenib in patients with locally advanced HCC, overall survival outcomes were not different between treatment arms. However, patients in radioembolization arm exhibited better quality of life and improved toxicity profile (5,6).
   (4) Personalized dosimetry aiming at delivering a radiation dose of at least 205 Gy has been found to be significantly associated with higher response rates. These findings encourage adoption of personalized dosimetry in future randomized controlled trial and question the interpretations of recent trials comparing radioembolization versus sorafenib (4).
2. Metastatic colorectal disease to the liver
   a. First-line setting
      (1) Combination with chemotherapy has been recently studied. The addition of radioembolization to FOLFOX-based first-line chemotherapy in patients with liver-dominant or liver-only metastatic colorectal cancer did not improve progression-free survival but it significantly delayed disease progression in the liver (7,8).
   b. Second-line setting
      (1) Currently a phase III trial (EPOCH) is evaluating radioembolization in patients with metastatic colorectal carcinoma of the liver who have failed first-line chemotherapy (9).
   c. Salvage setting
      (1) Median survival in the salvage setting (after failing at minimum second-line systemic therapies) is approximately 10.5 months (10)
3. Cholangiocarcinoma
   a. Median survival approaches 11 months, similar to systemic therapy (gemcitabine and cisplatin). Peripheral (mass-forming) cholangiocarcinoma may respond, whereas infiltrative tumors often have poor prognosis.

Adverse Events

1. Post-radioembolization syndrome
   a. Fatigue
   b. Abdominal pain
   c. Nausea
   d. Anorexia
   e. Fevers
2. Idiosyncratic reaction: During the immediate postprocedural time following radioembolization, patients may experience a rare and unusual reaction, nearly identical to that obtained in patients receiving urokinase, with clinical symptoms of rigors and alterations in hemodynamics.
3. Complications
   a. Abscess
   b. Biloma

   c. Gastritis/ulceration

   d. Radiation cholecystitis

Management of Complications

1. Postradioembolization syndrome: The typical side effects of radioembolization are managed conservatively. If required, over-the-counter analgesics can be utilized.

2. Idiosyncratic reaction

   a. Management is supportive, including fluids if hypotensive, as well as diphenhydramine and meperidine.

   b. This reaction is short-lived and usually lasts less than 1 hour.

3. Complications

   a. Abscess: Pyogenic liver abscesses require antibiotic therapy directed at the causative organism(s) and, in most cases, drainage. For a small abscess, antibiotic therapy without drainage may suffice.

   b. Biloma: Percutaneous treatments include biloma drainage, percutaneous transhepatic biliary drainage, or biliary leak site embolization/sclerosis.

   c. Gastritis/ulceration: Treatment options include acid suppression. A nonhealing ulcer may ultimately require surgery if symptoms are severe/persistent.

   d. Radiation cholecystitis: The majority of patients whose cystic artery is directly exposed to radioactive particles recover asymptomatically or with minimal supportive care despite abnormal radiographic findings. Antibiotics and/or cholecystectomy may be warranted in certain instances.

References

1. Lewandowski RJ, Gabr A, Abouchaleh N, et al. Radiation segmentectomy: potential curative therapy for early hepatocellular carcinoma. *Radiology*. 2018;287(3):1050–1058.
2. Salem R, Gordon AC, Mouli S, et al. Y90 radioembolization significantly prolongs time to progression compared with chemoembolization in patients with hepatocellular carcinoma. *Gastroenterology*. 2016;151(6):1155–1163.e2.
3. Salem R, Gabr A, Riaz A, et al. Institutional decision to adopt Y90 as primary treatment for hepatocellular carcinoma informed by a 1,000-patient 15-year experience. *Hepatology*. 2018;68(4):1429–1440.
4. Garin E, Tzelikas L, Guiu B, et al. Major impact of personalized dosimetry using 90Y loaded glass microspheres SIRT in HCC: final overall survival analysis of a multicenter randomized phase II study (DOSISPHERE-01). *J Clin Oncol*. 2020;38(4_suppl):516.
5. Vilgrain V, Pereira H, Assenat E, et al. Efficacy and safety of selective internal radiotherapy with yttrium-90 resin microspheres compared with sorafenib in locally advanced and inoperable hepatocellular carcinoma (SARAH): an open-label randomised controlled phase 3 trial. *Lancet Oncol*. 2017;18(12):1624–1636.
6. Chow PKH, Gandhi M, Tan SB, et al. SIRveNIB: selective internal radiation therapy versus sorafenib in Asia-Pacific patients with hepatocellular carcinoma. *J Clin Oncol*. 2018;36(19):1913–1921.
7. van Hazel GA, Heinemann V, Sharma NK, et al. SIRFLOX: Randomized phase III trial comparing first-line mFOLFOX6 (plus or minus bevacizumab) Versus mFOLFOX6 (plus or minus bevacizumab) plus selective internal radiation therapy in patients with metastatic colorectal cancer. *J Clin Oncol*. 2016;34(15):1723–1731.
8. Wasan HS, Gibbs P, Sharma NK, et al. First-line selective internal radiotherapy plus chemotherapy versus chemotherapy alone in patients with liver metastases from colorectal cancer (FOXFIRE, SIRFLOX, and FOXFIRE-Global): a combined analysis of three multicentre, randomised, phase 3 trials. *Lancet Oncol*. 2017;18(9):1159–1171.
9. Chauhan N, Mulcahy MF, Salem R, et al. TheraSphere Yttrium-90 glass microspheres combined with chemotherapy versus chemotherapy alone in second-line treatment of patients with metastatic colorectal carcinoma of the liver: protocol for the EPOCH phase 3 randomized clinical trial. *JMIR Res Protoc*. 2019;8(1):e11545.
10. Hickey R, Mouli S, Kulik L, et al. Independent analysis of albumin-bilirubin grade in a 765-patient cohort treated with transarterial locoregional therapy for hepatocellular carcinoma. *J Vasc Interv Radiol*. 2016;27(6):795–802.

24 Uterine Fibroid Embolization

James B. Spies, MD, MPH

Introduction

Uterine fibroid embolization (UFE) was first reported in 1995 and rapidly became accepted into practice around the world. There has been extensive study of the outcomes from embolization of fibroids, including several randomized trials comparing UFE to surgery, leading the American College of Obstetricians and Gynecologist Practice Bulletin on Alternatives to Hysterectomy in the Management of Leiomyomas states that uterine artery embolization is a safe and effective option for women with uterine fibroids (1). This finding was confirmed in the most recent systematic review by the Cochrane Collaborative (2).

Indications

1. Heavy menstrual bleeding
   a. Fibroids typically cause heavy menstrual bleeding without interperiod bleeding. The exception is submucosal fibroids, which may, in addition, cause interperiod bleeding and metrorrhagia. In nearly all cases, fibroids must be deep within the uterus distorting the endometrial cavity to cause heavy bleeding. If only serosal fibroids or small intramural fibroids are present and there is heavy menstrual bleeding, consider other possible causes prior to proceeding with embolization.
2. Pelvic pressure
   a. The most common bulk-related symptoms are pressure, heaviness, or bloating. These symptoms typically are worse around the time of the menstrual period. They respond well to UFE. It is important to remember that some perimenstrual bloating is normal, which will likely persist despite a successful UFE.
3. Pelvic pain
   a. Fibroids usually cause menstrual cramps or low-grade aching pain. Less frequently, they may cause shooting or severe pain. When severe pain is the predominant symptom, it is important to consider other causes of female pelvic pain such as endometriosis. Also, patients often will experience pain or tenderness over one particular fibroid. If the fibroids are mostly on one side of the pelvis and the patient has pain on the other, consider them as source
4. Urinary urgency, frequency, incontinence, retention, and hydronephrosis
   a. Uterine fibroids commonly compress the urinary bladder causing urgency and frequency, which respond well to embolization. Urinary incontinence is less common, and in women who have had prior vaginal deliveries, the incontinence may be of multifactorial origin. Hydronephrosis may be caused by a substantially enlarged fibroid uterus and usually resolves after UFE. However, a follow-up renal sonogram is needed 3 to 6 months after treatment to ensure resolution.

Contraindications

Absolute
1. Pregnancy
2. Suspected leiomyosarcoma or endometrial, cervical, or ovarian malignancy
   a. Preoperative embolization is occasionally requested prior to surgical resection of a suspected malignancy and this is an acceptable use of embolization, but UFE should never be considered as a sole therapy for a suspected leiomyosarcoma.

Relative

Many of these relative contraindications are circumstances that can be managed with additional care and should not exclude the use of embolization.

1. Coagulopathy or requirement for continuous anticoagulation
   a. Similar and greater risks of bleeding are present with surgery. The risks can be reduced or eliminated with the use of an arterial closure device at the puncture site, or radial artery access.
2. Renal insufficiency
   a. Contrast use should be limited and the patient should be well hydrated prior to the procedure.
3. Prior severe allergic reaction to iodinated contrast material
   a. Corticosteroid premedication can ameliorate this risk. It is important that appropriate drugs and equipment be immediately available and that there be secure intravenous (IV) access. Anesthesia support may be helpful for those with previous airway compromise during allergic reaction.
4. Desire for pregnancy within 2 years.
   a. Although patients can become pregnant and carry pregnancies to term, the relative likelihood of that occurring after UFE may be less than with myomectomy, at least within the first 2 years after treatment (3). However, the evidence supporting this is weak and therefore not definitive. In addition, fertility outcomes after repeat myomectomy are quite poor and therefore embolization may be the better choice. Also for those who are poor surgical risks or who have declined surgery, embolization may be a good option, with a clear understanding that reproductive outcomes are uncertain.

Preprocedure Preparation

1. Preprocedure history, physical examination, and consultation with an interventional radiologist
   a. Gynecologic examination by a gynecologist within 1 year
   b. Assessment of uterine size (by weeks of pregnancy) helpful during abdominal examination
2. Imaging evaluation
   a. Contrast-enhanced magnetic resonance imaging (MRI) is the preferred imaging assessment because it allows accurate assessment of fibroid number, size, and location as well as detection of adenomyosis.
   b. Transabdominal and transvaginal ultrasound examination of good quality may be a suitable substitute for an MRI in a resource-limited practice environment.
3. Laboratory evaluation
   a. Current Pap smear, which should be normal or indicating enhanced routine surveillance. For Pap smear findings indicating the need for colposcopy or cone biopsy, these should be completed if possible before proceeding with UFE.
   b. Endometrial biopsy when menstrual bleeding is markedly prolonged or when there is intermittent bleeding between cycles. A useful rule of thumb is biopsy for menstrual periods that are routinely longer than 10 days or when there is bleeding more frequent than every 21 days.
   c. Complete blood count, serum electrolytes (including serum creatinine), and a urine or serum pregnancy test in those at risk of pregnancy before the procedure. Given the importance of excluding pregnancy, we obtain a urine pregnancy test in all premenopausal women immediately prior to the procedure.
   d. Coagulation panel only in patients suspected of having a coagulopathy or who are anticoagulated prior to the procedure.
4. Patient preparation
   a. Patient should have nothing by mouth except normal medications with a sip of water for at least 6 hours prior to the procedure.

b. Foley catheter in the bladder prior to the procedure can be considered. This is for patient comfort and to keep bladder empty, which will reduce fluoroscopic dose, but with a small but real risk of catheter-associated urinary tract infection.

c. The patient should have the anticipated postprocedure recovery explained to them and they should be instructed on the anticipated postprocedure pain and the plan for its management.

d. Many interventionalists give a single dose of prophylactic antibiotics such as cefazolin 1 g IV, although there is no evidence that this has any impact on infection rates postprocedure.

e. The medications needed for postprocedure management should be prepared and ready to administer immediately at the end of the procedure.

f. Some interventionalists use dexamethasone 10 mg intravenously just prior to the procedure, which decreases periprocedural inflammation, pain, and nausea.

g. An IV line should be placed and the patient should be hydrated. One approach is to infuse 500 mL of normal saline over the 2 hours just before and during the procedure, with the rate reduced to 125 mL per hour thereafter.

h. Patient is sedated at the beginning of the procedure, with continuous monitoring by an anesthesia provider or a nurse trained in moderate sedation.

Procedure

Uterine Artery Catheterization

1. Femoral approach

    a. Either unilateral or bilateral femoral puncture can be used, with a 4-Fr or 5-Fr sheath typically used at each puncture site.

    b. A Cobra, Rösch Inferior Mesenteric (RIM), or other curved 4-Fr or 5-Fr catheter is passed from the right femoral sheath across the bifurcation of the aorta into the left hypogastric artery.

    c. Either that same 4-Fr or 5-Fr catheter, or, more commonly, a 0.027-in diameter microcatheter, is advanced into the uterine artery using a digital road map for guidance. The uterine artery usually arises as either the first branch off the inferior gluteal artery or as part of a genitourinary trunk at the level of the bifurcation of the superior gluteal and inferior gluteal arteries. Oblique positioning of the angiographic unit is essential for best visualization of the vessel because it is important to have good visualization of the uterine artery origin to allow easy access. Often the left anterior oblique is used for both uterine arteries. If one oblique does not show the origin of the vessel well, then the opposite oblique should be used.

    d. A popular alternative approach is to use the Roberts Catheter (Cook Inc, Bloomington, IN) for selection of the uterine artery. This long-armed recurved catheter is retracted at the groin entry site, which advances the tip into the uterine artery. It may also be used with a microcatheter.

    e. The uterine artery in patients with fibroids is typically tortuous, with a general U-shaped configuration. It descends to the level of the cardinal ligament, turns medially along that ligament, and courses to the uterine margin where it ascends along the side of the uterus. The microcatheter (or catheter) is advanced well into the uterine artery. Ideally, it would be advanced beyond any identifiable branches in the transverse segment of the vessel to avoid misembolization into branches to adjacent structures. However, due to severe tortuosity, advancing the catheter so far into the vessel may cause spasm in many patients. Thus, a balance between the ideal position and the avoidance of spasm is needed, and more proximal placement may be preferred. Spasm should be avoided because it may lead to a false end point, with recanalization shortly after catheter removal.

f. If a bilateral approach is to be used, the above process should be repeated from the opposite side into the right uterine artery prior to filming and embolization to allow simultaneous treatment.

g. If a unilateral approach is used, uterine arteriogram and embolization are done on the left, and then a Waltman loop is used to move the catheter into the right hypogastric artery. Alternatively, a RIM catheter can just be pulled back until its end engages the origin of the right hypogastric artery and a microcatheter used to cannulate the uterine artery with the same technique used on the left.

2. Radial approach

Radial access (see Chapter 1) for UAE is growing in popularity and has advantages of early ambulation and high patient satisfaction. There is a small risk of hand injury and stroke, given that the catheter does cross the origin(s) of cerebral vessels.

Embolization Technique

1. Embolic choice and technique

a. There are several embolic materials currently available for use in the United States and Europe. The two best studied are particle polyvinyl alcohol (PVA) (Contour, Boston Scientific, Natick, MA; Bearing, Merit Medical, South Jordan UT: Polyvinyl Alcohol Particles, Cook Inc, Bloomington, IN) and tris-acryl gelatin microspheres (Embosphere Microspheres, Merit Medical, South Jordan, UT) (4,5). Spherical PVA (Contour SE, Boston Scientific, Natick, MA) has been shown to be *inferior* in fibroid infarction and should not be used for fibroid embolization (5,6). Other embolic materials that have been cleared by the U.S. Food and Drug Administration (FDA) for embolization include acrylamide PVA hydrogel spheres (Bead Block, Boston Scientific, Natick, MA), Polyzene F-coated hydrogel spheres (Embozene Microspheres, Varian Medical Systems, Palo Alto, CA), and polyethylene glycol (PEG) spheres (Hydropearl, Terumo Interventional Systems, Somerset, NJ).

b. The embolic material is injected in small aliquots using the flow in the uterine vessels to carry the embolic material to the fibroid arterial supply. Fibroid branches are recognized as large, generally curvilinear branches that surround each fibroid before penetrating it. These are the targets for occlusion. The goal is *not* to occlude the entire uterine artery but to leave it with slow flow or near stasis, depending on the type of embolic material used. Supplemental gelatin sponge plugs or coils should not be used as this causes significantly greater pain due to enhanced myometrial ischemia and because these may completely occlude the uterine arteries permanently. This will prevent repeat embolization if the patient develops new fibroids.

2. Ovarian supply and embolization

a. There is occasionally additional supply to the uterus and fibroids from the ovarian arteries. Although only present in about 5% of patients, this can impact outcome. Because it can be difficult to determine whether there is supply to fibroids from ovarian arteries, assessment preprocedure by MRI or at the end of the embolization procedure with aortography is indicated in most patients, particularly in cases where there is a disproportionately small uterine artery, when there is clearly nonperfused tissue seen on uterine arteriography or in repeat embolization procedures.

b. Ovarian embolization is not well studied, and although there is some evidence that ovarian artery embolization does not significantly increase the risk of ovarian injury (7), consulting with the patient about possible ovarian injury may be appropriate prior to proceeding.

c. Selective catheterization of the ovarian artery may be best accomplished with a Mikaelsson catheter (AngioDynamics, Queensbury, NY). A microcatheter should be used and advanced into the vessel about one-third the distance to the ovary to ensure no reflux occurs into the aorta.

d. Ovarian embolization is performed with particulate or spherical embolic material until the fibroid branches are occluded. Flow is generally very sluggish because of severe spasm typically seen with ovarian catheterization.

Postprocedure Management

1. General care of the patient
   a. Most interventionalists observe the patient in hospital overnight, although it is increasingly common to discharge same day. The postprocedure treatment is usually the same for overnight or same-day patients.
   b. Diet advanced slowly as tolerated. Nausea can be an issue if advanced too quickly.
   c. The Foley catheter (if used) can be removed as soon as the patient is ambulatory.
   d. IV hydration should be continued until oral liquids are well tolerated.

2. Pain management
   a. There is usually moderate pain for 2 to 6 hours after embolization due to transient myometrial ischemia. The severity of pain is likely dependent on the degree of occlusion of the uterine arteries—overembolization should be avoided.
   b. Intraarterial preservative-free lidocaine injected into the uterine arteries at the end of embolization significantly reduces pain after UFE (8). This represents an "off label" use, but based on the extensive history of intraarterial use in angiography, appears to be safe.
   c. Hypogastric nerve block has also been demonstrated to significantly reduce pain after embolization (4). It is an invasive procedure, and great care should be exercised to avoid intravenous injection, which can cause seizures. There also have been rare cases of osteomyelitis and discitis, and avoiding the intervertebral disc is important.
   d. While the mainstay of intravenous pain management is IV narcotics, intravenous nonsteroidal antiinflammatory agents, and acetaminophen are important components of a balanced pain management plan. Ketorolac is typically given 15 to 30 mg IV every 6 hours regardless of pain and the PCA narcotics are administered by PCA pump to supplement. In the first few hours, the typical PCA dose may be inadequate, regardless of the medication used. Supplemental doses may be needed. IV acetaminophen at a dose of 1 g is also a powerful adjunct pain medication to address incompletely controlled pain.
   e. At the time of discharge, the patient is transitioned to oral medications. Typically, an oral nonsteroidal antiinflammatory such as ibuprofen or naproxen is used at regular interval dosing for 4 days or 5 days. This is supplemented by oral oxycodone/acetaminophen or hydrocodone/acetaminophen for intermittent use as needed for more severe pain. The peak pain after discharge is usually on postembolization days 2 and 3.
   f. Most patients will experience intermittent cramping, fatigue, and malaise, with one-third having a low-grade fever for several days. Usually, 7- to 10-day recovery is required to resume full activity.

3. Nausea
   a. The second most common symptom needing medical management is nausea. This may be prevented to a large degree by prophylactic doses of ondansetron (4 mg IV at the time of the procedure with an additional 4 mg IV 6 hours later). Additional doses can be given, along with oral or rectal promethazine or other antiemetics.

Results

1. Short-term outcomes
   a. Both menorrhagia and bulk-related symptoms (pain, pressure, and urinary symptoms) are improved in 80% to 95% of patients, depending on the study reviewed.
   b. Reintervention is needed in approximately 5% to 10% of patients within the first year due to lack of symptom improvement.
2. Long-term outcomes
   a. UFE has been demonstrated to be effective compared to hysterectomy in randomized trials at 5 years (5) and 10 years (6).
   b. UFE has a similar level of symptom control compared to myomectomy.
   c. There are insufficient data to determine whether myomectomy or UFE is preferred for women seeking to become pregnant, although results from one comparative trial suggest that there are better outcomes with myomectomy in the first 2 years in women who have not had prior fibroid surgery (3).

Complications

1. Fibroid passage
   a. Fibroid passage, which occurs in about 5% of cases, is the most common serious complication and presents as severe menstrual cramping, with or without discharge, tissue passage, or heavy bleeding (9). It may also have a more chronic presentation, with persisting vaginal discharge, often described as watery or clear mucous, which may become superinfected. This occurs most commonly 3 weeks to 6 months after the procedure and most frequently with large intracavitary fibroids or large fibroids with a large submucosal interface.
   b. Diagnosis may be made by vaginal examination if there is either tissue in the vagina or a dilated cervix. Impending passage may have the same symptoms but with a negative vaginal examination. Pelvic MRI examination will show tissue descending in the endometrial cavity, pointing to the cervix with occasional dilation of the internal cervical os. With more advanced passage, the cervix may be dilated with tissue extending from the endometrial cavity into the vagina.
2. Pulmonary embolus
   a. The most common life-threatening complication, with an incidence of about 1 in 400.
   b. Transient hypercoagulability occurs after UFE (similar impact but to a lesser degree than the hypercoagulability after surgery).
   c. Use of intermittent pneumatic compression devices on the legs may reduce the risk. For high-risk patients, low–molecular-weight heparin prophylaxis should be considered.
3. Misembolization
   a. Due to embolic material occluding the vascular supply to adjacent organs. Injury to other organs (other than the ovaries) or to the skin occurs very rarely, likely less than 1 in 1,000 patients for experienced interventionalists.
4. Myometrial injury
   a. Myometrial injury is also rare, about 1 in 500. Diagnosis should be suspected when pain is persisting and not improving after 4 to 5 days postembolization or when pain is severe enough to require readmission. Contrast-enhanced MRI will show nonenhancing areas of myometrium.
5. Loss of ovarian reserve/ovarian failure
   a. May occur as a result of uterine embolization and is age-dependent. Approximately 5% of women over 45 years old may have temporary or permanent amenorrhea after UFE. At age 40, the likelihood is closer to 1%.

Management of Complications

1. Fibroid passage: This is the most common complication requiring reintervention.
   a. Can be managed with observation if uncomplicated, although if infection occurs, oral or IV antibiotics are given.
   b. Dilation and curettage/hysteroscopic resection or manual extraction of the fibroid is often necessary. If the fibroid cannot be extracted, hysterectomy may be required.

2. Misembolization
   a. Management is usually conservative, with local wound care for minor skin injuries. Plastic surgery consult can be considered for more severe injuries that result in skin ulceration.
   b. Bladder injuries may require urologic evaluation and occasionally intervention.

3. Myometrial injury
   a. Initial management is conservative, with reinstitution of IV narcotics while assessing myometrial repair with serial contrast-enhanced MRI studies.
   b. If there is severe uterine injury, hysterectomy may be needed.

4. Loss of ovarian reserve/ovarian failure
   a. Treatment is conservative, with some women regaining menstrual cycles several months after embolization.
   b. For bothersome menopausal symptoms, the patient's gynecologist should be consulted to consider managing symptoms with hormone replacement therapy.

R e f e r e n c e s

1. American College of Obstetricians and Gynecologists. ACOG practice bulletin. Alternatives to hysterectomy in the management of leiomyomas. *Obstet Gynecol.* 2008;112(2 Pt 1): 387–400.
2. Gupta JK, Sinha A, Lumsden MA, et al. Uterine artery embolization for symptomatic uterine fibroids. *Cochrane Database Syst Rev.* 2012;5:CD005073.
3. Mara M, Maskova J, Fucikova Z, et al. Midterm clinical and first reproductive results of a randomized controlled trial comparing uterine fibroid embolization and myomectomy. *Cardiovasc Intervent Radiol.* 2008;31(1):73–85.
4. Yoon J, Valenti D, Muchantef K, et al. Superior hypogastric nerve block as post-uterine artery embolization analgesia: a randomized and double-blind clinical trial. *Radiology.* 2018;289(1):248–254.
5. Moss JG, Cooper KG, Khaund A, et al. Randomised comparison of uterine artery embolisation (UAE) with surgical treatment in patients with symptomatic uterine fibroids (REST trial): 5-year results. *BJOG.* 2011;118(8):936–944.
6. de Bruijn AM, Ankum WM, Reekers JA, et al. Uterine artery embolization vs hysterectomy in the treatment of symptomatic uterine fibroids: 10-year outcomes from the randomized EMMY trial. *Am J Obstet Gynecol.* 2016;215(6):745.e1–745.e12.
7. Hu N, Kaw D, McCullough M, et al. Menopause and menopausal symptoms after ovarian artery embolization: a comparison with uterine artery embolization controls. *J Vasc Interv Radiol.* 2011;22(5):710–715.
8. Noel-Lamy M, Tan KT, Simons ME, et al. Intraarterial lidocaine for pain control in uterine artery embolization: a prospective, randomized study. *J Vasc Interv Radiol.* 2017;28(1):16–22.
9. Shlansky-Goldberg RD, Coryell L, Stavropoulos SW, et al. Outcomes following fibroid expulsion after uterine artery embolization. *J Vasc Interv Radiol.* 2011;22(11):1586–1593.

Splenic and Renal Embolization

Sebastian Kos, EBIR, FCIRSE, David M. Liu, BSc, MD, FRCPC, and Stephen G.F. Ho, MD, FRCPC

Introduction

Embolotherapy of solid organs in the nontrauma patient can be performed for many indications (tumor, aneurysm, hypersplenism, and preoperative). Embolization for trauma, visceral aneurysms, and hepatic malignancies is covered elsewhere in this book. This chapter discusses splenic embolization for hypersplenism and renal embolization for angiomyolipoma (AML), nonfunctioning kidney/nephrotic syndrome, and prior to surgery or renal cell carcinoma (RCC).

Indications

1. Splenic artery embolization for hypersplenism and pancytopenia
   a. Hematologic disorders (idiopathic thrombocytopenic purpura, thalassemia, hereditary spherocytosis)
   b. Cirrhosis with portal hypertension
   c. Primary malignancies (lymphoma, leukemia)
   d. Congenital disease (e.g., Gaucher disease, atresia of bile ducts)
   e. Idiopathic hypersplenism
   f. Chemotherapy-associated splenomegaly
2. Renal artery embolization
   a. Total embolization
      (1) End-stage renal failure with intractable secondary hypertension
      (2) End-stage renal failure with intractable protein loss/nephrotic syndrome
      (3) End-stage renal failure with hydronephrosis and intractable secondary flank pain (1)
      (4) Failing kidney transplants with graft intolerance syndrome
      (5) Inoperable large RCC causing paraneoplastic syndromes
      (6) Preparation for surgery in patients refusing blood transfusions
      (7) Intractable neoplasm-induced hematuria in the nonsurgical patient
   b. Partial embolization
      (1) Small RCC with hematuria or paraneoplastic syndromes in the inoperable patient
      (2) Large RCC with hematuria or paraneoplastic syndromes in the inoperable patient with a single kidney
      (3) AML. Active or recurrent hemorrhage. Data guiding prophylactic embolization based on size is inconclusive (2)
      (4) Preparation for radiofrequency or cryoablation of RCC (3)
      (5) Preparation for surgery in patients refusing blood transfusions

Contraindications

Absolute
There are no absolute contraindications for renal and splenic artery embolization. Because these procedures usually involve other clinical disciplines, namely oncologists, nephrologists, urologists, hematologists, etc., a multidisciplinary consensus should be obtained prior to these treatments.

Relative
1. Contraindications to angiography
   a. Severe anaphylactoid reaction to iodinated contrast media

b. Uncorrectable coagulopathy
c. Renal insufficiency
2. Pregnancy
3. Acute or chronic infection of spleen/kidney
4. Acute hyperthyroidism
5. Thyroid carcinoma and planned radioiodine therapy
6. For renal artery embolization: solitary kidney

Preprocedure Preparation

1. Preprocedural assessment
   a. Informed consent must be obtained prior to the procedure.
   b. Computed tomographic angiography (CTA) or magnetic resonance angiography (MRA) should be obtained prior to the procedure to depict vascular anatomy, extent, and location of the disease (e.g., tumor), size of targeted organs (spleen).
   c. Recent laboratory data including partial thromboplastin time (PTT), international normalized ratio (INR), creatinine, glomerular filtration rate (GFR), complete blood count (CBC), platelet count, and C-reactive protein (CRP).
2. Patient preparation
   a. Patient preparation and preoperative management vary widely between centers and even operators. For splenic artery embolization, in 1979, Spigos et al. (4) described a regimen, which is still accepted by some authors (5). This includes antibiotic prophylaxis (e.g., cefazolin 1 g; 12 hours before and 1 to 2 weeks after the procedure), additional local antibiotics (e.g., gentamicin) applied with the embolic solution. *Note:* Other regimens including broad-spectrum coverage (e.g., Zosyn, 3.375 mg intravenously [IV] every 12 hours × 3 days posttreatment) and penicillin V 5 million units, coadministered with the embolic agent, have been applied but no evidence exists for "best practice" recommendation. Strict sterility (broad surgical scrub and/or povidone-iodine bath) is emphasized to minimize concerns relating to postembolic infection.
   b. For splenic embolization, a (14-valent) pneumococcal vaccine should be given days before the procedure. There is controversy on this subject.
   c. Patient on nil per os (NPO) for at least 6 hours prior to the procedure.
   d. Establish IV access.
   e. Supportive therapy (e.g., volume, oxygen).
   f. Establish patient monitoring (electrocardiogram [ECG], respiratory rate [RR] heart rate [HR], pulse oximetry).
   g. Administer conscious sedation. *Note:* For total renal embolization, general anesthesia may be required (especially when utilizing liquid embolics [cyanoacrylates or Onyx] or liquid sclerosants [alcohol]) due to severe pain.
   h. Administer IV antiemetics (e.g., diphenhydramine 50 mg, dexamethasone 10 mg, ondansetron 2 to 4 mg).
   i. Standard sterile preparation and draping should be applied.
   j. Transfemoral or transradial access may be used. In particular, for patients with abnormal coagulation parameters, transradial access may be preferred (6).

Procedure

1. Splenic artery embolization
   a. Following establishment of arterial access, selective catheterization of the celiac trunk and splenic artery is performed. For this, 5-Fr selective catheters (e.g., Cobra, Sidewinder) are commonly used in combination with a hydrophilic guidewire.
   b. Arteriogram is performed and related to individual anatomy (anatomic variations must be considered); the catheter is advanced such that nontarget

vessels can be safely avoided (*for splenic:* embolization of dorsal pancreatic, pancreatica magna and short gastric branches, or reflux into aorta; *for renal:* adrenal, spinal, and lumbar collaterals). However, the selective catheter should not be advanced into vessels that are less than twice the catheter's diameter, to avoid stasis and occlusion. Size of targeted vessels and splenic artery tortuosity often make usage of a coaxial system mandatory. Coaxial microcatheters safely allow engagement of splenic arteries even distal to the hilum.

Ensure that the embolic agent and microcatheter are compatible. This includes embolization coils, both controlled release and uncontrolled deployment systems.

Off-label intraarterial injection of lidocaine hydrochloride (50 to 100 mg) may be performed prior to embolization (based on anecdotal evidence) to decrease patient discomfort and abdominal pain during and after the procedure. (Slow injection and ECG monitoring *are mandatory* as cardiac arrhythmia may be induced.)

c. The embolic material to be used can be chosen according to operator's experience and preference. Different embolic agents have been described and applied for splenic artery embolization in the literature (e.g., autologous clot, Gelfoam pledgets [Pfizer, New York, NY], polyvinyl alcohol particles, microspheres, microcoils, ethanol, glue [isobutyl-2-cyanoacrylate]). However, no differences in complication rate, efficacy, or outcome have been demonstrated. More important than the actual choice of the embolic agent is the distal (hilar/posthilar) deployment of the embolic agent, as central embolization may not result in sufficient infarction due to collateral flow from pancreatic and gastric branches. (It is important to note that Gelfoam and nonspherical particles may clog within microcatheters, resulting in uncontrolled embolization or requirement to reselect the vessel and replace the catheter.)

d. More relevant for the procedural outcome than the actual embolic agent is the applied embolization concept (5).

   (1) **Complete** splenic embolization was initially described in 1973, but severe complications may occur and this should **not** be performed (7).

   (2) **Partial** splenic embolization was shown to have best results and a significantly lower complication rate. Any embolization for hypersplenism should be performed as a partial embolization. Two major techniques (selective vs. unselective) have been described.

      (a) Using the selective technique, splenic artery branches are selectively engaged and embolized to complete stasis. Intermittent angiographic runs (in parenchymal phase) document the actual extent of infarction.

      (b) For the nonselective approach, the catheter is positioned in the main splenic artery distal to the pancreatic branches and embolization is performed. As an objective end point, 50% to 80% decrease in parenchymal blush during digital subtraction angiography (DSA) arteriography may be used.

   3. **Partial sequential** embolization is a concept that should be applied for embolic treatment of massive splenomegaly, as single-step embolization may be more prone to complications (e.g., postembolic syndrome). In these cases, some authors recommend performing stepwise partial embolization (two to three treatments).

   4. Currently, no evidence is available regarding the optimal ratio of splenic tissue to be infarcted. Practice suggests that embolization of 50% to 80% of splenic tissue results in better outcome than embolization of <50% tissue and fewer complications than embolization of >80% splenic tissue.

2. Renal artery embolization
   a. Selective injection of the renal arteries is performed. For most cases, a coaxial approach using a combination of 5- to 6-Fr standard sheath or guide sheath of 5- to 6-Fr internal diameter (ID) (e.g., renal double curve), a 4- to 5-Fr diagnostic catheter (e.g., Sos-Omni, Cobra, Vertebral, Angled taper), and a hydrophilic guidewire should be used. Additional usage of microcatheters may be mandatory for superselective embolization of small renal tumors.
   b. Selective angiography should be performed with gantry angulation calculated from CT or MR to obtain optimal depiction of the renal vasculature.
   c. *Note:* Especially in patients with RCC, if the angiogram reveals arteriovenous fistulas, these should be embolized first, prior to any total or partial renal embolization to avoid paradoxical venous embolization and its complications (e.g., renal vein thrombosis, pulmonary embolism, stroke).
   d. Two main technical concepts have been described:
      (1) **Total** renal embolization
         (a) For total devascularization of the kidney, many therapeutic agents have been proposed and applied (e.g., ethanol, glue, small particles, coils, AMPLATZER vascular plug [AGA Medical Corp, Plymouth, MN]). Lacking significant evidence for a specific embolic agent to be superior, many institutions use ethanol due to its cost-effectiveness. For ethanol embolization,
            i. Proximal balloon occlusions should be performed to minimize nontargeted delivery and to maximize dwell time.
            ii. General anesthesia is essential for the management of potential hemodynamic instability resulting from systemic release of intraarterial ethanol as well as for the management of profound pain.
            iii. Following proximal occlusion, a single-contrast injection may determine the individual filling volume of the renal arterial tree.
            iv. Following deflation of the balloon, washout of the contrast media, and reinflation of the balloon, the assessed volume of medical strength ethanol can be safely injected (<20 mL on average).
            v. The balloon should remain inflated for several minutes and prior to deflation, remaining ethanol should be aspirated through the balloon catheter.
            vi. When using a technique without an occlusion balloon, 4 to 10 mL of ethanol should be slowly injected over several minutes.
            vii. Angiography should demonstrate stasis as an end point of the procedure.
      (2) **Partial** renal embolization
         (a) Partial embolization is mostly performed for the treatment for renal tumors (RCC, AML) prior to or instead (e.g., inoperable patient) of any surgical or locoregional therapy (e.g., radiofrequency ablation [RFA], cryoablation). Precise depiction of vascular anatomy and tumor-feeding vessels is crucial for selective embolotherapy.
         (b) For small tumors, coaxial usage of microcatheters is usually necessary to allow superselective engagement of feeding branches, thereby sparing healthy tissue from infarction.
         (c) For superselective embolization of feeding branches, mostly small particles, microcoils, and glue are used. Small, calibrated microspheres <300-μm diameter are preferred in order to assure adequate terminal embolization.

Postprocedure Management

1. Splenic artery embolization
   a. IV antibiotics (cefazolin 500 mg to 1 g every 8 hours; adapted to renal function).
   b. Analgesic therapy (perchlorpromazine and acetaminophen). In most cases, a patient-controlled analgesia (PCA) pump is required.

c. Antiemetic therapy (ondansetron and dexamethasone).
d. Prior to discharge, or after 1 month, CT or MRI should be performed to assess the actual amount of infarcted tissue.
e. The length of hospital stay depends on the underlying disease, the degree of postembolization syndrome, and the presence of complications. In our experience, most patients can be discharged 3 to 6 days after the procedure.
f. Provide specific instructions to minimize the chance, in the acute and subacute phases (3 to 6 months), of potential splenic rupture.
g. Follow-up hematologic assessment at 2 and 4 weeks.
2. Renal artery embolization
   a. Severe pain may result from total renal embolization; therefore, general anesthesia and anticipated multiday admission for management of postembolization syndrome are warranted.
   b. For further postprocedural care, see recommendations for splenic embolization.

Results

1. Splenic artery embolization—the described data on clinical benefit from splenic artery embolization are based on limited clinical trials with relatively low numbers of patients.
   a. Following splenic artery embolization, increase in platelets is noted within 2 weeks of procedure in up to 90% of patients. Transient hyperthrombocythemia may occur, and normal platelet counts may even be seen years after the procedure.
   b. Lower success rates of up to 70% were noted in 35 patients with portal hypertension due to biliary atresia, extrahepatic portal obstruction, and idiopathic cirrhosis (1,8).
   c. For partial splenic embolization in patients with portal hypertension, frequency of bleeding episodes from esophageal varices may be significantly reduced and hemoglobin, leukocytes, and platelets increased. However, it should be emphasized that data on the effect of splenic artery embolization on variceal bleeding risk are controversial. Repeat embolization may be considered for those patients with only partial response as a complete response is possible.
   d. Compared with surgical total splenectomy and the related risk of overwhelming postsplenectomy infection (OPSI), even current surgical literature advocates partial splenic embolization as a safe and efficient procedure (9).
   e. No significant difference in outcome has been shown when comparing embolic agent (coils vs. gelatin particles).
2. Renal artery embolization
   a. There is no evidence that renal embolization has a therapeutic benefit for RCC (10). However, preoperative selective embolization may facilitate laparoscopic tumor surgery.
   b. In patients with renal pathologies (e.g., arteriovenous malformation, AML, recurrent bleed) and high operative risk for surgical nephrectomy, clinical success with respect to management of acute bleeding (defined as resolution of presenting symptoms without need for further interventions) of transarterial embolization is comparable to complete nephrectomy.
   c. In end-stage renal disease, secondary hypertension and nephrotic syndrome may be successfully treated by bilateral total renal embolization.
   d. In patients with graft intolerance, total graft embolization may be clinically successful in greater than 50% of patients.
   e. Renal embolization in patients with polycystic kidney disease may result in decreased kidney size and improved quality of life (1).
   f. Embolization for AML is efficient, safe, and renal function may be preserved. Volume of reduction in size of an AML remains high, >70%.

Complications

1. Splenic artery embolization
   a. Local arterial puncture site complications.
   b. Pain, nausea, reactive pleural effusion, atelectasis, and postembolization fever are considered side effects of therapy rather than complications.
   c. Splenic abscess (<10%) on the basis of infarcted tissue and backflow of digestive bacteria through the flow-reversed splenic vein.
   d. The risk of other potential major complications (e.g., splenic perforation, necrosis of gastric wall, pancreatitis) can be minimized by meticulous technique and selective embolization.
2. Renal artery embolization
   a. Local complications at the arterial puncture site.
   b. As for splenic embolization, the risk of major complications, particularly nontarget embolization (e.g., aortic reflux, adrenal infarction, colonic and peripheral embolization), can be minimized by meticulous technique and selective embolization.
   c. Postembolization syndrome is commonly seen as a side effect, as described earlier.

Management of Complications

1. Pneumonia and pleural effusion: antibiotic therapy and pleural drainage
2. Splenic/renal abscess: antibiotic therapy, percutaneous drainage, splenectomy if refractory to treatment
3. For postembolization syndrome: symptomatic treatment with hydration and antiemetic and analgesic drugs

References

1. Ubara Y, Tagami T, Sawa N, et al. Renal contraction therapy for enlarged polycystic kidneys by transcatheter arterial embolization in hemodialysis patients. *Am J Kidney Dis.* 2002; 39(3):571–579.
2. Murray TE, Lee MJ. Are we overtreating renal angiomyolipoma: a review of the literature and assessment of contemporary management and follow-up strategies. *Cardiovasc Intervent Radiol.* 2018;41(4):525–536.
3. Tocke I, Mahnken A, Bücker A, et al. Nephron-sparing percutaneous ablation of a 5 cm renal cell carcinoma by superselective embolization and percutaneous RF ablation. *Rofo* 2001;173(11):990–983.
4. Spigos DG, Jonasson O, Mozes M, et al. Partial splenic embolization in the treatment of hypersplenism. *AJR Am J Roentgenol.* 1979;132(5):777–782.
5. Madoff DC, Denys A, Wallace MJ, et al. Splenic arterial interventions: anatomy, indications, technical considerations, and potential complications. *Radiographics.* 2005;25(suppl 1): S191–S211.
6. Naritaka Y, Shiozawa S, Shimakawa T, et al. Transradial approach for partial splenic embolization in patients with hypersplenism. *Hepatogastroenterology.* 2007;54(78):1850–1853.
7. Maddison FE. Embolic therapy of hypersplenism [abstract]. *Invest Radiol.* 1973;8:280–281.
8. Nio M, Hayashi Y, Sano N, et al. Long-term efficacy of partial splenic embolization in children. *J Pediatr Surg.* 2003;38(12):1760–1762.
9. Amin MA, el-Gendy MM, Dawoud IE, et al. Partial splenic embolization versus splenectomy for the management of hypersplenism in cirrhotic patients. *World J Surg.* 2009;33(8): 1702–1710.
10. May M, Brookman-Amissah S, Pflanz S, et al. Pre-operative renal arterial embolisation does not provide survival benefit in patients with radical nephrectomy for renal cell carcinoma. *Br J Radiol.* 2009;82(981):724–731.

26 BPH: Prostatic Artery Embolization

Francisco Cesar Carnevale, PhD, Airton Mota Moreira, MD, PhD, and André Moreira de Assis, MD

Benign prostatic hyperplasia (BPH) is the most common benign neoplasia in males, and moderate or severe lower urinary tract symptoms (LUTS) will occur in approximately one-half of men in their 80s. Men with BPH can present with prostatic enlargement, bladder outlet obstruction, or both. LUTS due to BPH, such as hesitancy, poor and/or intermittent stream, straining, prolonged micturition, feeling of incomplete bladder emptying, dribbling, or irritative symptoms such as frequency, urgency, urge incontinence and nocturia can significantly impact patient quality of life (QoL) and may be only partially relieved by medical management. Invasive therapies for BPH include transurethral resection of prostate (TURP), open prostatectomy or laser enucleation. Prostatic artery embolization (PAE) has emerged as an effective alternative for men who wish to avoid the associated significant morbidities of these procedures (including retrograde ejaculation, a major concern to many men seeking PAE) (1). Previous studies have established its safety and effectiveness with significant prostate volume reduction, as well as urodynamic, LUTS, and QoL improvements. These results have been reproducible across multiple centers and endorsed by major international societies (2). It is critical that the interventional radiologist (IR) be familiar with the pathophysiology of, and full array of treatments for, BPH!

Indications

1. LUTS due to BPH with no improvement from, or intolerance to, medical treatment (5-alpha-reductase inhibitors and/or selective alpha-blockers)
2. LUTS due to BPH
3. Urinary retention (UR) with indwelling catheter

Contraindications

Absolute
1. Active urinary tract infection (UTI)
2. Bladder atonia
3. Neurologic bladder dysfunction or other neurologic disorder impacting bladder function
4. Large bladder diverticula or stones requiring surgery
5. Urethral stricture
6. Renal failure

Relative
1. Confirmed or suspected malignant neoplasm
2. Detrusor muscle hypocontractility
3. Coagulation disorders

Preprocedure Preparation

1. Involvement of a multidisciplinary team of IRs, diagnostic radiologists, and urologists in patient selection and follow-up is mandatory.
2. The International Prostate Symptom Score (IPSS), (scored as mild, moderate, or severe); the International Index of Erectile Function, (scored as severe, moderate, mild-to-moderate, mild, or no dysfunction); and the IPSS-QoL questionnaire are used as assessment tools.

3. All patients undergo digital rectal examination and prostatic-specific antigen (PSA) blood sample analysis. Transrectal prostate biopsy is indicated if there is suspicion of cancer.
4. If necessary, a urodynamic study is performed to confirm presence of infravesical obstruction and to evaluate bladder function. Some patients can remain obstructed on follow-up urodynamic testing, despite clinical improvement of LUTS.
5. Pelvic magnetic resonance imaging (MRI) allows detailed evaluation of the total and zonal prostate volumes, BPH nodules, lobe symmetry, median lobe protrusion and lesions suspicious for malignancy.
   a. Postcontrast sequences demonstrate prostatic parenchymal enhancement patterns and atherosclerotic changes in pelvic arteries.
   b. Bladder wall thickness, diverticula, polyps, stones, or disorders of other pelvic structures can be assessed.
   c. An endorectal coil is not necessary in most cases.
6. An ultrasound may assess upper urinary tracts, prostate volume, bladder wall, post void residual (PVR) and, if available, prostate elastography.
7. A proton-pump inhibitor, nonsteroidal antiinflammatory, and other symptomatic medications including urinary analgesics are administered. Prophylactic antibiotics such as ciprofloxacin or a third-generation cephalosporin are prescribed starting 24 hours preprocedure. (Ciprofloxacin 400 mg IV preprocedure and 500 mg orally twice a day for 7 days after PAE.)

Procedure (3,4)

1. Obtain informed consent.
2. PAE is generally performed under local anesthesia and intravenous sedation on an outpatient basis.
3. A Foley catheter with balloon filled with a mixture of saline and 10% to 20% iodinated contrast medium will provide an anatomic landmark. This helps beginners to be more confident but may result in urethral trauma (pain and bleeding), median lobe trauma, or urinary tract infection.
4. Angiographic equipment with cone-beam computed tomography (CBCT) is essential.
5. Just as the prevalence of BPH increases with age, so do atherosclerosis and other comorbidities. PAE can be a technically challenging procedure with high radiation exposure to both the medical team and patient. Deep familiarization with materials and devices, intraprocedure imaging techniques, microcatheterization skills, and accurate knowledge of the pelvic vascular anatomy are required. Identifying and catheterizing target arterial branches are among the most critical and time-consuming steps.
   a. Pelvic aortoiliac digital subtraction angiography (DSA) may be useful to assess the arterial anatomy (pigtail catheter in distal aorta, 20 mL contrast, 10 mL per second, 600 psi).
   b. The aortic bifurcation is crossed and the IIA is catheterized using a 5-Fr diagnostic catheter. The most common diagnostic catheters used through the femoral approach are the Cobra C2, Vertebral, Robert's uterine catheter (RUC]—Cook Inc, Bloomington, IN) and Carnevale prostate catheter (CPC—Merit Medical System, Inc, South Jordan, UT). The RUC and CPC catheters can be used for both internal iliac arteries (IIAs). Due to its long curve, the RUC may reduce the microwire torqueability and pushability when used in a coaxial system. The CPC catheter (5-, 10-, and 15-cm tip) is chosen according to the distance between the aortic bifurcation and the IIA. Simmons I or II, or vertebral catheters can be used if necessary.
   c. Although common femoral puncture is more common, radial access is safe and feasible. The IIA is accessed under fluoroscopic or roadmap guidance using a 125-cm 5-Fr Berenstein catheter and 0.035-in hydrophilic wire.

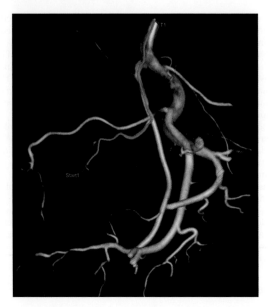

FIGURE 26.1 • Internal iliac artery 3D angiographic image can be used as a roadmap for accurate identification of the prostatic artery.

d. After selecting the IIA trunk, a CBCT is performed (2 mL/sec, with 4 to 6 seconds delay) to identify the vascular anatomy, avoid multiple DSA series and reduce radiation exposure. To avoid missing a proximal branch, it is essential that the 5-Fr catheter is positioned at the IIA common trunk. The images provide a rich source of anatomical information that helps to identify the prostatic arteries and nontarget branches. After imaging reconstruction, a computed 3D pelvic angiographic roadmap allows the identification of, and route of access to, the prostatic artery (Fig. 26.1).

e. An IIA DSA can also be performed (12 mL; 4 mL/sec; 300 psi; 20 to 50 degrees ipsilateral oblique, and /or 10 to 20 degrees caudal angulation).

f. The PROVISO acronym (internal Pudendal, middle Rectal, Obturator, Vesical Inferior and vesical Superior arteries under Oblique view) is a useful trick to remember the pelvic arterial anatomy (Fig. 26.2).

g. Identification of the target arteries can be difficult due to common variations of the prostatic origin. de Assis proposed an angiographic classification used by the authors (5): **type I**, origin from a common trunk with the superior vesical artery (SVA) (28.7%); **type II**, origin from the anterior division of the IIA, inferior to the SVA (14.7%); **type III**, origin from the obturator artery (18.9%); and **type IV**, origin from the internal pudendal artery (IPA) (31.1%). Less common origins are classified as type 5 (5.6%), the most relevant being origin from the accessory IPA (2.1%). Unilateral duplication was seen in 8.0%. Each type of anatomy presents a specific technical challenge. A type I with atherosclerotic changes may be the hardest to catheterize. In such cases, making a double curve in the microwire ("C" or Cobra shape), using curved microwires or advancing the 5-Fr catheter near to the prostatic artery origin can help (3).

h. In some cases protective embolization with coils or gelatin sponge is necessary to avoid distal nontarget embolization, most commonly high-flow anastomosis to penis, bladder, and rectum.

i. Because these branches are small and tortuous, we suggest prostatic artery catheterization with small-diameter hydrophilic microcatheters (2.0 to 2.4 Fr)

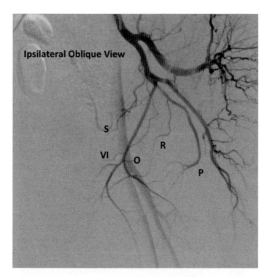

FIGURE 26.2 • Internal iliac artery angiography demonstrating the internal Pudendal, middle Rectal, Obturator, Inferior and Superior Vesical arteries under the Oblique ipsilateral view to explain the PROVISO acronym.

and a 0.014- or 0.016-in shapeable hydrophilic microwire. The 0.016″ Fathom wire (Boston Scientific, Natick, MA) has good trackability in tortuous vessels and its tip can be easily reshaped, if necessary.

j. Device improvements designed to reduce reflux and nontarget embolization include microcatheters with a mounted compliant balloon or other antireflux system. They prevent reflux by lowering the proximal pressure and reversing the flow in distal vascular anastomoses, however improved clinical outcomes have not been reported with any specific kind of microcatheter.

k. After prostatic artery catheterization, a DSA run is obtained to visualize the central gland (anteromedial) and peripheral zone (posterolateral) branches (Fig. 26.3).

l. Nitroglycerin, 100 to 200 μg diluted in saline is injected to prevent vasospasm and facilitate distal catheterization. Vascular spasm can be managed with additional vasodilators.

m. Embolization is performed using a 1-mL syringe and slow injections of a highly diluted Embosphere (Merit Medical Systems, Inc, South Jordan, UT) 100 to 500 μm solution or polyvinyl alcohol particles, 50 to 250 μm until complete vascular stasis, avoiding reflux to undesired branches (3,6).

n. After stasis, wait 3 to 5 minutes to assess early recanalization. Flush the microcatheter with saline frequently during embolization. If any forward flow is observed, continue embolizing. If venous filling and total stasis is observed, consider stopping (target endpoint).

o. Withdraw the catheter proximally and perform a final angiographic run to check for additional prostatic branches. If accessory prostatic branches are not embolized, clinical LUTS recurrence may occur (7).

p. The contralateral IIA is catheterized using a Waltman loop if a cobra or vert catheter is used, or the RUC or CPC catheters, and embolization is performed using the same steps. Bilateral embolization has better clinical outcomes compared to unilateral embolization and is endorsed by a multisociety position statement (2).

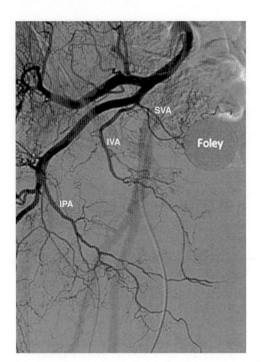

FIGURE 26.3 • Internal iliac artery angiography (ipsilateral oblique image) obtained during PAE showing the branches of the anterior division as the superior vesical artery (SVA), the inferior vesical artery (IVA) and the internal pudendal artery (IPA), and their relationships to the Foley balloon. The central gland and capsular branches can be seen arising from the IVA.

q. Important technical considerations:
   (1) The PErFecTED technique (Proximal Embolization First, Then Embolize Distal) is a bilateral two-step embolization protocol resulting in greater prostate infarction rates, significant increase in IPSS and Qmax and a lower symptom recurrence rate. Carnevale et al. showed a 1-year recurrence rate of 22.0% for standard embolization versus 5.3% for PErFecTED technique ($p < 0.01$) (8).
      (a) After standard proximal embolization (first step), the microcatheter is advanced further into intraprostatic branches, in order to continue embolizing (second step). The use of a 2.0-Fr microcatheter is strongly recommended. Slow injection of the microspheres is essential to achieve parenchymal ischemia.
      (b) Angiographic runs should be performed a few minutes after completing embolization.
      (c) CBCT is strongly recommended either to differentiate prostatic branches from rectal or bladder branches, and to confirm that the whole prostatic lobe has been embolized (Fig. 26.4).
      (d) Attention to anatomy demonstrated on CBCT and conventional angiography is essential before selective embolization is performed (Fig. 26.5).
      (e) When facing intra high-flow prostatic artery anastomoses to clinically relevant territories, two main strategies can be employed: navigate the microcatheter distal to the origin of the anastomosis before starting embolization with microparticles, or perform selective protective

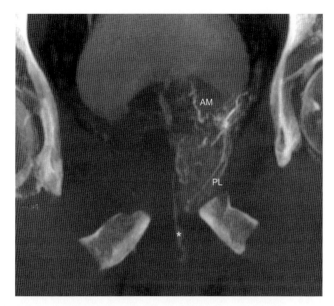

FIGURE 26.4 • Cone-beam computed tomography (CBCT) performed during PAE shows contrast enhancement of the entire left prostatic lobe via the anteromedial (AM) and the posterolateral (PL) branches. Venous phase enhancement is seen at the apex of the prostate (*asterisk*).

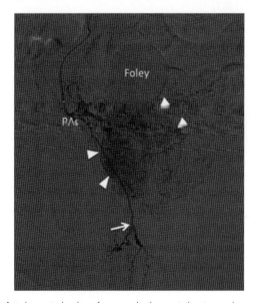

FIGURE 26.5 Anterior–posterior view of a superselective prostatic artery angiogram showing the microcatheter positioned at the origin of the right prostatic arteries (PAs). Right intraprostatic branches and partial left lobe opacification are observed (*arrowheads*). A collateral arterial shunt to the penis (*white arrow*) is seen.

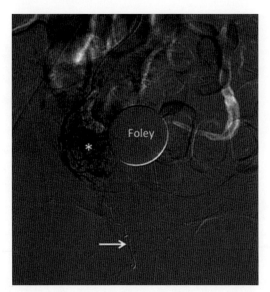

FIGURE 26.6 • Superselective angiography showing the capsular shunt occluded after coil embolization.

embolization of the anastomosis with coils or gelatin sponge (Figs. 26.6 and 26.7).

   (f) When performing protective embolization, it is important to navigate the microcatheter as far as possible into the intraprostatic anastomosis.

  (2) Although migration of small amounts of microspheres through anastomoses to the obturator territory or other pelvic parietal structures may occur, clinical complication is not expected. There is no need for coiling these connections. In addition, particle reflux to seminal vesicle branches does not seem to cause complications.

Postprocedure Management

1. Indwelling catheters, if used exclusively as a guide during PAE should be removed right after the procedure. Patients with long-term catheters should be instructed to return 2 weeks later for trial of spontaneous voiding. If urinary symptoms persist and the catheter cannot be removed, another attempt is tried every 7 days.

2. Patients should be discharged 3 to 6 hours after PAE. We encourage the use of closure devices to reduce hospital stay.

3. Antibiotics are maintained until 7 days post PAE. During the first week, patients will also receive proton-pump inhibitors, antiemetics, nonopioid analgesics, and nonsteroidal antiinflammatories. Alpha 1-adrenergic receptor antagonist is maintained for 2 to 4 weeks, to mitigate post-PAE syndrome. Opioids and steroidal antiinflammatory drugs may also be used whenever necessary. Dysuria, frequency, and urgency have been observed in all patients treated by PAE and are related to ischemic prostatitis. Similar to any other visceral embolization, symptoms such as nausea, fever in the absence of infection, urethral burning, peri prostatic or pelvic pain, minor blood in urine and/or mixed in the stool with mucus for 3 to 5 days may be expected (post-PAE syndrome) (9).

4. A 24-hour postprocedure PSA measurement seems to correlate to the degree of ischemia. The higher the PSA, the greater the glandular ischemia.

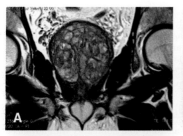
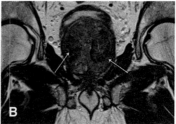
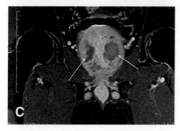

FIGURE 26.7 • A: T2-weighted coronal MRI demonstrating an enlarged prostate due to BPH nodules in the central gland. **B:** MRI 3 months postembolization showing prostatic volume reduction in low-signal areas in the central gland (infarcted areas). **C:** Infarcted nodules (*white arrows*) seen as avascular regions (fat-suppressed postcontrast sequence).

5. Patients are advised to contact the IR team with any concerns during the first week.
6. Follow-up is scheduled at 3 and 12 months and then annually to access clinical outcome including the IPSS and the IPSS-QoL questionnaire, US with PVR assessment, prostate MRI, uroflowmetry, and serum PSA.

Results (2,4,8,10)

1. Technical success, if defined as bilateral embolization, varies from 75% to 94.3%. When including unilateral embolization as technical success, published rates reach 95% to 100%.
2. Clinical success can be defined in multiple ways, primarily related to freedom from Foley catheter, and IPSS and QoL improvements.
   a. For patients with chronic UR, clinical success can be defined as removal of the indwelling catheter and varies from 80.5% to 91%.
   b. The authors consider clinical success achieved when IPSS decreases by 8 and QoL by 3.
   c. Others define clinical success as improved symptoms (IPSS ≤15 points and a decrease of at least 25% from the baseline score), improved QoL (QoL score ≤3 points or a decrease of at least 1 point from baseline), and no need for medical or other therapy after PAE.
   d. Published mean 12-month results include: 15-point drop in IPSS, a mean decrease of QoL score of 2.2, and a mean change of 5.5 points in maximum urinary flow rate (Qmax) at 12 months.
   e. The authors' results reported after median follow-up of 72 months (10) include improvement in: IPSS, 16 points +/− 7; QoL score, 4 points +/− 1; prostatic volume reduction, 39 cm³ +/− 39 (39% +/− 29); maximum urinary flow rate, 6 mL/sec +/− 10 (155% +/− 293); and PVR, 70 mL +/− 121 (48% +/− 81) (p <0.05 for all). Symptomatic recurrence was seen in 23%.

3. Prostate volume reduction ranges from 20% to 40% (mean of 30%) (Fig. 26.7A–C).
   a. Ischemic changes occur exclusively in the transition zone on the side of embolization, initially as hemorrhagic necrosis and after 12 months most become shrunken infarcts. Infarcts are not seen in the peripheral zone.
4. Clinical outcomes including IPSS and QoL values, peak urinary flow, and PVR are comparable between PAE and TURP at 12- and 24-month follow-up. TURP has best results at 1 and 3 months; however, hospital stay is significantly shorter with PAE.

Complications and Management (9)

1. Detailed knowledge of pelvic arterial anatomy and familiarity with advanced microcatheterization techniques are essential to optimize outcomes and avoid complications.
2. Postembolization syndrome, including nausea, vomiting, hematuria, and fever is expected and should be managed with prophylactic antibiotics, analgesics, non-steroidal antiinflammatory drugs (NSAIDs) or steroids, antiemetics, antipyretics, and alpha blockers.
3. Minor events include proctalgia with dysuria, acute UR, urinary, rectal or seminal bleeding (usually minor), UTI or infectious prostatitis, and access site complications. Fortunately, most are self-limited or managed with medical treatment.
   a. The use of smaller microspheres may be related to a higher incidence of minor adverse events, although the data are not conclusive.
4. Major complications related to nontarget embolization are rare. To date, one case of bladder wall necrosis requiring surgical resection has been reported. Others include transient bladder and rectal wall ischemia, bone infarction, and radiodermatitis.

References

1. Manov JJ, Mohan P, Kava B, et al. Benign prostatic hyperplasia: a brief overview of pathogenesis, diagnosis, and current state of therapy. *Tech Vasc Interv Radiol.* 2020;23(3):10068.
2. Young S, Golzarian J. Prostate artery embolization: state of the evidence and societal guidelines. *Tech Vasc Interv Radiol.* 2020;23(3):100695.
3. Carnevale FC, Antunes AA. Prostatic artery embolization for enlarged prostates due to benign prostatic hyperplasia. How I do it. *Cardiovasc Intervent Radiol.* 2013;36(6):1452–1463.
4. Bhatia S, Harward SH, Sinha VK, et al. Prostate artery embolization via transradial or transulnar versus transfemoral arterial access: technical results. *J Vasc Interv Radiol.* 2017;28(6):898–905.
5. de Assis AM, Moreira AM, de Paula Rodrigues VC, et al. Pelvic arterial anatomy relevant to prostatic artery embolisation and proposal for angiographic classification. *Cardiovasc Intervent Radiol.* 2015;38(4):855–861.
6. Maclean D, Harris M, Drake T, et al. Factors predicting a good symptomatic outcome after prostate artery embolisation (PAE). *Cardiovasc Intervent Radiol.* 2018;41(8):1152–1159.
7. de Assis AM, Moreira AM, Carnevale FC. Angiographic findings during repeat prostatic artery embolization. *J Vasc Interv Radiol.* 2019;30(5):645–651.
8. Carnevale FC, Moreira AM, Harward SH, et al. Recurrence of lower urinary tract symptoms following prostate artery embolization for benign hyperplasia: single center experience comparing two techniques. *Cardiovasc Intervent Radiol.* 2017;40(3):366–374.
9. Moreira AM, de Assis AM, Carnevale FC, et al. A review of adverse events related to prostatic artery embolization for treatment of bladder outlet obstruction due to BPH. *Cardiovasc Intervent Radiol.* 2017;40(10):1490–1500.
10. Carnevale FC, Moreira AM, de Assis AM, et al. Prostatic artery embolization for the treatment of lower urinary tract symptoms due to benign prostatic hyperplasia: 10 years' experience. *Radiology.* 2020;296(2):444–451.

27 Temporary Central Venous Access: Peripherally Inserted Central Catheters and Nontunneled Central Venous Catheters

Sidney Regalado, MD and Brian Funaki, MD

Introduction

Central venous (CV) access devices can be placed faster, more safely, and with fewer complications when imaging guidance (IG) is utilized than when placed with reliance on external anatomic landmarks (1). The placement of a nontunneled CV catheter has certain advantages over the placement of a tunneled CV catheter or implantable subcutaneous chest port. Nontunneled CV catheters are commonly placed using local anesthesia only, often at the bedside in an ICU setting when patients are too ill to be transported. As these temporary catheters are placed without subcutaneous tunneling, less stringent adherence to coagulation parameters can be observed. When the indication for these CV catheters no longer exists, these devices can be easily removed at the bedside.

Indications (2)

1. Therapeutic indications
   a. Administration of chemotherapy, TPN, blood products, intravenous medications and fluids
   b. Performance of hemodialysis and plasmapheresis
2. Diagnostic indications
   a. To confirm a diagnosis or establish a prognosis.
   b. To monitor response to treatment.
   c. For repeated blood sampling.

Contraindications

Absolute
1. Cellulitis at insertion site
2. Allergy to catheter material

Relative
1. Uncorrectable coagulopathy
2. CV occlusion
3. PICC lines are contraindicated in patients who are at risk for chronic renal failure or who have chronic kidney disease due to concern for damage to potential future dialysis fistula sites

Preprocedure Preparation

The preprocedure preparation is similar irrespective of the access device that is chosen.

1. Review of medical history to:
   a. Establish an indication.
   b. Obtain a history of concurrent or prior CV access devices and history of related complications, such as extremity or facial swelling.
   c. Identify pertinent allergies.
2. Review of prior imaging studies to assess for anatomic variants and vessel patency. A quick ultrasound (US) survey is recommended.
3. Physical examination of extremities, including pulses.
4. Informed consent.
5. *NPO status is not needed as the procedure is typically performed with local anesthesia only.*
6. Guidelines for *coagulation parameters* should be followed. PICCs and nontunneled CV access are considered to be low risk for bleeding which is easily detected and controllable (3).
   a. INR should be checked in patients on Coumadin. INR goal is less than 2.0.
   b. PTT is recommended in patients receiving intravenous unfractionated heparin. PTT should be less than 1.5 times control.
   c. Platelet count not routinely recommended, but, transfusion is recommended for counts less than 50,000/μL. Others utilize a platelet count ≥25,000 (4).
   d. Plavix and aspirin do not need to be withheld.
   e. Low–molecular-weight heparin (therapeutic dose) should be withheld for one dose before procedure.
7. Prophylactic antibiotics are not given before nontunneled CV catheter placement.

Procedure

General Considerations

1. Nontunneled CV catheters and PICCs are placed in the IR suite or at the bedside (with or without fluoroscopic guidance) depending on operator preference and the clinical status of the patient.
2. The skin is sterilized with a 2% chlorhexidine-based preparation. Standard surgical scrub protocol for the operator includes hand scrubbing, gloves, mask, cap, and gown.
3. Local anesthesia with 1% lidocaine is utilized for all line placements.
4. Choice of line:
   a. CV catheters differ in composition, length, number of lumens, and size. A large internal lumen is optimal for infusions of viscous liquids, whereas multiple lumens facilitate infusion of incompatible infusates. Generally speaking, increasing the number of lumens in the catheter will increase the size of the catheter. For multilumen catheters, if one lumen increases in size, the other lumens may have to decrease in size to maintain a reasonable catheter outer diameter. The choice of catheter size and number of lumens is significant, as the risk of vessel thrombosis and infection increases as the size of the catheter and number of lumens increase.
   b. Power injectable PICC lines and nontunneled CV catheters are available and can be identified by the catheter tubing which indicate the injection rate parameters. The Bard Power PICC has a maximum injection rate of 5 mL/sec at 300 psi (Bard Access Systems, Salt Lake City, UT).

5. Guidance technique
   a. US guidance is always recommended for venipunctures to avoid inadvertent arterial puncture.
   b. When the patient can medically tolerate movement to an angiographic suite, fluoroscopic guidance is used for visualization of guidewires, catheters, and venography. A spot fluoroscopic image at the conclusion is used to document the catheter tip.
   c. When bedside CV lines are placed, only US guidance is used. Thus, a follow-up radiograph is obtained to verify catheter tip position.
6. Catheter tip position
   a. Superior vena cava—right atrial junction is ideal.
   b. Catheter tips can migrate with respirations, retraction due to pendulous breast tissue, and with movement from the supine to upright position (1).
   c. Preexisting CV stenoses or fibrin sheaths may necessitate placement either higher in the SVC or deeper in the right atrium.

PICC Line Placement

1. Choice of vein
   a. Either arm can be used, but the nondominant arm is preferred.
   b. Some operators will choose the largest vein in the upper arm above the elbow as their access vein, while others will routinely select the basilic vein, as it is not adjacent to the brachial artery and nerve.
      (1) The cephalic vein may be used but is prone to spasm and thrombosis.
      (2) The brachial vein travels alongside the brachial artery increasing the risk of arterial puncture.
2. A tourniquet is placed in the upper arm to distend the veins.
3. US guidance and a micropuncture needle (typically 21 G), is used for venous access The access vein can also be punctured using fluoroscopic guidance after injection of contrast medium.
4. A 0.018-in (60-cm) mandril guidewire is advanced centrally under fluoroscopic guidance or until resistance is felt, if fluoroscopy is not available.
5. A skin nick is made and an appropriately sized peel-away sheath is placed.
6. Using fluoroscopy, the required catheter length is measured using the guidewire and the PICC line is cut to length. If the procedure is performed bedside, catheter length is estimated.
7. The PICC line is advanced using a stiffening stylet or a guidewire to the desired position.
8. PICC function is checked by injection of saline and the peel-away sheath is removed.
9. Catheter is anchored to the skin with an adhesive catheter lock or nonabsorbable suture.
10. Dilute heparinized saline is instilled in the lumens and catheter caps are placed.
11. Sterile dressing is applied.
12. Completion spot fluoroscopic image (or chest radiograph) is obtained to document catheter tip position for future reference.
13. Tips for puncturing veins
    a. For inadvertent arterial puncture with a skinny needle, simply remove the needle and apply manual compression to achieve hemostasis.
    b. If the wire does not advance easily through the needle, the needle tip is either against the wall or a double wall puncture may have occurred. Pull the wire back into the needle. Withdraw the needle into the lumen and gently advance the wire with fluoroscopic guidance until the wire advances easily.

c. If the wire tip becomes significantly deformed, consider removing the wire and needle together (as a unit) in order to prevent shearing of the wire.

d. If it is difficult to advance the wire further along the course of the vein, vasospasm may be present. This can be confirmed with a gentle flush of contrast. Wait a few minutes for vasospasm to resolve spontaneously or consider administering nitroglycerin locally (100- to 200 mcg). Alternatively, choose a new vein.

e. Stenosis/occlusion: A tortuous vein or an anatomic variant may be present. Venography will define anatomy. A digital roadmap and a properly selected wire and catheter will help in navigating past the problem.

Central Venous Catheter Placement

1. Choice of vein
   a. The right internal jugular vein (IJV) is the preferred site. Access into this vein has the lowest risk of complications, including pneumothorax (PTX) and thrombosis (5). It has a straight course toward the right atrium simplifying catheter placement.
   b. The left IJV is a more challenging access site since it drains into the brachiocephalic vein, which may be tortuous and enter the SVC at a right angle, necessitating additional manipulation for central access. The wire has a natural tendency to enter the azygous arch or the right ventricle when directed from the left side. In such situations, curved catheters (such as an MPA; Boston Scientific, Natick, MA) and floppy-tip wires (e.g., J-wire or a hydrophilic glidewire) are helpful to access the IVC.
   c. If internal jugular access cannot be achieved, the external jugular veins are acceptable targets (1).
   d. Subclavian veins are often targeted by nonradiologists as they can be catheterized using external landmarks. However, subclavian vein access is associated with a higher risk of CV thrombosis and PTX (1,2,5). Given the risk of thrombosis and stenosis, due to pinching of this vein between the clavicle and first rib, subclavian vein access is contraindicated in patients who are at risk for chronic renal failure, who have chronic kidney disease or who are on dialysis.
   e. The femoral veins are often catheterized in patients who are uncooperative or coagulopathic, or when access is obtained in emergency situation as these veins can be easier to cannulate. The groin is more tolerant to complications such as bleeding when compared to the neck. Femoral veins are less optimal sites of venous access as there is an increased risk of infection and worse patency (1).
   f. After a medical course necessitating multiple catheters, patients are predisposed to developing CV occlusions. When conventional veins have been exhausted, unconventional venous access should be attempted (1,6). Unconventional routes to the central veins include recanalization of collateral neck or chest veins, translumbar access into the IVC, transhepatic venous access, or a surgically placed direct right atrial venous access.

2. Access: Using US guidance and a micropuncture needle, the vein is accessed (Fig. 27.1).

3. The microwire (0.018-inch) is advanced centrally under fluoroscopic guidance or until resistance is felt, if fluoroscopy is not available. A transitional dilator is placed (typically 5-Fr).

4. A working guidewire (typically 0.035-in) is advanced into the IVC (Fig. 27.2).

5. Serial dilators are advanced over the wire.

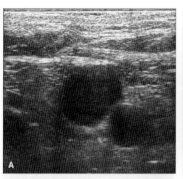
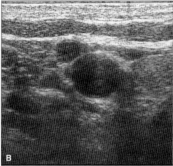
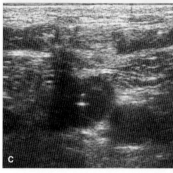

FIGURE 27.1 • Ultrasound evaluation of the internal jugular vein. **A:** Internal jugular vein (*left*) and carotid artery (*right*). **B:** Compression of the internal jugular vein (*left*) shows patency of the vessel. **C:** Echogenic needle tip in the center of the internal jugular vein (*left*).

6. An appropriate length catheter is advanced over the wire. A 15-cm long catheter is commonly used when accessing the right IJV and a 19-cm long catheter is used when accessing the left IJV. The wire is then removed.
7. Catheter tip position is assessed when possible and function is verified.
8. Catheter is sutured to the skin.
9. Catheter flushing and dressings are placed per hospital protocol.

Device Removal

1. Nontunneled central lines and PICC lines can be removed at bedside or in the recovery room using local anesthesia and manual traction.
2. If the device is removed for suspected catheter infection, the catheter tip is sent for culture.

Postprocedure Management

1. With the use of IG, catheter malposition is rare. If the catheter was not placed under fluoroscopic guidance a chest x-ray is obtained following the procedure to document position.
2. Patients are given written instructions that describe proper care of the catheter and catheter exit sites. Signs and symptoms of complications are discussed and contact information provided.
3. The care of CV catheters is dictated by hospital protocol and includes instructions for line flushing and dressing changes. This is discussed in Chapter 29.

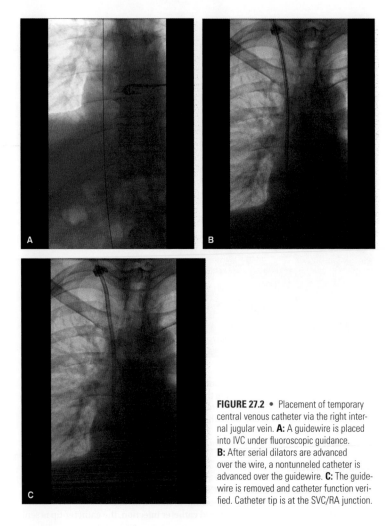

FIGURE 27.2 • Placement of temporary central venous catheter via the right internal jugular vein. **A:** A guidewire is placed into IVC under fluoroscopic guidance. **B:** After serial dilators are advanced over the wire, a nontunneled catheter is advanced over the guidewire. **C:** The guidewire is removed and catheter function verified. Catheter tip is at the SVC/RA junction.

Results

Successful placement of a CV access device requires a catheter placed into the venous system with the tip in the desired location. The catheter must also function appropriately for its intended use (i.e., medication administration vs. dialysis) (2). The reported placement success rates are between 95% and 96%. The threshold for successful placement in the IJV is 95% and in the subclavian or peripheral route is 90% (2).

Complications

Complications are defined as early (within 30 days of placement) or late (occurring after 30 days). Early complications are subdivided into those within 24 hours (procedurally related) and those that occur beyond that time window. Image-guided insertions are associated with lower complication rates when compared to placement using external landmarks (2,5). The overall, complication rate is 7% (2,5). The overall procedure threshold for major complications is 3% (4). Radiologic placement results in fewer early complications (5% to 10%), lower infection rates (9.7 vs. 14 per 1,000 catheter days), and fewer late complications (20% vs. 30%) when compared to surgical placement (7). Several of the more common complications are described below.

1. Malposition
   a. Catheter malposition immediately after placement is rare with the use of IG. Tip malposition occurs in 3% to 32% *without* image guidance, versus 0% to 4% *with* image guidance (7). Fluoroscopic guidance is used to confirm the proper positioning of the catheter and immediate adjustments can be made at the time of placement. If the catheter position is uncertain, venography can also be performed. Routine chest radiographs are not needed after image-guided catheter placement. If a PICC line is inserted at the bedside, a follow-up chest radiograph is obtained to verify catheter tip position.
   b. Catheter tips may lodge in a variety of locations due to anatomic variants including a left SVC, duplicated SVC, anomalous pulmonary vein, a collateral vein or retrograde within a vein.

2. Pneumothorax
   a. The incidence of PTX and accidental arterial puncture is low when US guidance is used for IJV access (1% to 2%). The risk of PTX is higher when only external anatomical landmarks are used for direct subclavian vein access (1). The risk is 0% for PICC placements.
   b. Most PTX remain asymptomatic, especially if the visceral pleura is displaced less than 2 to 3 cm from the parietal pleura. PTX is usually apparent immediately on postprocedure imaging. Rarely, a delayed PTX can develop several days later (1,8–10).

3. Air embolus
   a. Air embolus is a rare complication that occurs, if intrathoracic pressure drops, during catheter insertion into the vein through a peel-away sheath (1%). Air entry can be minimized by having the patient maintain a positive intrathoracic pressure by continuously humming and by manually crimping the external portion of the sheath immediately after removing the dilator and guidewire. The sheath should remain crimped until the catheter is advanced into it. Tiny air emboli declare themselves less frequently as patients remain asymptomatic. Large air emboli can be symptomatic. With cough and respiratory distress, or can even be fatal. In those cases, air luceny in the right atrium or pulmonary outflow can be seen on fluoroscopy. A peel-away sheath with a valve can help minimize this risk (10).

4. Great vessel or cardiac perforation
   a. Perforation is a rare complication (<1%) that may occur if dilator is advanced over a kinked guidewire or if the wire is not in the IVC (1,10). Catheters placed in the right subclavian vein are more prone to this as the vessel enters perpendicular to the SVC. Signs of hemodynamic instability, hemothorax, mediastinal hematoma, or cardiac tamponade may be present.

5. Late complications such as infection, fibrin sheath formation, venous thrombosis and catheter fracture, and their management will be discussed in Chapter 29. These are more often the consequence of long-term access.

Management of Complications

Malposition

1. A malpositioned catheter at the time of placement can be adjusted using fluoroscopic guidance and a guidewire.

2. If a catheter tip has migrated after the initial placement, many corrective options exist. For instance, if a catheter tip has migrated into the azygous arch, the catheter can be repositioned into the SVC using a pigtail catheter or an endovascular snare from a femoral approach. If catheter is too short, a catheter exchange may be indicated. If catheter is too long, catheter can be pulled back.

3. Poor aspiration of a PICC line may indicate that the catheter may be kinked. This can be corrected using a guidewire to straighten out the catheter. If any catheter will not aspirate when the tip is central, the tip may be against the wall of the RA. The catheter can slowly be withdrawn until free flow is achieved.

4. If a small-bore catheter is accidentally placed in the arterial system, catheter removal with manual compression can be attempted. If a large-diameter catheter is placed in the arterial system, removal may need to be performed in the operating room with a cut down. Other options upon removal of an arterial catheter include balloon tamponade, deployment of a covered-stent or closure device.

Pneumothorax

1. Small pneumothoraces are managed conservatively.

2. A large or symptomatic PTX, can be treated with a small-bore chest tube attached to a Heimlich valve (Becton Dickinson, Franklin Lakes, NJ).

3. If a Heimlich valve is insufficient, the catheter can be attached to a Pleur-Evac (Teleflex, Inc., NC) system or wall suction.

4. Rarely would a conventional surgical large-bore chest tube need to be placed.

Air Embolus

1. Not treated if emboli are small or patient is asymptomatic.

2. If symptomatic, place patient in the left lateral decubitus position (left side down) and administer 100% oxygen.

Great Vessel or Cardiac Perforation

1. Catheter removal in the operating room, as needed.

2. Catheter can be removed in the angiography suite. However, the equipment for balloon tamponade or stenting should be readily available. A surgical team may need to stand by for high-risk cases.

References

1. Funaki B. Central venous access: a primer for the diagnostic radiologist. *Am J Roentgenol.* 2002;179(2):309–318.

2. Lewis CA, Allen TE, Burke DR, et al. Quality improvement guidelines for central venous access. *J Vasc Interv Radiol.* 2003;14(9 Pt 2):S231–S235.

3. Malloy PC, Grassi CJ, Kundu S, et al. Consensus guidelines for periprocedural management of coagulation status and hemostasis risk in percutaneous image-guided interventions. *J Vasc Interv Radiol.* 2009;20(7 Suppl):S240–S249.

4. O'Connor SD, Taylor AJ, Williams EC, et al. Coagulation concepts update. *Am J Roentgenol.* 2009;193(6):1656–1664.

5. Silberzweig JE, Sacks D, Khorsandi AS, et al. Reporting standards for central venous access. *J Vasc Interv Radiol.* 2003;14(9 Pt 2):S443–S452.

6. Funaki B, Zaleski GX, Leef JA, et al. Radiologic placement of tunneled hemodialysis catheters in occluded neck, chest, or small thyrocervical collateral veins in central venous occlusion. *Radiology.* 2001;218(2):471–476.

7. McBride KD, Fisher R, Warnock N, et al. A comparative analysis of radiological and surgical placement of central venous catheters. *Cardiovasc Intervent Radiol.* 1997;20(1):17–22.

8. Tyburski JG, Joseph AL, Thomas GA, et al. Delayed pneumothorax after central venous access: a potential hazard. *Am Surg.* 1993;59(9):587–589.

9. Vescia S, Baumgartner AK, Jacobs VR. Management of venous port systems in oncology: a review of current evidence. *Ann Oncol.* 2008;19(1):9–15.
10. Bhutta ST, Culp WC. Evaluation and management of central venous access complications. *Tech Vasc Interventional Rad.* 2011;14(4):217–224.

28 Long-Term Central Venous Access: Tunneled Catheters and Subcutaneous Ports

Sidney Regalado, MD and Brian Funaki, MD

Introduction

Long-term central venous (CV) access devices are comprised of tunneled catheters and subcutaneous chest ports. Tunneled catheters are used for weeks to months (or even years) and are most commonly placed for chemotherapy, TPN, plasmapheresis, and hemodialysis. Implantable subcutaneous ports are used for access if the indication remains for months to years. Most commonly, ports are placed for chemotherapy. Generally speaking, tunneled catheters are easier/quicker to place and exchange, but, have a higher risk of infection and are more lifestyle limiting (overall cosmetic appearance and ease of hygiene) when compared to subcutaneous ports. All of these devices can be removed when they are no longer needed (1).

Indications (2)

1. Administration of chemotherapy, TPN, blood products, intravenous medications, and fluids
2. Performance of hemodialysis and plasmapheresis.

Contraindications

Absolute (1)
1. Bacteremia or sepsis
2. Cellulitis at insertion site
3. Allergy to catheter material

Relative (1)
1. Uncorrectable coagulopathy
2. Central venous occlusion

Preprocedure Preparation

Preprocedure preparation is similar to the placement of temporary CV access catheters described in the prior chapter. Notable differences are described below.
1. In addition to local anesthesia, patients often require conscious sedation. Patients must remain NPO for 6 hours, or per institutional protocol.
2. Guidelines to *coagulation parameters* should be followed to prevent bleeding complications (3). Tunneled CV access and subcutaneous ports are considered to be procedures with moderate risk of bleeding.

a. Routine INR should be obtained in all patients. INR goal is less than 1.5.
b. PTT is recommended in patients receiving intravenous unfractionated heparin. Normal range is 25 to 35 seconds. PTT should be less than 1.5 times control.
c. Platelet count not routinely recommended, but, transfusion is recommended for counts less than 50,000 per µL. Others utilize a platelet count ≥25,000 (4).
d. Plavix is withheld for 5 days before procedure. Aspirin not withheld.
e. Low–molecular-weight heparin (therapeutic dose) should be withheld for one dose before procedure.
3. *Prophylactic antibiotics* before central line placement is controversial as several studies support and refute their utility (5). If prophylaxis is desired for tunneled catheter or port placement, 1-g cefazolin or 500-mg clindamycin can be administered within 45 minutes of skin incision.

Procedure

General Considerations
1. All tunneled catheters and ports are placed in a fluoroscopy suite.
2. The skin is sterilized with a 2% chlorhexidine-based preparation. Standard surgical scrub protocol for the operator includes hand scrubbing, gloves, mask, cap, and gown.
3. Local anesthesia with 1% lidocaine is used for all line placements.
4. Conscious sedation with fentanyl citrate and midazolam hydrochloride is routinely administered. The nurse must continuously monitor vital signs.
5. Choice of device. As with temporary catheters, the smallest catheter size and minimum number of lumens to satisfy the indication for the access is important to decrease thrombotic complications. Power injectable devices permit their use for contrast injection during CT examination.
6. Guidance technique:
   a. Ultrasound (US) guidance is always recommended for venipunctures.
   b. Fluoroscopic guidance is used for visualization of guidewires, catheters, and venography.
7. Choice of vein
   a. The jugular veins are the preferred access site for tunneled catheters and subcutaneous ports. Subcutaneous ports can be placed through an arm vein, similar to a PICC line, however, arm ports are associated with higher risk of complications such as thrombosis (1).
   b. Femoral veins are less optimal sites of venous access as there is an increased risk of infection and worse patency (1,6).
   c. When conventional veins are exhausted, nonconventional access is considered.

Tunneled Central Venous Catheters

1. For women with large breasts, the breast should be taped inferiorly to relieve sagging and to prevent excessive retraction (with cephalad catheter-tip movement) when the patient resumes an upright posture.
2. The placement of tunneled catheters using conventional veins is essentially the same for all indications. Access to the jugular vein is made similarly to nontunneled access (Fig. 28.1A–C).
3. A working guidewire is placed from access site to the IVC (Fig. 28.1D).
4. The intended subcutaneous path of the tunnel is anesthetized with lidocaine using a long needle and preferably a single skin entry.

5. A skin nick is made in the chest wall at the desired catheter entry site so as to create a subcutaneous tunnel of 8 to 10 cm in length, and a tunneling device is advanced through this nick toward the neck venotomy site making a gentle curve in the tract (Fig. 28.1E). Some devices have a preformed curve.

6. An appropriately sized peel-away sheath is placed through the jugular access over the existing stiff 0.035″ wire.

7. The tunneled catheter is pulled through the tunnel so that the proximal retention cuffs are at least 2 cm within the entry to the tunnel (Fig. 28.1F).

8. Then the catheter is briskly advanced through the jugular peel-away sheath positioning the tip at the SVC/RA junction (Fig. 28.1G). See tips for avoiding air embolism.

9. The neck venotomy site is closed with skin glue (Dermabond; Ethicon, Mokena, IL) or a suture.

10. The tunneled catheter is anchored to the skin with a nonabsorbable suture.

11. Function is verified by aspiration and flushing of ports with saline.

12. Heparin is instilled in the lumens and caps are placed according to hospital policy.

13. Sterile dressing is applied.

14. Completion spot fluoroscopic image is saved to document tip position.

Chest Port

1. After gaining access to the jugular vein, a working guidewire is placed from access site to the IVC (Fig. 28.2A).

2. The intended port placement site and the tunnel tract are generously anesthetized with lidocaine with a minimal number of skin entries.

3. Using a No. 15 scalpel, a single 3 cm-long skin incision is made in the chest wall parallel to the sensory dermatomes. A subcutaneous pocket is made using blunt dissection. The pocket should be large enough to contain the port without excessive skin tension. If the port is placed too deeply, access with the Huber (B. Braun Medical, Inc., Bethlehem, PA) needle can be difficult. If the pocket is too superficial, skin erosion and breakdown can occur. If the pocket is too capacious, the port can flip over. If pocket is too small, excessive tension may lead to dehiscence of the wound.

4. The tunneling device is then advanced from the pocket to the neck venotomy site making a gentle curve in the tract (Fig. 28.2B). The catheter is pulled through the subcutaneous tunnel (Fig. 28.2C).

5. An appropriate peel-away sheath is placed over the wire at the IJV entry site.

6. The catheter tubing is advanced through the peel-away sheath and positioned at the SVC/RA junction. The endhole of the peel-away tubing outside of the patient must be clamped in order to prevent air embolism and bleeding.

7. The catheter tubing is cut at the level of the port pocket and is then attached to the port reservoir and secured by the hub (done in nonattached systems only). Care is required in allowing for enough catheter length within the pocket to attach it to the port, but not so much that it kinks. The port is lowered into the pocket.

8. Pocket is closed with a two-layer closure. The deep layer is closed with 3-0 absorbable sutures (Ethicon, Mokena, IL). A recent report suggests that barbed absorbable suture can be used for the deep layer closure with good success and potentially better outcomes than traditional absorbable suture. The cutaneous layer is closed with skin glue or a running subcuticular 4-0 absorbable suture.

9. The port is accessed with noncoring needle, aspirated, flushed with saline to check for leaks, and instilled with heparin volume as specified.

10. The venotomy site is closed with skin glue or 4-0 absorbable suture.

11. A sterile dressing is applied.

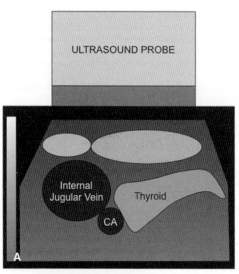

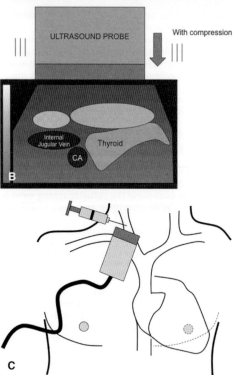

FIGURE 28.1 • Tunneled catheter placement. **A:** Transverse sonographic assessment of right internal jugular vein. **B:** Vein is compressible which suggests patency of the vessel. **C:** Ultrasound guidance for skinny needle puncture of right internal jugular vein. *(Continued)*

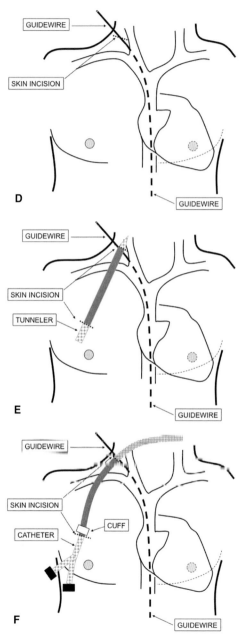

FIGURE 28.1 • *(Continued)*
D: Guidewire is advanced into the IVC (*solid portion* is external to the vessel and *long-dashed portion* is intravascular). **E:** Skin incisions are made in the right chest wall and at the neck venotomy sites (*short-dashed lines*). A tunneler is advanced to the puncture site in the neck (*polka dot portion* is external to the skin and the *solid portion* is in the subcutaneous tunnel). **F:** Catheter is pulled through the tunnel and the retention cuff is under the skin (*polka dot portion* is external to skin, *solid portion* is in the tract, and the *grid pattern* is going to enter the vessel through a peel-away sheath).

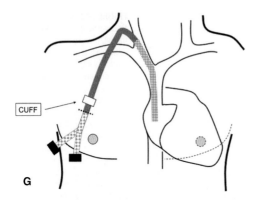

FIGURE 28.1 • *(Continued)*
G: Tip of tunneled catheter is at the SVC/RA junction (*polka dot portion* is external to skin, *solid portion* is in the tract, and the *grid pattern* is intravascular). CA, carotid artery.

CUFF

G

12. Follow-up spot fluoroscopic image is obtained to document catheter-tip position.
13. If needed, the Huber needles are placed and secured for the clinical service.

Device Removal

1. Tunneled central lines can be removed at bedside or in the recovery room using local anesthesia and manual traction. The retention cuff is freed from the sub-cutaneous tissues by using blunt and/or sharp dissection. Tunneled catheters can break during removal. The catheters will typically break at the junction of the catheter tubing and the cuff. If possible, the catheter is clamped to prevent air embolus and bleeding. If this is not possible, extrinsic compression on the catheter over the clavicle is performed to prevent bleeding and air embolus. An incision is made proximal to the cuff and the catheter is removed using blunt dissection and clamped.
2. Port removal is performed in the procedure room using sterile conditions. The majority of port removals are performed with local anesthesia only.
   a. An incision is made and the port is removed using blunt dissection. The port, hub, and catheter are removed. If the pocket is clean, the pocket is closed with absorbable sutures and skin glue.
   b. If the pocket is infected, copious irrigation is performed. The pocket is packed with iodoform packing strips and allowed to close secondarily.
   c. If the device is removed for suspected catheter infection, the catheter tip is sent for culture.

Exchanging a Nonfunctioning Tunneled Catheter

1. A tunneled catheter may not be functioning due to malposition of the catheter tip, fibrin sheath formation, or clotting of the catheter. Exchange of a tunneled catheter can be done using the same tract. Preprocedure protocol detailed above is followed.
2. A stiff hydrophilic wire is advanced into each lumen of the old tunneled catheter and into the IVC using fluoroscopic guidance. The old catheter is removed after dissecting the cuff out of the subcutaneous tissues (as described earlier). The old catheter is removed over the wires (as described earlier).
3. If a pericatheter fibrin sheath is suspected, angioplasty can be performed using an 8- to 12-mm balloon to disrupt it.
4. A new catheter is advanced over the wires.
5. The catheter is secured and function is verified.
6. Spot fluoroscopic image and sterile dressing are placed.

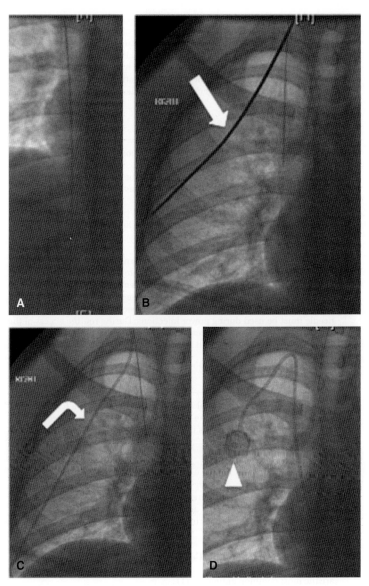

FIGURE 28.2 • Placement of a tunneled CV catheter or subcutaneous chest port. A: A guidewire is placed into the IVC under fluoroscopic guidance. B: During the placement of a port, a pocket is created using blunt dissection after making a 2 to 3 cm skin incision. A subcutaneous tunnel is made using a tunneler device (*arrow*). C: The catheter (*bent arrow*) is pulled through the tunnel to the neck venotomy site. D: The catheter is advanced through a peel-away sheath. Most ports still have to be assembled by connecting the catheter tubing, locking hub, and the port together. Port (*arrowhead*) is buried in the pocket and the pocket is closed. Catheter tip at the SVC/RA junction.

7. Occasionally, the new catheter may be difficult to advance through the tract, which can be due to an immature tract or sharp angulation at the venotomy entry site. The tract and venotomy site can be stretched with dilators or angioplasty balloons. The catheter can be advanced through a peel-away sheath placed in the tract to provide stiffness and support while manual compression is placed over the venotomy site to help direct the catheter inferiorly. Many catheters have either tapered distal ends or have guidewire stylets which can help facilitate catheter exchanges.

Postprocedure Management

1. With the use of imaging guidance, catheter malposition is rare. A spot radiographic is obtained to document tip position.
2. Patients are given written instructions that describe proper care of the catheter and wound. Signs and symptoms of complications are discussed and contact information provided.
3. The care of tunneled catheters and subcutaneous ports is dictated by hospital protocol and includes instruction for line flushing and dressing changes. This is discussed in Chapter 29.
4. Power injectable catheters
   a. Power injectable tunneled catheters have external identifying labels on the catheter which indicate maximum injection rates.
   b. Power injectable ports have multiple safety identifiers. Certain devices can be identified by shape or palpation points on the septum. Identifiers are also present on scout CT or plain radiographs. A special power injectable Huber needle must be used during power injections. During routine access of the port, nonpower injectable Huber needles may be used.
   c. Patients should be given written information to document the type of device that has been placed.

Results

As with temporary access, successful fluoroscopic placement of a CV access device into the venous system, with the tip of the catheter in the desired location and functioning appropriately for its intended use, is accomplished in nearly all cases (95%).

Complications

Early complications of CV access were described in the previous chapter and are directly applicable to long-term CV access. Unique late complications do arise with long-term CV catheters as their implantation time is longer than temporary catheters.

1. Infection
   a. Most common complication. Coagulase-negative Staphylococcus species, *Staphylococcus aureus*, aerobic gram-negative bacilli and *Candida albicans* are the most common pathogens (1).
      (1) In general, ports have the lowest infection rate, followed by tunneled catheters, and then nontunneled catheters. (7,8). The infection rate of ports has been reported at 0.21/1,000 catheter days, while for tunneled lines it has been reported at 2.77/1,000 catheter days (1,9).
      (2) Rate of catheter site infection is 0.26/1,000 catheter days. Rate of bloodstream infections is 0.19/1,000 catheter days (1,8,9).
      (3) In cases of suspected line infection, patients are treated with broad-spectrum antibiotics to cover the most common pathogens. The

antibiotic choice is tailored based on results of blood cultures, wound cultures, or catheter-tip cultures.

2. Fibrin sheath formation
   a. Most common cause of catheter dysfunction. The classic complaint is that the catheter can infuse but will not aspirate.
   b. A fibrin sheath is a proteinaceous coat of eosinophilic material and scattered inflammatory cells that envelop the catheter tubing and tip that can be identified on venography by contrast puddling at the tip or traveling in a retrograde direction along catheter tubing, rather than flowing directly in the central veins (1,10).
   c. Catheter dysfunction by a thrombus near the tip of the catheter can mimic the symptoms of a fibrin sheath as both can cause a one-way valve disrupting proper function.

3. Catheter-related CV thrombosis
   a. Manifestations of SVC syndrome such as arm swelling and face swelling can develop due to catheter-related CV thrombosis. Often there is a preexisting stenosis which is exacerbated by superimposed acute clot. Catheter-tip malposition increases the risk of thrombosis (10).
   b. Incidence is ~4% (2).

4. Catheter pinch-off
   a. Complications related to catheters passing through the subclavian vein do not occur with RIJV access.
   b. Catheters that are placed too medially are chronically compressed by the right rib and clavicle by the costoclavicular ligament and subclavius muscle (1,10). Repetitive compression can lead to fatigue and fracture. The catheter fragment may then embolize to the heart or pulmonary artery (~1%) (10).

Management of Complications

1. Infections
   a. Not every catheter suspected of being infected should be removed immediately. Consider catheter salvage if patient is stable and/or lacks other sites for potential venous access.
   b. Exit site or wound infections are initially treated with antibiotics.
   c. Tunnel infections or port pocket infections require catheter removal and antibiotics.
   d. If bacteremia is present, antibiotics are given. If blood cultures are negative for 48 hours, catheter exchange over a guidewire can be performed for PICC lines or tunneled central lines.
   e. If patient is septic, emergent catheter removal is indicated.
   f. Infected tunneled lines are removed by manual traction after dissection of the cuff. Catheter exit site closes by secondary intention. The catheter tip is sent for culture and sensitivity.
   g. Ports are excised and pocket irrigated. If pocket is clean, it can be closed primarily. If port pocket is purulent, the pocket is packed with iodoform packing gauze until pocket is clean and closes by secondary intention. Catheter tips are sent for culture and sensitivity. Extensive port pocket infections may require plastic surgery consultation.

2. Fibrin sheath formation
   a. First-line treatment is administering tissue plasminogen activator (tPA) into the lumens (1,10). Success rate is 87% to 93% for catheter clearance (10).
      (1) Alteplase (Cathflo; Genentech, San Francisco, CA) is reconstituted by injecting 2.2 mL of sterile water into the alteplase powder.
      (2) Administer the appropriate amount of alteplase based on the specified volume of the catheter.

(3) Allow 30 minutes of dwell time and reassess for patency.

(4) If still occluded, allow an additional 90 minutes of dwell time (120 minutes total) and recheck for patency.

(5) If still occluded, readminister a repeat dose of alteplase and repeat dwell times.

(6) An alternative protocol for pharmaceutical fibrin sheath disintegration involves administering an alteplase drip. A sample infusion protocol is to administer 2- to 4-mg alteplase mixed with 50-mL saline and infused over 3 to 4 hours (10).

b. If thrombolytics fail, exchange of catheter over a guidewire, with or without balloon angioplasty, can be performed (1,10).

c. Exchange of a port is more involved compared to exchanging a tunneled catheter. Therefore, fibrin sheath stripping using a loop snare is recommended.

3. Catheter-related CV thrombosis

a. Anticoagulation is the initial treatment.

b. If catheter is no longer needed, removal is indicated.

c. If catheter is needed, anticoagulation is continued. If anticoagulation is insufficient, thrombolytic therapy may be instituted.

d. If patient has an underlying SVC stenosis, angioplasty and/or stenting is needed to relieve symptoms.

e. A small amount of thrombus is often seen around catheter tips by CT. If asymptomatic and small clot burden, manage conservatively. If thrombus is large, consider anticoagulation.

4. Catheter pinch-off

a. A compressed, unfractured, subclavian catheter is followed with serial radiographs.

b. If catheter is partially fractured or has embolized, removal of the device is indicated. The embolized fragment can be retrieved using a loop snare.

c. Fragments can get chronically "endothelialized" into the right heart wall and this would preclude removal.

References

1. Funaki B. Central venous access: a primer for the diagnostic radiologist. *Am J Roentgenol.* 2002;179(2):309–318.

2. Lewis CA, Allen TE, Burke DR, et al. Quality improvement guidelines for central venous access. *J Vasc Interv Radiol.* 2003;14(9 Pt 2):S231–S235.

3. Malloy PC, Grassi CJ, Kundu S, et al. Consensus guidelines for periprocedural management of coagulation status and hemostasis risk in percutaneous image-guided interventions. *J Vasc Interv Radiol.* 2009;20(7 Suppl):S240–S249.

4. O'Connor SD, Taylor AJ, Williams EC, et al. Coagulation concepts update. *Am J Roentgenol.* 2009;193(6):1656–1664.

5. Covey AM, Toro-Pape FW, Thornton RH, et al. Totally implantable venous access device placement by interventional radiologists: are prophylactic antibiotics necessary? *J Vasc Interv Radiol.* 2012;23(3):358–362.

6. Zaleski GX, Funaki B, Lorenz JM, et al. Experience with tunneled femoral hemodialysis catheters. *Am J Roentgenol.* 1999;172(2):493–496.

7. Yip D, Funaki B. Subcutaneous chest ports via the internal jugular vein. *Acta Radiol.* 2002;43(4):371–375.

8. Moureau N, Poole S, Murdock MA, et al. Central venous catheters in home infusion care: outunneled catheteromes analysis in 50,470 patients. *J Vasc Interv Radiol.* 2002;13(10):1009–1016.

9. Groeger JS, Lucas AB, Thaler HT, et al. Infectious morbidity associated with long-term use of venous access devices in patients with cancer. *Ann Intern Med.* 1993;119(12):1168–1174.

10. Bhutta ST, Culp WC. Evaluation and management of central venous access complications. *Tech Vasc Interv Radiol.* 2011;14(4):217–224.

29 Central Venous Access Management

Rakesh Navuluri, MD, FSIR and Brian Funaki, MD

Introduction

Complications associated with central venous catheters (CVC) include:
- infection
- bleeding
- fibrin sheath
- thrombosis
- central venous stenosis or occlusion
- catheter malpositioning
- air embolism
- cardiac arrhythmia

Minimizing these complications starts with proper site care, but interventional radiologists should also be aware of how to identify and resolve these issues.

Site Care

A major source of catheter-associated blood stream infections (CLABSI) is contamination at the catheter entrance site. Use of best practice guidelines can reduce colonization at the catheter entrance site and consequently incidence of CLABSI.

1. Use of skin antiseptic solution during dressing changes, and when performing dressing changes every 7 days.
2. Skin damage at CVC insertion, whether preexisting or as a consequence of CVC insertion from adhesive dressing or chemical irritants, can further impair skin integrity and lead to infection. Dressing changes should be performed using aseptic nontouch technique which entails proper hand washing, use of gloves, and handling of catheter at the nonsterile portions away from the lumen. Additional recommendations include the use of proper site hygiene, clear transparent dressing to allow for monitoring of the entrance site, and proper catheter securement with suture and/or catheter stabilization device.
3. Chlorhexidine gluconate dressings have been shown to reduce the rate of catheter-related infections in the intensive care setting (1). However, there is insufficient data to support the use of antibiotic locking solution or prophylactic use of systemic antibiotics. Unnecessary use of antibiotics may potentially lead to antimicrobial resistance, allergic reaction or toxicity (2). Consider prophylactic antibiotic lock only in patients with long-term catheters who have a history of multiple CLABSI despite optimal maximal adherence to aseptic technique.
4. Anticoagulant locking solution should be used to prevent thrombosis. Low-concentration heparin (1,000 U per mL) is most commonly used. Alternatives include 4% trisodium citrate and 0.9% saline, or even tPA. There is no role of systemic anticoagulation as routine prophylactic therapy in patients without a history of recurrent thrombosis or known hypercoagulable state.
5. Appropriate catheter utilization is also important to maintain catheter functionality and minimize infections. Temporary lines in the internal jugular vein should be used for no more than 3 weeks, and no longer than 1 week for femoral vein lines. Ports use should be limited to intermittent therapy such as for chemotherapy, antibiotic infusions in cystic fibrosis or factor infusions for

hemophilia. Administration of TPN via ports is strongly discouraged due to risk of infection and the associated complexities involved with removal of a totally implantable device relative to a tunneled catheter. Lipids from TPN solution and some drugs can precipitate inside the port catheter lumen and cause obstruction (3).

Catheter Evaluation

Physical examination is the first line of catheter evaluation.
1. The catheter entrance site should be assessed for signs of infection including erythema, warmth, swelling, pain, fluctuance, or pus.
2. Catheter functionality should be interrogated using a saline syringe. The ability to flush saline but not aspirate blood may indicate a ball-valve effect that can be due to a catheter tip abutting a vessel wall, thrombus at the catheter tip, or a fibrin sheath. It may also reflect a catheter fracture which can be seen as leakage of saline in extracorporeal portion of catheter. However, fracture of the intracorporeal portion cannot be confirmed by physical examination.

Catheter malfunction should be further assessed by radiography. Imaging can reveal kinking or fracture, or even malpositioning of the catheter with the tip deflected into the azygous or ascending lumbar vein. A linogram or portogram, performed with injection of contrast under fluoroscopy, is best to confirm the presence of catheter fracture, fibrin sheath, thrombus, or even vessel stenosis or occlusion.

Catheter Malfunction

1. Infection
   a. Catheter-associated infection within 10 days of placement is typically related to skin flora with the most common organisms being *Staphylococcus aureus* and *Staphylococcus epidermidis*. These are introduced either during catheter placement or subsequent catheter access. Infection that occurs after 10 days is typically associated with intraluminal colonization. The incidence of infection also increases exponentially with the period of catheter use. Other risk factors for catheter-associated infection include neutropenia, malignancy, steroid use, thrombosis, TPN, and frequent use. There is also a greater incidence with temporary nontunneled catheters.
   b. Blood cultures, from both the CVC and a peripheral vein, should be obtained before starting systemic antibiotic therapy. Superficial or exit site infection (cellulitis) may be treated with antibiotics alone without need for catheter removal. Most other cases, including infection of a tunneled tract or subcutaneous pocket, require removal of the CVC. The distal catheter tip, and reservoir septum in the case of port catheters, should be sampled once removed.
   c. Port pocket infection that is associated with gross purulent material should be closed by secondary intention. This can be accomplished by daily packing of the open wound with iodiform gauze, and subsequent transition to saline-soaked gauze changed every 2 to 3 days once the wound appears clean.
      Criteria for catheter replacement vary by institution. At the authors' institution the patient must be afebrile and blood cultures must demonstrate no growth for 48 hours prior to replacement of a tunneled catheter or port. Replacement of catheter at a new site, different from that of a recently removed infected CVC, may be preferable.
2. Fibrin sheath
   A fibrin sheath is a connective tissue sleeve that envelops the catheter and represents a reaction to the presence of a foreign body. It typically develops from

the vein entry site along the catheter toward the tip, though it may also develop at the catheter tip where it contacts the vessel wall. Consequently, higher CVC tip position within the superior vena cava rather than in right atrium may be a predisposing factor. Fibrin sheaths can develop as soon as 24 hours after catheter insertion.

a. The first-line treatment is instillation of tPA, as it is noninvasive and can be performed at bedside. Two milligrams of tPA (in 2-mL saline) should be slowly instilled into each catheter lumen then allowed to sit for 30 minutes, after which the catheter is flushed with saline. If necessary, the procedure may be repeated.

b. More invasive options include catheter exchange, disruption of the fibrin sheath with balloon angioplasty, or stripping of the fibrin sheath using a snare. There is some evidence to suggest that longer patency rates may be achieved with simple line exchange rather than fibrin sheath stripping and this is generally the first-line therapy. However, simple catheter exchange could potentially result in placement of the new catheter within the existing fibrin sheath. Concurrent balloon disruption of the fibrin sheath with catheter exchange may be considered in refractory cases. It should be noted that there is some evidence that angioplasty of the central veins can predispose to central vein stenosis (4) and therefore should be performed sparingly.

3. Thrombosis

Catheter-associated thrombus can be intrinsic or extrinsic. Intrinsic thrombus occurs within or immediately surrounding the catheter, whereas extrinsic thrombus is external to the catheter and/or attached to the vessel intima (5). Thrombus may cause partial or complete catheter occlusion including a ball valve-like effect that prevents aspiration from the catheter, and even increased infection risk. Only 1% to 5% of catheter-related thrombosis is symptomatic, and typically presents beyond 2 weeks. With routine screening by venography, the incidence of CVC-associated thrombus in cancer patients has been reported between 27% and 66% (6). Many cases are incidentally noted on CT. There is a greater incidence of catheter-associated thrombus with:

- higher catheter tip position
- subclavian vein and left internal jugular vein access
- longer duration of catheter placement
- larger catheter diameter
- smaller central vein diameter
- greater number of lumens
- catheter material (polyurethane > silicon)
- type of solution instilled within catheter lumen
- hypercoagulable state
- associated medical comorbidities (malignancy, obesity) (5)

Potential long-term consequences of catheter-associated thrombus include central venous occlusion, upper extremity swelling, and SVC syndrome.

Anticoagulation is the first-line treatment of catheter-associated thrombus. Alternatively, small catheter tip thrombus may be dislodged with forceful saline flush, or advancing and rotating a J-tipped guidewire through the catheter lumen. Intraluminal thrombolytic instillation or infusion has also been reported. Catheter exchange may resolve catheter functionality issues but will inevitably result in dislodgement and embolization of thrombus. In most cases this is asymptomatic and well tolerated in the setting of anticoagulation. Large thrombus burden or septic thrombus may be addressed with aspiration thrombectomy.

4. Central venous stenosis

Central venous stenosis is a long-term complication of CVCs. The true incidence is difficult to ascertain as most cases are asymptomatic due to development of collaterals. However, stenosis may present as superior vena cava syndrome which is characterized by facial or upper extremity swelling. In these cases, further evaluation by CT venogram with subsequent endovascular treatment including possible stent placement should be undertaken.

In rare instances catheter entrapment can occur with in-growth of vessel endothelium or even endocardium into the catheter lumen. However, routine tunneled catheter exchange to prevent this complication is not recommended.

5. Catheter malposition
   a. Spontaneous catheter malpositioning can occur due to changes in body position during normal daily activities. In some instances, malpositioning may reflect suboptimal catheter length. Catheter retraction due to downward shifting of chest soft tissue in an upright position reflects a catheter of inadequate length and often requires replacement with a longer CVC. Conversely, catheters that are too long may lead to arrhythmias from catheter tip irritation of the right atrial wall and necessitate catheter replacement with a shorter CVC.
   b. Kinking or redundance of a catheter may be resolved by placing a stiff wire through the lumen under fluoroscopic guidance or by forceful injection of saline. The catheter tip may also be repositioned with the use of a snare.
   c. Pinch-off syndrome can result from subclavian-placed CVCs which are weakened and fractured at the thoracic inlet between the clavicle and first rib. Immediate removal of the central line and retrieval of any migrated fracture fragment is necessary. Catheter fracture can also occur as a complication during catheter removal. This is associated with catheters that have become scarred in from prolonged implantation time or that have degraded with time or extensive use. The retained catheter should be immediately clamped to prevent air embolism. Various maneuvers have been described to remove the retained catheter including cut-down with soft-tissue dissection, or using a snare under fluoroscopic guidance.

References

1. Timsit JF, Schwebe LC, Bouadma L, et al. Chlorhexidine-impregnated sponges and less frequent dressing changes for prevention of catheter-related infections in critically ill adults: a randomized controlled trial. *JAMA.* 2009;301(12):1231–1241.

2. Schiffer CA, Mangu PB, Wade JC, et al. Central venous catheter care for the patient with cancer: American society of clinical oncology clinical practice guideline. *J Clin Oncol.* 2013;31(10):1357–1370.

3. Tabatabaie O, Kasumova GG, Eskander MF, et al. Totally implantable venous access devices: a review of complications and management strategies. *Am J Clin Oncol.* 2017;40(1):94–105.

4. Ni N, Mojibian H, Pollak J, et al. Association between disruption of fibrin sheaths using percutaneous transluminal angioplasty balloons and late onset central venous stenosis. *Cardiovasc Intervent Radiol.* 2009;31:114–119.

5. Gunawansa N, Sudusinghe DH, Wijayaratne DR. Hemodialysis catheter-related central venous thrombosis: clinical approach to evaluation and management. *Ann Vasc Surg.* 2018;51:298–304.

6. Verso M, Agnelli G. Venous thromboembolism associated with long-term use of central venous catheters in cancer patients. *J Clin Oncol.* 2003;21:3665–3675.

30 Dialysis Fistulae

Aalpen A. Patel, MD, MBA and Scott O. Trerotola, MD

Introduction

An estimated 4 million patients worldwide receive renal replacement therapy and is forecast to increase to 5.4 million patients by 2030. Approximately 520 thousand of those patients are from the United States (1,2). In the mid-1990s, the National Kidney Foundation began to give evidence-based guidance to the teams caring for dialysis patients. The Disease Outcomes Quality Initiative (DOQI) recommendation document was published in 1997. In 2000, the scope was expanded to include chronic kidney disease even before the need for dialysis arises. This effort is now termed the Kidney Disease Outcomes Quality Initiative (NKF-KDOQI). The Vascular Access section was last updated in 2019 (3).

Long-term dialysis access is created via the construction of an arteriovenous (AV) shunt. This connection between an artery and a vein may be created by using native conduits (native arteries and veins), artificial conduits (grafts), or hybrid conduits. This chapter will address native arteriovenous fistulae (AVF). There are two new devices (Ellipsys endovascular arteriovenous fistula [endoAVF] system by Medtronic, Dublin, Ireland and WavelinQ endoAVF system by Becton, Dickinson and Company, Franklin Lakes, New Jersey) that allow endovascular creation of AVF. As more evidence accumulates and more dialysis teams are educated in the cannulation nuances for fistulae created by these devices, they may play an important role in access creation for appropriately selected patients.

The traditional fistula first approach has given way to a patient-centric approach that considers the individual patient's needs, circumstances, and preferences in developing an End-Stage Kidney Disease (ESKD) Life-Plan. The creation of an ESKD Life-Plan allows for an open discussion of access complications and the plan for the next access; it also encourages a comprehensive evaluation of lifetime access needs for kidney replacement therapy (KRT). The NKF-KDOQI 2019 update guides that the choice of access be considered in the context of ESKD Life-Plan (3).

Regular assessment of AVF should be performed to detect hemodynamically significant stenosis. It has been proven in a randomized trial that treatment of hemodynamically significant anatomic stenoses in fistulae reduces the incidence of access thrombosis and improves patency (4). The following complementary methods may be used as part of a quality assurance (QA) program. Physical examination and evaluation for such findings as arm swelling, development of collateral veins, prolonged bleeding, change in flaccidity of fistula, and change in outflow vein should be performed by a qualified health care professional on a monthly basis, which is termed *monitoring*. If special instrumentation is used to perform evaluation of the AVF at periodic intervals, it is termed *surveillance*. The NKF-KDOQI 2019 update does not recommend routine direct flow measurements, pressure measurements, or imaging for surveillance due to insufficient evidence (3).

Indications (for Diagnostic Imaging and Intervention)

1. Failure of the AVF to mature. The first access evaluation should occur 4 to 6 weeks after creation.
    a. Diagnostic fistulogram, if
        (1) Flow <600 mL/min (in the usable segment)
        (2) Draining vein <6 mm in diameter (usable segment)
    b. Angioplasty of stenosis anywhere in circuit up to the central veins; there is no evidence that central venous stenosis affects maturation.

c. Embolization or ligation of "competing" veins. This is a controversial issue because there is little evidence that treatment of such vessels helps with maturation.
2. Failing AVF. An AVF is thought to be failing when there is inadequate flow (<600 mL per minute or inadequate diameter of the usable venous segment of less than 6 mm. This failing behavior is usually due to inflow or outflow stenosis(es) greater than 50% associated with
   a. Decreased flow (decreased clearance)
   b. Increased static venous pressure
   c. Pseudoaneurysm
   d. Prolonged bleeding after needle removal
   e. Arm swelling
   f. Recirculation
   g. Abnormal physical examination
3. Clotted AVF

Contraindications

Absolute
a. Uncorrectable coagulopathy
b. Fistula infection. *Note*: Fistula infection is very unusual. As opposed to AVGs, erythema and warmth over a clotted AVF nearly always represents thrombophlebitis and not an infection.

Relative
a. Right-to-left cardiopulmonary shunt (for declotting procedures due to the risk of paradoxical emboli)
b. History of contrast reaction
c. Significant cardiopulmonary disease. During declotting procedures, pulmonary emboli can occur. Most of the time, they are without clinical consequences; however, in patients with right ventricular failure, pulmonary hypertension, and cardiac dysrhythmias, fatal pulmonary emboli have been reported.
d. Ischemia distal to the AV anastomosis. Increasing the flow through a fistula may further divert blood from the ischemic area and result in worsening of the steal syndrome.
e. Systemic infection

Preprocedural Preparation

1. Informed consent. This encounter also helps establish a rapport with the patient and helps to ease anxiety.
2. Intravenous (IV) antibiotics should be administered prior to thrombectomy/thrombolysis (cefazolin 1 to 3 g IV [weight based] or vancomycin 0.5 to 1.5 g IV [weight based] because the contents of a clotted fistula may be colonized) (5).
3. Obtaining a history of the current fistula (along with physical examination) is a critical step in preprocedural assessment. The following should be assessed and documented:
   a. When the fistula was created
   b. Type of fistula
   c. The method used for fistula creation
   d. If failure to mature, has there been any prior successful use
   e. When the dysfunction or clotting occurred
   f. Presence of steal symptoms
   g. Arm, face, or breast swelling
   h. Fever or chills
   i. History of prior interventions

4. Regardless of the type of access, the following should be assessed by physical examination and documented:
   a. Pulses: radial, ulnar, and brachial pulses (use Doppler if not palpable)
   b. Capillary refill and warmth of the arm/hand
   c. Chest wall collaterals
   d. Cardiac and pulmonary examination: to assess the patient's ability to safely tolerate moderate sedation and the procedure. Patients with existing pulmonary edema may require preprocedure dialysis via a temporary hemodialysis catheter.
   e. Physical evaluation of the AVF should be performed prior to each intervention.
      (1) Type and condition of access (radiocephalic fistula, brachiocephalic fistula, basilic or cephalic vein transposition, Gracz fistula or endovascular fistula), presence of aneurysms, pseudoaneurysms, or hematoma and the location of the anastomosis. This information helps in the choice of fistula access site(s) for intervention.
      (2) Presence or absence of thrill/pulse
      (3) An assessment of whether the fistula is tense or flaccid (even with thrill)
5. Review of the images from prior interventions is critical (especially when there is early failure after a prior procedure). In particular, determine if the previous intervention was optimal. This is a crucial step and should not be omitted.
6. Coagulation parameters (international normalized ratio [INR], partial thromboplastin time [PTT], and platelet count) should be assessed. An INR ≤ 2, PTT <40 seconds, and platelets $>25,000$ are acceptable.

Procedure

Interventions performed in AVFs include fistulography and angioplasty in nonmaturing or failing fistulae and clearing of clot from occluded fistulae (*declotting procedures*). Each will be described separately.

Fistulography and Percutaneous Transluminal (Balloon) Angioplasty for Nonmaturing Fistulae

1. Assemble the appropriate tools and equipment prior to the procedure:
   a. For fistula access: 18-gauge Angiocath or a micropuncture set
   b. Guidewires: Roadrunner (Cook Medical, Bloomington, IN) (preferred), Bentson wire, or long-tapered (8 cm taper) Glidewire.
   c. Sheaths: high-flow 6-Fr and/or 7-Fr short sheaths (4 to 6 cm long) with sidearm
   d. Balloons: Ultrahigh-pressure balloons: High pressures are often needed for percutaneous transluminal (balloon) angioplasty (PTA), especially in AVF. Short shaft balloons may be more convenient in fistula intervention.
   e. Inflation system (either of the following two):
      (1) 1-mL polycarbonate syringe, 10-mL syringe, and a flow switch. When a high-pressure balloon is used, this system is cost-effective and can generate more pressure than an inflator (6).
      (2) Dedicated inflator.
   f. Other equipment as needed:
      (1) Stents (covered and uncovered, self-expanding, and balloon expandable)
      (2) Catheters: Berenstein or Kumpe catheter (40 or 65 cm), Binkert, left internal mammary artery (LIMA), Rösch inferior mesenteric (RIM), or Cobra I catheter, depending on the type of fistula and anatomy.
2. Heparin 3,000 units is given IV at the beginning of the procedure and more as needed, guided by activated clotting time, as nonmaturing fistulae are prone to spasm and thrombosis. Nitroglycerin (NTG, 100 µg per mL) should be available for treatment of spasm.

3. For nonmaturing fistulae, the first access should be via the arterial side. Retrograde brachial or radial access is obtained by ultrasound-guided direct puncture using the 3-Fr inner dilator of a micropuncture set. This method reduces the risk of venous spasm and the need for inflating a blood pressure cuff to reflux contrast across the anastomosis, as is necessary with puncture of the venous side of the fistula. A fistulogram via brachial artery injection will demonstrate the "true" flow dynamics of the fistula and any hemodynamically significant stenoses that might be the reason for nonmaturation of the fistula. Venous spasm is common in a nonmaturing fistula and responds well to NTG, although rarely will require PTA to treat it. The brachial artery access may also be used for administration of NTG and heparin as needed in the procedure.

4. If there are stenoses requiring treatment, entry sites into the fistula from the venous side are chosen based on the fistulogram. Angioplasty should be performed via the venous side of the fistula to avoid arterial complications. If dilation of all stenosis is not possible via only one access, a second ultrasound or palpation-guided access to the fistula may be performed with a micropuncture set or an Angiocath.

5. Every stenosis ≥50%, potentially compromising inflow or outflow, should be treated with PTA.
   a. Usually a balloon 1 mm larger than the size of the adjacent normal vein is adequate in the primary outflow vein (7-mm and 8-mm balloons are common), with an inflation time of 90 seconds.
   b. For radiocephalic anastomosis, 5- to 6-mm balloons usually suffice. The authors strive for 6 mm, whenever possible.
   c. If the initial results are not satisfactory, progressive oversizing of balloons is performed as well as prolonged inflations of 5 minutes or more.
   d. Endografts are used for venous rupture refractory to prolonged PTA or for elastic recoil in locations not easily amenable to surgical intervention. Stents or endografts should not be used in lesions where the stenosis waist cannot be effaced with a balloon. Of note, there is little if any role for bare metal stents in hemodialysis access interventions due to their inferior results compared to endografts.

6. A completion fistulogram should be performed by hand injection of contrast through the arterial access or via the sidearm of the venous sheath to assess residual stenoses and exclude rupture. The maximum acceptable residual stenosis is less than 30%. Restoration of a nonpulsatile thrill is the best predictor of long-term results; this should be the goal in all cases (7).

7. In the complete absence of significant stenoses, if veins are present that are considered to possibly be diverting blood from the primary conduit, consideration should be given to surgical/percutaneous ligation (preferred for cost) or embolization of these veins. Proof that such veins are truly competing can be done by temporarily occluding the vein by external compression and determining if there is an improvement in the physical examination or, ideally, directly measuring flow. Truly competing veins will be extremely rare, less than 1% in most practices (8).

8. Treatment of "competing" veins should not be done at the same time as PTA of significant stenosis because the PTA will result in maturation in the vast majority of nonmaturing fistulae (8).

9. The puncture site may be closed in several ways, taking care not to thrombose the fistula:
   a. For arterial access and all punctures in nonmaturing fistulae, manual compression is recommended by the authors. Ultrasound-guided compression may aid in preventing hematoma in patients with large arms.
   b. Manual compression with a clotting agent.
   c. Purse-string suture, with a temporary device holding the strings or knot.

Fistulography and PTA for Failing AVFs

1. Equipment: as for nonmaturing fistulae.
2. For most interventions in nonoccluded mature fistulae with diminished function, heparin is not required unless flow is seen to be markedly reduced on fistulography.
3. The puncture site can usually be chosen based on presenting symptoms and physical examination, augmented by ultrasound. This initial evaluation will help avoid puncturing in the wrong direction and at the wrong site.
   a. If a low flow is suspected and the fistula is flaccid, inflow stenosis is likely the culprit and requires a venous puncture directed toward the AV anastomosis.
   b. If high pressure is the presenting complaint and the fistula is tense, the stenosis is likely on the venous side, and the venous puncture should be made in the downstream direction.
   c. An alternative option of entry site into the fistula for fistulogram and intervention in failing and clotted fistula is a transradial approach (9). It has been shown to reduce procedure time while maintaining similar contrast use and fluoroscopy time. It is another option available in the tool kit for fistula intervention (10).
4. A diagnostic fistulogram is vital and should opacify the anatomy from the arterial inflow to the right atrium before any intervention. The fistulogram provides a picture of both static stenoses and dynamic flow diverted via venous collaterals. The arterial inflow can be evaluated using a reflux maneuver. For forearm fistulae, an upper arm blood pressure cuff is inflated to suprasystolic pressure to occlude the outflow veins and direct the contrast back toward the anastomosis rather than through the venous outflow.
5. Any stenosis ≥50% that explains the presenting symptoms should be identified and treated with PTA.
   a. The occlusion or stenosis is crossed with a guidewire using standard techniques.
   b. Usually, a balloon 1 mm larger than the size of the vessel is adequate (typically 6 mm for a radiocephalic anastomosis, for the remainder of the fistula, 7- and 8-mm balloons are typical) with an inflation time of 90 seconds and up to 5 minutes for prolonged PTA. A randomized trial showed that a 3-minute inflation yielded better immediate result than a 1-minute inflation; however, this did not translate into improved long-term patency (11).
   c. Ultrahigh-pressure balloons have virtually eliminated the "resistant" stenosis.
   d. If the initial result after dilation is inadequate, progressive oversizing of balloons and prolonged inflation of 5 minutes are used to achieve a satisfactory result.
   e. KDOQI recommends avoiding bare-metal stent placement in the treatment of significant stenotic lesions in an AVF. Primary use of a stent-graft is recommended over angioplasty for in-stent stenosis in AVF circuit due to improved outcomes at 6 months. In addition, KDOQI recommends that any stent-graft placement decision consider the consequences of stent-graft placement on future accesses as planned in the ESKD Life-Plan (3). Other common indications for stent-graft placement are venous rupture refractory to prolonged PTA, elastic stenoses in locations where surgical intervention is not easily possible, and stenoses that recur within 3 months or less where no surgical options are available. The literature supports the surgical revision of accessible lesions when PTA fails (12,13). Whether stent-grafts are preferable to surgical revision remains an unanswered question.
   f. There is emerging evidence that there may be a role for drug-coated balloons (DCBs) in the treatment algorithm for stenoses in native fistulae. A recent single-blinded randomized trial by Lookstein et al. showed a statistically significantly higher patency in the DCB arm at 6 months compared to uncoated balloon arm, without any increased risk in the DCB arm. Future trials will provide insight into whether these results hold true for AV grafts for in-stent stenoses (2).

6. A postprocedural fistulogram should be performed to assess the effectiveness of angioplasty and to exclude vessel rupture. After maximal treatment, there should be less than 30% residual narrowing at all stenoses, ideally as close to 0% as possible. A continuous thrill (without significant pulsatility) is more indicative of a satisfactory outcome than a hemodynamic end point (7).

7. Residual stenosis due to recoil (i.e., successful waist effacement with residual stenosis >30%) is moderately common and almost always responds to prolonged PTA (two 5-minute inflations). If prolonged PTA fails, a stent or covered stent may be indicated. If there are no anatomic abnormalities on the postprocedural fistulogram and there are abnormalities on the physical examination (particularly a very weak thrill), a subclavian or innominate artery stenosis must be suspected and treated if present, working through the dialysis access.

Clearing of Thrombus from Occluded AVFs ("Declotting Procedure")

Equipment: as for nonmaturing fistulae

Systemic heparin is essential in declotting procedures because it helps to blunt any vasospastic or bronchospastic response to small pulmonary emboli, in addition to its role in preventing rethrombosis during the procedure. Prior to any declotting procedure on an AVF, heparin 3,000 units IV should be administered. Native fistula declotting procedures may be prolonged, requiring repeated heparin administration to maintain the activated clotting time above 250 seconds.

1. Mechanical thrombectomy: The authors use mechanical thrombectomy almost exclusively. Several mechanical thrombectomy devices are available for use; it is beyond the scope of this chapter to describe them all. The technique described in the following text has steps common to all types of mechanical devices. The steps described are in the sequence used for most cases, but it may be varied to suit a particular situation.

   a. Access: As in any hemodialysis access, the entry site into the fistula depends on the physical examination. Ultrasound findings are helpful to choose a site that is without clot or stenosis and as central as possible. Whenever possible, puncturing into or immediately adjacent to a stenosis should be avoided. This can help prevent the need for a second puncture. The access is made toward the anastomosis using Angiocath or a micropuncture set. Two punctures may be required, one toward the anastomosis and the other toward the primary venous outflow. A sufficient distance between each access site will allow the treatment of any intervening narrowed segments and eliminates sheath overlap, which may compromise flow. The 6-Fr or 7-Fr sheaths are placed depending on the size of balloons or devices to be used.

   b. Clot removal: After adequate heparin administration, a guidewire and catheter are used to cross the anastomosis. Achieving this step is essential for a successful declotting procedure. Rarely, brachial artery puncture may be required to cross the AV anastomosis; however, the authors do not advocate using brachial artery access for intervention. Via the sheaths directed toward the anastomosis or central veins, the thrombus is macerated with a balloon or a mechanical thrombectomy device in both directions and aspirated manually through the large sidearm or automatically by the device itself.

   c. Occasionally, an adherent chronic thrombus is difficult to fragment and remove, even with wall contact devices. Local massage (by hand or with an ultrasound transducer to monitor progress) may loosen the clot. If this maneuver is not successful, the clot may be loosened with a Fogarty adherent clot catheter (Edwards Lifesciences, Irvine, CA) and subsequently fragmented with a thrombectomy device and removed. Removal of wall adherent clots may result in better outcomes after declotting.

   d. Treatment of the anastomosis/perianastomotic stenosis: The key to successful thrombolysis in a dialysis access is the restoration of flow. This is usually achieved by treatment of the anastomotic plug/stenosis. Initially, this may be treated with a Fogarty balloon or a wall contact thrombectomy device, followed by PTA.

   e. Treatment of significant stenoses with angioplasty and/or stents: After carefully confirming antegrade flow in the fistula with a tiny injection of contrast, a diagnostic fistulogram can be performed. However, in order to prevent arterial emboli, forward flow must be documented before the diagnostic study is performed. Any stenoses identified are treated with PTA.

   f. Postprocedural fistulogram: A completion fistulogram is performed from the anastomosis to the right atrium, including the primary venous outflow. The arterial inflow may be visualized with outflow occlusion and contrast reflux (preferred), or by injection of contrast directly into the artery. The venous outflow may be occluded using a balloon or by external compression (manual or with a blood pressure cuff). Manual compression may increase the radiation dose to the operator. The same anatomic and clinical endpoints as for angioplasty of failing fistulae are used.

   g. Access site hemostasis: as for failing fistulae

2. Pharmaceutical thrombolysis (included for niche applications and historical purposes)

   a. Primary thrombolysis: The use of thrombolytic agents is another way patency can be achieved. Two catheters are placed from opposite directions without crossing the anastomosis. Lytic agents and heparin are pulsed into the clot until the clot is cleared. Any underlying stenoses that are uncovered are then treated in the standard fashion (14). Tissue plasminogen activator (tPA) doses vary between 3 mg and 20 mg. For resistant clots or when there is a large clot burden, infusion thrombolysis may also be performed.

   b. Adjunct thrombolysis: When there is very firm clot, large clot volumes, or in fistulae that have been clotted for over a week, some operators will instill lytic agents into the clot prior to mechanical thrombectomy. The lytic agent, tPA (2 to 4 mg) or reteplase (2 to 3 units), combined with heparin (3,000 to 5,000 units) is injected into the clotted fistula 0.5 to 2 hours prior to the procedure. In order to prevent central venous and arterial emboli due to pressurization of the fistula, both "limbs" of the fistula are occluded manually. The theory is that partial clot lysis prior to or during mechanical thrombectomy would shorten the procedure; however, in a prospective randomized trial, this was proven not to be the case (15).

Postprocedural Management

1. Postprocedural dialysis: The patient's condition, dialysis schedule, and preprocedure potassium levels will guide the decision to dialyze on the day of the procedure.
2. Distal pulses should be rechecked and documented.
3. For QA purposes, ensure that the access is usable for dialysis.

Results

1. Outcomes for AVF angioplasty when the failing AVF has *not* undergone mechanical thrombectomy or thrombolysis
   a. Technical success (less than 30% residual stenosis): 87%
   b. Primary patency after intervention: 66% at 6 months, 49% at 1 year, and 29% at 2 years (16)
   c. Secondary patency after intervention: 94% at 6 months, 84% at 1 year, and 79% at 2 years (16)
2. Outcome for AVF angioplasty when the AVF has undergone angioplasty following mechanical declotting or thrombolysis (using a transradial approach) (9)
   a. Technical success: 96% (9)

b. Primary patency after the intervention (varies with clot volume): 92% at 1 month, 77% at 3 months, 55% at 6 months, and 44% at 12 months. The primary patency of short segment thrombosis versus long segment was 57% versus 19%, respectively

c. Secondary patency after the initial intervention: 96% at 1 month, 93% at 3 months, 89% at 6 and 12 months

Complications

Major
1. Vein rupture resulting in a nonfunctioning access
2. Death related to sepsis
3. Volume overload from fluids administered during the procedure
4. Bleeding complications of thrombolysis
5. Pulmonary emboli
6. Arterial emboli (can be major or minor)

Minor
1. Venous rupture has been reported in up to 10% of transposed fistulae. This usually will not result in loss of the access if it is recognized and treated
2. Fistula thrombosis during PTA
3. Bacteremia
4. Pseudoaneurysm formation

Management of Complications

1. Arterial emboli
   a. If symptomatic, the embolus must be removed. Initial treatments should include back bleeding, Fogarty catheter technique, or thromboaspiration.
   b. Thrombolysis may be tried next. A surgical thrombectomy is an option of last resort.
   c. Puncture of the radial artery may be used to push the clot in a retrograde direction out of the artery.
   d. In an asymptomatic patient, the back bleeding technique may be tried because it does not risk further impaction of the clot. For this technique to work effectively, the fistula flow must be established first. If the clot is not cleared by this method, further treatment may not be required, particularly in light of the risk of clot impaction or more distal embolization associated with other techniques.
2. Venous rupture
   a. Approximately 70% of venous ruptures will respond to prolonged balloon tamponade (two 5-minute inflations).
   b. In the 30% of ruptures in which tamponade fails, covered stents can be used successfully to salvage the access (13,17).

References

1. Liyanage T, Ninomiya T, Jha V, et al. Worldwide access to treatment for end-stage kidney disease: a systematic review. *Lancet.* 2015;385(9981):1975–1982. doi:10.1016/S0140-6736(14)61601-9.
2. Lookstein RA, Haruguchi H, Ouriel K, et al. Drug-coated balloons for dysfunctional dialysis arteriovenous fistulas. *N Engl J Med.* 2020;383(8):733–742. doi:10.1056/NEJMoa1914617
3. Lok CE, Huber TS, Lee T, et al. KDOQI clinical practice guideline for vascular access: 2019 update. *Am J Kidney Dis.* 2020;75(4 Suppl 2):S1–S164. doi:10.1053/j.ajkd.2019.12.001
4. Tessitore N, Mansueto G, Bedogna V, et al. A prospective controlled trial on effect of percutaneous transluminal angioplasty on functioning arteriovenous fistulae survival. *J Am Soc Nephrol.* 2003;14(6):1623–1627.

5. Ayus JC, Sheikh-Hamad D. Silent infection in clotted hemodialysis access grafts. *J Am Soc Nephrol.* 1998;9(7):1314–1317.
6. Foering K, Chittams JL, Trerotola SO. Percutaneous transluminal angioplasty balloon inflation with syringes: who needs an inflator? *J Vasc Interv Radiol.* 2009;20(5):629–633.
7. Trerotola SO, Ponce P, Stavropoulos SW, et al. Physical examination versus normalized pressure ratio for predicting outcomes of hemodialysis access interventions. *J Vasc Interv Radiol.* 2003;14(11):1387–1394.
8. Liang H, Fu J, Wang P, et al. Endovascular salvage of immature autogenous hemodialysis fistulas. *Cardiovas Intervent Radiol.* 2014;37(3):671–678.
9. Wu CC, Wen SC, Chen MK, et al. Radial artery approach for endovascular salvage of occluded autogenous radial-cephalic fistulae. *Nephrol Dial Transplant.* 2009;24(8):2497–2502.
10. Shamimi-Noori S, Sheng M, Mantell MP, et al. Diagnosis and treatment of nonmaturing fistulae for hemodialysis access via transradial approach: a case-control study. *J Vasc Interv Radiol.* 2020;31(6):993–999.e1. doi:10.1016/j.jvir.2020.01.023.
11. Forauer AR, Hoffer EK, Homa K. Dialysis access venous stenoses: treatment with balloon angioplasty—1- versus 3-minute inflation times. *Radiology.* 2008;249(1):375–381.
12. Quinn SF, Schuman ES, Demlow TA, et al. Percutaneous transluminal angioplasty versus endovascular stent placement in the treatment of venous stenoses in patients undergoing hemodialysis: intermediate results. *J Vasc Interv Radiol.* 1995;6(6):851–855.
13. Gray RJ, Horton KM, Dolmatch BL, et al. Use of Wallstents for hemodialysis access-related venous stenoses and occlusions untreatable with balloon angioplasty. *Radiology.* 1995;195(2):479–484.
14. Cohen MA, Kumpe DA, Durham JD, et al. Improved treatment of thrombosed hemodialysis access sites with thrombolysis and angioplasty. *Kidney Int.* 1994;46(5):1375–1380.
15. Vogel PM, Bansal V, Marshall MW. Thrombosed hemodialysis grafts: lyse and wait with tissue plasminogen activator or urokinase compared to mechanical thrombolysis with the Arrow-Trerotola percutaneous thrombolytic device. *J Vasc Interv Radiol.* 2001;12(10):1157–1165.
16. Neuen BL, Gunnarsson R, Baer RA, et al. Factors associated with patency following angioplasty of hemodialysis fistulae. *J Vasc Interv Radiol.* 2014;25(9):1419–1426. doi:10.1016/j.jvir.2014.05.020.
17. Dale JD, Dolmatch BL, Duch JM, et al. Expanded polytetrafluoroethylene–covered stent treatment of angioplasty-related extravasation during hemodialysis access intervention: technical and 180-day patency. *J Vasc Interv Radiol.* 2010;21(3):322–326.

31 Dialysis Grafts

Aalpen A. Patel, MD, MBA and Scott O. Trerotola, MD

Introduction

Long-term dialysis access is created via the surgical construction of a connection between an artery and a vein using only the native vessels or nonnative conduits. Nonnative conduits include synthetic grafts (polytetrafluoroethylene or polyurethane), biologic grafts (bovine heterograft, bovine mesenteric vein, cryopreserved femoral vein, or human umbilical cord vein), or hybrid grafts (with self-sealing composite material or cryopreserved vein). This chapter will address the endovascular management of nonnative arteriovenous grafts (AVGs).

The Kidney Diseases Outcomes Quality Initiative (NKF-KDOQI) recommendations state that the construction of dialysis access should consider a patient-centric approach using an ESKD Life-Plan and patient access needs. An ESKD Life-Plan allows a comprehensive yet individualized plan for access through the expected span of the patient's life. Access type is then determined with ESKD Life-Plan, patient preferences, the support structure in mind. Of course, the ultimate goal is dialysis access success with high usability and minimal complications. In this way, the new guidelines are less prescriptive. If an AVG fits in the ESKD Life-Plan and patient preference, the distal first to proximal approach should be used (1). The preferred order for AVG creation is a forearm graft (loop graft preferred over straight graft), upper arm graft, and chest wall prosthetic graft ("necklace graft"). Lower extremity AVG is an access of last resort.

The rationales for monitoring and surveillance methods are the same as for dialysis fistulae and are discussed in Chapter 30.

Indications

1. Failing AVG. Clinical or hemodynamic abnormality and associated vessel/graft stenosis of greater than 50%, leading to
   a. Decreased flow (decreased clearance)
   b. Increased venous pressure
   c. Pseudoaneurysm
   d. Prolonged bleeding after needle removal
   e. Arm swelling
   f. Recirculation
   g. Abnormal physical examination
2. Clotted AVG

Contraindications

Absolute
1. Uncorrectable coagulopathy
2. Graft infection

Relative
1. Right-to-left cardiopulmonary shunt (for declotting procedures due to risk of paradoxical emboli)
2. History of contrast reaction
3. Systemic infection
4. Significant cardiopulmonary disease. During declotting procedures, pulmonary emboli can occur. Most of the time, they are without clinical consequences; however, in patients with right ventricular failure, pulmonary hypertension, or cardiac dysrhythmias, fatal pulmonary emboli have been reported.
5. Ischemia distal to the arteriovenous (AV) anastomosis. Increasing the flow through a graft may further divert blood from the ischemic area and result in worsening of the steal syndrome.
6. AVGs inserted less than 30 days prior to intervention have not formed sufficient perigraft scar tissue and may bleed when punctured. The resulting hematoma may lead to loss of the hemodialysis access altogether or local infection. Patency associated with declotting in this situation is exceedingly poor.

Preprocedural Preparation

1. A physician (preferably the one performing the procedure) or an advanced practitioner (depending on hospital policy or state law) must obtain informed consent. This encounter also helps establish a rapport with the patient and helps to ease anxiety.
2. Intravenous (IV) antibiotics should be considered prior to thrombectomy (cefazolin or vancomycin, based on weight) because the contents of a clotted graft are often colonized (2).
3. Obtaining a history of the current AVG (along with physical examination) is one of the most important steps in the preprocedural assessment. The following should be assessed and documented:

a. When the access was created
b. Type of access
c. When the dysfunction or clotting occurred
d. Presence of steal symptoms
e. Arm, face, or breast swelling
f. Warmth or erythema of the access site
g. Fevers or chills
h. History of prior interventions

4. Regardless of the type of access, the following should be assessed by physical examination and documented:
   a. Pulses: radial, ulnar, and brachial pulses (dorsalis pedis, posterior tibial, popliteal, and femoral pulses for lower extremity grafts). Use a Doppler device if the pulses are not palpable.
   b. Capillary refill and warmth of the arm/hand
   c. Chest wall collaterals
   d. Cardiac and pulmonary examination. Assessment of the patient's ability to safely tolerate moderate sedation and the procedure. Patients with pulmonary edema may require preprocedural dialysis via a temporary hemodialysis catheter.
   e. Physical evaluation of the graft should be performed prior to each intervention.
      (1) Graft site: for warmth and erythema that might indicate graft infection or cellulitis. A graft infection is an *absolute* contraindication to percutaneous intervention.
      (2) Type of access: straight or loop, the direction of inflow and outflow, presence of aneurysmal graft degeneration, and the location of anastomoses. This information helps in the determination of the access site(s).
      (3) Presence or absence of a thrill or pulse. Rarely, a patient may be referred with a "clotted graft" that is actually not clotted but has very low flow. In these cases, an inflow lesion should be sought and corrected.
      (4) A review of the images from prior interventions is vital (especially when there is early failure after a prior procedure). In particular, determine whether the outcome of the previous intervention was optimal.
      (5) Coagulation parameters (international normalized ratio [INR], partial thromboplastin time [PTT], and platelet count) should be assessed. INR <2.0, PTT <40 seconds, and platelets >25,000 per μL are acceptable.

Procedure

Interventions performed on AVGs include fistulography and angioplasty in failing grafts and clearing of clot from occluded grafts ("declotting procedures").

Fistulography and Angioplasty for Failing AVGs
1. Assemble the appropriate equipment.
   a. For access: 18-gauge Angiocath or micropuncture set
   b. Guidewires: stiff hydrophilic wire or a Bentson wire
   c. Sheaths: high-flow 6-Fr and/or 7-Fr short sheaths (4- to 6-cm long) with a sidearm
   d. Balloons: high-pressure angioplasty balloons
   e. Inflation system
      (1) Dedicated inflator or
      (2) 1-mL polycarbonate syringe, 10-mL syringe, and a flow switch (3)
   f. Other equipment as needed: stents (covered self-expanding, and balloon expandable)
2. The puncture site can usually be chosen based on presenting symptoms and physical examination, occasionally augmented by ultrasound. This initial evaluation will help avoid puncturing in the wrong direction. For example, if a low flow is suspected and the graft is flaccid, the arterial limb upstream from the

flaccid segment, or the inflow arteries, maybe the culprit lesion. This would require puncture toward the arterial anastomosis. Conversely, if high pressure is the chief complaint and the graft is tense, the puncture should be made toward the venous anastomosis.

3. A diagnostic fistulogram is critical and should be performed from the arterial inflow to the right atrium prior to any intervention. The fistulogram gives both a picture of static stenoses and of dynamic flow as a result of the stenosis, diverted via the venous collaterals. The arterial inflow may be evaluated with a reflux maneuver. A common technique is to compress the graft downstream from the access to direct the contrast back toward the inflow.

4. Any stenosis ≥50% that explains the presenting symptoms should be identified and treated with percutaneous transluminal (balloon) angioplasty (PTA). Stent-graft placement should be considered over PTA alone for certain lesions as noted below.

   a. The occlusion or stenosis is crossed with a guidewire using standard techniques.

   b. Usually, a balloon 1 mm larger than the size of the graft is adequate, with an inflation time of 90 seconds.

   c. If the initial result is inadequate, progressive oversizing of balloons is performed as well as prolonged inflations of 5 minutes or more, in order to achieve a satisfactory result.

   d. KDOQI recommends that bare-metal stents should be avoided in the treatment of significant stenotic lesions in an AVG (1).

   e. KDOQI recommends using self-expanding stent-grafts over angioplasty alone for treatment of graft-venous anastomotic stenosis and in-stent stenoses as it has been shown to have improved patency at 6 months (1,6). Of course, any stent-graft placement should consider the consequences of future AV access plans noted in the patient's ESKD Life-Plan; the access team should be consulted as needed (1). The most common other indications for stent-graft placement are venous rupture refractory to prolonged PTA, elastic stenoses in locations where surgical intervention is not easily possible, and stenoses that recur within 3 months or less where no surgical options are available. The literature has supported surgical revision of accessible lesions for failed PTA (4).

   f. There is increasing evidence for AVF that drug-coated balloons use lead to higher patency of the treated site than use of conventional balloons in treatment of stenoses in fistulae. Future trial will determine if these results translate to AVG and in-stent stenosis (5).

5. A completion fistulogram (from the arterial anastomosis to the right atrium, including the venous outflow) is performed to assess the effectiveness of angioplasty/stent-graft placement and to exclude vessel rupture. The arterial inflow may be visualized with outflow occlusion and contrast reflux (preferred) or cannulating the artery (via the graft) and performing the fistulogram from the artery. The venous outflow may be occluded by a balloon (preferred) or manual compression.

6. After maximal treatment, there should be less than 30% residual narrowing at all stenoses (6), ideally as close to 0% as possible. Restoration of a thrill on a physical examination is the best predictor of long-term results; thus, a thrill should be sought in all cases (7).

7. The site of puncture may be closed in several ways. Care must be taken not to thrombose the graft.

   a. Manual compression

   b. Manual compression with a clotting agent (8)

   c. Purse-string suture (with a temporary device that holds the strings or a knot)

Clearing of Thrombus from Occluded AVGs (Declotting Procedures)

1. Equipment: same as for the treatment of failing AVGs; additional equipment as noted in the following text.

2. Mechanical thrombectomy. The authors use mechanical thrombectomy almost exclusively for declotting procedures. There are several mechanical thrombectomy devices available; it is beyond the scope of this chapter to describe them all. The technique described in the following text has steps common to all types of mechanical devices. The steps described are in the sequence used for most cases, but it may be varied to suit a particular situation. If using a rheolytic device, PTA of the outflow should be performed earlier to reduce the chance of increasing pressure in the access and the likelihood of arterial emboli.

   a. Access: The choice of access site depends on graft configuration.
      (1) Loop AVG: The first puncture is made near the apex directed toward the venous anastomosis and a second puncture (2 cm from the venous anastomosis) is directed toward the arterial anastomosis. Choosing a graft access site in this manner allows maximum flexibility in clot access, sufficient distance between each access site to treat any narrowed segments between them and reduces the chances of sheath overlap that may impede flow.
      (2) Straight AVG: The first puncture is made 1 to 2 cm from the arterial anastomosis in the direction of the venous anastomosis and the second 1 to 2 cm from the venous anastomosis directed toward the arterial anastomosis.

   b. Systemic heparin is essential in declotting procedures because it helps to blunt any physiologic response to small pulmonary emboli, in addition to its role in preventing rethrombosis during the procedure. Prior to any declotting procedure on an AVG, heparin 3,000 units IV should be administered.

   c. An angled catheter (Berenstein or Kumpe) is advanced across the occlusion and into the central veins. A pullback venogram is performed from the right atrium to the venous anastomosis, being careful not to inject into the clotted graft because this may result in arterial emboli.

   d. A 7-Fr short sheath (preferably 4 to 6 cm) with a radiopaque tip and large-bore side arm (suitable for aspiration) is inserted via the puncture directed toward the venous anastomosis.

   e. A 6-Fr or 7-Fr sheath is placed at the second puncture directed toward the arterial anastomosis. The clot is not aspirated prior to the second access because doing this may lead to the collapse of the graft, making the second access difficult.

   f. Clot removal. The thrombus is macerated with a mechanical thrombectomy device in both directions and aspirated manually via the sheath or fragmented and aspirated automatically with a rheolytic device. Balloon maceration alone may result in an unacceptable high pulmonary embolic load.

   g. Treatment of the arterial plug: This can be performed with a Fogarty balloon (over the wire or non-over the wire) or a mechanical thrombectomy device (only one device, the Arrow-Trerotola percutaneous thrombolytic device [PTD] is U.S. Food and Drug Administration [FDA] approved for this, however).
      (1) A Fogarty balloon should be advanced beyond the arterial anastomosis; then under fluoroscopy, the balloon should be inflated and pulled back through the anastomosis. The plug is often firm and adherent and may require several passes for adequate treatment.
      (2) If using a mechanical thrombectomy device (in particular the PTD), it is passed beyond the arterial anastomosis and deployed in the artery. The device is pulled back until it is seen to deform the arterial plug and then activated, and mechanical thrombectomy is performed, treating the arterial plug and the arterial limb. It is important that the device not be deployed at the anastomosis but rather in the artery because inadvertent forward motion of the basket during deployment might cause an arterial embolus.

    (3) Regardless of the method used to break up the clot, aspiration of the fragmented thrombus through the sheaths is performed.

    (4) Diagnostic fistulography can be performed; however, in order to prevent arterial emboli, antegrade flow in the graft must first be documented with a tiny injection of contrast. Any residual clot must be treated.

3. Treatment of significant stenoses with angioplasty and/or stent-graft and postprocedural fistulogram are performed in the same manner as described earlier for failing grafts.

4. Access site hemostasis is obtained.

5. Chemical thrombolysis. Primary and secondary thrombolysis can be performed in the same manner as described for dialysis fistulae.

Postprocedural Management

1. Postoperative dialysis: The patient's condition, dialysis schedule, and preoperative potassium levels will guide the decision to dialyze on the day of the procedure.

2. Distal pulses should be rechecked and documented.

3. For quality assurance (QA) purposes, ensure the graft is usable for dialysis.

Results

1. Outcomes for graft angioplasty when the graft has not undergone mechanical thrombectomy or thrombolysis
   a. Clinical success (ability to perform dialysis for at least one session): 86% to 98% (9,10)
   b. Primary patency after angioplasty: 85%, 53%, 29% at 3, 6, and 12 months, respectively (10)
   c. Primary-assisted patency of grafts after PTA: 56% to 86% and 37% to 63% at 6 and 12 months depending on conventional versus cutting balloon (9)
   d. The primary AVG patency for stent-graft: when focusing only on the graft-venous anastomosis, at 6 months, the primary patency of the treatment is 51% for the stent-graft group and only 23% for the PTA group (6)

2. Mechanical declotting or thrombolysis
   a. Successful clearing of thrombus: 89% to 100% (10–12)
   b. Primary patency after intervention: 40% to 63% at 3 months and in the vicinity of 20% to 26% at 12 months (10,13)

Complications and Management of Complications

As described for dialysis fistulae.

References

1. Lok CE, Huber TS, Lee T, et al. National kidney foundation. KDOQI clinical practice guideline for vascular access: 2019 update. *Am J Kidney Dis.* 2020;75(4 Suppl 2):S1–S164. doi:10.1053/j.ajkd.2019.12.001.

2. Ayus JC, Sheikh-Hamad D. Silent infection in clotted hemodialysis access grafts. *J Am Soc Nephrol.* 1998;9(7):1314–1317.

3. Foering K, Chittams JL, Trerotola SO. Percutaneous transluminal angioplasty balloon inflation with syringes: who needs an inflator? *J Vasc Interv Radiol.* 2009;20(5):629–633.

4. Anaya-Ayala JE, Smolock CJ, Colvard BD, et al. Efficacy of covered stent placement for central venous occlusive disease in hemodialysis patients. *J Vasc Surg.* 2011;54(3):754-9. doi:10.1016/j.jvs.2011.03.260

5. Lookstein RA, Haruguchi H, Ouriel K, et al. Drug-coated balloons for dysfunctional dialysis arteriovenous fistulas. *N Engl J Med.* 2020;383(8):733–742. doi:10.1056/NEJMoa1914617

6. Haskal ZJ, Trerotola S, Dolmatch B, et al. Stent graft versus balloon angioplasty for failing dialysis-access grafts. *N Engl J Med.* 2010;362(6):494–503.

7. Trerotola SO, Ponce P, Stavropoulos SW, et al. Physical examination versus normalized pressure ratio for predicting outcomes of hemodialysis access interventions. *J Vasc Interv Radiol*. 2003;14(11):1387–1394.
8. Wang DS, Chu LF, Olson SE, et al. Comparative evaluation of noninvasive compression adjuncts for hemostasis in percutaneous arterial, venous, and arteriovenous dialysis access procedures. *J Vasc Interv Radiol*. 2008;19(1):72–79.
9. Saleh HM, Gabr AK, Tawfik MM, et al. Prospective, randomized study of cutting balloon angioplasty versus conventional balloon angioplasty for the treatment of hemodialysis access stenoses. *J Vasc Surg*. 2014;60(3):735–740.
10. Turmel-Rodrigues L, Pengloan J, Baudin S, et al. Treatment of stenosis and thrombosis in haemodialysis fistulas and grafts by interventional radiology. *Nephrol Dial Transplant*. 2000;15(3);2029–2036.
11. Beathard GA, Welch BR, Maidment HJ. Mechanical thrombolysis for the treatment of thrombosed hemodialysis access grafts. *Radiology*. 1996;200(3):711–716.
12. Uflacker R, Rajagopalan PR, Vujic I, et al. Treatment of thrombosed dialysis access grafts: randomized trial of surgical thrombectomy versus mechanical thrombectomy with the Amplatz device. *J Vasc Interv Radiol*. 1996;7(2):185–192.
13. Turmel-Rodrigues L, Pengloan J, Bourquelot P. Interventional radiology in hemodialysis fistulae and grafts: a multidisciplinary approach. *Cardiovasc Intervent Radiol*. 2002;25(1):3–16.

32 Dialysis Catheter Management

Peter R. Bream, Jr., MD, FSIR

Introduction

In 2019, the National Kidney Foundation revised their Guidelines for Vascular Access (Kidney Disease Outcomes Quality Initiative [NKF-KDOQI]) (1). All proceduralists placing dialysis catheters should be familiar with this document. The new guidelines focus on developing an End-Stage Kidney Disease (ESKD) Life-Plan that is personalized for each patient, revised annually, and should be reviewed when deciding where to place a dialysis catheter.

Hemodialysis catheters can be categorized by duration of use (acute or chronic catheters) and method of insertion (tunneled or nontunneled catheters). Tunneled catheters are appropriate for most clinical situations. Nontunneled, temporary catheters are used primarily for hospitalized patients without an existing functional access, either for initiation of hemodialysis or temporary dialysis. Central venous catheters have advantages when compared to arteriovenous fistulae (AVFs) and prosthetic grafts, including simplicity of insertion, immediate utility, access without needle cannulation, and ease of replacement and removal.

Proceduralists placing dialysis access should practice vein preservation in all patients. This means thoughtful selection of access site, deliberate placement of catheter tip location, and liberal use of previous access via catheter exchange or cut down.

Indications

1. Urgent need of renal replacement therapy but no functional AVF or graft
2. Stage 5 chronic kidney disease (CKD5) requiring acute hemodialysis but no usable hemodialysis access
   a. Long-term (tunneled) catheters should be used, as outlined in the NKF-KDOQI guidelines, while awaiting placement or maturation of an arteriovenous AVF or prosthetic graft.

3. Permanent vascular access in rare cases, for example, patients with cardiac failure who cannot tolerate a left-to-right shunt, upper extremity vascular anomalies or disease precluding placement of a graft or fistula, and patients with diffuse dermatologic conditions that would complicate surgical placement or recurrent needle cannulation of fistula.
4. Patients with a limited lifespan (e.g., malignancy).
5. Failed AVF or prosthetic graft while awaiting surgical revision or creation of a new vascular access.
6. Exhaustion of all surgical options for an AVF or graft placement.
7. Dysfunctional or infected peritoneal dialysis catheter.
8. Patients without renal failure who have metabolic disturbances, uncorrectable without hemodialysis, undergoing plasmapheresis, or stem cell harvest.

Contraindications

Absolute
1. Sepsis. A temporary nontunneled catheter can be inserted
2. Uncorrectable coagulopathy. Consider a nontunneled catheter placed with ultrasound guidance.

Relative
1. Coagulopathy. Abnormal coagulation parameters or low platelet counts should be corrected prior to access placement. Uremia causes platelet dysfunction that can result in bleeding, which may require therapy such as desmopressin acetate (DDAVP) administration.
2. Electrolyte abnormalities. Uremic patients may have hyperkalemia and cardiac irritability. Serum potassium measurement is recommended for patients with acute renal failure. Elevated potassium can induce arrhythmias manifested by peaked T-waves, flattened P-waves, and prolonged QRS. All patients with hyperkalemia, particularly if acute should have an electrocardiogram (ECG), and measures should be taken to decrease serum potassium. Interventions include oral Kayexalate (sodium polystyrene sulfonate), intravenous (IV) insulin and glucose, and inhaled albuterol.
3. Orthopnea. Patients with congestive heart failure, pulmonary edema, or sleep apnea may not be able to remain supine during a procedure. Optimization of oxygenation and judicious sedation are required. A lower extremity temporary or tunneled catheter can be considered.

Preprocedure Preparation

Basic Considerations
1. Assessment of the current and recent medical history including review of patient's ESKD Life-Plan (1)
   a. Current lab values: only in patients with risk factors.
   b. Knowledge of prior central venous access procedures and complications.
   c. Drug allergies including contrast agents.
2. Informed consent should be obtained and documented.
3. IV sedation with appropriate monitoring is often needed.
4. The recent update of procedural guidelines for interventional procedures places both tunneled and nontunneled catheter placement, exchange, and removal as *low risk*. Antiplatelet therapy such as clopidogrel or aspirin does not require discontinuation (2,3).
5. Antibiotics do not decrease the incidence of postprocedural catheter-related infections (4).

Selection of Catheter Insertion Site

1. Vein preservation is a guiding principle when choosing an access site. The preferred access sites in order are right internal jugular vein, right external jugular vein then left internal jugular vein.
2. A tunneled catheter should *not* be inserted on the same side as a maturing hemodialysis fistula or graft.
3. Avoid subclavian (sole venous outflow of ipsilateral upper extremity) vein access due to risk of central venous stenosis and thrombosis. It should only be used when surgical options in the ipsilateral upper extremity have been exhausted.
4. Femoral vein catheters:
   a. Have a higher incidence of infection and dislodgement and shorter patency times (5).
   b. When nontunneled, should only be used for bed-bound patients.
   c. Due to the risk of iliac vein stenosis, should only be used after thoughtful discussion with transplant surgery, with consideration of the patient's ESKD Life-Plan.
   d. Should extend to the IVC due to the tortuosity of the iliac veins and subsequent risk of stenosis.

Evaluation of Catheter Insertion Site

1. The neck, chest wall, and shoulder region should be examined for:
   a. Skin conditions or scars that may interfere with catheter insertion or creation of a subcutaneous tunnel.
   b. Superficial collateral veins indicative of central venous obstruction.
   c. Implanted pacemaker or cardioverter-defibrillator devices.
2. The location and patency of the access vein should be evaluated with ultrasound prior to draping the patient. Images should be recorded to satisfy compliance requirements.

Selection of a Hemodialysis Catheter

1. Criteria for selecting a hemodialysis catheter
   a. Duration of use: Nontunneled hemodialysis catheters are for short-term use (<14 days). A tunneled (cuffed) hemodialysis catheter should be used when the anticipated duration of hemodialysis treatment is >1 week. Inpatients who will need central venous access beyond dialysis should have a triple-lumen dialysis catheter placed to allow concomitant central venous access and dialysis.
   b. Catheter performance: Despite reported differences there is currently no proven advantage of one catheter through over another. Catheter choice should be based on local experience, goals for use, and cost.
   c. Catheter length: The distal tip of a hemodialysis catheter should *not* be cut or trimmed. Hemodialysis catheters are available in several standard lengths, measured in tip to cuff in centimeters, and correct catheter length is determined by patient size and the site of insertion. Rigid nontunneled catheters should have the distal tip positioned at the junction of the superior vena cava and right atrium. Soft tunneled catheters can be positioned with the catheter tip in the right atrium. Femoral catheters should be positioned with the catheter tip in the inferior vena cava (IVC), cephalad to the confluence of the common iliac veins.

Procedure

Insertion of Tunneled Hemodialysis Catheter

1. All procedures require maximal sterile technique (1,4).
2. When using the internal or external jugular vein, the neck should be slightly extended and the head rotated to provide optimal exposure.

3. Moderate sedation with IV fentanyl and midazolam is typical for insertion. Sedation or analgesics are not often needed for catheter exchange or removal.

4. The vein entry site should be located near the base of the neck to avoid kinking of the catheter. The surrounding tissue is infiltrated with 5 to 10 mL of 1% to 2% buffered lidocaine with or without epinephrine. A short dermatotomy is cut and spread with Kelly forceps down to the vein. When placing a tunneled catheter, create a large enough pocket for the catheter to turn into the vein by spreading the tissues caudally toward the anticipated tunnel. This will facilitate easier passage of the tunneler and prevent kinking of the catheter.

5. Ultrasound guidance should be used for venous puncture (1,6). There are two methods:

   a. In-plane: In general, catheter placement should be done using this method. The transducer is placed transversely across the lower internal jugular vein and then rotated slightly so that a line drawn through the ultrasound plane points toward the opposite nipple. This slight oblique angle will facilitate the wire coursing caudally instead of cranially. The needle is then inserted adjacent to the transducer and the ultrasound adjusted to allow visualization of the needle from the skin to the vein entry site.

   b. Out-of-plane: This method may promote catheter kinking due to its high entry point into the vein and should not be used for tunneled catheter insertion.

6. A micropuncture set decreases puncture-related complications.

7. After vein puncture, the 0.018-in guidewire is advanced into the central vein over which the dilator from the set is inserted to its hub.

8. The 0.018-in guidewire can be used to measure the intravascular distance from the puncture site to the right atrium. Localize the carina on the supine fluoroscopic image. The cavoatrial junction is approximately 2 to 2.5 vertebral bodies below the carina (7).

9. Catheter exit site and the length of the subcutaneous tunnel are determined by the length of the hemodialysis catheter. The choice of the length of catheter is determined by several factors:

   a. Measurement of the intravascular distance (as defined above).

   b. The cuff of the catheter should be at least 4 cm from the jugular vein entry site.

   c. The catheter exit site should be 2 cm from the cuff, to facilitate removal without requiring a cut down.

   d. Most patients will require a 19- or 23-cm catheter for the right side and a 23- or 27-cm catheter for the left side. Table 32.1 helps determine catheter choice and tunnel length.

10. Using the measurements described, the catheter exit site and course of the subcutaneous tunnel are determined and infiltrated with local anesthetic. The tunnel should be in the deltopectoral groove at an approximately 45 degrees angle from the entry site.

11. A 1- to 1.5-cm incision is made at the catheter exit site.

Table 32.1 **Measurements to Determine Tunneled Dialysis Catheter Length**

Measured Intravascular Length	Catheter Length (TTC, cm)[a]	Tunnel Length (cm)
≤15 cm	19	6
>15 cm to 19 cm	23	6–9
>19 cm to 23 cm	27	6–9
>23 cm to 27 cm	31	6–9

[a]Tip to cuff length.

12. The tunneler, with hemodialysis catheter attached, is inserted into the catheter exit site, advanced to the venotomy site to create the subcutaneous tunnel and pulled through so that the Dacron cuff is positioned at least 2 cm within the subcutaneous tunnel.

13. Disconnect the tunneler and both lumens of the hemodialysis catheter should be filled with sterile saline and locked. Verify that both pinch clamps are closed.

14. A stiff 0.038-in guidewire is inserted through the dilator at the venotomy and advanced under fluoroscopy to the IVC. This assures that the azygous vein is not inadvertently catheterized, thus the peel-away sheath will be in the SVC.

15. The venotomy site is sequentially dilated, each dilator is advanced only 2 to 3 cm into the central vein.

16. A peel-away introducer sheath is advanced over the stiff guide into the central vein with fluoroscopic guidance. The guidewire and inner dilator are simultaneously removed from the peel-away sheath; the sheath is immediately occluded with the thumb if not equipped with a hemostatic valve to prevent air embolism. Alternatively, the table can be tilted head down to increase intrathoracic pressure. The hemodialysis catheter is quickly inserted through the introducer sheath.

17. Adjust the catheter tip to the level of the cavoatrial junction or into the right atrium to ensure optimal blood flow (1). Correct orientation of the catheter tip is important for optimal performance. In staggered tipped or split tip catheters, the distal end hole of the arterial (red) lumen should be oriented medially, and the distal end hole of the venous (blue) lumen laterally. In symmetric tip catheters, the tip is in the mid right atrium.

18. Hold the hemodialysis catheter firmly at the venotomy site as the peel-away introducer sheath is removed.

19. Fluoroscopy is used to determine the position of the catheter tip and to check for kinks
    a. The catheter can be adjusted by applying gentle traction.
    b. A stiff guidewire can be inserted into one lumen for advancement of the catheter or to remove kinks.
    c. A final fluoroscopic image should be recorded.

20. The venotomy site is closed using absorbable suture or sterile adhesive. The catheter is secured either by a sandal tie suture or by suturing the wings of the catheter.

21. A sterile occlusive dressing should be applied to cover the catheter exit site. If there is bleeding at the site, a gauze dressing can be placed under occlusive dressing.

Removal of a Tunneled Hemodialysis Catheter

As a general guideline, the catheter can be removed when the fistula or graft has been successfully used for three hemodialysis sessions, the peritoneal dialysis catheter is functional, or the patient no longer requires hemodialysis. Coagulation status does not have a bearing on bleeding risk and should not be routinely assessed before catheter removal (8).

1. Cut and remove retention sutures to allow thorough cleaning of the catheter and exit site.

2. Place sterile drape over the exit site. Catheter hub and Luer connectors are excluded from the sterile field.

3. Infiltrate catheter exit site with buffered lidocaine (1% to 2%) and around the Dacron cuff if it is deep within the subcutaneous tunnel.

4. The ease of catheter removal is dependent on how long the catheter has been in place and location of the Dacron cuff. The cuff becomes incorporated into the surrounding tissue within 2 to 3 weeks, if not fully incorporated the catheter can be removed by applying firm traction. If the catheter is difficult to remove, Kelly forceps can be inserted into the catheter exit site and to bluntly

dissect the Dacron cuff from the surrounding tissue. If the cuff is too deep, a separate incision adjacent to the cuff may be needed for blunt dissection. Do not use sharp dissection to avoid catheter puncture or severing.

5. As the catheter is withdrawn apply manual compression on the subcutaneous tunnel to prevent air embolism and bleeding. Inspect the catheter to verify it has been completely removed.

6. Apply a sterile gauze bandage and occlusive dressing.

Exchange of a Tunneled Hemodialysis Catheter

Exchange may be necessary for improving catheter function, changing position of the catheter tip, replacing a damaged catheter, or removing a colonized or infected catheter.

1. Aspirate and discard the lock solution should be aspirated from both lumens of the hemodialysis catheter. Remove retention sutures to allow more thorough cleaning of the catheter and exit site.

2. Conscious sedation or preprocedural antibiotics are not typically necessary.

3. Assess the course and tip position of the existing hemodialysis catheter and determine appropriate length of catheter by fluoroscopy.

4. Fill and lock both lumens of the new catheter with sterile saline and close both pinch clamps.

5. The catheter cuff is released as detailed previously.

6. Under fluoroscopy, a 0.035-in guidewire (most commonly stiff hydrophilic) is advanced through the venous (blue) lumen into the IVC. While maintaining the guidewire position(s) the hemodialysis catheter is withdrawn. As it is removed from the exit site, apply manual compression on the subcutaneous tunnel to prevent air embolism and bleeding. Inspect the catheter to verify it has been completely removed.

   a. Venography can be performed if there is concern of a fibrin sheath.

   b. The catheter is retracted so that the arterial (red) lumen is still in the vein and contrast injected.

   c. To disrupt a fibrin sheath, a 10 mm × 40–80 mm angioplasty balloon is inflated inside the vein just inside the entry site and then advanced all the way into the IVC while inflated. Take care not to angioplasty the vein, just disrupt the sheath.

7. Insert the new hemodialysis catheter. Most tunneled hemodialysis catheters have a side hole in the distal tip of the venous (blue) lumen to allow "weaving" of the guidewire through the distal tips of both the venous and arterial lumens, to provide increased catheter tip stability. The guidewire is held in position as the new hemodialysis catheter is positioned with the distal tip in the right atrium, with care to assure appropriate orientation of the arterial and venous lumens.

   a. After removal of an infected or colonized catheter, consider wiping the guidewire with alcohol-soaked gauze.

8. The catheter is secured and dressed in a similar manner to a newly placed line.

Postprocedure Management

1. Document the final catheter tip position with fluoroscopy or chest x-ray.

2. The catheter should be locked with a solution between use as per local protocol.

3. Some patients may need oral analgesics for 24 to 48 hours.

4. Each patient should have a plan for a permanent vascular access which minimizes duration of hemodialysis catheter use.

Results

1. With imaging guidance a catheter can be inserted into nearly every patient. Alternative routes of venous access (translumbar, transhepatic) can be used for patients with occluded central veins.
2. The National Kidney Foundation's NKF-KDOQI Guidelines for Vascular Access have redefined catheter dysfunction. Previously guidelines were provided for blood flow rates, now catheter dysfunction is defined as "failure to maintain the prescribed extracorporeal blood flow required for adequate hemodialysis without lengthening the prescribed HD treatment." (1)
3. Long-term tunneled catheter survival may be dependent on the catheter insertion site. Catheters inserted from the left internal jugular vein have a tendency to kink and exhibit greater movement of the catheter tip when compared to catheters inserted from the right internal jugular vein.

Complications/Management

Catheter-related complications are a significant cause of hospitalization, morbidity, and mortality in hemodialysis-dependent patients. Excellent catheter management is vital. Complications should be classified by occurrence timing; insertion (<24 hours), early (24 hours to 30 days), and late (> 30 Days) and severity; major (requiring escalation of care) and minor (no escalation of care), and these should be reported consistently.

1. Insertion-related and early complications from a jugular or subclavian approach—overall threshold should not exceed 4% by Society Interventional Radiology (SIR) guidelines (9,10). Actual complication rates in practice are as follows:
   a. Malposition (3%). Most will require repositioning or exchange.
   b. Pneumothorax (1% to 3%). Can be treated with a chest tube if symptomatic.
   c. Hemothorax (1%). This should be evaluated with contrast-enhanced CT preferably with arterial phase and delayed imaging. If active extravasation is present, open surgical or endovascular intervention is indicated. A chest tube may be indicated in some cases.
   d. Hematoma (1% to 3%). Treat with direct pressure and possibly reversal of anticoagulation.
   e. Venous perforation (0.5% to 1%). Can be immediately fatal (usually hemopericardium) Nonfatal perforation generally requires immediate surgical intervention. A large balloon can be inflated to temporize until percutaneous or surgical intervention is possible.
   f. Air embolism (<1%). Place patient left lateral decubitus to trap air in the right side of the heart. A 100% nonrebreather is used for oxygen delivery. Most instances resolve with these maneuvers. Appropriate personnel should be summoned to prepare for the possibility of cardiac arrest.
   g. Wound dehiscence (1%). Generally requires catheter removal and replacement at a second site if infection is suspected. Antibiotics are necessary in the majority of cases.
   h. Central Line Associated Blood Stream Infection (CLABSI) (1% to 3%). If the central catheter is tunneled, it should be removed and a temporary catheter inserted. Sepsis otherwise should be treated as in any other case, with appropriate escalation of clinical care.
   i. Catheter-associated venous thrombosis (4%). Treatment depends on the venous access capital of the patient. If there are other access options, removal of the existing catheter and replacement at a second site with anticoagulation is appropriate, especially if symptomatic. If asymptomatic, then treatment with anticoagulation and preservation of the access is preferred.

2. Long-term complications of hemodialysis catheters
   a. Catheter occlusion related to venous thrombosis or fibrin sheath (8%). It is often preferable to maintain access at the site of occluded catheter. This can sometimes be maintained by removal over a wire with venoplasty and potentially stent placement if the venous access is salvageable. Simple catheter exchange is not successful in the majority of cases because removing the catheter does not necessarily disrupt the fibrin sheath that is present in chronic catheter placement.
   b. Venous stenosis. A nearly inevitable consequence of long-term indwelling venous catheterization, especially large hemodialysis catheters. This can be treated with angioplasty and stent placement.
   c. Infection is a significant cause of hospitalization, morbidity, and mortality in hemodialysis-dependent patients. The broad range of reported infection rates may be due to variations in clinical practice. *Staphylococcus epidermidis* and *Staphylococcus aureus* are responsible for the majority of catheter-related infections. In some cases, the catheter should be removed and either the patient should have a line holiday with concurrent antibiotic treatment or a temporary catheter should be placed until blood cultures are clear.

References

1. Lok CE, Huber TS, Lee T, et al. KDOQI clinical practice guideline for vascular access: 2019 update. *Am J Kidney Dis.* 2020;75(4):S1–S164.
2. Davidson JC, Rahim S, Hanks SE, et al. Society of interventional radiology consensus guidelines for the periprocedural management of thrombotic and bleeding risk in patients undergoing percutaneous image-guided interventions—Part I: Review of anticoagulation agents and clinical considerations. *J Vasc Interv Radiol.* 2019;30(8):1155–1167. Available from: https://doi.org/10.1016/j.jvir.2019.04.016
3. Patel IJ, Rahim S, Davidson JC, et al. Society of interventional radiology consensus guidelines for the periprocedural management of thrombotic and bleeding risk in patients undergoing percutaneous image-guided interventions—Part II: Recommendations: Endorsed by the Canadian Association for Interventional Radiology and the Cardiovascular and Interventional Radiological Society of Europe. *J Vasc Interv Radiol.* 2019;30(8):1168–1184.e1. Available from: https://doi.org/10.1016/j.jvir.2019.04.017
4. Miller DL, O'Grady NP. Guidelines for the prevention of intravascular catheter-related infections: recommendations relevant to interventional radiology. *J Vasc Interv Radiol.* 2003;14(2 Pt 1):133–136.
5. Fry AC, Stratton J, Farrington K, et al. Factors affecting long-term survival of tunnelled haemodialysis catheters–a prospective audit of 812 tunnelled catheters. *Nephrol Dial Transplant.* 2008;23(1):275–281. Available from: http://www.ncbi.nlm.nih.gov/pubmed/17890252
6. Dexheimer Neto FL, Teixeira C, de Oliveira RP. Ultrasound-guided central venous catheterization: what is the evidence? *Rev Bras Ter Intensiva.* 2011;23(2):217–221. Available from: http://www.scielo.br/scielo.php?script=sci_arttext&pid=S0103-507X2011000200015&lng=pt&nrm=iso&tlng=en
7. Song YG, Byun JH, Hwang SY, et al. Use of vertebral body units to locate the cavoatrial junction for optimum central venous catheter tip positioning. *Br J Anaesth.* 2015;115(2):252–257. Available from: http://www.ncbi.nlm.nih.gov/pubmed/26170349
8. Patel IJ, Davidson JC, Nikolic B, et al. Consensus guidelines for periprocedural management of coagulation status and hemostasis risk in percutaneous image-guided interventions. *J Vasc Interv Radiol.* 2012;23(6):727–736. Available from: http://dx.doi.org/10.1016/j.jvir.2012.02.012
9. Dariushnia SR, Wallace MJ, Siddiqi NH, et al. Quality improvement guidelines for central venous access. *J Vasc Interv Radiol.* 2010;21(7):976–981. Available from: http://dx.doi.org/10.1016/j.jvir.2010.03.006
10. Vesely TM, Beathard G, Ash S, et al. Classification of complications associated with hemodialysis vascular access procedures a position statement from the American Society of Diagnostic and Interventional Nephrology. *J Vasc Access.* 2008;9(1):12–19.

33 Venography

Rulon L. Hardman, MD, PhD

Introduction

Diagnostic venography is performed only when noninvasive imaging is nondiagnostic or prior to a contemplated intervention. It is an infrequent first-line modality because of the accuracy of noninvasive imaging—both for peripheral (Doppler ultrasound) and central (computed tomography venography [CTV]/magnetic resonance venography [MRV]) veins. Preintervention venography is discussed in the appropriate chapters. The discussion here is restricted to the careful technique required for performing high-quality, diagnostic venography.

Indications

Lower Extremity Venography
1. Planning for catheter-directed venous thrombolysis
2. Evaluation of venous malformations
3. Assessment of superficial and perforator anatomy in complex endovascular therapies (1)
4. Evaluation of venous reflux and valvular incompetency by descending lower extremity venography
5. Diagnosis of deep vein thrombosis (DVT) following nondiagnostic or incomplete ultrasound examination; also, when there is a high clinical suspicion for DVT but an extremity ultrasound study is negative

Upper Extremity Venography
1. Evaluation of superior vena cava (SVC) or subclavian vein obstruction or stenosis (2)
2. Evaluation for external compression of the axillary–subclavian vein secondary to clavicular fracture, thoracic outlet syndrome, or neoplastic compression
3. Presurgical mapping for hemodialysis access including percutaneous fistula creation (3)
4. Planning for complicated central venous access or evaluation following a complication of central venous access
5. Diagnosis of superficial thrombosis or DVT following nondiagnostic or incomplete ultrasound or MRV

Contraindications

Relative
1. Previous contrast reaction (premedicate if necessary)
2. Renal insufficiency
3. Pregnancy—only perform in extreme cases where duplex ultrasound and MRV are nondiagnostic. Use lead shielding over pelvis during fluoroscopy
4. Severely compromised cardiopulmonary status

Preprocedure Preparation

1. Clarify the indication for the procedure
2. Review all prior ultrasounds, noninvasive testing, and available cross-sectional imaging
3. Obtain informed consent
4. Consider assessing renal function if large volumes of contrast are to be used

Procedure

Lower Extremity Ascending Venography (4,5)

1. Patient is positioned on a fluoroscopic table, preferably with tilt and digital subtraction angiography (DSA) capabilities. Some perform ascending venography with the patient supine but tilting may provide additional physiologic information. A 6- or 12-in footrest is used to support the contralateral leg. The knee of the extremity being studied can be supported in 30 degrees of flexion with a foam pad to improve flow through the popliteal vein. Avoid excessive external compression, which can obstruct the popliteal vein.
2. Access a vein on the dorsum of the foot with a 20- or 21-gauge butterfly needle or small peripheral IV catheter. Direct the needle toward the toes if possible, to aid in filling the deep veins. If extravasation is seen, leave the catheter in place and select another location for access.
   a. A swollen foot can lead to compression of the superficial veins
      (1) Elevate the extremity for several hours prior to the procedure, and/or
      (2) Wrap the foot in elastic bandage for 30 to 60 minutes or longer, as necessary
   b. Collapsed, poorly visible veins
      (1) Keep the extremity in a dependent position, and/or
      (2) Apply warm compresses to the dorsum of the foot
      (3) Ultrasound guidance will aid difficult access
3. Infusion setup. Attach a three-way stopcock, with inputs for a contrast syringe and heparinized saline syringe or bag
4. High concentration (350 mg per mL) contrast may not mix as well with blood as a lower concentration. Routine venography usually requires between 50 mL and 100 mL of contrast.
5. Standard imaging
   a. Preferably with the table upright at 45 to 60 degrees, gently inject contrast by hand and periodically assess the vein puncture site for extravasation. Barring none, follow the IV contrast column intermittently with fluoroscopy until contrast reaches the popliteal vein (about 50 mL).
   b. Obtain anteroposterior (AP) and lateral images of the lower leg by manually rotating the extremity or the C-arm. Obtain magnified images at any area of discontinuous or clot-filled vein.
   c. Take AP and bilateral oblique images of the popliteal vein with the table at 30 to 45 degrees.
   d. AP images of the thigh are obtained with a decrease tilt to 15 to 30 degrees. Flow may be brisk through the thigh and imaging at one to two frames per second may be required.
   e. Continue venography through the pelvic veins, to the confluence at the inferior vena cava (IVC). An AP view is taken of the pelvis. Bilateral obliques are recommended to evaluate the internal iliac veins. If a positive diagnosis of thrombus is made at a lower level, especially in pregnant patients, examination of the pelvis is not necessary.
   f. To improve visualization of the iliac veins and IVC, use DSA imaging at two or three frames per second combination with one of the following:
      (1) Have patient compress his/her femoral vein below the inguinal ligament during contrast injection to fill the extremity veins. Release compression just prior to imaging of the pelvis.
      (2) Manually compress the calf and thigh veins (if no large clots are seen in large veins on fluoroscopy) while imaging more central veins.
      (3) Raise leg or tilt table to horizontal position prior to quickly imaging pelvic veins.

6. Preferential filling of superficial veins
    a. Placement of both an above-ankle and above-knee tourniquet improves deep venous filling. Using tourniquets may cause venous spasm or artifact at the tourniquet site. Imaging can be performed with and without tourniquets in place.
    b. A blood pressure cuff inflated to 50 mm Hg just above the ankle may afford uniform compression and avoid the artifacts associated with tourniquets.
7. Interpretation
    a. Note normal lower extremity venous anatomy (Figs. 33.1 and 33.2). Interpretation should include assessment of the deep veins of the calf, thigh, and pelvis; filling of incompetent perforating veins (deep to superficial filling) is noted.
    b. Visualization of thrombus as a filling defect within the vein is diagnostic of acute DVT. Outlining thrombus with contrast passage along the vein wall is referred to as "tram-tracking."
    c. Quantitative estimation of clot burden and its change following treatment can be described using grading systems (6). These are rarely used in daily practice.

Upper Extremity Venography (7)
1. Patient is positioned supine with arm extended, approximately 70 degrees from the body, palm up (anatomic position) on an arm extension board.
    a. Ninety-degree or greater angulation of the arm relative to the body can cause compression of the axillary vein.
    b. A small pillow behind the shoulder may facilitate contrast opacification of central veins.

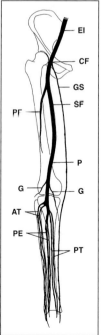

FIGURE 33.1 • Lower extremity veins. The lower extremity is composed of superficial, deep, and perforating veins. The calf veins are paired. The paired anterior tibial veins arise from the venous plexus at the dorsum of the foot. The peroneal veins join with the posterior tibial veins—both are paired. The posterior tibial veins arise from the ventral foot veins. The greater saphenous is the dominant superficial vein, which arises at the medial foot and continues along the medial calf and medial thigh. The lesser saphenous vein courses along the lateral ankle and to the lateral calf. The lesser saphenous may empty into the popliteal vein or greater saphenous. Perforating branches are not named but can be seen along the thigh and calf. *EI*, external iliac; *CF*, common femoral; *GS*, greater saphenous; *SF*, superficial femoral; *PF*, profunda femoral; *P*, popliteal; *G*, gastrocnemius veins; *AT*, anterior tibial; *PE*, peroneal; *PT*, posterior tibial. (Reprinted with permission from Dyer R. *Handbook of Basic Vascular and Interventional Radiology.* Churchill Livingstone; 1993:188.)

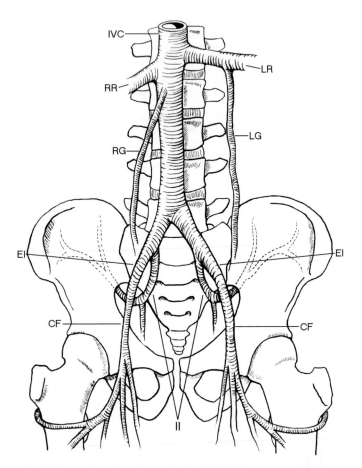

FIGURE 33.2 • Deep pelvic and abdominal veins. The left gonadal vein has confluence with the left renal vein. The right gonadal vein usually drains into the IVC directly. The internal iliac vein arises from the confluence of the superior gluteal, inferior gluteal, pudendal, obturator, lateral sacral, middle hemorrhoidal, vesical, uterine, and vaginal veins. *IVC*, inferior vena cava; *LR*, left renal; *RR*, right renal; *LG*, left gonadal; *RG*, right gonadal; *EI*, external iliac; *CF*, common femoral; *II*, internal iliac. (Figure art by Sharon A. Vogl.)

2. Place a 22- or 25-gauge butterfly needle or 21-gauge IV catheter into a dorsal hand vein. Confirm access by injecting saline.
3. Venography is performed with contrast with concentrations between 200 and 300 mg per mL. Hand injection usually consists of 2 to 4 mL per second, for a total injection volume of 8 to 20 mL. Power injection can be used if access is suitable. Extravasation is evaluated between runs.
4. Inflating an upper arm blood pressure cuff to 50 mm Hg facilitates filling of the deep venous system. The forearm veins can be filled with contrast and spot images obtained.
   a. Avoid use of a tourniquet because this can lead to vasospasm or artifact.

5. Standard images
   a. Obtain AP (palm up) and lateral images of the hand and forearm, including paired ulnar, interosseous, and radial veins. The patient can hold a bag of saline or tape the hand to an arm support to maintain a palm-up position. Spot images are usually sufficient for diagnosis.
   b. Obtain an AP image of the upper arm, including paired brachial, basilic, and cephalic veins. Flow can be brisk. DSA at one or two frames per second can capture the best vein opacification.
   c. A central venogram is obtained documenting the axillary vein, subclavian vein, and SVC. Obtain upper extremity and central venous images as you slowly deflate the blood pressure cuff and/or reduce arm elevation.
   d. Place a 4-Fr or 5-Fr catheter into an upper extremity vein if venography of the central veins is too dilute following hand injection. Following contrast injection with a 20-mL saline "chaser" may also facilitate central opacification. DSA at two or three frames per second is utilized.
   e. In patients being evaluated for thoracic outlet syndrome, images should also be obtained with the arm in abduction and external rotation (ABER) positioning.
6. Interpretation
   a. Note status of upper extremity venous anatomy (Fig. 33.3). Comment on both the deep and superficial veins of the forearm, arm, and chest.

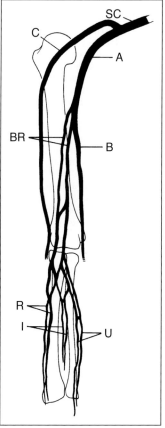

FIGURE 33.3 • Upper extremity veins. The upper extremity veins are paired into deep and superficial drainage. The superficial veins tend to be larger and the dominant system of the upper extremity. The superficial system comprises the cephalic and basilic veins at the forearm. The cephalic vein extends along the lateral forearm. The cephalic vein joins the axillary vein at the humeral head or clavicle. The cephalic vein can be paired. The basilic vein runs through the medial forearm and continues to the upper arm. The basilic vein joins the brachial vein at the mid-upper arm to form the axillary vein. The median antebrachial vein runs on the ventral forearm and drains the palmar venous plexus. The deep veins (radial and ulnar veins) are small, paired, communicate with each other, and accompany the forearm arteries. *SC*, subclavian; *C*, cephalic; *A*, axillary; *BR*, brachial; *B*, basilic; *R*, radial; *I*, interosseous; *U*, ulnar. (From Dyer R. *Handbook of Basic Vascular and Interventional Radiology.* Churchill Livingstone; 1993:160, with permission.)

b. Hemodialysis access planning (mapping): Assess the superficial veins including the condition and size of the cephalic vein in both the forearm and arm and the basilic vein in the arm. Comment on any discontinuous segments. Note central venous stenoses.

c. Evaluation for superficial thrombosis or DVT: An intraluminal defect within the vein confirms acute venous thrombosis similarly to lower extremity findings. Well-formed collaterals around the obstruction are more common in chronic venous thrombosis.

d. Thoracic outlet obstruction: Evaluate the length and location of venous stenosis/occlusion when assessing central obstruction. Note anatomic variants, for example, cervical ribs. Note venous collaterals around the obstruction.

CO_2 Venography (7,8)

CO_2 venography is a reasonable alternative in patients with contrast allergy or renal insufficiency. Patients with renal insufficiency but not yet on dialysis may be best imaged for dialysis access planning with CO_2 (9).

1. Characteristics of CO_2 are described in Chapter 91.

2. Care must be taken to use a self-contained (airtight) system while administering CO_2. Various CO_2 tank options are available, including purpose built systems for vascular imaging. No matter which system is used, exquisite care must be taken to avoid injecting room air at all costs.

   a. *60-mL syringe.* Attach a 60-mL syringe with a one-way valve and a three-way stopcock to the line from a CO_2 canister. Fill the syringe with CO_2 and briskly clear the syringe three times. Lock CO_2 into the syringe with the one-way stopcock. Attach the stopcock to catheter's Luer lock.

   b. *Disposable canisters with a K-Valve switch* (AngioAdvancements, LLC, Ft. Myers, FL). A K-Valve switch is a closed system allowing for flow of CO_2 from a small disposable cartridge into a "reservoir" syringe. The gas is then pushed from the reservoir syringe into the "administration" syringe. One-way valves between the connections allow for a continuous closed airtight system.

3. Venography

   a. DSA images are acquired at high imaging rates, for example, six frames per second. Most digital angiography systems have CO_2-imaging software that permits sequential images to be stacked (summed) to enhance image contrast.

      (1) Injection of 5 to 20 mL in the forearm and lower leg is usually sufficient for imaging.

      (2) Injection of 10 to 30 mL is usually needed at the upper arm and thigh.

      (3) Injection of 30 to 40 mL is needed to evaluate the IVC.

   b. Wait 30 to 60 seconds between injections to allow absorption of the injected gas.

   c. CO_2 displaces the gas blood to give a negative contrast image (white veins on grayscale background).

4. Imaging considerations

   a. CO_2 is buoyant and will rise to the nondependent part of the vessel, unless the gas displaces the entire blood volume in the vessel. This principle should be considered if there is a dependent thrombus or vessel abnormality. A 90-degree obliquity will demonstrate if the entire vessel area is being imaged.

   b. CO_2 best defines the anatomy in small and medium vessels

   c. CO_2 gas defects should disappear within 30 seconds. If gas persists, there is likely room air contamination of the CO_2.

5. Safety

   a. A total dose of up to 1.6 mL per kg of CO_2 can be administered safely during a study (8).

   b. "Air lock." Gas can be trapped in a nondependent branch vessel, blocking blood flow and causing ischemia. Avoid air lock by waiting at least 60 seconds between injections for the gas to wash away.

c. Unlike contrast, CO_2 is a compressible gas. A 20-mL syringe can hold up to 200 mL of gas through compression. A highly pressurized injection can cause pain. This can be avoided by using a large syringe to avoid excessive compression (60 mL).

d. Contamination. CO_2 can be easily contaminated. Do not leave CO_2-filled syringes sitting for long because the CO_2 will slowly be replaced with room air. Exchange CO_2 tanks/reservoirs regularly.

e. Do not use CO_2 in the coronary arteries, thoracic aorta, or cerebral vessels due to risk of stroke.

Postprocedure Management

1. Postprocedure observation is not required following venography performed without sedation.

2. Postprocedure hydration is important following large volumes of contrast to avoid renal toxicity, especially if the patient has preexisting renal impairment. Encourage oral fluid intake for patients who can drink; otherwise hydrate with IV fluids.

3. Wash out contrast from extremity veins at end of the study by infusion of heparinized saline (1,000 units per L) for several minutes.

Results

1. In extremity evaluation for DVT, sensitivity is 100% for clots larger than 0.5 cm. Specificity is 95% using the strict criteria of a filling defect noted on more than one view (6).
   a. False-positive examinations can occur as a result of:
   (1) Underfilling of a vein, creating a pseudothrombus
   (2) Inadvertent injection of air
   (3) Extrinsic defects that may be due to compression by adjacent muscles or positional entrapment

2. CO_2 has been shown to have sensitivity and specificity of 97% and 85%, respectively, compared to contrast venography (7).

Complications

1. Postvenography thrombophlebitis (incidence <3%)
   a. Occurs with contrast, indicating irritation and most often resolves without sequelae

2. Extravasation of contrast into subcutaneous tissue
   a. Stop infusion immediately
   b. Assess size of extravasation: Less than 10 mL in a patient without peripheral arterial or venous disease is considered clinically insignificant
   c. Treat significant extravasation with analgesic and warm compresses for 24 hours
   d. Surgical consultation is warranted if there is neurologic or vascular compromise

3. Contrast reactions (see Chapter 65)

References

1. Varcoe RL, Thomas SD, Bourke V, et al. Utility of adjunctive digital subtraction venography for the treatment of saphenous vein insufficiency. *J Endovasc Ther.* 2017;24(2):290–296.

2. Desjardins B, Rybicki FJ, Kim HS, et al. ACR appropriateness criteria suspected upper extremity deep vein thrombosis. *J Am Coll Radiol.* 2012;9(9):613–619.

3. Lok CE, Huber TS, Lee T, et al; KDOQI Vascular Access Guideline Work Group. KDOQI clinical practice guideline for vascular access: 2019 update. *Am J Kidney Dis.* 2020;75 (4 suppl 2):S1–S164.

4. Sidhu PS, Alikhan R, Ammar T, Quinlan DJ. Lower limb contrast venography: a modified technique for use in thromboprophylaxis clinical trials for the accurate evaluation of deep vein thrombosis. *Br J Radiol*. 2007;80(959):859–865.

5. Andrews RT. Contrast peripheral phlebography and pulmonary angiography for diagnosis of thromboembolism. *Circulation*. 2004;109(12 Suppl 1):I22–I27.

6. Navin P, O'Sullivan GJ. What is the definition of successful lysis: reporting standard? *Phlebology*. 2016;31(1 Suppl):15–23.

7. Heye S, Maleux G, Marchal GJ. Upper-extremity venography: CO$_2$ versus iodinated contrast material. *Radiology*. 2006;241(1):291–297.

8. Sharafuddin MJ, Marjan AE. Current status of carbon dioxide angiography. *J Vasc Surg*.2017; 66(2):618–637.

9. Hawkins IF, Cho KJ, Caridi JG. Carbon dioxide in angiography to reduce the risk of contrast-induced nephropathy. *Radiol Clin North Am*. 2009;47(5):813–825.

34 Pulmonary Embolism: Endovascular Interventions

Andrew Kesselman, MD, RPVI, Ronald S. Winokur, MD, FSIR, RPVI and Akhilesh K. Sista, MD, FSIR, FAHA

Introduction

Pulmonary embolism (PE) remains an important cause of morbidity and mortality worldwide and is associated with increased mortality rates for up to 3 months after the index PE event (1). Risk stratification of the PE patient as characterized by the American Heart Association (AHA) and European Society of Cardiology (ESC) definitions (Table 34.1) is important for guiding management (2,3). Acute PE can be categorized as low risk, submassive/intermediate risk, or massive/high risk. The optimal management of submassive/intermediate and massive/high risk PE is heavily debated in the literature and has not yet been defined. In this chapter we will review workup, current trends, and available therapies.

Table 34.1 **Societal Definitions of Acute Pulmonary Embolus (PE)**

1. American Heart Association (AHA) definitions (2):
   a. Massive—Sustained hypotension (systolic blood pressure <90 mm Hg for at least 15 minutes or requiring inotropic support, not due to a cause other than PE, such as arrhythmia, hypovolemia, sepsis, or left ventricular [LV] dysfunction); pulselessness; or persistent profound bradycardia (heart rate <40 bpm with signs or symptoms of shock).
   b. Submassive—Without systemic hypotension (systolic blood pressure ≥90 mm Hg) but with either RV dysfunction or myocardial necrosis.
   c. Low risk—Without hypotension or RV dysfunction/myocardial necrosis.
2. European Society of Cardiology (ESC) definitions (3):
   a. High risk—With hemodynamic instability, clinical parameters of PE severity and/or comorbidity including high Pulmonary Embolism Severity Index (PESI) scores, RV dysfunction on TTE or CTPA and elevated cardiac troponin levels
   b. Intermediate risk
      1. Intermediate-low risk—High PESI score but does not require RV dysfunction or elevated cardiac troponin levels, although one of these may be present
      2. Intermediate-high risk—High PESI scores and requires RV dysfunction on TTE or CTPA *and* elevated cardiac troponin levels
   c. Low risk—lacking these indicators of risk

Diagnosis of Pulmonary Embolism

Advances in less invasive radiographic modalities, such as computed tomography pulmonary angiography (CTPA), alone or in combination with clinical risk scores, venous ultrasound, echocardiography, and biomarkers (e.g., serum D-dimer), have diminished the diagnostic role of catheter angiography for PE (4). For the remainder of this chapter, pulmonary angiography will be described in conjunction with intervention or prior to surgery. CTPA offers many advantages including increased accessibility, short performance time, and high accuracy. It allows adequate visualization of the pulmonary arteries to the subsegmental branches and may provide alternative diagnoses if PE is excluded. The Prospective Investigation On Pulmonary Embolism Diagnosis (PIOPED) II study reported that CTPA had a sensitivity of 83% and a specificity of 96% and a positive predictive value between 92% and 96% in patients with higher clinical probability (4). VQ scintigraphy can still play a role in indeterminate cases and in specific patient situations (e.g., renal insufficiency, severe contrast allergy).

Treatment of Pulmonary Embolism

The standard treatment for all patients diagnosed with acute PE is anticoagulation (5). Systemic thrombolytic treatment (TT) of patients with PE has been available for more than 30 years, and its risks and benefits have been assessed in several randomized and nonrandomized trials. The information regarding catheter-directed thrombolysis (CDT) and/or catheter thrombectomy is more limited. The American College of Chest Physicians suggests catheter-directed therapy as an alternative to TT for patients who cannot receive IV thrombolysis but require therapeutic escalation (6). The ESC recommends that catheter-directed treatment (CDT) be considered as an alternative to rescue thrombolytic therapy for patients who deteriorate hemodynamically at institutions with access to CDT (4). Endovascular techniques discussed in this chapter are mostly off-label applications of approved devices due to rapid change in technology, though several have been approved for PE in the last 5 years.

To address this public health crisis related to PE morbidity and mortality, pulmonary embolism response teams (PERTs) have been created around the world in an effort to immediately and simultaneously engage multiple specialists to determine the best course of action and coordinate the clinical care for patients with acute PE. Preliminary results from early adopters suggest that PERTs are feasible and facilitate access to advanced therapies (7). Research is needed to determine if the PERT approach improves survival, reduces long-term complications, and is cost effective.

Pulmonary Thrombolysis and Thrombectomy

1. **Systemic thrombolysis** for PE reduces clot burden rapidly and improves hemodynamic parameters in patients with shock or systemic hypoperfusion (5). One randomized trial showed a survival advantage and one demonstrated a significant favorable change in RV systolic pressure and improved exercise tolerance in patients receiving heparin plus fibrinolysis versus heparin alone (3). However, TT has not been proven to reduce mortality or risk of recurrent PE in patients who are hemodynamically stable (3). The risk of bleeding from systemic thrombolysis increases with age and body mass index. Proper patient selection for TT based on risk stratification should reduce potential harm and maximize patient benefit. Systemic thrombolytic drugs are administered via a peripheral IV line. Streptokinase, urokinase (UK), and tissue plasminogen activator (tPA) (alteplase) are approved by the U.S. Food and Drug Administration (FDA) for the treatment of massive PE. The major risks of thrombolytic therapy are hemorrhage and stroke. A review of the literature reported a major hemorrhage rate of 11.9% and a risk of intracranial hemorrhage of 1.2% to 1.9% (5). Both full-dose

(100 mg) tPA and half-dose (50 mg) tPA regimens have been described. Recent evidence suggests that half-dose thrombolysis for PE may provide similar efficacy with reduced bleeding risk compared with full-dose therapy, but comparative studies are lacking.

2. **Surgical embolectomy** is often offered as a last therapeutic resort for patients with fulminant PE who are too unstable, have failed, or have contraindications to thrombolytic therapy. In addition, findings of right heart thrombi in the setting of massive PE, may change treatment considerations from thrombolysis to surgical embolectomy (5). Surgical embolectomy has a high morbidity and mortality in these severely ill patients. A meta-analysis of 597 patients undergoing pulmonary embolectomy with heart–lung bypass showed an overall mortality of 29%, which increased to 58% in patients requiring cardiopulmonary resuscitation (5). These numbers are lower in dedicated centers; however, surgical embolectomy is not widely available, and only a few centers have extensive experience with this procedure (5).

3. **Endovascular treatment**
   a. Pharmacologic. Treating acute PE with intrathrombus delivery of thrombolytic drug attempts to maximize the thrombolytic effects and minimize the required dose of the drug and its complications. This assumption is based on the experience with CDT of peripheral arterial bypass grafts and dialysis fistulas, supported by results from animal models of PE showing superiority of the direct intrathrombus delivery (5). The required dose of the thrombolytic agent is much lower than that required for systemic thrombolysis protocols. In the setting of hemodynamic shock from massive PE, CDT is a potentially lifesaving treatment for patients who have not responded to or cannot tolerate systemic thrombolysis or when emergency surgical embolectomy is unavailable or contraindicated (3,5).
   b. Mechanical. Catheter-based systems can be divided into devices that remove thrombus and those that fragment existing thrombus into smaller pieces. Fragmentation decreases pulmonary vascular resistance and improves pulmonary perfusion. The explanation is that a central occlusive thrombus prevents perfusion of a larger portion of the distal bed than do the smaller fragments dispersed peripherally. Such dispersion by mechanical clot fragmentation also increases the efficacy of subsequent CDT by increasing the thrombus surface area for enzymatic action (5).

Indications

1. Select cases of submassive PE in which the PERT decides that there is high risk of progression to massive PE. Most of these patients will be intermediate-high risk PE by ESC criteria.
2. Cases of massive PE with hemodynamic compromise when systemic thrombolysis is contraindicated and/or surgical embolectomy is not available. At institutions where endovascular practitioners are quickly available and there is rapid ability to engage in catheter-based thrombectomy techniques, these techniques can be considered as part of the PERT discussion.

Contraindications

1. Left bundle-branch block on electrocardiogram (ECG). Consider placing a transvenous pacing catheter to treat complete heart block in the event that catheter-induced right bundle branch block (RBBB) occurs.
2. Severe prior documented contrast reaction. Consider emergent premedication regimen per institutional protocol.
3. Uncorrectable coagulopathy.
4. Prior intracranial hemorrhage.[a]
5. Ischemic stroke within 3 months.[a]

6. Brain or spine primary or metastatic neoplasm.[a]
7. Recent major surgery within 10 days.[a]
8. Significant head or facial trauma within 3 months.[a]

Preprocedure Preparation

1. Perform standard preprocedural preparation for angiography.
2. Check cardiopulmonary status (history, physical examination, diagnostic tests, etc.)—including brain natriuretic peptide (BNP) and troponins, transthoracic echocardiography (TTE).
3. Review imaging: Chest x-ray, VQ scan, CTPA, and/or venous Doppler studies.
4. Check serum electrolytes, blood urea nitrogen (BUN)/creatinine (Cr), coagulation parameters (INR < 1.8), and platelets (>50,000 per μL).

Procedure

Venous Access
1. Access can be obtained via the femoral vein, brachial vein or the internal jugular vein for all types of endovascular procedures. Internal jugular or femoral vein access will be needed for large-bore thrombectomy devices. Up to 14% of patients undergoing pulmonary angiography can have thrombus in the IVC (5). If in doubt, perform limited ultrasound of the femoral veins prior to puncture and perform venography of pelvis and/or IVC.
2. Sheath placed and secured to skin—5- to 22-Fr (based on device used) with lengths up to 70 cm (longer lengths can allow pressure measurements via the main PA and assist with catheter stability in a dilated right ventricle).

Selective Catheters
1. Femoral access: Preshaped catheters (e.g., Grollman, APC) or pigtail catheters maneuvered with a tip-deflecting wire may be used to access the main pulmonary artery.
2. Internal jugular or brachial access: Preshaped catheters (e.g., C2) are available that enter the PA without a need for tip-deflecting wire.
3. Balloon-tipped catheters (e.g., Swan-Ganz, Fogarty) can be filled with CO_2 gas and floated through the right ventricle to the pulmonary artery. This can help avoid injury to the valvular complex or corda tendineae, an important consideration when using large-bore devices. This catheter can be exchanged over a wire for another diagnostic catheter, if necessary.

Measure Right Heart Pressures
1. If the PA systolic pressure is >70 mm Hg, the mortality associated with pulmonary angiography is increased (approximately 2% to 3%) (2). In such cases, use subselective injection (with balloon occlusion technique, if necessary) and nonionic contrast media. These safety measures are even more important if cardiac output is impaired (5).

Arteriographic Technique
1. Contrast agents: *Nonionic low osmolality* contrast agents (e.g., visipaque) are preferred and considered mandatory for patients with elevated right-sided pressures. Low-cost alternative agents are acceptable when right-sided pressures are normal.
2. Injection rates
   a. Main PA injection: 30 mL at 15 mL per second, for the anatomic evaluation of central pulmonary arteries

---

[a]Considerations with thrombolysis.

b. Selective arteriography: right or left PA, 20 to 30 mL at 10 to 15 mL per second
c. Subselective arteriography: Use the CTPA or VQ scan as guide, especially for patients with pulmonary hypertension. Hand injections usually performed via flush catheter.
3. Imaging: Using CTPA or VQ scan as a road map may allow for more selective angiographic evaluation and fewer angiographic images resulting in lower-contrast volumes.

Catheter-Directed Thrombolysis

Depending on thrombus distribution, unilateral or bilateral pulmonary arterial catheters maybe placed with side holes spanning the involved segments. Typical infusion rates consist of 1 mg per hour through a single infusion catheter, 0.5 to 1 mg per hour through each infusion catheter or a weight-based total dose of 0.01 mg/kg/hour tPA, over 12 to 24 hours duration. The need for concomitant full-dose anticoagulation is controversial as it may increase bleeding risk however protocols involving 300 to 500 Units of Heparin per hour without adjustment for aPTT have been described (8).

Thrombolysis Catheters

1. Standard infusion catheters—Various vendors, 4- or 5-Fr infusion catheters with or without tip occluding wires or valves.
2. *Ekos Endovascular System* (Boston Scientific, Natick, MA)—5.2-Fr infusion catheter that contains ultrasonic elements that have been hypothesized to aid in thrombolysis. This device has FDA clearance for the treatment of PE.

Catheter Thrombectomy, Aspiration, and Maceration

Novel catheter thrombectomy and aspiration devices are increasing in number and availability ranging from 8- to 24-Fr sizes. They all primarily function by engaging the catheter tip in thrombus and using continuous high-pressure aspiration. Maceration devices are available for each device to break the thrombus into smaller fragments and to prevent against device occlusion. It is important to administer anticoagulation when removing thrombus and monitor for therapeutic activated clotting time (ACT) and blood loss.

Thrombectomy Devices

1. *Guiding catheter technique:* An 8- or 9-Fr coronary guiding catheter (without side holes) is placed through a 10-Fr sheath (tip left in PA). Aspiration is performed with a 60-mL syringe, removing small amounts of clot during each pass. It remains a simple and cost-effective means for thrombus removal.
2. *Indigo Aspiration System* (Penumbra, Alameda, California): Continuous aspiration mechanical thrombectomy system designed to remove clot. This system utilizes the pump (ENGINE) to deliver continuous vacuum suction (−29 in Hg) to the Indigo System Aspiration Catheters to address thrombus in vessels of various sizes (CAT6, CAT8, or CAT12 lightning). The Indigo Separators are designed to be used in tandem with the corresponding catheters to break up resistant clot in the catheter lumen. FDA cleared for use in PE.
3. *FlowTriever system* (Inari Medical, Irvine, California): A 16-, 20-, and 24-Fr trackable, large lumen catheter, and large-bore syringe designed to extract large volumes of clot. Can be combined with a catheter containing three self-expanding nitinol mesh disks that are designed to engage, disrupt, and deliver clot to the aspiration device. FDA cleared for use in PE.
4. *ASPIREX* (Straub Medical, Wangs, Switzerland): An 8-Fr mechanical thrombus aspiration device specifically designed for the treatment of PE. The catheter is introduced over a 0.018-in guidewire to the site of proximal occlusion of the PA or with the greatest thrombus content, where it is activated. A motor rotates a spiral located in the body of the catheter at 40,000 rpm, creating negative

pressure—thrombus is macerated and removed through an L-shape aspiration system. The device has been successfully used in PE, but is not FDA cleared.
5. *AngioVac* (AngioDynamics, Albany, NY) is a large-bore (22-Fr) cannula approved by the FDA for venous drainage during extracorporeal bypass for up to 6 hours to include removal of fresh, soft thrombi, or emboli. This device requires a clinical perfusionist and general anesthesia in addition to an interventional radiology team.
6. *JETi* (Walk Vascular, Irvine, CA): This 6- or 8-Fr thrombectomy device combines clot fragmentation with catheter aspiration. It is not FDA cleared for use in PE.
7. *AngioJet Peripheral thrombectomy system* (Boston Scientific, Natick, MA): A high-velocity saline solution jet from a dedicated drive unit creates a strong Venturi effect at the tip of a 6- or 8-Fr catheter. This results in the fragmentation of the thrombus into microparticles that are aspirated through the catheter. Successful use of this device has been reported (8). However, the AngioJet device has also been associated with bradyarrhythmias and deaths when used in the pulmonary arteries and carries an FDA black box warning. Therefore, its use should be avoided by most practitioners in the pulmonary circulation.

Postprocedure Management

Catheter-Directed Thrombolysis
1. Continuation of therapy in monitored unit (ICU). Fibrinogen can be checked Q6 hours; however, this is not routinely performed by all providers.
2. Repeat pulmonary angiography and pressure measurements can be performed in the IR suite prior to catheter removal at the conclusion of lytic infusion. Bedside pressure measurements without pulmonary angiography is also acceptable to document the change mean pulmonary pressure.
3. Outpatient follow-up should be performed by the interventional provider or a member of the PERT following hospital discharge. If there are persistent symptoms of shortness of breath or an abnormal TTE, referral to a pulmonary hypertension specialist should be considered.

Catheter Thrombectomy, Aspiration, and Maceration
1. Immediate postprocedure care could involve a monitored unit bed or an intensive care location based on hemodynamics and necessity for continued CDT.
2. Massive PE patients who fail CDT and continue to deteriorate, can be considered for extracorporeal membrane oxygenation (ECMO).
3. Outpatient follow-up should be similar to the description above.

Data and Complications

Catheter-Directed Thrombolysis
Analysis of 2,392 patients in International Cooperative Pulmonary Embolism Registry (ICOPER) demonstrated that PE remains an important clinical problem with high mortality rate and served as a basis for subsequent trials (9). Recent studies have noted relatively low rates of major bleeding and overall high rates of technical success. The PERFECT registry data of 101 patients from 7 sites demonstrated that CDT improved clinical outcomes including clinical success in 86% of patients with acute PE, improvement in right heart strain in 89% of patients on repeat echocardiography; and no major procedure-related complications with minor bleeding events in 12.9% of patients (10). The SEATTLE II trial (A Prospective, Single-Arm, Multicenter Trial of EkoSonic Endovascular System and Activase for Treatment of Acute Pulmonary Embolism) of 150 patients required at least a 12-hour infusion and 24-mg alteplase demonstrating decreased mean right ventricular (RV)/left ventricular (LV) diameter ratio, decreased mean pulmonary artery systolic pressure

(51.4 mm Hg vs. 36.9 mm Hg) and improved modified Miller Index score (22.5 mm Hg vs. 15.8) however had an alarming 10% major bleeding rate and lacked a control arm for comparison (11). The ULTIMA trial provided prospective data on 59 randomized patients supporting CDT over anticoagulation alone for reversing RV dilatation (i.e., reduction in RV/LV ratio) at 24 hours with minimal bleeding complications (12). More high-quality data is needed to identify the optimal dose, duration and protocol for CDT to improve short-term and long-term clinical outcomes.

Catheter Thrombectomy, Aspiration, and Maceration

FLARE was a prospective, single-arm, multicenter study that evaluated the safety and effectiveness of the Inari Flowtriever device in 106 patients across 18 centers. The device was associated with a reduction in the RV/LV ratio of 0.38 at 48 hours after the intervention. The adverse event rate was 3.8% (13).

EXTRACT-PE was a prospective, single-arm, multicenter trial conducted under an Investigational Device Exemption (IDE) from the U.S. FDA that evaluated the safety and efficacy of the Indigo Aspiration System in the treatment of acute PE enrolling 119 participants across 22 U.S. study centers. The primary efficacy endpoint was met with a significant mean reduction in RV/LV ratio of 0.43, corresponding to a 27.3% reduction at 48 hours after intervention. The composite major adverse event rate was 1.7% within 48 hours (14).

Chronic Pulmonary Thromboembolic Disease

Advances in endovascular and surgical techniques have opened new avenues in the treatment of *chronic thromboembolic pulmonary hypertension (CTEPH)*.

1. Careful interpretation of pulmonary angiograms in the setting of CTEPH is essential for determining operability. The angiographic findings of chronic PE can be subtle; they include pouching defects, webs, mural irregularities, luminal narrowing, and occlusion.
2. For CTEPH patients with technically inoperable disease or with an unfavorable risk-to-benefit ratio for surgical pulmonary endarterectomy, balloon pulmonary angioplasty (BPA), also called percutaneous transluminal pulmonary angioplasty, is emerging as a possible alternative therapy (15).

Conclusions

1. Given the paucity of rigorous clinical trials of CDT, the decision to proceed with percutaneous treatment of PE is facilitated by a multidisciplinary team consisting of interventional radiologists, pulmonologists, cardiologists, and cardiothoracic surgeons who are familiar with all available treatment options for PE. The makeup of the PERT may vary by institution and can also include specialties such as Vascular Medicine, Internal Medicine, and Vascular Surgery.
2. If possible and when appropriate, cardiac surgical backup should be arranged prior to intervention in case of a need to convert to surgical embolectomy. This is of most concern in cases of right atrial thrombus or massive PE.
3. Currently, there is no single technique that is clearly established as superior, and therefore, the choice of techniques depends on the individual physician's and institutional experience as well as PERT consensus. In the setting of massive PE, a combination of strategies, including mechanical thrombectomy, maceration, and/or CDT can be used to improve flow across the pulmonary circulation to restore systemic pressures.
4. More rigorous data (randomized control trials and large multicenter registries) are needed to drive evidence-based medicine and individualized care in PE. Endovascular techniques show promise however studies focusing on long- and short-term term clinical outcomes will help support increased access and utilization.

R e f e r e n c e s

1. Chatterjee S, Chakraborty A, Weinberg I, et al. Thrombolysis for pulmonary embolism and risk of all-cause mortality, major bleeding, and intracranial hemorrhage: a meta-analysis. *JAMA*. 2014;311(23):2414–2421. doi:10.1001/jama.2014.5990
2. Giri J, Sista AK, Weinberg I, et al. Interventional therapies for acute pulmonary embolism: current status and principles for the development of novel evidence: a scientific statement from the American Heart Association. *Circulation*. 2019;140(20):e774–e801.
3. Konstantinides SV, Meyer G, Becattini C, et al. ESC guidelines for the diagnosis and management of acute pulmonary embolism developed in collaboration with the European Respiratory Society (ERS). *European Heart Journal*. 2019;41(4):543–603.
4. Stein PD, Woodard PK, Weg JG, et al. Diagnostic pathways in acute pulmonary embolism: recommendations of the PIOPED II investigators. *Radiology*. 2007;242(1):15–21.
5. Turba UC, Hagspiel KD. The treatment of pulmonary arterial thrombectomy and thrombolysis. In: K. Kandarpa, L. Machan, eds. *Handbook of Interventional Radiologic Procedures*. 4th ed. Lippincott, Williams & Wilkins; 2011:338–345.
6. Guyatt GH, Eikelboom JW, Gould MK, et al. Approach to outcome measurement in the prevention of thrombosis in surgical and medical patients: Antithrombotic Therapy and Prevention of Thrombosis, 9th ed: American College of Chest Physicians Evidence-Based Clinical Practice Guidelines. *Chest*. 2012;141(2 suppl):e185S–e194S.
7. Rivera-Lebron B, McDaniel M, Ahrar K, et al. Diagnosis, treatment and follow up of acute pulmonary embolism: consensus practice from the PERT consortium. *Clin Appl Thromb Hemost*. 2019;25:1076029619853037. doi:10.1177/1076029619853037
8. Kuo WT, van den Bosch MA, Hofmann LV, et al. Catheter-directed embolectomy, fragmentation, and thrombolysis for the treatment of massive pulmonary embolism after failure of systemic thrombolysis. *Chest*. 2008;134(2):250–254
9. Goldhaber SZ, Visani L, De Rosa M. Acute pulmonary embolism: clinical outcomes in the International cooperative pulmonary embolism registry (ICOPER). *Lancet*. 1999;353(9162):1386–1389
10. Kuo WT, Banerjee A, Kim PS, et al. Pulmonary embolism response to fragmentation, embolectomy, and catheter thrombolysis (PERFECT): Initial results from a prospective multicenter registry. *Chest*, 2015;148(3):667–673.
11. Piazza G, Hohlfelder B, Jaff MR, et al. A prospective single-arm multicenter trial of ultrasound-facilitated catheter-directed low-dose fibrinolysis for acute massive and submassive pulmonary embolism: the SEATTLE II study. *JACC Cardiovasc Interv*. 2015;8(10):1382–1392.
12. Kucher N, Boekstegers P, Müller OJ, et al. Randomized controlled trial of ultrasound-assisted catheter-directed thrombolysis for acute intermediate-risk pulmonary embolism. *Circulation*. 2014;129:479–486.
13. Tu T, Toma C, Tapson VF, et al. A prospective, single-arm, multicenter trial of catheter-directed mechanical thrombectomy for intermediate-risk acute pulmonary embolism. *J Am Coll Cardiol Intv* 2019;12(9):859–869.
14. National Library of Medicine 2020, ClinicalTrials.gov NIH, last accessed July 2020, https://clinicaltrials.gov/ct2/show/NCT03218566.
15. Godinas L, Bonne L, Budts W, et al. Balloon pulmonary angioplasty for the treatment of nonoperable chronic thromboembolic pulmonary hypertension: Single-center experience with low initial complication rate. *J Vasc Interv Radiol*. 2019;30(8):1265–1272. doi:10.1016/j.jvir.2019.03.023.

35 Vena Caval Filters

Leonardo A. Campos, MD and John A. Kaufman, MD, MS

Introduction

Vena caval filters are intravascular devices designed to prevent pulmonary embolus (PE) by trapping venous emboli. Filters do not prevent formation of new thrombus or promote lysis of a preexisting thrombus or embolus. The primary means of therapy and prophylaxis for deep vein thrombosis (DVT) and PE are pharmacologic.

There are three basic classes of filters.

1. Permanent filters: Permanent vena caval filters are the oldest class of filters and were not designed to be repositioned or retrieved. Using special techniques, these devices may be retrieved percutaneously if indicated.

2. Optional filters: Permanent filters designed to provide the option of percutaneous removal or conversion to a nonfiltration state. The two basic types are retrievable and convertible filters.

    a. Retrievable filters can be retrieved or repositioned percutaneously during a device-specific time window. Manufacturers suggest ranges of retrievability on the basis of clinical trials and experience. In practice, filter retrievability times may vary by device and are typically longer than manufacturers recommend. Filters should be retrieved once they are no longer indicated to prevent complications of long-term indwelling filters.

    b. Convertible filters have the potential to open to a stent-like configuration after implantation so that they no longer function as filters. After conversion, some or all of the filter remains in the patient's vena cava without providing protection from PE. Conversion may be mechanical, requiring a second procedure, or automatic (bioconvertible) based upon absorbable components.

3. Temporary filters: Temporary filters are devices that must be removed in their entirety or dissolve completely after a certain period of time.

    a. Tethered devices have an attached catheter or wire that is extravascular at the access site, allowing the filter to be easily retrieved. Permanent filtration requires the removal of the temporary filter and placement of a different device.

    b. Absorbable filters are implanted devices without tethers that completely dissolve after a predetermined length of time. These are in clinical trial at the time of this publication.

Filter Placement

Indications

There remains significant controversy over the appropriate indications for vena cava filter placement among professional medical societies (1).

All Filter Types

1. Accepted: documented venous thromboembolism (VTE) with one or more of the following:

    a. A contraindication to anticoagulation, such as active gastrointestinal bleeding (not fecal occult blood), recent intracranial hemorrhage or surgery, or vascular brain metastases.

    b. Documented progression or recurrence of VTE while anticoagulated. In general, anticoagulation with a different agent should be tried first.

c. A complication of anticoagulation, such as massive retroperitoneal hemorrhage, that requires interruption or termination of anticoagulation.

d. Chronic PE requiring thromboendarterectomy.

2. Routine placement in the following conditions is currently *recommended against* (1):

a. Prophylactic IVC filter placement in trauma patients without known acute VTE or patients who are to undergo major surgery without known acute VTE.

b. Routine IVC filter placement in patients who develop recurrent DVT while on anticoagulation is not recommended. Instead, pursue alternative anticoagulation and investigation into the cause of the recurrent DVT.

c. Routine placement of an IVC filter in a patient who develops VTE and can be anticoagulated.

d. Routine IVC filter placement during interventions for lower extremity and iliocaval DVT.

Optional and Temporary Filters

There are no unique indications for optional or temporary filters. These filters should be utilized when nonpermanent protection from PE is anticipated at the time of filter placement.

Contraindications

1. There are no absolute contraindications to filter placement but rare circumstances exist in which filters may be contraindicated, including:

a. Total thrombosis of the vena cava

b. Inability to gain access to the vena cava

c. Inability to image during filter placement

d. Vena cava too small or too big to safely accommodate the filter

e. Confirmed allergy to a component of the filter

f. Localized muscular vein thrombus or focal nonocclusive thrombus in an axial vein that can be easily monitored for progression with ultrasound (US) while awaiting anticoagulation

2. The following are *not contraindications* to filter placement:

a. Ongoing sepsis

b. Inability to document residual peripheral thrombus in a patient with who cannot be anticoagulated. Current imaging techniques cannot fully evaluate all possible sources of emboli, and more thrombus may form and embolize after imaging

Preprocedure Preparation

1. The consent for the placement of a vena caval filter should *include all of the usual risks associated with percutaneous venous procedures* as well as the following:

a. Recurrent PE

b. Symptomatic caval thrombosis

c. Filter embolization, fracture, or malposition

d. Symptomatic perforation by a filter element

e. Pericardial tamponade for superior vena cava (SVC) filter placement

2. Laboratory values (2)

a. Preprocedure PT/INR not routinely recommended, yet may be considered in special circumstances:

(1) Coagulation studies and blood counts for patients on therapeutic anticoagulation

(2) Serum creatinine in patients with impaired renal function

b. International normalized ratio (INR) less than 3.0

c. Platelets greater than 20,000 per μL

3. Patient evaluation

a. Review available cross-sectional imaging of the abdomen for anomalous caval anatomy and presence of thrombus

b. Assess for availability of venous access (trauma patients with neck braces, pelvic fixation, existing lines, etc.)

Procedure

1. Obtain access: Vena cava filters can be placed from the femoral veins, jugular veins (internal or external), subclavian veins, upper extremity veins, or directly into the IVC via translumbar approach. The access site will depend on the device and patient factors such as venous patency and anatomy. The right femoral or internal jugular vein is the preferred approach for filters with a rigid design or not delivered over a guidewire.

2. Imaging: High-quality imaging during filter placement maximizes the likelihood of a satisfactory outcome. Poor imaging increases the chance of filter misplacement and other operator errors.

   a. Goals of preplacement imaging
      (1) Define vena caval and renal vein anatomy.
         (a) Duplicated IVC occurs in less than 1% and usually joins at the left renal vein but may also join lower.
         (b) Left-sided IVC is found in less than 1%.
         (c) Circumaortic left renal vein is found in 3% to 4%. The lower component of the venous ring lies behind the aorta and drains into the IVC lower than a normal left renal vein.
         (d) Retroaortic left renal vein occurs in 2% to 3% and usually drains into the IVC below the right renal vein or rarely at the confluence of the iliac veins.
         (e) Duplicated SVC occurs in less than 1%.
         (f) Persistent left SVC drains into the coronary sinus.
         (g) Left-sided SVC is extremely rare.
      (2) Determine vena cava size.
         (a) "Mega cava" (IVC diameter >28 mm) is found in less than 1%.
         (b) IVC is typically oval in cross-section, so measurements in a single plane may not be accurate.
      (3) Confirm patency of vena cava.

   b. Cavography
      (1) For IVC, position pigtail catheter (4-Fr or greater) at the confluence of the iliac veins.
      (2) For SVC, inject from a brachiocephalic vein.
      (3) Use the same positioning and field of view that you will employ during filter deployment.
      (4) Injection rate for iodinated contrast of 15 to 20 mL per second for 2 seconds.
      (5) CO_2 cavography can be performed by hand injection of 30 to 40 mL CO_2.
      (6) Digital subtraction angiography (DSA) filming at three to six frames per second during suspended respiration in anterior–posterior projection. Additional projections can be obtained as needed. Contralateral iliac vein and renal veins are identified as inflow of unopacified blood or by reflux of contrast into orifices of veins.
      (7) If veins cannot be localized, try the following: Reposition pigtail catheter closer to the expected location of tributaries, increase rate and volume of contrast injection, use oblique projection, selectively catheterize veins, and use intravascular ultrasound (IVUS).

   c. IVUS: Alone or combined with fluoroscopy, IVUS can be used to guide filter placement in gravid patients, patients with contraindications to all contrast agents and for bedside filter placement (3). An IVUS catheter with a large axial field (e.g., 60 mm or more) is necessary.
      (1) Femoral venous access is easiest when using IVUS alone (avoids negotiating right atrium).

(a) Tandem ipsilateral access, bilateral access, or single puncture technique
(2) Determine IVC dimensions and patency.
(3) Localize renal vein orifices and iliac confluence.
(a) Note locations with fluoroscopy or measure distance from venous access site.
(4) Deploy filter using fluoroscopic guidance if available.
(5) Obtain plain radiograph of the abdomen to document filter position and configuration.
d. US: Transabdominal US guidance for filter placement can be performed at the bedside. This approach has the following limitations:
(1) The IVC is not always easy to image in large patients or those with significant bowel gas.
(2) Variant renal vein and IVC anatomy may not be detected.
3. Filter placement
a. General principles
(1) After performing initial imaging, note the level of renal vein inflow and confluence of iliac veins relative to a fixed reference point, such as the spine, a radiopaque ruler, or other measuring device.
(2) Without moving the patient or image intensifier, exchange the pigtail catheter over a guidewire for a filter delivery sheath.
(3) Watch under fluoroscopy when reinserting the guidewire into the pigtail catheter to avoid malpositioning the guidewire (e.g., into an ascending lumbar vein).
(4) Serial dilation may be required for large delivery systems. A stiff or exchange-length guidewire may be needed for difficult or remote access.
(5) Position the delivery sheath central to the desired final location of the filter when placing from the femoral approach; position the sheath peripheral to the renal veins when access is from above.
(6) Leave guidewire in place for over-the-wire delivery system (make sure to use a straight guidewire to avoid guidewire entanglement in the filter post deployment).
(7) Before advancing filter into delivery sheath, inspect to be sure that the orientation of the filter is correct for the chosen access route (i.e., femoral or jugular).
(8) Advance filter to the end of the delivery sheath. Reposition the entire system so that the constrained filter is in the desired location.
(9) Deploy the filter per manufacturer's instructions.
(10) Withdraw the delivery sheath several centimeters below the filter when access is from the groin; leave the sheath at the top of the filter when deployed from above.
(11) Repeat cavogram through the delivery sheath using the same injection and filming rate as described earlier.
b. Filter location (Fig. 35.1)
(1) Normal IVC
(a) The top of a single-level cone-shaped filter should be just at or slightly above the lower edge of the orifice of the lowest renal vein. This minimizes potential "dead space" above the filter should filter occlusion occur.
(b) The top of a bi-level cone-shaped filter (a device with upper arms and lower legs) should be below the orifice of the lowest renal vein to prevent prolapse of one of the arms into a renal vein.
(c) Filters that are not cone shaped should be placed below the renal vein orifices.
(d) All filters should be placed so that there is adequate wall contact between the stabilizing filter elements and the IVC.

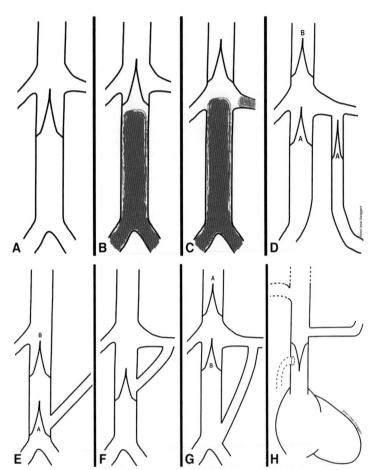

FIGURE 35.1 • Suggested VC filter placement locations for (**A**) a normal infrarenal IVC with no intraluminal thrombus; (**B**) infrarenal IVC thrombus, not quite approaching renal veins and with adequate room for filter legs to attach; (**C**) infrarenal and renal vein thrombus; (**D**) duplicated IVC—either two infrarenal filters *(A)* or a single filter *(B)* in suprarenal segment; (**E**) retroaortic (low insertion) of a left renal vein *(A or B)*; (**F**) circumaortic left renal vein; (**G**) left renal vein insertion at confluence of left iliac vein and IVC *(A or B)*; (**H**) SVC placement to confine upper extremity emboli.

    (e) When a filter is already present and does not contain thrombus and the indication is recurrent PE, a second filter can be placed below the first if sufficient room is present. Otherwise, place a second filter above the first (including suprarenal if necessary).
  (2) Thrombus in IVC
    (a) Thrombus does not extend to the renal veins: Place the filter as low as possible in the infrarenal IVC but above thrombus, even if the body of the filter lies entirely within the intrarenal IVC. If there is little room for infrarenal attachment of the filter, consider a cone-shaped device or a suprarenal placement.

    (b) Thrombus extends to or originates from the renal veins: Place the filter in the suprarenal segment, either just above the renal veins or in the intrahepatic IVC. Use a short filter (i.e., not Bird's Nest, as wires may prolapse into the right atrium and cause arrhythmia).

    (c) Thrombus extends above the existing filter: Place a second filter above thrombus, usually in the suprarenal IVC.

(3) Duplicated IVC

    (a) Place one filter in each IVC, just below the renal veins.

    (b) Place a single suprarenal filter.

    (c) If the second IVC is an *accessory cava*, in that it is small and communicates with the main IVC at the levels of both the common iliac and renal veins, consider occluding the accessory cava with coils or plugs and place one filter in the normal location in the main IVC.

(4) Circumaortic left renal vein

    (a) Theoretical concern is embolization via the venous ring if the filter is placed between the two vein orifices. If a sizeable retroaortic component is present, place the filter feet below the orifice of the retrocaval portion of the ring.

    (b) If the retoroaortic component is small and inserts very low on the IVC, place filter in usual location relative to the main renal veins.

      i. If the small retroaortic component still concerning as a collateral pathway for an embolus, occlude with coils or plugs.

(5) Retroaortic left renal vein

    (a) Place the filter below the orifice of the left renal vein if sufficient room exists.

    (b) In case of a very low left renal vein orifice, place the filter with its apex at the level of the right renal vein.

(6) Mega cava

    (a) The VenaTech LP (B. Braun Medical, Bethlehem, PA) is approved in Europe for IVC diameters up to 35 mm.

    (b) Bird's Nest filter (Cook Medical Inc, Bloomington, IN) is approved for IVC diameters up to 40 mm.

    (c) If neither (a) nor (b) are possible, place filters in each common iliac vein.

(7) SVC

    (a) Use a short filter, ideally single level cone shaped without arms.

    (b) The feet of the filter should be superior to the azygos vein if possible but still in the SVC.

    (c) Avoid placing the filter arms in the right atrium.

    (d) Placed too low in the SVC, filter elements can perforate into the pericardial space and possibly cause hemopericardium and tamponade.

c. Pregnancy

  (1) Female with current pregnancy:

    (a) Suprarenal location minimizes fetal radiation exposure during fluoroscopic guidance.

    (b) IVUS can be used for placement without ionizing radiation.

  (2) Woman with upcoming planned pregnancy: Fetal wastage due to IVC filter or trauma to mother due to compression of the filter by the uterus is a theoretical but unsubstantiated concern. Nevertheless, suprarenal filter placement should be discussed with the patient.

    (a) In a gravid patient with indwelling IVC filter, caesarean section minimizes the length of anticoagulation cessation compared to vaginal delivery. In addition, this mitigates concern of filter impingement or other complications secondary to uterine contractions.

d. Problem solving during deployment

  (1) *Kinked sheath*: This occurs most often with left-sided access, tortuous vessels, and filters not delivered over a guidewire. Pushing the filter against a kink can result in perforation of the sheath and extrusion of the filter.

    (a) Gently advance the filter and sheath as a unit 1 to 2 cm. This moves the kink central to the acute angle in the vessel. Attempt to resume delivery.

    (b) If this fails, withdraw the filter and sheath as a unit just peripheral to the acute angulation. This may allow the kink to straighten but frequently results in formation of a new kink.

    (c) If this fails, withdraw the filter and sheath to the skin access site as a unit, leaving as much empty sheath in the vessel as possible. Cut the sheath and insert a guidewire. Options at this point include:

        i. Inserting a new sheath that is large enough to accommodate the filter delivery sheath and long enough to cross the point of kinking. Coaxially advance the filter and delivery sheath through the larger sheath, which should provide the support necessary to prevent kinking.

        ii. Changing to a more flexible filter design.

    (d) If this fails, abandon the access site and select a more direct alternate access if possible.

(2) *Incompletely opened filter:* manifests in different ways depending on the filter designs. For example, with cone-shaped filters, as clustered or crossed legs.

    (a) Usually of little clinical consequence, unless there is incomplete coverage of the IVC, the filter will not function properly or the filter has been misplaced into a small branch.

    (b) If any question, perform cavogram or other imaging.

        i. Confirm location and stability of filter.

        ii. Evaluate for thrombus.

    (c) When intervention is warranted,

        i. Ask patient to cough several times (this rarely works but is quick).

        ii. Gently manipulate the filter with an angled catheter.

        iii. For retrievable and temporary filters, remove and insert fresh device.

        iv. If permanent or convertible filter fails to open completely and migration is a concern, place a second filter central to the first or consider reposition or removal of the unopened filter.

(3) *Severely tilted filter (>15 degrees):* More common with conical-shaped filters and is associated with difficult retrieval and/or failure as the tip is prone to become embedded in the vessel wall (4). Theoretically, a significant tilt may also compromise thromboembolic filtration.

    (a) Advance a reverse curve catheter over a guidewire to gently manipulate the filter to correct the tilt. Caution should be taken to avoid filter migration.

    (b) If the above does not resolve the severe tilt, then retrieve the filter and place a new filter.

Postprocedure Management

1. Permanent filters
   a. Routine monitoring in immediate postprocedure period for venous access procedures.
   b. Alert patient and other caregivers to observe for limb edema, which may indicate caval thrombosis or DVT.
   c. Primary pharmacologic treatment or prophylaxis for VTE should commence at the first safe opportunity.
   d. Regular abdominal films (every 3 to 5 years) to monitor filter position and integrity. Multiple projections are helpful for identifying tilt, fracture, or limb migration.
2. Retrievable filters
   a. The same as items **a.** through **c.** for permanent filters.

b. These patients require tracking and routine follow-up evaluation to assess anticoagulation status and continuing need for filter. The most influential factor enhancing IVC filter retrieval/mechanical conversion is a plan for follow-up at the time of filter placement.
  (1) Initial follow-up should occur at standard interval (e.g., 1 to 3 months) to assess appropriate conditions for retrieval (see following text) and allow filter retrieval as soon as clinically safe.
  (2) Primary physicians may require guidance regarding the timing of filter retrieval.
  (3) The physician who placed the filter should perform the follow-up.
c. Factors that affect filter retrieval should be anticipated at the time of placement and addressed during the follow-up period (5):
  (1) Patient factors (socioeconomic/demographic)
    (a) Age >80 years old, considerable distance from a health care facility, insurance coverage, education
  (2) Medical factors
    (a) Comorbidities that may limit eligibility for retrieval
  (3) Systemic factors
    (a) Methods to increase patient contact for follow-up have shown to increase retrieval rates:
      i. Scheduling automatic patient follow-up at time of placement, physician education, patient tracking databases, implementation of a dedicated IVC filter clinic, and systems that periodically contact patients and referring physicians have all demonstrated the ability to increase filter retrieval rates
  (4) Technical factors:
    (a) Increase likelihood of failed retrieval attempts:
      i. Tilt, apposition of the hook to IVC wall, leg perforation, and dwell time

Results
1. Successful deployment: 99%
2. Postfilter recurrent PE: 0.5% to 6%

Complications
Concerns have been raised that retrievable filters may have a higher incidence of adverse events than permanent filters (6).
1. Major procedural: less than 1%
2. Access site thrombosis (asymptomatic): 2%
3. Caval thrombosis: 0.6% to 8%
4. Filter fracture: 2% to 10%
5. Filter migration (major): 1%
6. Filter infection: greatly less than 1%
7. IVC penetration/perforation (most asymptomatic): 0% to 86%
8. Thirty-day mortality due to filter: less than 1% (*Note*: overall 30-day mortality rate of 17% is primarily due to concurrent diseases.)

Management of Complications
1. Suspected recurrent PE
  a. Document PE with objective testing
    (1) No PE, stop
  b. If PE is found
    (1) Image filter
      (a) Contrast-enhanced CT for filter location, position in IVC, and patency
      (b) Abdominal plain film with US or magnetic resonance imaging (MRI) (nonferromagnetic filters) is alternative for patients who should avoid iodinated contrast agents

   c. If patient can be anticoagulated

     (1) Initiate anticoagulation

   d. If patient cannot be anticoagulated

     (1) If the filter is obviously damaged, incompletely opened, malpositioned, or migrated, place a second filter.

       (a) For retrievable filters, also consider removal of original filter.

     (2) Determine source of PE, including new lower extremity DVT, thrombus extending through the filter, renal vein thrombus, ovarian vein thrombus, or upper extremity DVT.

     (3) When the source is the lower extremities or due to propagation of thrombus through the filter, place a second filter. If the first filter is free of thrombus, a second filter can be placed above or below. If the first filter contains trapped thrombus, place a second filter above (in suprarenal IVC if necessary).

     (4) If the source is upper extremity thrombus, consider an SVC filter.

     (5) If no source can be found, assume that the most likely source is lower extremity DVT and place a second filter.

2. Suspected occlusion of filter or caval thrombosis

   a. Document with objective testing

     (1) If filter and IVC are patent, no further evaluation is needed

   b. Filter or IVC occlusion is found

     (1) Treatment beyond anticoagulation is not indicated if the patient is asymptomatic

   c. If the patient is symptomatic, document acuity and the level of occlusion

     (1) Evaluate for DVT with imaging modality of choice.

     (2) If no lower extremity thrombus is present, image the IVC and filter with computed tomography (CT), MRI, or cavogram.

     (3) If the patient no longer has contraindication to anticoagulation, consider thrombolysis and/or long-term anticoagulation.

     (4) If the patient has a contraindication to anticoagulation, consider mechanical thrombectomy. Be sure to use a device that cannot become entangled in the filter. The goal is not to clean up the filter completely but to restore flow.

     (5) If thrombus extends above the filter, place a second filter central to the first if indicated.

     (6) Chronic IVC occlusion with filter in place can be recanalized with angioplasty and stents.

       (a) Remove filter at time of recanalization.

       (b) If filter cannot be removed, stent through the filter or push filter aside with stents.

       (c) Patient will not be protected against PE and may require long-term anticoagulation.

3. Suspected filter migration

   a. Confirm that the filter has moved by comparison to old imaging studies.

     (1) If the filter remains in a position that protects the patient from PE, then perform no intervention but continue follow-up.

       (a) Reimage in 1 to 3 months.

       (b) If filter continues to move, consider second filter central to the first.

         i. If first filter is a retrievable device, consider removing and placing a new device.

     (2) If the filter has migrated into the common iliac vein and continued protection is required, place a second filter central to the first.

       (a) If first filter is retrievable device, consider removal.

     (3) If the filter has migrated to the heart or pulmonary circulation, migration may have been caused by massive embolus.

(a) Patient is no longer protected from PE, and new filter may be indicated.

(b) Intracardiac filters should be removed. Percutaneous repositioning or retrieval may be feasible, but great care must be exercised to avoid cardiac trauma. Surgical removal may be necessary.

(c) Limited experience with pulmonary arterial filters suggests that removal is not necessary in asymptomatic patients.

4. Fracture of filter element

    a. If fracture results in compromise of filter function, place a second filter.

      (1) Consider removal if retrievable filter.

    b. Expectant management is exercised for asymptomatic patients.

    c. If filter fragment migrates into adjacent tissues, no therapy is necessary unless the patient is symptomatic.

      (1) If the patient is symptomatic, confirm the precise location of the fragment with CT.

      (2) Consider surgical removal if the patient is symptomatic and surgery is feasible.

    d. If filter fragment has embolized to the heart

      (1) Assess patient for arrhythmia, perforation, or chest pain. Urgent intervention is required for symptomatic patients.

        (a) Some fragments may be retrieved percutaneously with low complication rates via the use of a snare through a directional guiding catheter (7).

          i. Fragments perpendicular to the ventricular wall appear to be more likely to cause symptoms and are more likely to be retrieved percutaneously, if an adequately sized portion of the fragment is intravascular. However, the available literature is limited.

        (b) Surgical removal is required if percutaneous retrieval is not possible or there is a perforation.

      (2) If asymptomatic

        (a) Cross-sectional imaging to localize fragment

        (b) Consultation with cardiology and cardiac surgery

    e. If filter fragment has embolized to the pulmonary artery

      (1) Complications are rare.

      (2) Expectant management.

      (3) Percutaneous snare retrieval if fragment is considered high risk.

    f. If filter fragment is partially intravascular in the IVC

      (1) Percutaneous snare retrieval if there is risk of fragment embolization

      (2) Expectant management

      (3) Trap filter against IVC wall with stent if considered high risk for migration but cannot be retrieved.

5. Penetration of IVC by filter element

    a. Majority of patients are asymptomatic and can be followed expectantly.

    b. If the patient is symptomatic.

      (1) Confirm the location of penetrated elements by CT, endoscopy, and angiography as necessary.

      (2) Exclude other etiologies of symptoms, such as lumbar spine disease or gastrointestinal processes.

      (3) Treat symptoms with nonaddictive analgesics.

      (4) If retrievable filter, consider removal.

      (5) Consider surgical exploration and removal of extracaval filter elements, if necessary.

      (6) For all of the above, assess patient's VTE status and need for protection from PE.

      (7) Antibiotic prophylaxis that covers gastrointestinal flora should be considered prior to removing a filter with gastrointestinal perforation (8).

Optional Filter Retrieval or Mechanical Conversion

Vena caval filtration may be discontinued when the risk of clinically significant PE is reduced to an acceptable level and is estimated to be less than the risk of leaving the filter in place. Remember: All optional filters are approved as permanent implants.

Indications
1. Absolute
   a. The filter is a documented source of major morbidity that will be relieved by retrieval (e.g., unmanageable pain secondary to limb perforation).
2. Relative
   a. Adequate primary therapy of VTE or prophylaxis is achieved, and filtration is no longer deemed necessary.
   b. The patient is no longer deemed at risk for VTE; thus, filtration is no longer deemed necessary.
   c. The filter is no longer protective as a result of a change in position or loss of structural integrity.
   d. Patient is on life-long anticoagulation solely because of the filter.

Contraindications
1. The patient continues to have an indication for vena caval filtration.
2. Significant retained thrombus within the filter. Small filling defects adherent to the filter elements are not a contraindication to retrieval. Visual aids to estimating the size of retained thrombus are available.
3. The patient is unable to achieve adequate anticoagulation or primary prophylaxis (occasionally, this is a patient compliance issue).
4. The patient is anticipated to return to a high-risk state for PE in the future.
5. Life expectancy of the patient is less than 6 months (unlikely that the patient will realize the presumed benefits of filter removal).
6. Lack of vascular access for retrieval
7. The patient wants the filter to remain in place.

Preprocedure Preparation
1. Recommended conditions prior to filter retrieval or conversion
   a. An indication for permanent filtration is not present.
   b. The risk of clinically significant PE is acceptably low as a result of a change in clinical status or achievement of sustained appropriate anticoagulation or prophylaxis.
   c. The patient is not anticipated to return to a condition at high risk for PE.
   d. The patient's life expectancy is long enough so that the presumed benefits of filter removal can be realized.
   e. The filter can be safely retrieved or converted.
2. A focused history and physical should be performed to assess signs and symptoms of new, recurrent, or progressive VTE.
3. The performing physician should discuss with the patient the rationale for discontinuing filtration and the voluntary nature of filter retrieval or conversion.
4. Laboratory studies
   a. Routine preprocedural use of laboratory studies is not recommended except in select scenarios:
      (1) Coagulation studies and blood counts for patients on therapeutic anticoagulation.
      (2) Patients on warfarin should have stable laboratory values, with no evidence of bleeding for at least 7 days. For patients taking warfarin, measure INR on the day of the procedure to ensure it is within the appropriate range.
      (3) Serum creatinine in patients with impaired renal function.

5. Imaging (1)
   a. Routine preprocedural imaging of the filter prior to removal is recommended against except in select situations:
      (1) Patients suspected of having new, recurrent, or progressive VTE, diagnostic imaging for DVT or PE should be performed prior to filter retrieval. Conversely, if a patient is therapeutically anticoagulated and has no signs or symptoms of new, recurrent, or progressive VTE, no additional imaging is required.
      (2) Patients with filters placed for VTE prophylaxis should undergo imaging of the lower extremity veins (duplex venous US) prior to filter retrieval to detect interval development of VTE.
      (3) Patients who are being planned for retrieval with filters placed at outside facilities with no prior imaging available or those with filters in place >180 days are recommended to undergo CT imaging with contrast to evaluate for factors associated with difficult retrieval—tilt, embedded tip, fracture, or penetration.
   b. Review available prior imaging to assess filter type, location, presence of trapped thrombus, filter integrity, caval penetration, and filter migration.
   c. Goals of reviewing preretrieval imaging
      (1) Evaluate the presence of trapped thrombus in the filter.
      (2) Define the position of the filter in the vena cava.
      (3) Assess for complicating factors such as an embedded retrieval tip/hook, fracture or limb penetration.
6. Anticoagulation status
   a. The recommended duration of anticoagulation for VTE prior to filter retrieval is 2 to 3 weeks.
   b. Patients taking warfarin should have a stable INR and no evidence of bleeding for at least 7 days.
   c. Do *not* interrupt anticoagulation for filter retrieval or conversion.
   d. Do *not* attempt to remove or convert filter if the patient meets criteria for therapeutic anticoagulation and is not therapeutically anticoagulated.
   e. Retrieval may be postponed for INR >3.5 or platelets <20,000 per μL.
7. The consent for retrieval or conversion of a vena caval filter includes all of the usual risks associated with percutaneous venous procedures as well as the following:
   a. Failure to retrieve the filter 5% to 50%
      (1) Failure rate increases with the duration of dwell time and specific filter.
   b. Filter migration <1%
   c. Filter fracture <1%
   d. Symptomatic laceration or perforation of the vena cava <1%
   e. Vena caval thrombosis <1%
   f. Hemodynamically significant arrhythmia <1%

Procedure
1. Access
   a. Dependent on filter design; usually jugular or femoral vein
2. Imaging: High-quality imaging during filter retrieval maximizes the chance of successful filter retrieval and minimizes the chances of complication or a prolonged or difficult retrieval.
   a. Goals of preretrieval imaging are the same as mentioned above in Section 5c of preprocedural imaging:
      (1) Evaluate the presence of trapped thrombus in the filter.
      (2) Define the position of the filter in the vena cava.
      (3) Assess for complicating factors such as an embedded retrieval tip/hook, fracture, or limb penetration.

(4) If other imaging methods (CT, MRI, US) have accomplished these goals within 24 hours of the procedure, catheter-based cavography is optional but strongly recommended.

b. Cavography
   (1) For IVC, position pigtail catheter (5 to 7 Fr) below the filter. Take care not to dislodge the filter or entrap catheters or guidewires in the filter.
   (2) For SVC, inject from a brachiocephalic vein.
   (3) Injection rate for iodinated contrast of 15 to 20 mL per second for 2 seconds.
   (4) DSA filming at four to six frames per second during suspended respiration in anterior–posterior projection. Additional projections can be obtained as needed to evaluate the status of the filter.
   (5) Consider cone-beam CT cavogram.
   (6) CO_2 cavography is a safe alternative in patients with renal failure or contrast allergies.

c. IVUS: In patients with contraindications to all contrast agents, IVUS can be utilized, in conjunction with fluoroscopy, to evaluate the filter prior to retrieval.
   (1) Evaluate presence of thrombus.
   (2) Assess for tip/hook embedment in the caval wall.
   (3) Identify limb penetration.

3. Retrieval
   a. Retrieval devices
      (1) Endovascular snares or snare variants
      (2) Proprietary grasping devices
      (3) Biopsy forceps
      (4) Excimer laser sheath
   b. General technique
      (1) Filter elements in contact with the wall of the IVC may be covered with a layer of fibrocellular matrix, neointima, or pseudointima. Elements that perforate the wall of the IVC are usually encapsulated (unless they enter another lumen) with tissue that is in continuity with the IVC adventitia.
      (2) Adequate sheath size positioned close to the intended site of engagement with the filter apex. Refer to manufacturer's documentation regarding appropriate sheath size—it is often larger than delivery sheath size.
         (a) When difficult retrievals are anticipated because of the incorporation of filter elements into the wall of the IVC, consider coaxial sheaths of similar length. For complex retrievals, sheaths from 16 to 20 Fr may be required.
      (3) Introduce a snare and catheter or other recommended retrieval device through the sheath and grasp the filter.
      (4) The technique used to remove filters varies by device. Always refer to the manufacturer's instructions. There are two basic approaches.
         (a) Peeling the filter away from the IVC
            i. Maintain the filter in stable position with countertraction grasping device and push the retrieval sheath over the filter until the filter is entirely captured within the sheath.
         (b) Extracting the filter from the IVC
            i. Maintain the sheath in stable position providing counterpressure on the IVC wall and pull the filter into the retrieval sheath.
      (5) Once the filter is entirely within the sheath, retrieve the filter through it, taking care to avoid sheath damage from sharp filter edges. Inspect the filter for integrity, making sure all pieces were removed.
      (6) Postretrieval cavography is recommended when the patient reports pain during or after the procedure or after a prolonged or difficult retrieval.

c. Advanced techniques: In general, advanced techniques are any technique beyond the standard sheath and snare technique. Advanced techniques are employed as a form of escalation at the time of a difficult retrieval, or after a failed retrieval using standard techniques. Cavography is recommended after a retrieval with these techniques.

(1) Appropriately sized occlusion balloons and stent-grafts should be readily available to manage immediate complications when employing advanced techniques.

(2) Loop snare

(a) Advance a reverse curve catheter through the filter, taking care to stay above any secondary struts. Advance an exchange-length nitinol-based (i.e., low risk of kinking) hydrophilic guidewire through this catheter, snare the guidewire from the same venous access site, and pull the distal end of the wire through the sheath to form a loop snare. Capture the filter using an appropriately sized sheath and the loop snare or track a snare over both limbs of the loop snare to capture the filter.

(3) Hangman technique (9)

(a) Form a loop snare around the filter apex, running the wire *between* the filter elements and the caval wall but not through the filter elements. Apply traction on the loop snare to separate the filter apex from the wall of the cava.

(4) Endobronchial forceps (off-label)

(a) Following detailed venography, advance the endobronchial forceps (model 4162; Lymol Medical, Woburn, MA) through a 16- or 18-Fr sheath.

i. Prior to insertion into the sheath, the forceps can be gently bent with a light angle to allow the forceps to engage the filter tip.

(b) If there is encapsulating tissue, gently grasp and remove the tissue surrounding the filter tip.

(c) Once the encapsulating tissue is removed, grasp the filter tip and remove the filter through the sheath.

(5) Excimer laser sheath assistance

(a) Connect the laser-tipped sheath to the laser system (Cava Clear, Philips, Cambridge, MA) and calibrate per protocol to 60 mJ per mm^2.

(b) Place a 16- or 18-Fr sheath with the tip just cranial to the tip of the filter. Insert the 14-Fr or 16-Fr laser-tipped sheath over a wire coaxially through the 16- or 18-Fr sheath respectively until resistance is encountered.

(c) While maintaining gentle traction on the filter with a snare, activate the laser and advance the sheath. The larger outer sheath can be used for additional blunt dissection while holding counter traction on the filter, and the laser deactivated.

(d) Once the adhered components are free, advance the sheaths over the filter while maintaining counter traction with the snare.

(e) Laser-assisted retrieval is 99.4% successful in removing embedded filters that are refractory to high force retrieval via other advanced techniques and with significantly lower force as it utilizes photothermal tissue ablation while tension is applied to the filter (10)

(6) Factors that are associated with difficult retrieval

(a) Significant filter tilt

(b) Embedded filter cap

(c) Prolonged filter dwell time

(d) Leg penetration

4. Troubleshooting difficult retrieval (see Chapter e-83, Retrieval of Intravascular Foreign Bodies)

a. Difficult retrievals often require escalation to the use of advanced retrieval techniques, simply defined as involving more than a retrieval snare and sheath.

b. It is recommended to have appropriately IVC-sized occlusion balloons and stent grafts immediately ready if attempting these techniques.

c. *Difficulty grasping hook or other locus for engaging the filter*—this is often related to filter tilt or tortuosity of the vena cava (e.g., a patient with scoliosis).

   (1) A curved catheter can be advanced to engage the filter and then manipulated to move the filter more centrally within the vein.

   (2) A directional guide catheter can be used to advance the snare to the appropriate location on the filter.

   (3) Use a second wire (buddy wire) to direct the retrieval device to the filter. Thread a 5-Fr catheter through the filter adjacent to the hook or engagement site and remove the catheter over a stiff guidewire. Advance a snare over (track the loop over the wire) or adjacent to the stiff guidewire to capture the filter.

   (4) Use the loop snare technique.

   (5) Gently inflate a balloon within the filter to attempt to straighten the filter within the vein.

d. *Filter tip adherent to the caval wall.* The critical imaging feature is an unopacified tissue cap around the filter tip or projection of the filter tip outside the opacified venous lumen.

   (1) Attempt Hangman technique (see advanced techniques above).

   (2) Gently inflate a balloon within the filter to attempt to free the filter apex from the caval wall and straighten the filter within the vein.

   (3) Very cautiously use rigid endobronchial forceps to dissect the embedded filter apex free.

e. *Filter is firmly adhered to the wall of the cava.* This is usually diagnosed after capturing the filter while attempting to sheath the filter.

   (1) When using a coaxial sheath system, the outer and inner sheaths can be sequentially advanced over the filter.

   (2) If the filter hook becomes straightened during forceful snare retrieval, consider using endobronchial forceps to grasp the filter hook and oversheath the filter. Alternatively, the loop snare technique can also be used in this scenario.

   (3) Advance a balloon catheter from a separate access and attempt to pry the filter struts off the caval wall by gentle balloon inflation.

   (4) Advance excimer laser sheath over filter to disrupt adherent tissue.

f. Retrieval attempt is abandoned.

   (1) Perform cavogram to assess the status of filter and IVC.

      (a) Consider short course of anticoagulation if IVC injury or thrombus is seen.

      (b) Routine anticoagulation for the presence of an IVC filter without additional indication is not recommended (1).

      (c) If filter is no longer protective against PE, communicate this information to the patient and the primary physician.

   (2) If filter remains collapsed and causes IVC stenosis, perform angioplasty on the filter, with balloon sized to the IVC, to push filter against the wall.

5. Conversion

   a. General technique

      (1) Determine the mechanism of conversion for the patient's device.

         (a) For example, snare removal of a constraining apical cap.

      (2) Perform assessment and imaging of the patient as described for retrieval procedures earlier.

      (3) Utilize appropriate sheaths and endovascular devices for triggering conversion of the filter.

(4) Confirm removal of all extractable components from the patient.
(5) Perform cavogram to document status of IVC and converted device.

Postprocedure Management

1. Routine monitoring in immediate postprocedure period for venous access procedures.
2. Primary treatment or prophylaxis for VTE should continue until no longer clinically indicated.

Results (11)

1. 98.2% total success rate of retrieval when combining both routine (73.2%) and advanced (94.7%) techniques.

Complications (11,12)

Overall complication rate is 1.7% when using both routine and advanced techniques. Risks are higher with advanced retrieval techniques when compared to routine (5.3% vs. 0.4%). However, these techniques are only employed for removal of filters with suboptimal retrieval conditions (significant tilt, embedded components, penetrated or fractured components, etc.) so a direct comparison of the complication rate of standard versus advanced techniques is not feasible.

1. Filter or filter fragment embolization
2. Caval injury
   a. Laceration
   b. Pseudoaneurysm
   c. Intussusception
3. Caval thrombosis

Management of Complications (11,12)

1. Filter or fragment embolization
   a. See above Sections 3 and 4 under Management of Complications for filter placement.
2. Caval laceration or pseudoaneurysm
   a. Consider reversing anticoagulation.
   b. Maintain wire access across injury.
   c. Most mild cases self-resolve given low-pressure state of the IVC, it is reasonable to repeat cavogram to check for resolution.
   d. For more severe episodes or mild episodes that do not self-resolve, then proceed to temporary balloon occlusion with appropriately sized balloon.
   e. If refractory to balloon occlusion may require placement of appropriately sized stent graft.
3. Intussusception or IVC stenosis
   a. If non flow limiting and asymptomatic then no intervention necessary.
   b. If flow limiting or symptomatic then venoplasty and/or stent.
4. Caval thrombosis
   a. Can be treated with percutaneous thrombectomy and venoplasty.
   b. See Chapter 36 regarding venous thrombectomy and thrombolysis.

References

1. Kaufman JA, Barnes GD, Chaer RA, et al. Society of Interventional Radiology Clinical Practice Guideline for Inferior Vena Cava Filters in the Treatment of Patients with Venous Thromboembolic Disease. *J Vasc Interv Radiol.* 2020;31:1529–1544.
2. Patel IJ, Rahim S, Davidson JC, et al. Society of Interventional Radiology Consensus Guidelines for the Periprocedural Management of Thrombotic and Bleeding Risk in Patients Undergoing Percutaneous Image-Guided Interventions-Part II: Recommendations: Endorsed by the Canadian Association for Interventional Radiology and the

Cardiovascular and Interventional Radiological Society of Europe. *J Vasc Interv Radiol.* 2019;30(8):1168–1184.e1.

3. Harris SA, Velineni R, Davies AH. Inferior vena cava filters in pregnancy: a systematic review. *J Vasc Interv Radiol.* 2016;27(3):354–360.

4. Dinglasan LA, Oh JC, Schmitt JE, et al. Complicated inferior vena cava filter retrievals: associated factors identified at preretrieval CT. *Radiology.* 2013;266(1):347–354.

5. Crumley KD, Hyatt E, Kalva SP, et al. Factors affecting inferior vena cava filter retrieval: a review. *Vasc Endovascular Surg.* 2019;53(3):224–229.

6. Andreoli JM, Lewandowski RJ, Vogelzang RL, et al. Comparison of complication rates associated with permanent and retrievable inferior vena cava filters: a review of the MAUDE database. *J Vasc Interv Radiol.* 2014;25(8):1181–1185.

7. Trerotola, SO, Stavropoulos SW. Management of fractured inferior vena cava filters: outcomes by fragment location. *Radiology.* 2017;284(3):887–896.

8. Kesselman A, Oo TH, Johnson M, et al. Current controversies in inferior vena cava filter placement: AJR Expert panel narrative review. *AJR Am J Roentgenol.* 2021;216(3):563–569.

9. Al-Hakim R, McWilliams JP, Derry W, et al. The hangman technique: a modified loop snare technique for the retrieval of inferior vena cava filters with embedded hooks. *J Vasc Interv Radiol.* 2015;26(1):107–110.

10. Kuo WT, Doshi AA, Ponting JM, et al. Laser-assisted removal of embedded vena cava filters: a first-in-human escalation trial in 500 patients refractory to high-force retrieval. *J Am Heart Assoc.* 2020;9(24):e017916.

11. Al-Hakim R, Kee ST, Olinger K, et al. Inferior vena cava filter retrieval: effectiveness and complications of routine and advanced techniques. *J Vasc Interv Radiol.* 2014;25(6):933–939.

12. Grewal S, Lewandowski RJ, Ryu RKW, et al. Inferior vena cava filter retrieval: patient selection, procedural planning, and postprocedural complications. *AJR Am J Roentgenol.* 2020;215(4):790–794.

36 Acute Extremity DVT: Thrombectomy and Thrombolysis

Suresh Vedantham, MD

Introduction

Acute deep vein thrombosis (DVT) occurs in approximately 300,000 persons per year in the United States alone (1). Because pulmonary embolism (PE) can be fatal, its prevention using anticoagulant therapy has been the mainstay of DVT therapy for over 50 years (2). However, anticoagulant drugs do not actively eliminate venous thrombus, so in many cases, their use is not sufficient to prevent serious DVT complications. Early thrombus progression occurs in a minority of anticoagulated DVT patients and can threaten life, limb, or organ function; prolong hospitalization; and exacerbate DVT symptoms such as limb pain, swelling, and ambulatory difficulties. Despite use of anticoagulant therapy, 25% to 50% of proximal DVT patients will develop significant quality-of-life (QOL) impairment from the postthrombotic syndrome (PTS), a debilitating late DVT complication characterized by chronic leg fatigue or heaviness, swelling, pain, paresthesias, venous claudication, stasis dermatitis, and/or skin ulceration (3,4). PTS can also affect the upper extremity, particularly when the subclavian vein from the dominant arm is involved with the initial DVT episode. The development of PTS is incompletely understood, but at a macroscopic level appears to involve at least two components, the development of which are mediated by a thrombosis-triggered inflammatory process: (a) residual thrombus and/or venous fibrosis block blood flow ("obstruction") and (b) thrombosis directly damages the venous valves, causing valvular incompetence ("reflux"). When reflux and/or obstruction is present, ambulatory venous hypertension develops and ultimately leads to the edema, tissue hypoxia and injury, progressive calf pump dysfunction, subcutaneous fibrosis, and skin ulceration of PTS (5).

Catheter-directed thrombolysis (CDT) was pioneered by interventional radiologists in the early 1990s. CDT has shown the ability to remove venous thrombus and has been hypothesized to provide a range of early and late clinical benefits, but also carries safety risks. During recent years, the completion of pivotal randomized clinical trials has yielded substantial insight into the short-term and long-term effects of CDT and related procedures, and greater confidence in defining appropriate patient selection characteristics and treatment expectations (6).

Indications

1. **Urgent first-line CDT** is performed as an adjunct to anticoagulant therapy to prevent life-, limb-, or organ-threatening complications of acute DVT.
   a. In patients with acute limb-threatening circulatory compromise (i.e., phlegmasia cerulea dolens).
   b. In patients with extensive inferior vena cava (IVC) thrombosis who are deemed to be at high risk for fatal PE.
   c. In patients with acute renal failure from thrombus extension into the suprarenal IVC and/or renal veins.
2. **Nonurgent second-line CDT** can be performed for patients with symptomatic extensive DVT who exhibit clinical and/or anatomic progression of DVT on anticoagulant therapy.
   a. Rapid iliocaval or subclavian/brachiocephalic thrombus extension
   b. Exacerbation or persistence of major lower or upper extremity symptoms
   c. Failure to experience sufficient symptom improvement to permit ambulation or normal arm function
3. **Nonurgent first-line CDT** can be performed as an adjunct to anticoagulant therapy in patients with symptomatic, acute extensive DVT.
   a. Patients with acute iliofemoral DVT may experience greater improvement in early leg symptoms, reduction in PTS severity, and improvement in venous QOL.
   b. Patients with acute axillosubclavian DVT related to Paget–Schroetter syndrome also appear to be excellent candidates for a combined surgical-interventional approach in which CDT-mediated thrombus removal is the first step.

Contraindications

1. Active internal bleeding
2. Recent (<3 months) gastrointestinal bleeding
3. Recent stroke (<6 months)
4. Intracranial or intraspinal bleeding, tumor, vascular malformation, or aneurysm
5. Severe liver dysfunction
6. Severe thrombocytopenia or other bleeding diathesis
7. Pregnancy
8. Severe uncontrolled hypertension
9. Recent (<10 days) major surgery, trauma, cardiopulmonary resuscitation, obstetric delivery, lithotripsy, or other major invasive procedure
10. Recent (<3 months) eye operation or hemorrhagic retinopathy
11. Bacterial endocarditis or acute bacterial septic thrombophlebitis
12. Moderate-to-severe renal dysfunction
13. Severe acute illness that precludes adequate sedation or proper positioning on the table
14. Patients with isolated femoral–popliteal or calf DVT are not likely to benefit
15. Patients >65 years of age may be less likely to benefit and more likely to have a major bleed

Preprocedure Preparation

1. Obtain clinical history and perform physical examination to confirm the presence of a symptom and/or clinical manifestation that merits aggressive therapy. Know the patient's risk factors for bleeding complications, his or her baseline ambulatory status, and his or her life expectancy. Patients who are chronically nonambulatory or who have very short life expectancy may not experience meaningful benefits from CDT. If a patient has a compelling reason for treatment and is at high risk for bleeding, stand-alone percutaneous mechanical thrombectomy can be considered (without administration of thrombolytic drugs).

2. Review duplex venous ultrasound to confirm the diagnosis of DVT, evaluate the extent of thrombus, and plan the therapeutic approach. If needed, evaluation of central veins may be performed with computed tomography (CT) scan, magnetic resonance (MR) venography, or injection venography.

3. Laboratory evaluation: serum creatinine, hemoglobin (Hgb)/hematocrit (Hct), platelet count, international normalized ratio (INR), partial thromboplastin time (PTT). Pregnancy test should be performed in women of childbearing potential.

4. Provide a balanced discussion of the risks, benefits, alternatives to, and uncertainties surrounding CDT and obtain informed consent. Discuss the use of adjunctive measures such as angioplasty and stent placement to treat stenotic lesions that are uncovered.

5. For most patients, ensure that the INR is below 2.0 (preferably 1.5) before starting CDT and stop any nonheparin anticoagulants at least 24 hours before CDT. These parameters can be modified for patients with severe clinical manifestations or for patients with renal dysfunction (the latter may require longer periods of oral anticoagulation cessation). If the patient has mild-to-moderate contrast allergy, premedicate with steroids and histamine antagonists.

6. In selected patients with lower extremity DVT, a retrievable IVC filter may be placed prior to starting CDT. Because PE rates have been low when infusion-first CDT (see Complications section) is used, IVC filter placement is probably unnecessary when this method is used.

Procedure

1. Select a venous access site, ideally peripheral to the extent of the thrombus.
   a. Usual sites for lower extremity DVT treatment are the popliteal vein or posterior tibial vein. Other veins that can be used include the internal jugular vein, small saphenous vein, and other ipsilateral tibial veins. Use of the contralateral common femoral vein is not recommended (to avoid causing contralateral DVT), but can be used if necessary.
   b. For upper extremity DVT, usual sites are the brachial or basilic veins.
   c. In choosing an access site, it is important to consider the sheath size needed to accommodate the planned infusion catheter/device. For example, it may not be wise to select a distal posterior tibial vein access site if an 8-Fr sheath will be needed. In some situations when the thrombus extends through the popliteal vein and into the calf, additional access sites may be used (e.g., popliteal vein and posterior tibial vein).

2. Administer conscious sedation with appropriate monitoring, perform sterile preparation, and inject local anesthetic (e.g., 1% lidocaine) into the skin over the selected vein(s).

3. Perform an ultrasound-guided puncture to obtain catheter access into the selected vein(s). A 5- to 7.5-MHz linear array transducer is routinely used. A 21-gauge micropuncture needle is ultrasound visible, and its use may help to minimize bleeding. Pass a 0.018-in guidewire and exchange for a transition dilator and then advance a diagnostic catheter (4 Fr or 5 Fr) into the venous system

over a 0.035-in hydrophilic guidewire. Real-time fluoroscopic monitoring should be used throughout the procedure.

4. Perform a venogram through the diagnostic catheter to define the thrombus extent. This should be done with serial hand injections of 5- to 10-mL iodinated contrast, diluted as needed with 0.9% normal saline, and digital subtraction imaging.

5. Exchange the diagnostic catheter for a 7- to 8-Fr vascular sheath.

6. Decide whether to perform "infusion-first CDT" or "single-session pharmacomechanical CDT (PCDT)" and select a drug delivery catheter. If single-session PCDT will be used, skip to step 8. If only percutaneous mechanical thrombectomy (PMT) will be used, skip to step 9.

7. Patients undergoing infusion-first CDT

   a. Select a multi–side-hole infusion catheter with an infusion segment that matches the length of the thrombosed venous segment. For infusion-first CDT, either a traditional multi–side-hole infusion catheter or an ultrasound-emitting infusion catheter (Ekos, Boston Scientific, Natick, MA) may be used. Ultrasound-assisted CDT is hypothesized to loosen fibrin strands, facilitate drug dispersion, and enable faster therapy with a reduced thrombolytic dose; however, it is much costlier and does not appear to provide superior results compared with CDT using a standard multi–side-hole catheter (7).

   b. Advance catheter into position over the guidewire and start infusing the thrombolytic drug. *Note:* None of these drugs is approved by the U.S. Food and Drug Administration (FDA) for DVT therapy—all are approved for other indications but are used off-label for DVT (6). By far, the largest published experience, which includes rigorous multicenter randomized controlled trials (RCTs) (8,9), has used tissue plasminogen activator.

      (1) Recombinant tissue plasminogen activator (rt-PA) at 0.01/mg/kg, not to exceed 1.0 mg per hour (8,9)

      (2) Urokinase (UK) at 120,000 to 180,000 U per hour (10,11)

      (3) Reteplase at 0.50 to 0.75 U per hour

      (4) Tenecteplase (TNK) at 0.25 to 0.50 mg per hour

   c. If ultrasound-assisted CDT is being performed, press the Start button on the machine to administer low-power ultrasound energy during drug delivery.

   d. Simultaneously administer concomitant anticoagulant therapy by either (a) infusing subtherapeutic unfractionated heparin (UFH) through the vascular sheath at an hourly dose that is sufficiently low to prevent the PTT from becoming supratherapeutic—either one can target the PTT to 1.2 to 1.7 times control or to less than 60 seconds, or simply use a dose in the range of 6 to 12 units/kg/h (8,9), or (b) administering low–molecular-weight heparin (LMWH) such as enoxaparin at 1 mg per kg subcutaneous injections every 12 hours (9). The use of fondaparinux, rivaroxaban, dabigatran, apixaban, and edoxaban is discouraged because there are few prospective studies of concomitant use with thrombolytic drugs.

   e. If treating lower extremity DVT, elevate the symptomatic leg during the infusion.

   f. Monitor the patient in a stepdown unit or intensive care unit (ICU) during the infusion and obtain peripheral blood laboratory studies at least every 8 to 12 hours (Hct/Hgb, PTT). Follow these levels closely because elevated PTT levels during thrombolysis have been associated with bleeding complications, and a rapid drop in hematocrit may be a sign of occult bleeding (e.g., retroperitoneal bleeding).

   g. The nurse and/or the treating physician should clinically evaluate the patient frequently to assess for sentinel bleeding (e.g., epistaxis, ear bleeding, profuse access site bleeding) that may indicate a systemic thrombolytic state of greater intensity than desired.

h. The fibrinogen level may also be monitored, although there are little data to support its usefulness for preventing complications of DVT thrombolysis procedures.

i. After 6 to 18 hours of infusion, bring the patient back to the angiographic suite and repeat the venogram. Skip to step 9.

8. Patients undergoing single-session pharmacomechanical CDT: Patients in whom the goal is to complete DVT treatment in a single-procedure session may have the thrombolytic drug administered via one of several catheter/devices. A detailed description of the exact method of use of each of these very different devices is beyond the scope of this handbook. However, here are key differences between single-session PCDT and infusion-first CDT:

a. The single-session PCDT techniques involve the delivery and rapid dispersion of a significant dose of the thrombolytic drug as the first step in thrombus removal. Typically, 5 to 25 mg of rt-PA (or the equivalent) is administered during this procedure session. Different devices rely on different methods to achieve rapid drug dispersion within the thrombus. One commonly used technique is described below.

b. Power-pulse thrombolysis using the AngioJet Rheolytic Thrombectomy System (Boston Scientific Corp, Minneapolis, MN): An AngioJet Solent Proxi or Xelante catheter is advanced to and from within the thrombus with the device in power pulse mode (i.e., the outflow port is occluded). This results in powerful pulse-spray delivery of the thrombolytic drug into the clot. After a dwell period of 30 minutes, the AngioJet is used in aspiration mode to remove the softened residual clot.

c. Because single-session PCDT may be more mechanically aggressive than infusion-first CDT, most physicians anticoagulate the patient to therapeutic levels during PCDT.

9. Percutaneous mechanical thrombectomy—if thrombolytic drugs are not given, one of several devices can be used to attempt thrombectomy. However, the efficacy and safety of these devices has not been evaluated in well-designed prospective studies. Anecdotal reports suggest that traditional smaller-bore devices (i.e., 5 to 8 Fr) do not reliably provide sufficient thrombus removal to enable effective treatment of extensive DVT. In recent years, large-bore devices (i.e., 12 to 20 Fr) have been made available and may provide a useful tool for special situations (e.g., thrombus in the right atrium or suprarenal IVC), but prospective studies are not available to shed light on their safety or clinical effectiveness.

10. Clean-up of residual thrombus: After the initial thrombolytic drug infusion (infusion-first CDT) or injection/dispersion (single-session PCDT), repeat venogram is performed. If near-complete lysis and good anterograde flow are observed (by visual estimation) with no venous stenosis or obstruction, treatment may be stopped. If residual thrombus is present, the physician may use one or more of the following adjunctive measures to remove it.

a. *Balloon maceration* of the thrombus: Advance a standard angioplasty balloon catheter (6 to 10 mm for the femoral vein, 10 to 12 mm for the common femoral vein or iliac vein) over the guidewire into the thrombus. Inflate the balloon within the thrombus. Deflate the balloon. Repeat these steps as needed with the balloon positioned in different parts of the thrombus. Remove the angioplasty balloon catheter over the guidewire.

b. *Catheter aspiration thrombectomy*: Advance a standard 7- to 8-Fr catheter over the guidewire to the cephalad aspect of the thrombus. Attach a large (30 to 60 mL) syringe to the catheter. Vigorously aspirate with the syringe during withdrawal of the catheter through the thrombus. Repeat these steps as needed and then remove the catheter.

c. *Device-mediated thrombus aspiration* may be performed using one of several thrombectomy devices.

11. Infusion end point: After each of the preceding measures is used, perform a repeat venogram to assess progress. If significant residual obstructing thrombus is still present, position a multi—side-hole infusion catheter within the thrombus and perform infusion CDT in the same manner as earlier. The drug may be infused until near-complete thrombolysis is observed, clinically overt bleeding becomes evident, or until minimal progress is seen on two subsequent venograms. Keep the thrombolytic infusion as short as possible to avoid bleeding issues—less than 24 hours to treat unilateral DVT and less than 36 hours for bilateral DVT are suggested, although these guidelines have not been prospectively validated.

12. Treatment of obstructive lesions: After all thrombus removal steps are completed, perform a repeat venogram. It is also ideal to perform intravascular ultrasound (IVUS) at this time to ensure that venographically occult thrombus or stenosis is identified.

   a. Balloon angioplasty and stent placement may be performed to correct areas of venous stenosis or obstruction that persist since these lesions, when not treated, have been associated with high rates of immediate rethrombosis.

   b. Self-expanding stents with radial flexibility may be used in the iliac vein and extended into the common femoral vein if needed.

   c. Stents in the femoral or popliteal vein are not likely to remain patent, so balloon angioplasty is a better choice for femoropopliteal stenotic lesions.

   d. Stent placement is contraindicated in the subclavian vein; patients with Paget–Schroetter syndrome should have their thoracic outlet decompressed surgically at some point soon after CDT.

   e. At present, it is not clear what stent is best to use. As of this writing, the FDA has approved multiple venous stents for iliac vein use while others are under clinical trial investigation. However, published experienced is limited and it is not clear if patencies are superior to legacy (off-label) self-expandable stents.

13. Perform a final venogram, remove the sheath, and achieve hemostasis by direct compression.

Postprocedure Management

1. It is important to realize that rethrombosis (symptomatic or occult) is a major challenge after CDT. In the ATTRACT trial, despite favorable initial thrombus clearance, venous noncompressibility was very common at 1 month and 12 months postintervention, and correlated with more PTS, more moderate-or-severe PTS, and poorer QOL (12). Therefore, close monitoring to ensure excellent anticoagulation is crucial in the postprocedure period.

2. Therapeutic-level anticoagulation should be resumed immediately after hemostasis is obtained using either UFH or LMWH. For most patients, transition to an oral agent may begin either the same evening or the next day. If the patient is felt to be at particularly high risk for rethrombosis, then LMWH may be continued and the transition to oral therapy delayed. Oral aspirin 81 mg daily may be used in patients with stents.

3. Patients with a lower extremity access site should remain at bed rest with the treated leg immobile for at least 4 hours. After that, early ambulation is desirable.

4. For patients who will receive warfarin, continue heparin (UFH or LMWH) until the INR exceeds 2.0 for 2 consecutive days. Exception: In patients with cancer-related DVT, LMWH monotherapy (not warfarin) is superior to warfarin.

5. For subjects in whom a retrievable IVC filter was placed, the filter may be removed at any time after PCDT is completed. There is no need to stop anticoagulation for filter retrieval unless it is supratherapeutic. In general, the patient should be therapeutically anticoagulated and should not have significant ($\geq$25% of the filter's volume) thrombus within the filter.

6. If the patient has significant lower extremity swelling, offer the patient the option of wearing graduated compression stockings (either 20 to 30 mm Hg or 30 to 40 mm Hg) on a daily basis. Although their use does not appear to prevent PTS or to reduce lower extremity pain, they may help to reduce extremity swelling. If the leg is initially too tender for stockings, consider using wraps first, then transitioning to stockings after 7 to 14 days.

7. The patient should be seen in follow-up within 1 month of the procedure. In the meantime, extra attention is needed to ensure adequacy of anticoagulation.

Results

1. **Infusion CDT** (with no thrombectomy device component) has been shown to dissolve acute thrombus in over 80% of patients with acute (symptom duration ≤14 days) proximal DVT in a 473-patient prospective multicenter registry, a multicenter RCT, and in a pooled analysis of observational studies (6,7,11). Disadvantages include the need for prolonged drug infusions (i.e., around 48 hours), ICU care, and repeated laboratory and venographic monitoring. In the randomized Catheter-directed Venous Thrombolysis in acute iliofemoral vein thrombosis—[CaVenT] study, the use of infusion CDT with anticoagulant therapy in patients with DVT involving the iliac and/or upper femoral venous system was associated with a 26% relative reduction in the risk of PTS over 2-year follow-up (41.1% vs. 55.6%, $p = 0.04$) compared with anticoagulant therapy alone (8). The difference in PTS rates increased at 5-year follow-up, but there was no QOL benefit at 2 or 5 years. Factors which limited the generalizability of CaVenT include its modest sample size (outcomes reported in 189 patients, of whom 92 patients received CDT) and geographical limitation (Southern Norway).

2. In a pilot randomized trial (BERNUTIFUL), **ultrasound-assisted CDT** (UA-CDT) appeared to provide comparable results as infusion CDT without the additional ultrasound. The degree of thrombus removal, venous patency, and PTS at 1-year was similar in the two groups (7). In the randomized CAVA trial, 184 patients with acute iliofemoral DVT were randomized to receive UA-CDT with standard therapy versus standard therapy alone. UA-CDT was found to provide substantial thrombus removal but did not reduce PTS or improve QOL at 1 year (10).

3. **Pharmacomechanical CDT** (PCDT) refers to thrombus dissolution via the combined use of CDT and device-based PMT. The ATTRACT (Acute Venous Thrombosis: Thrombus Removal with Adjunctive Catheter-Directed Thrombolysis) trial, a National Institutes of Health (NIH)–funded multicenter randomized clinical trial, evaluated the ability of PCDT to prevent PTS in 692 patients with acute proximal DVT that extended above the popliteal vein. Key findings:
   a. PCDT successfully eliminated venous thrombus, restoring immediate venous patency, and resulting in less residual venous thrombus (9,12)
   b. PCDT did not prevent PTS or reduce the occurrence of valvular reflux (9,12). Patients ≥65 years of age were more likely to develop PTS with PCDT than younger patients.
   c. In patients with iliofemoral DVT, PCDT increased the degree of improvement in leg pain and swelling over the first 30 days, and reduced the severity of PTS over 2 years (but that was not the case for patients with isolated femoral–popliteal DVT) (13,14)
   d. In patients with iliofemoral DVT (but not isolated femoral–popliteal DVT), PCDT improved venous disease-specific QOL—the effect was of substantial size within the first 6 months, and was relatively small between 12 and 24 months (15)
   e. In patients with iliofemoral DVT, greater thrombus clearance correlated with reduced PTS severity (16). Hence, optimization of thrombus removal and venous flow are worthwhile.

Complications

1. The rates of additional major bleeding (beyond the control arms) in three pivotal randomized trials were 3.2% (CaVenT—infusion CDT), 1.4% (ATTRACT—PCDT), and 5.6% (CAVA—UA-CDT) (8–10). No fatal or intracranial bleeds were observed in these studies, though several patients required surgical or interventional therapy. In ATTRACT, five of six major bleeds occurred in patients ≥65 years of age, with none occurring in patients <60 years old. These findings suggest that in the clinical trial setting with careful patient selection and a defined technique, CDT and related methods may be reasonably safe. However, real-world use of CDT as illustrated by registry data suggests that around 10% of patients undergoing CDT may suffer a major bleed, with 0.4% to 0.9% suffering an intracranial bleed (11). These findings certainly argue for careful patient selection and diligent monitoring.

2. Periprocedure symptomatic PE has occurred in approximately 1% of patients during/after CDT in large studies (8–11). Periprocedure fatal PE occurred in 0.2% of patients in the urokinase registry, and in no patients in ATTRACT (9,11).

3. Prevention of complications
    a. Close monitoring and diligent communication with nursing staff is crucial during CDT.
    b. Nonheparin anticoagulants should be avoided during CDT or PCDT (except for patients with heparin-induced thrombocytopenia who may require an alternative to heparin). If the patient was on warfarin, the INR should ideally be reduced to 1.5 or less before thrombolysis. Close monitoring of dosing and administration of UFH and LMWH is essential. The PTT should not be allowed to become supratherapeutic during lysis.
    c. During CDT or PCDT, the physician should reduce the drug dose or stop it entirely at his or her discretion if there are safety concerns.
    d. If serious bleeding occurs at the venous access site (uncontrolled by sheath upsizing or compression), the drug administration should be stopped. If sheath upsizing and/or compression are effective in stopping the bleeding, the drug may be restarted at a lower dose with careful repeat evaluations of the access site to ensure no recurrence.
    e. If serious bleeding occurs in a distant location, or if a severe or life-threatening reaction occurs, administration of the thrombolytic drug should be permanently stopped.
    f. If serious bleeding occurs, infusion of heparin should also be stopped and, at physician discretion, protamine and/or cryoprecipitate may be given.

References

1. Heit JA, Cohen AT, Anderson FA, et al. Estimated annual number of incident and recurrent, non-fatal and fatal venous thromboembolism (VTE) events in the US [abstract]. *Blood.* 2005;106(11):267a.

2. Kearon C, Akl EA, Ornelas J, et al. Antithrombotic therapy for VTE disease: CHEST guideline and expert panel report. *Chest.* 2016;149(2):315–352.

3. Kahn SR, Shrier I, Julian JA, et al. Determinants and time course of the postthrombotic syndrome after acute deep venous thrombosis. *Ann Intern Med.* 2008;149(10):698–707.

4. Kahn SR, Shbaklo H, Lamping DL, et al. Determinants of health-related quality of life during the 2 years following deep vein thrombosis. *J Thromb Haemost.* 2008;6(7):1105–1112.

5. Nicolaides AN, Hussein MK, Szendro G, et al. The relation of venous ulceration with ambulatory venous pressure measurements. *J Vasc Surg.* 1993;17(2):414–419.

6. Vedantham S, Sista AK, Klein SJ, et al. Society of Interventional Radiology and Cardiovascular and Interventional Radiological Society of Europe Standards of Practice Committees. Quality Improvement Guidelines for the Treatment of Lower-Extremity Deep Vein Thrombosis With Use of Endovascular Thrombus Removal. *J Vasc Interv Radiol.* 2014;25(9):1317–1325.

7. Engelberger RP, Stuck A, Spirk D, et al. Ultrasound-assisted versus conventional catheter-directed thrombolysis for acute iliofemoral deep vein thrombosis: 1-year follow-up data of a randomized-controlled trial. *J Thromb Haemost.* 2017;15(7):1351–1360.

8. Enden T, Haig Y, Kløw NE, et al. Long-term outcomes after additional catheter-directed thrombolysis versus standard treatment for acute iliofemoral deep vein thrombosis (the CaVenT study): a randomised controlled trial. *Lancet.* 2012;379(9810):31–38.

9. Vedantham S, Goldhaber SZ, Julian J, et al. Pharmacomechanical catheter-directed thrombolysis for deep-vein thrombosis. *N Engl J Med.* 2017;377(23):2240–2252.

10. Notten P, ten Cate-Hoek AJ, Arnoldussen CWKP, et al. Ultrasound-accelerated catheter-directed thrombolysis versus anticoagulation for the prevention of post-thrombotic syndrome (CAVA): a single-blind, multicentre, randomised trial. *Lancet Haematol.* 2020;7(1):e40–e49.

11. Mewissen MW, Seabrook GR, Meissner MH, et al. Catheter-directed thrombolysis for lower extremity deep venous thrombosis: report of a national multicenter registry. *Radiology.* 1999;211(1):39–49.

12. Weinberg I, Vedantham S, Salter A, et al. Relationships between the use of pharmacomechanical catheter-directed thrombolysis, sonographic findings, and clinical outcomes in patients with acute proximal DVT: results from the ATTRACT multicenter randomized trial. *Vasc Med.* 2019;24(5):442–451.

13. Comerota AJ, Kearon C, Gu C, et al. Endovascular thrombus removal for acute iliofemoral deep vein thrombosis: analysis from a stratified multicenter randomized trial. *Circulation.* 2019;139(9):1162–1173.

14. Kearon C, Gu C, Julian JA, et al. Pharmacomechanical catheter-directed thrombolysis for acute femoral-popliteal deep-vein thrombosis: analysis from a stratified randomized trial. *Thromb Haemost.* 2019;119(4):633–644.

15. Kahn SR, Julian JA, Kearon C, et al. Quality of life after pharmacomechanical catheter-directed thrombolysis for proximal deep vein thrombosis. *J Vasc Surg Venous Lymphat Disord.* 2020;8(1):8–23.

16. Razavi MK, Salter A, Goldhaber SZ, et al. Correlation between post-procedure residual thrombus and clinical outcome in DVT patients receiving pharmacomechanical thrombolysis in a multicenter randomized trial. *J Vasc Interv Radiol.* 2020;31(10):1517–1528.e2.

37 Endovascular Management of Chronic Deep Venous Obstructive Disease

Kush R. Desai, MD, FSIR

Introduction

Chronic deep venous obstructive diseases of the lower and upper extremities are clinically and epidemiologically distinct processes. While there are pathologic similarities between these two entities, there are significant differences in disease course, approach, and management.

Chronic Lower Extremity Deep Venous Disease

Lower extremity deep venous occlusive disease can largely be separated into postthrombotic and nonthrombotic etiologies. Postthrombotic syndrome (PTS) occurs with varying severity in nearly 50% of all patients following acute deep vein thrombosis (DVT) (1). Involvement of the iliofemoral (common femoral, external iliac, and common iliac) venous segments and inferior vena cava (IVC) have been shown to be associated with more severe PTS symptoms that can include pain/fatigue, severe edema, dermatitis, and soft tissue ulceration (2,3). The pathophysiology of PTS consists of a combination of luminal obstruction from organization of thrombus and inflammation that damages venous valves leading to reflux; together, these two processes result in the clinical sequelae of ambulatory venous hypertension (4). Postthrombotic obstruction can be treated with the placement of self-expanding venous stents, which can reduce pain, edema, and promote ulcer healing (5). Treatment of superficial reflux is also an important component in the endovascular management of PTS, and is discussed elsewhere in this book (Chapter 44).

Nonthrombotic venous obstruction is caused by external compression of deep veins by arteries. Left iliac vein compression syndrome (commonly known as "May–Thurner syndrome") is the most commonly encountered type, where there is compression of the left common iliac vein (CIV) between the right common iliac artery and vertebral body. Although compression syndromes can result in acute iliofemoral DVT, they can also cause venous stasis symptoms in the absence of thrombus, including pain/fatigue, edema, ulceration, and in females, symptoms of female pelvic venous disease (commonly known as pelvic congestion syndrome); these lesions are commonly referred to as nonthrombotic iliac vein lesions (NIVL). However, accurate estimates of the incidence of clinically significant nonthrombotic deep venous disease is difficult as it can be asymptomatic in a significant portion of the population (6); thus, a thorough clinical evaluation to exclude other causes is mandatory prior to intervention. Self-expanding venous stents are placed when treatment is indicated.

Chronic Upper Extremity Deep Venous Disease/Thoracic Central Venous Obstruction

Unlike lower extremity venous obstruction, upper extremity deep venous disease resulting from thoracic central venous obstruction (TCVO) can result from several different etiologies, including indwelling central venous devices (catheters, cardiac device leads), extrinsic compression from malignancy, and infectious or inflammatory processes. Anatomic compression of the subclavian vein between the first rib/clavicle or anterior scalene muscle/first rib can result in chronic occlusion typical of venous thoracic outlet syndrome; when there is associated acute axillosubclavian DVT, this is known as "Paget–Schroetter syndrome." Given the myriad causes and the variety of anatomy that can be affected by TCVO, the epidemiology is poorly understood; similarly, the clinical course and management can vary significantly (7). Patients can present with severe symptoms such as pain, facial edema, and respiratory distress resulting from superior vena cava (SVC) syndrome, or can be relatively asymptomatic. Thus, an individualized approach is necessary to effectively treat patients with TCVO.

Indications

Postthrombotic Lower Extremity Deep Venous Obstruction

1. Patients with moderate-to-severe PTS have a history of DVT in the index limb and most frequently have a component of iliofemoral and/or iliocaval venous occlusion on noninvasive imaging studies.
2. PTS symptoms that include the following symptoms/findings to varying degrees:
   a. Pain that limits or prevents normal activities of daily living and worsens with short periods of activity or standing (venous claudication).
   b. Edema that involves the calf and thigh where compression therapy is less effective.
   c. Distal lower extremity stasis dermatitis including eczema, subcutaneous fibrosis, lipodermatosclerosis, and/or atrophie blanche.
   d. Venous stasis ulceration involving the distal lower extremity. Venous stasis ulcers are frequently present above the malleoli and pretibial soft tissues and should be distinguished from ulceration secondary to arterial disease.
   e. Significant impact on both overall and venous-specific quality of life (QOL).

3. Undiagnosed iliac vein compression that was previously clinically silent may suddenly present with acute iliofemoral DVT. Management of this clinical scenario is addressed in Chapter 36.

Nonthrombotic Lower Extremity Deep Venous Obstruction

1. Patients with NIVL may present with symptoms that include:
   a. Asymmetric lower extremity edema.
   b. Pain, heaviness, and/or fatigue of the affected extremity with activity or prolonged standing (venous claudication).
   c. Asymmetrically advanced superficial venous disease in the affected limb, including venous stasis ulceration.
   d. Pelvic symptoms in females suggesting of pelvic venous disease (see Chapter 43).
2. Patients with NIVL, by definition, have no known history of antecedent DVT.

Thoracic Central Venous Obstruction

1. Symptoms of TCVO are highly variable and depend on anatomical segment involved, causative factors, and comorbidities.
2. SVC syndrome is most commonly secondary to malignant compression, though can be due to device- or catheter-related occlusion.
   a. Patients can present with respiratory distress, severe facial/upper extremity edema, and inability to tolerate oral secretions.
   b. Urgent endovascular intervention and/or external radiation therapy is frequently indicated.
3. Venous thoracic outlet syndrome (TOS)/Paget–Schroetter syndrome is due to extrinsic compression of the subclavian vein by a cervical rib or muscular hypertrophy.
   a. Known as "effort-induced" thrombosis when DVT occurs ipsilateral to the compression, often seen in athletes.
   b. Present with sudden onset, unilateral upper extremity edema.
   c. May be coincident with other thoracic outlet syndromes (arterial, neurogenic).
4. Other TCVO.
   a. Catheter- and device-related occlusions are the most common, and can include dialysis patients or patients with cardiac leads.
   b. Infectious/inflammatory processes that result in venous occlusion, including fibrosing mediastinitis.
5. TCVO can be asymptomatic or minimally asymptomatic.

Contraindications

1. Absolute
   a. For PTS and TOS intervention, there should be no contraindication to anticoagulation.
   b. Active systemic infection.
   c. Severe contrast reaction refractory to steroid and antihistamine medications.
   d. Pregnancy.
   e. Known allergies to stent material (i.e., nickel allergy).
   f. Nondialysis-dependent oliguria where contrast nephropathy is a concern; alternatively, carbon dioxide contrast can be used based on operator experience.
2. Relative
   a. Anemia and thrombocytopenia, should be correctable.
   b. Short life expectancy; palliative treatment of SVC syndrome can be considered in appropriate procedural candidates.

Preprocedure Preparation

Postthrombotic Lower Extremity Deep Venous Obstruction
1. Obtain a thorough history and physical. Specifically review the following:
   a. Venous thromboembolism history, including prior episodes of acute DVT.
   b. Use and compliance with conservative measures, including compression stockings, venous return assist devices, and venoactive medications (none of which are approved by the U.S. Food and Drug Administration [FDA]).
   c. Anticoagulation history; assess for potential risk factors for bleeding from anticoagulation and expected level of patient compliance.
   d. Assess for comorbid conditions that may impact the success or safety of an intervention. Further, many PTS patients have phlebolymphedema, which is chronic lymphatic damage that results from chronic venous obstruction and does not typically improve following endovascular intervention.
   e. Evaluate overall QOL; if patients are unlikely to derive benefit from PTS symptom reduction, intervention may not be indicated. For example, selection of patients that are nonambulatory or have a limited life expectancy may not be appropriate candidates for intervention.
   f. Obtain index limb measurements for comparative purposes following intervention. Typically, measure ankle circumference 5 cm above the medial malleolus, calf circumference 5 cm below the tibial tubercle, thigh measurement above patella.
   g. If a prior or current venous stasis ulcer is present, assess length of time it was or has been present. If active ulcer present, obtain measurements of the ulcer and assess for infection. If infected, prescribe appropriate antibiotic therapy. If involving muscular, tendinous, or osseous structures, obtain wound care/ surgical consultation for further management.
2. Evaluate patients according to venous disease scoring systems to guide decision making.
   a. Clinical, Etiologic, Anatomic, Pathologic (CEAP) score; 2020 update. Patients should at a minimum have C3 disease (edema) though most will have more advanced disease.
   b. Venous Clinical Severity Score (VCSS). Patients often have a score of 8 or greater.
   c. Villalta score. Patients often have a score of 10 or greater.
3. Review noninvasive imaging studies.
   a. Evaluate abdominopelvic venous structures with computed tomographic or magnetic resonance venography (CTV, MRV, respectively) or IVC/iliac duplex ultrasonography. The choice of imaging study will be dependent on local practice/physician preference and expertise. Assess for presence of >50% luminal stenosis or occlusion, length of stenosis, and predisposing factors that resulted occlusion (i.e., left iliac vein compression/May–Thurner syndrome, or in an iliocaval occlusion, an obstructed IVC filter).
   b. Assess venous inflow at level of common femoral vein (CFV) with venous duplex ultrasound. If the CFV is occluded or severely stenotic, assess the femoral vein and profunda femoris vein (PFV) for flow and stenosis. The PFV in particular is critical in maintenance of stent patency in the absence of a normal CFV.
   c. Evaluate superficial veins for reflux (see Chapter 44) as they may require treatment after successful deep venous recanalization. In patients with stasis ulceration, foam sclerotherapy of the ulcer bed is frequently necessary.
4. Provide a balanced discussion of the benefits, risks, potential complications, and conservative alternatives to endovascular therapy. Discuss expectations and potential outcomes (see Results section in this chapter).
5. In patients undergoing recanalization, initiate anticoagulation prior to the procedure. In the periprocedural and immediate postprocedural period,

low–molecular-weight heparin (LMWH) is preferred due to consistent anti-thrombotic activity and theoretical antiinflammatory properties. Anticoagulation is generally continued through the procedure.

6. Evaluate anesthetic needs. Patients with extensive disease may require more than moderate sedation; monitored anesthesia care or general anesthesia may be necessary due to the length of the procedure.

Nonthrombotic Lower Extremity Deep Venous Obstruction

1. Obtain a thorough history and physical, focusing on venous disease-specific symptoms. Specifically, assess whether superficial venous disease workup and treatment has occurred (see Chapter 44). Review if above-described conservative measures have been used and their effect along with compliance.

2. Assess for alternative explanations for symptoms. For example, lower extremity edema can be caused numerous disorders, including lymphedema, heart failure, hypoalbuminemia, and various medications including calcium channel blockers.

3. Evaluate imaging for venous compression.
   a. CTV/MRV and/or IVC/iliac duplex to assess for venous compression syndromes. Evaluate ipsilateral internal iliac vein for flow reversal, which increases confidence that compression is cause of patient's symptoms.
   b. Insufficiency examination to assess for the presence of deep venous reflux (typically, >1 second) or nonphasic flow. Presence of deep venous reflux or nonphasicity, particularly in the CFV, adds to diagnostic confidence.

4. Provide a balanced discussion of benefit, potential risks, and expected outcomes. For female pelvic venous disease patients without extremity symptoms where compression is thought to be causing pelvic symptoms, refer to Chapter 43.

Thoracic Central Venous Obstruction

1. Obtain a thorough history and physical, specifically evaluating:
   a. Cause and risk factors for occlusion.
   b. Time course and severity of symptoms, which will dictate urgency of intervention.
   c. Expected improvement from intervention, as many TCVO can be minimally symptomatic.

2. Evaluate imaging for extent of disease and causative factors.
   a. SVC syndrome: Assess extent of SVC occlusion and cause (tumor, catheter/device).
   b. TOS/Paget–Schroetter: Identify compression lesion, presence of associated acute thrombus.
   c. Other TCVO: Assess causative factors (devices/catheters, inflammation/infection).
   d. For all TCVO, assess inflow vessels to optimize patency of intervention. Patients with extensive occlusion involving axillary and subclavian veins or brachial veins are likely to have poorer patency.

3. Plan for procedure.
   a. SVC syndrome: Obtain anesthesia support given concern for airway preservation.
   b. TOS: Paget–Schroetter: Assess need for concomitant thrombectomy, obtain surgical consultation for future rib resection/scalenectomy.
   c. Catheter/device-related occlusion: Evaluate for ongoing need for devices (i.e., dialysis catheters, cardiac leads), involve necessary subspecialists to assist in decision making regarding necessity of intervention and/or device placement following recanalization.

4. For patients with asymptomatic or minimally symptomatic TCVO, consider regular surveillance for symptom progression instead of intervention.

Procedure

Postthrombotic Lower Extremity Deep Venous Obstruction

1. Select a venous access site.
   a. If the CFV is uninvolved, either CFV or great saphenous vein adjacent to the saphenofemoral junction may be used.
   b. If the CFV is involved, either popliteal, small saphenous, posterior tibial, mid-thigh femoral, or internal jugular vein access may be used per operator preference.
   c. For iliocaval or other complex occlusions, multiple accesses are necessary.
2. Perform sterile preparation and initiate sedation/anesthesia.
3. Using a linear high-frequency ultrasound transducer for guidance, administer local anesthetic to the soft tissues and obtain access with a 21-gauge micropuncture needle.
4. Under real-time fluoroscopic guidance, advance a 0.018-in wire and place a transitional dilator in the vessel. Place a 0.035-in hydrophilic wire into the vessel; once sufficient wire access has been obtained, place a 9- or 10-Fr sheath into the vessel.
5. Using a 5-Fr diagnostic catheter, perform venography with digital subtraction technique to assess the extent of the occlusion.
6. Traverse the occlusion with a stiff hydrophilic wire and catheter. Attempt to identify the occluded vein, which may be obscured by collaterals. Note, a crossing/support catheter (i.e., TriForce, Cook Medical, Bloomington, IN; QuickCross, Philips, Andover, MA; NaviCross, Terumo, Somerset, NJ) may be necessary to provide sufficient support for crossing the occlusion. The use of sharp/radiofrequency techniques is common but carries increased procedural risk and should only be performed by experienced operators and will not be discussed further here.
7. Confirm traversal into a normal venous segment by venography. Care must be taken to ensure that collateral vessels/azygos system is not mistaken for the IVC.
8. Once the occlusion has been traversed, exchange for a stiff 0.035-in working wire.
9. Perform intravascular ultrasound (IVUS) to assess the length of the occlusion (using both markers on the catheters and imaging findings), the inflow vessels (i.e., PFV) in the event of CFV compromise, and cranial/caudal stent landing zones. Note, IVUS is of limited utility in selecting stent diameter in PTS given that there frequently is not a suitable "normal" reference vessel to measure.
10. Administer systemic anticoagulation prior to predilation and stent placement; typically 70 to 100 units per kg unfractionated heparin or bivalirudin/argatroban in patients with heparin-induced thrombocytopenia. Monitor activated clotting time (ACT) through the remainder procedure at approximately 30-minute intervals, with a target of 200 to 300.
11. Sequentially predilate the occluded venous segments to the target stent diameter via balloon angioplasty; typically, 14 to 16 mm in iliac veins, 12 to 14 mm in the CFV. The diameter chosen will depend upon the stent model that is selected. In the event of an iliocaval occlusion, predilate to the target diameter of the selected stent. Consider balloon angioplasty of the inflow vessels as needed to optimize inflow.
    a. If an IVC filter was the cause for iliocaval occlusion, consider retrieval based on local filter retrieval expertise (8).
12. Select stent landing zones based on venographic and IVUS findings. Deploy on-label self-expanding venous stents in the occluded segments. Select stent lengths that will adequately cover the occluded segments without significant protrusion into normal venous anatomy. Stent placement below the inflow of the PFV (roughly at the level of the lesser trochanter) is rarely performed due to low patency rates.
    a. In the iliac veins, 14 to 16 mm diameters are typically used.
    b. In the CFV, 12 to 14 mm diameters are typically used.

c. Sizing of stents depends on whether nitinol stents (which deploy true to size) or elgiloy stents (Wallstent, which is a woven stent and has a variable diameter based on its deployed length) are chosen.

d. At press time, on-label iliofemoral stents are Vici and Wallstent (Boston Scientific, Marlborough, MA), Venovo (Becton Dickinson/Bard, Tempe, AZ), Zilver Vena (Cook Medical), and Abre (Medtronic, Minneapolis, MN). Several stents are in development.

e. There is currently no on-label IVC stent. Numerous off-label applications have been described, including stents designed for tracheobronchial applications, larger-diameter iliofemoral approved stents, and placement of iliofemoral stents in a "double-barrel" configuration.

13. Perform postdilation balloon angioplasty of each stent to its rated diameter.

14. Perform venography and IVUS to assess luminal restoration and determine if there is adequate flow. Ensure that there is adequate lesional coverage by the stents. Perform additional intervention if necessary to optimize flow.

15. Remove the sheath and achieve hemostasis with direct compression.

Variations to the Procedure for Nonthrombotic Lower Extremity Deep Venous Obstruction

1. Nonthrombotic lesions can typically always be treated from a groin (CFV, great saphenous) access.

2. Nonthrombotic lesions are not typically difficult to cross, in most cases, a 5-Fr diagnostic catheter and stiff hydrophilic wire are sufficient.

3. IVUS has a significantly different role in nonthrombotic disease as there is typically always a "normal" reference segment. Classic teaching has been to select patients with 50% area stenosis at the lesion site relative to a normal vein segment, newer data suggest that patients that improve with stent placement typically have a >61% minimum diameter stenosis relative to a normal vein segment (9). Ensure not to compare to a prestenotically dilated CIV; typically, the best segment for comparison is the external iliac vein. Similarly, use the EIV as the reference segment when selecting stent size for placement.

4. Baseline therapeutic anticoagulation is likely not necessary; these patients do not have thrombotic disease. Intraprocedural anticoagulation is likely sufficient.

5. With elgiloy stents, ensure not to place too short of a stent as there can be stent embolization.

Variations to the Procedure for TCVO

1. Typical access sites are basilic, brachial, or cephalic veins. If additional sites are needed for complex occlusions, femoral venous access can be used as necessary.

2. Many of the tools for traversal of chronic lower extremity postthrombotic occlusions apply here as well. Again, the use of sharp/radiofrequency techniques is common but carries increased procedural risk and should only be performed by experienced operators. Risks include mediastinal, lung, or cardiac injury, including tamponade. If using such techniques in close proximity to the heart, adequate surgical backup and preparation for emergent chest or pericardial drainage is mandatory.

3. For TOS/Paget–Schroetter syndrome with acute thrombus, see Chapter 36 for discussion of thrombectomy techniques. Notably, stent placement in these patients is not advised due to the high risk for stent fracture at the mechanical compression site. Stent placement in this location should be reserved for highly selected scenarios with limited options.

4. No stent is specifically approved for used in TCVO. Stent size selection is variable with minimal data to provide guidance. Typically, 12- to 14-mm stents in the innominate veins are sufficient. For focal SVC stenosis, consider using IVUS to measure the uninvolved portion of the SVC for guidance on stent selection.

5. For extensive reconstructions involving subclavian and innominate veins and SVC, ensure that the patient's symptoms are severe enough to dictate that an intervention is likely to be helpful, and that the inflow into the occluded segments appears sufficient to support stent patency.

Postprocedure Management

1. For patients with postthrombotic occlusions or extensive TCVO, including TOS/Paget–Schroetter syndrome, anticoagulation should be administered postprocedure.
   a. LMWH is preferable early in the postprocedural course, but can be transitioned to an oral agent a few weeks after.
   b. The duration of anticoagulation will depend on the nature and severity of disease, as well as the patient's prior thrombosis history. Consider comanagement with a hematologist.
   c. The use of antiplatelet agents in the setting of stents is controversial with little supporting data. Consider a short period of clopidogrel (3 months) followed by low-dose aspirin (81 mg) indefinitely.
   d. Nonthrombotic disease patients typically do not require anticoagulation or antiplatelet therapy.
2. Compression therapy for lower extremity disease should be encouraged for symptom reduction. Start at 20 to 30 mm Hg compression if compliance is a concern; for severe postthrombotic disease, consider 30 to 40 mm Hg or higher, as tolerated.
3. For patients with a component of phlebolymphedema, consider lymphedema therapy, including manual lymphatic drainage and pneumatic compression.
4. Imaging follow-up will be dictated by local preference and expertise, and can include duplex or CTV. MRV will be of limited utility for assessing stent patency.
5. Perform imaging and clinical follow-up at 1 month. Ongoing long-term follow-up should be considered for patients with extensive postthrombotic disease or complex TCVO, as reintervention may be needed to assist patency and address symptom recurrence.

Results

1. Postthrombotic recanalizations: A meta-analysis demonstrated a 1-year primary patency of 79% and 5-year projected patency of 60% (10). However, this data was with many stents being placed off-label, and before techniques for treatment of PTS were refined to the level used today. Further, several on-label venous stents are available; the data from the trials for these stents will be additive. The C-TRACT (Chronic Venous Thrombosis: Relief with Adjunctive Catheter-Directed Therapy) trial is a National Institutes of Health funded, multicenter randomized clinical trial evaluating the outcomes of stents in patients with moderate-to-severe iliac-obstructive PTS, and is expected to be the most rigorous assessment of endovascular PTS care.
2. Nonthrombotic recanalizations: Meta-analysis data suggest high primary patency rates at 1 year, approximately 96%, and projected 5-year patency rates of approximately 90% (10). These high patency rates are corroborated in numerous other trials.
3. General outcomes of TCVO recanalizations are difficult to assess, given the variety of anatomy that may be involved, the different contributing comorbidities, and the lack of systematic approaches to treatment. Limited data are available on the treatment of Paget–Schroetter syndrome, with a meta-analysis suggesting clinical improvement in approximately 90% following thrombectomy and surgical decompression (11).

Complications

1. Common procedural complications can occur, including bleeding from the access or intervention site, or infection related to an invasive procedure, including site infection or stent infection. Serious complications of this nature are rare with proper technique.
2. Stent occlusion is a complication that is not fully understood. The short-term consequences of loss patency and recurrence are known, however, the effect of a permanently implanted malfunctioning device is not known.
3. Patients with chronic venous disease often require long-term anticoagulation, which carries risk of bleeding diatheses. Ongoing assessment for the need for anticoagulation should occur in patients on long-term therapy.
4. Potentially catastrophic complications can occur with the use of sharp/RF recanalization techniques, particularly in TCVO procedures, and should only be performed by experienced operators that are prepared to manage potential complications.

References

1. Vedantham S, Goldhaber SZ, Julian JA, et al. Pharmacomechanical catheter-directed thrombolysis for deep-vein thrombosis. *New England J Med.* 2017;377(23):2240–2252.
2. Comerota AJ, Kearon C, Gu CS, et al. Endovascular thrombus removal for acute iliofemoral deep vein thrombosis. *Circulation.* 2019;139(9):1162–1173.
3. Strandness DE, Jr, Langlois Y, Cramer M, et al. Long-term sequelae of acute venous thrombosis. *JAMA.* 1983;250(10):1289–1292.
4. Shull KC, Nicolaides AN, Fernandes e Fernandes J, et al. Significance of popliteal reflux in relation to ambulatory venous pressure and ulceration. *Archives Surg.* 1979;114(11):1304–1306.
5. Neglen P, Hollis KC, Olivier J et al. Stenting of the venous outflow in chronic venous disease: long-term stent-related outcome, clinical, and hemodynamic result. *J Vasc Surg.* 2007;46(5):979–990.
6. Kibbe MR, Ujiki M, Goodwin AL, et al. Iliac vein compression in an asymptomatic patient population. *J Vasc Surg.* 2004;39(5):937–943.
7. Dolmatch BL, Gurley JC, Baskin KM, et al. Society Of Interventional Radiology Reporting Standards for Thoracic Central Vein Obstruction: Endorsed by the American Society of Diagnostic and Interventional Nephrology (ASDIN), British Society of Interventional Radiology (BSIR), Canadian Interventional Radiology Association (CIRA), Heart Rhythm Society (HRS), Indian Society of Vascular and Interventional Radiology (ISVIR), Vascular Access Society of the Americas (VASA), and Vascular Access Society of Britain and Ireland (VASBI). *J Vasc Interv Radiol.* 2018;29(4):454–460:e453.
8. Desai KR, Xiao N, Karp J, et al. Single-session inferior vena cava filter removal, recanalization, and endovenous reconstruction for chronic iliocaval thrombosis. *J Vasc Surg Venous Lymphat Disord.* 2019;7(2):176–183.
9. Gagne PJ, Gasparis A, Black S, et al. Analysis of threshold stenosis by multiplanar venogram and intravascular ultrasound examination for predicting clinical improvement after iliofemoral vein stenting in the VIDIO trial. *J Vasc Surg Venous Lymphat Disord.* 2018;6(1):48–56 e41.
10. Razavi MK, Jaff MR, Miller LE. Safety and effectiveness of stent placement for iliofemoral venous outflow obstruction: systematic review and meta-analysis. *Circ Cardiovasc Interv.* 2015;8(10):e002772.
11. Peek J, Vos CG, Unlu C, et al. Outcome of surgical treatment for thoracic outlet syndrome: systematic review and meta-analysis. *Ann Vasc Surg.* 2017;40:303–326.

38 Transvenous Biopsy

Ye Joon Kim, MD and Osman Ahmed, MD

Introduction

Histopathologic analysis of the liver and kidney remains the gold standard for the diagnosis and evaluation of acute and chronic liver disease and most renal parenchymal diseases. Percutaneous liver and kidney biopsies were initially described in 1883 and 1951, respectively, and developments in technique have improved procedural efficacy and safety (1,2). Despite these advancements, the approach of percutaneous biopsies (e.g., transection of hepatic/renal capsule) poses risks for certain patients. In patients with contraindications to percutaneous transabdominal biopsy, a transvenous approach is a well-established method to safely obtain diagnostic tissue. Recently, transvenous biopsy for perivascular masses, intravascular tumors, and tumor thrombi has emerged as a feasible method for obtaining tissue.

Indications

1. Transvenous liver biopsy (3)
   a. Diffuse liver disease
   b. Severe coagulopathy or thrombocytopenia
   c. Massive ascites
   d. Morbid obesity
   e. Need for hemodynamic assessment as part of their diagnostic workup (e.g., hepatic venography, transjugular intrahepatic portosystemic shunts)
   f. Vascular tumor/peliosis hepatis
2. Transvenous kidney biopsy (2)
   a. Severe coagulopathy
   b. Morbid obesity
   c. Failed percutaneous renal biopsy

Contraindications

Relative
1. Lack of suitable venous access (e.g., chronic central venous occlusion, Budd–Chiari syndrome)
2. Diagnosis of focal lesions
3. Uncorrectable coagulation parameters
4. Renal failure and/or history of adverse reaction to iodinated contrast material

Preprocedure Preparation

1. Indication for procedure, medical/surgical history, and pertinent imaging is reviewed. Transplantation anatomy is particularly pertinent.
2. Focused physical examination is performed.
3. Informed consent obtained detailing risks specific for the procedure with discussion regarding need for possible blood transfusion if periprocedural bleeding occurs. **Consent for possible percutaneous biopsy** when appropriate for all cases (i.e., particularly if biopsy being performed for purposes of obtaining concurrent wedged pressure measurements); anatomy may preclude safe biopsy in a minority of patients.

4. Prothrombin time (PT)/international normalized ratio (INR), partial thromboplastin time (PTT), platelet count, and serum creatinine level are obtained. Each institution should establish acceptable coagulation parameters; as a general guideline, INR <2.0 and platelets >50,000 per µL of blood are acceptable. If the clinical situation dictates biopsy, these parameters may be exceeded, for example, in patients with fulminant liver failure where correction may be impossible.
5. All patients receive peripheral intravenous (IV) access to facilitate sedation.
6. Patients are nil per os (NPO) following institutional guidelines for sedation: clear liquids 8 hours and NPO 4 hours prior to the procedure.

Procedure

1. Transvenous access
   a. Patient is positioned supine on the fluoroscopic table.
   b. Minimizing sedation initially is helpful for obtaining accurate and reproducible hepatic venous pressures. Additional sedation may be given prior to biopsy.
   c. Right internal jugular access is preferred, given direct anatomic alignment with superior vena cava/inferior vena cava (IVC).
   d. Common femoral and left internal jugular venous access are both safe and effective alternatives in situations where right internal jugular and/or hepatic vein is not accessible (e.g., occlusion, acute angle) (1)
   e. After local anesthesia with 1% lidocaine, internal jugular venous access is achieved using direct ultrasound guidance. A 5-Fr introducer catheter is replaced for a 9- or 10-Fr vascular sheath.
2. Liver biopsy
   a. Two U.S. Food and Drug Administration (FDA)-approved transjugular liver biopsy sets are available for use and include (a) TLAB-Patel Set (Argon Medical, Plano, TX)—available with an 18- or 19-gauge Flexcore biopsy needle and (b) LABS-100/200 set (Cook Medical, Bloomington, IN)—available with an 18- or 19-gauge Quick-Core biopsy needle.
   b. Using an angled 5-Fr multipurpose catheter (MPA) (Cook Medical, Bloomington, IN) and hydrophilic guidewire, cannulate the right hepatic vein (RHV). If the hepatic venous angle is acute, a cobra-2 catheter (Cook Medical, Bloomington, IN) or reverse curve catheter such as an SOS Omni selective catheter (AngioDynamics, Latham, NY) can be helpful to obtain access into the hepatic veins. The RHV is preferred because it is posterior in the liver and biopsy will be directed anteriorly. Selection of the RHV can be confirmed by rotating the fluoroscopic tube into an oblique orientation to confirm that the wire is directed posteriorly.
   c. Perform hepatic venography through the 5-Fr catheter to assess patency of selected vein (Fig. 38.1). Transvenous hepatic pressures can be obtained if indicated.
   d. Over a 0.035-in, 145-cm Amplatz wire (Cook Medical, Bloomington, IN), advance the stiff-angled guide cannula supplied in the transjugular biopsy kit distally into the RHV.
   e. Advance biopsy needle through guide cannula and before advancing the needle into the hepatic parenchyma, rotate angled guide cannula (positioned in RHV) anteriorly directed into the right hepatic lobe.
   f. Obtain samples from central portion of the liver, avoiding transcapsular punctures. Mild forward pressure on the cannula during needle exchanges will prevent retraction into the IVC. Caudal orientation of the needle specimen notch with respect to the guide cannula has been demonstrated to produce superior core biopsy specimens (4).

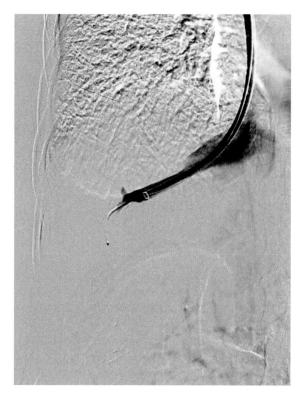

FIGURE 38.1 • Digital subtraction venography demonstrates a patent hepatic vein. The middle third of the vein is selected for the biopsy site.

    g. Deploy biopsy needle after advancing needle into parenchyma (Fig. 38.2). Remove needle from guide cannula and place specimen in formalin container; care should be taken to reduce sample fragmentation.
    h. Repeat biopsy until sample deemed adequate for diagnosis.
    i. Stiff-angled guide cannula and vascular sheath are now removed; manual pressure is applied at venotomy site until hemostasis achieved.
    j. Specimen is delivered to appropriate lab.
  3. Kidney biopsy
    a. Equipment: renal access and biopsy set (RABS-100, Cook Medical, Bloomington, IN)
    b. Using an angled 5-Fr MPA and hydrophilic guidewire, cannulate the right renal vein. Advance the catheter into the posterior lower pole branch of the right renal vein.
    c. Exchange hydrophilic wire for a 0.035-in, 145-cm Amplatz wire (Cook Medical, Bloomington, IN) and gently advance the 7-Fr sheath and inner stiffening cannula distally as possible into a peripheral cortical vein of the lower pole. Venography is performed through the sheath; when cortical staining occurs, the sheath is appropriately positioned.
    d. With gentle forward pressure on the 7-Fr sheath, advance the 19-gauge, 20-mm Quick-Core side cut biopsy needle (70 cm) into the renal parenchyma.

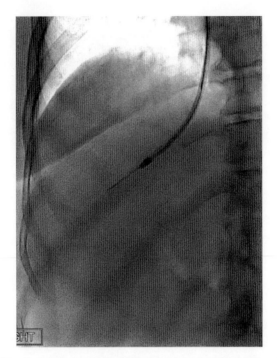

FIGURE 38.2 • Fluoroscopic image during biopsy demonstrates the transjugular cannula and needle being advanced into the hepatic parenchyma.

Deploy the needle cutting cannula. Four passes are usually adequate for histologic evaluation (2).
   e. After obtaining specimen, inject contrast medium through the 7-Fr sheath to identify any capsular perforation. If present, prophylactic embolization can be performed with Gelfoam or coils.
   f. Specimen can be evaluated by the pathology department for glomerular adequacy during procedure or delivered to appropriate lab in formalin.
4. Transvenous hepatic pressure measurement
   a. General: The hepatic venous pressure gradient (HVPG) is an indirect, minimally invasive method to measure portal perfusion pressure. It is obtained by subtracting the free hepatic venous pressure (FHVP), reflective of intraabdominal pressure, from the wedged hepatic venous pressure (WHVP), reflective of sinusoidal pressure. In cirrhosis caused by alcoholic liver disease, hepatitis B, and hepatitis C, however, intersinusoidal communications are lost due to fibrosis and WHVP accurately reflects portal pressure (5). This makes HVPG reflective of portal perfusion pressure. HVPG is normally ≤5 mm Hg. HVPG ≥10 mm Hg is considered clinically significant portal hypertension because it is predictive of the presence and development of varices, clinical decompensation in patients without varices, development of hepatocellular carcinoma (HCC), and decompensation at surgery for HCC (5). Strict technique is required in order to obtain accurate and reproducible results. Sweep speed of pressures should be set at 5 mm per second or slower so that changes in pressures over time are visually perceptible. A mean pressure line should also be recorded to help in interpretation (Fig. 38.3).

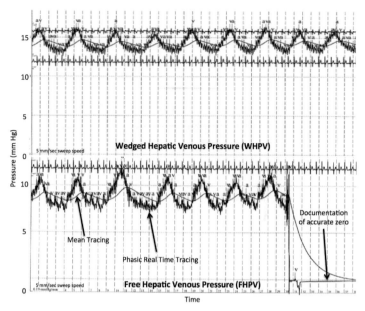

FIGURE 38.3 • This tracing represents excellent, stable wedged **(top)**, and free **(bottom)** hepatic venous pressures. Note how the oscillations in the tracing, which are due to respiration, are very regular due to very little anxiolysis with minimal Versed only. The mean tracing helps to visualize an average and the compressed waveform (5 mm per second sweep speed) is easy to read. For clinical studies, documentation of an accurate zero is also recorded.

b. Sedation: Moderate sedation with fentanyl and Versed induces substantial changes in respiration, which in turn makes measurement of HVPG unreliable and poorly reproducible. Over sedation is the most common error resulting in poorly obtained pressures. Ideally, only mild anxiolysis is provided with minimal Versed (0.02 mg per kg).

c. A pressure transducer is attached to the angiographic table with a zero level set at the midaxillary line.

d. FHVPs are typically obtained with the catheter 2 to 4 cm into the hepatic vein and near the confluence with the IVC. Fifteen to 20 seconds should be allowed for the pressure to equilibrate.

e. WHVP is measured by arresting hepatic venous outflow to create a static column of blood between the catheter and the hepatic sinusoids. This can be performed with a 5-Fr end-hole diagnostic catheter advanced and subsequently wedged into a small hepatic vein, or by the use of a balloon catheter. Although the use of a balloon catheter is recommended to improve the reliability and reproducibility of measurements the difference in WHVP measurements between the two systems is small (5). Use of a balloon catheter effectively samples a larger area of liver because there are often regional differences in fibrosis. This may be performed with a Fogarty balloon. WHVP may take 1 to 2 minutes to equilibrate. After the measurement has been recorded, a gentle wedged venogram is performed to ensure that the balloon has been occlusive (Fig. 38.4). Wedged venography should not be performed prior to measurement because the different viscosity of contrast as compared to blood may affect pressure measurements. Hepatic vein to

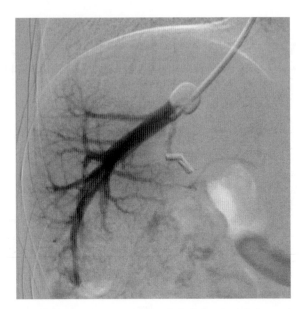

FIGURE 38.4 • Wedged hepatic venography. An occlusion balloon is relatively central, and gentle venography is performed until distal branches are visualized. Notice how large of an area is sampled by using the balloon; this improves reproducibility and reliability. These images document appropriate wedging of the balloon, ensuring that the wedged pressure was accurate.

    hepatic vein collaterals should be identified because these will falsely lower the HVPG.

f. Two sets of FHVP and WHVP should be obtained. Each subsequent measurement should be within 1 mm Hg of the previous or they should be repeated.

g. Select the infrahepatic IVC and obtain an IVC pressure. This pressure should be within 2 mm Hg of the free hepatic pressure. If it is not, this may be reflective of inaccurate measurement or hepatic venous outflow stenosis.

h. Right atrial pressure and infrahepatic IVC pressure are normally similar. Ascites can elevate intraabdominal pressure compared to right atrial pressure. For this reason, the infrahepatic IVC pressure rather than the right atrial pressure is used to reference the FHVP.

i. Documentation of right atrial pressure is important in the evaluation of patients following liver transplantation and patients being evaluated for Budd–Chiari syndrome to exclude hemodynamic IVC stenosis.

j. Proceed with additional conscious sedation and biopsy if indicated.

Transvenous Biopsy of Perivascular/Retroperitoneal Tumors (6)

1. Transvenous approach for biopsy of intravascular or perivascular masses requires an individualized approach given the variability in size and location of masses. In addition, operator experience using intravascular ultrasound, intracardiac echocardiography, and/or cone-beam CT is required.

2. Transvenous biopsies may be effective in procuring samples of tumor thrombi and perivascular tumors that may otherwise be difficult or risky to attain through a percutaneous approach.

3. Cone-beam CT guidance can also be used in conjunction with fluoroscopy to further increase the efficacy of sampling of masses present in the retroperitoneal space (e.g., pericaval tumors, peri-/pancreatic tumors).
4. Venous access from a jugular or femoral approach is obtained. Required equipment include a transjugular biopsy kit with intravascular imaging (echo or ultrasound) and/or cone-beam CT. Two access points are typically used to facilitate placement of biopsy equipment and imaging catheters, respectively.
5. Using either live intravascular imaging guidance or cone-beam CT, the cannula of the biopsy set is directed toward the target lesion and samples are acquired.

Postprocedure Management

1. General care of the patient
   a. These procedures are typically well tolerated, and patients can resume normal activity in 24 hours.
   b. Clear liquid diet for first hour; regular diet thereafter if tolerated.
   c. Monitor vital signs every 15 minutes for 1 hour, then every 30 minutes for 2 hours, and then every hour postprocedure until discharged.
   d. If vital signs are stable and pain is controlled, the patient may be discharged after bed rest period (2 hours for transvenous liver biopsies and 4 hours after transvenous kidney biopsies).
   e. Patients receive written instructions regarding follow-up for potential late complications.

Results

1. Transvenous liver biopsy
   a. Reported technical success is 97% with the most common cause of failure due to the inability to catheterize a suitable hepatic vein, more often seen in patients with liver transplants (1). Lack of transvenous access is another reason for technical failure; however, the use of the left internal jugular, external jugular, subclavian, or femoral veins may be utilized to complete the examination (1).
   b. Left or middle hepatic venous access is necessary in patients with left lobe-only transplants. Although this approach differs from the traditional approach of sampling via the RHV seen in patients with orthotopic whole liver transplants (OWLTs) and right lobe-only transplants, technical success and adequacy of sampling is comparable (7).
   c. Four complete portal tracts (CPTs) are usually considered the minimum for defining a liver transplant biopsy to rule out rejection, and six complete portal tracts are considered minimum for assessing the histologic diagnosis of diffuse liver disease (i.e., recurrence of viral liver disease). Frequently, one or two needle passes are adequate for histopathologic diagnosis; however, liver specimens of 20 mm in length containing 11 complete portal tracts are needed for grading and staging chronic hepatitis (8).
   d. Sample fragmentation is most often seen with liver cirrhosis and has been reported in 14% to 25% of transvenous liver biopsy samples. Fragmentation may interfere with diagnostic quality of the specimen (1).
   e. Adequate tissue is obtained in up to 96% of the time by reported experiences (9). A larger gauge needle (18 gauge) may provide better samples for staging liver fibrosis. Four cores are routinely submitted.
2. Transvenous kidney biopsy
   a. Technical success is 92% to 96% with most failures resulting from inability cannulating the renal veins (1,2).
   b. Tissue adequacy is 98% and comparable to percutaneous renal biopsy (1).

3. Hepatic venous pressure measurements
   a. Technical success is >95% and is only limited by lack of ability to catheterize the hepatic veins (1).
4. Transvenous biopsy of perivascular/retroperitoneal tumors
   a. Technical success in small retrospective case series ranges from 88% to 100% (6).
   b. Similarly, tissue adequacy ranged from 86% to 100%.

Complications

1. Transvenous liver biopsy (3,10): Overall complications (7.1%) are either related to liver puncture (3.5%) or other mechanism (3.3%). Most are minor complications and include fever, neck hematoma, abdominal pain, or minor bleeding around the liver capsule. Major complications including pneumothorax, intraperitoneal hemorrhage, and arrhythmias are seen in 0.6% of patients. Hemorrhagic complications are more common in patients with previous bone marrow transplants (2.9% vs. 0.6%). Mortality is rare (0.1%) resulting from intraperitoneal hemorrhage or ventricular arrhythmia.
2. Transvenous kidney biopsy (2): Major complications (1%) requiring blood transfusion or intervention are rare. Transient microscopic hematuria is more common.
3. Hepatic venous pressure measurement: Access site hemorrhage, vagal reactions, and arrhythmias may be encountered in a similar frequency to transjugular biopsy. Most other more serious complications are related to concurrent transvenous liver biopsy.
4. Perilesional hemorrhage from accidental puncture of renal arteries has been reported for transvenous biopsy of perivascular and peripancreatic masses (6). No major complications however resulted.

Management of Complications

1. Complications are mostly minor and can usually be treated with supportive measures including IV fluids and oral medications.
2. Patients with hemodynamic instability or clinical and/or laboratory features of intraabdominal bleeding should be immediately resuscitated with large-bore IV access, IV fluids, and/or transfusion. Immediate evaluation with either catheter angiography or CT angiography should be pursued.
3. If pain is out of proportion to the examination, parenchymal/subcapsular hemorrhage or bile peritonitis should be suspected. Intermittent, severe pain suggesting biliary colic may be seen with hemobilia. Cross-sectional imaging with computed tomography (CT) (+/− intravascular iodinated contrast) is a fast and reliable way to assess for clinically significant bleeding or other complication. If postprocedure pain is severe and unable to be controlled adequately, overnight admission to the hospital maybe necessary.
4. Capsular perforation of the liver can be effectively managed by transcatheter embolization. In situations of diffuse bleeding, nonselective embolization with Gelfoam can allow rapid control of hemorrhage.

References

1. Behrens G, Ferral H. Transjugular liver biopsy. *Semin Intervent Radiol*. 2012;29(2): 111–117.
2. Cluzel P, Martinez F, Bellin MF, et al. Transjugular versus percutaneous renal biopsy for the diagnosis of parenchymal disease: comparison of sampling effectiveness and complications. *Radiology*. 2000;215(3):689–693.
3. Kalambokis G, Manousou P, Vibhakorn S, et al. Transjugular liver biopsy—indications, adequacy, quality of specimens, and complications—a systematic review. *J Hepatol*. 2007; 47(2):284–294.

4. Smith TP, Kim CY, Smith AD, et al. Hepatic venous pressure measurements: comparison of end-hole and balloon catheter methods. *J Vasc Interv Radiol.* 2012;23(2):219–26.e6. doi:10.1016/j.jvir.2011.09.025

5. Berzigotti A, Seijo S, Reverter E, et al. Assessing portal hypertension in liver diseases. *Exper Rev Gastroenterol Hepatol.* 2013;7(2):141–155.

6. Sherk WM, Khaja MS, Majdalany BS, et al. Transvenous biopsy in the diagnosis of intravascular or perivascular neoplasm: a single-center retrospective analysis of 36 patients. *J Vasc Interv Radiol.* 2019;30(1):54–60. doi:10.1016/j.jvir.2018.08.002

7. Lee KA, Taylor A, Bartolome B, et al. Safety and efficacy of transjugular liver biopsy in patients with left lobe-only liver transplants. *J Vasc Interv Radiol.* 2019;30(7): 1043–1047.

8. Miraglia R, Maruzzelli L, Minervini M, et al. Transjugular liver biopsy in liver transplant patients using an 18-gauge automated core biopsy needle. *Eur J Radiol.* 2011;80(3): e269–e272.

9. Behrens G, Ferral H, Giusto D, et al. Transjugular liver biopsy: comparison of sample adequacy with the use of two automated needle systems. *J Vasc Interv Radiol.* 2011;22(3): 341–345.

10. Ahmed O, Ward TJ, Lungren MP, et al. Assessing the risk of hemorrhagic complication following transjugular liver biopsy in bone marrow transplantation recipients. *J Vasc Interv Radiol.* 2016;27(4):551–557.

39 Preoperative Hepatic Augmentation

Joshua Cornman-Homonoff, MD and David C. Madoff, MD

Introduction

Surgical hepatectomy is widely utilized in the management of primary and metastatic disease of the liver but can be accompanied by hepatic insufficiency when a large amount of liver is removed. In such cases, the volume of the future liver remnant (FLR) can limit the extent of resection as it has been shown to be an independent predictor of postoperative complications (1). Portal vein embolization (PVE) and its variants are thus essential tools for those patients with suboptimal FLR volumes. Preoperative embolization of the portal vein branches supplying the liver to be removed redirects blood flow to the nonoccluded liver, thereby inducing FLR hypertrophy and enabling more extensive resection. Although PVE remains the standard of care, several newer techniques have been described which may further augment the degree of hypertrophy (DH), chief among them combination portal and hepatic vein embolization (HVE), termed liver venous deprivation (LVD). As hepatobiliary surgical techniques continue to evolve and indications for curative hepatectomy expand, PVE and its variants will remain essential adjuncts to major hepatectomy given their high safety and proven efficacy.

Indications

Patients planned for hepatic resection with standardized future liver remnant (sFLR; see definition below) volumes less than the following:

1. 20% in those with normal underlying liver parenchyma.
2. 30% in those with liver injured by extensive chemotherapy.
3. 40% in those with advanced liver disease including cirrhosis/advanced fibrosis.

Contraindications

Absolute
1. Clinically significant portal hypertension (hepatic venous pressure gradient >12 mm Hg).
2. Tumor invasion of the portal vein precluding safe catheter manipulation and/ or optimal delivery of embolic material.
3. Complete lobar portal vein occlusion, as blood flow diversion has already occurred.

Relative
1. Extrahepatic metastatic disease, including portal lymphadenopathy.
2. Diffuse bilobar hepatic disease.
3. Tumor precluding safe access to the portal venous system.
4. Biliary dilatation within the FLR. When present, biliary decompression should be performed first.
5. Mild portal hypertension.
6. Uncorrectable coagulopathy.
7. Renal insufficiency.

Preprocedure Preparation

1. Confirm absence of clinically significant portal hypertension, which would preclude performance of the procedure.
2. Review available imaging with specific attention paid to tumor burden and location, portal vein patency, anatomic variants, biliary dilatation, and presence of ascites, the last of which may require concurrent paracentesis.
3. Estimate the size of the FLR.
   a. The FLR is directly measured on either MRI or CT. Volumes are assessed by contouring the hepatic segment of interest on each slice, multiplying by the slice thickness, and then summing individual slice volumes, as per the following formula: FLR = $\sum$ (contour area × slice thickness). Of note, some PACS systems now incorporate methods to simplify this process by interpolating contours on slices between those which are user-defined and then automatically calculating the volume of the defined portion of liver.
   b. Because liver volume correlates with body size, accuracy of FLR measurement can be increased by normalizing for patient size. This resulted in the development of the standardized FLR (sFLR), which is calculated as the ratio of the FLR to total estimated functioning liver volume (TELV): sFLR = FLR / TELV. TELV in turn is calculated as follows: TELV = −794.41 + 1267.28 × BSA, where BSA is the body surface area.
4. Determine anesthetic needs. Although PVE can generally be performed under moderate sedation using a combination of fentanyl and midazolam, general anesthesia is recommended for patients with multiple comorbidities or for those who cannot cooperate.

Procedure

1. Although embolization of either lobe is technically feasible, performance of left PVE is uncommon because the larger right hepatic lobe is generally of sufficient size to obviate the occurrence of postsurgical hepatic insufficiency. Even in patients who require an extended left hepatectomy, which involves resection of all but segments 6 and 7, the FLR is typically in the range of 33%. For these reasons, the ensuing discussion focuses on the approach to right PVE.
2. Antibiotic prophylaxis is generally not required. The exception is patients with biliary obstruction, who should receive ceftriaxone 1 g IV immediately before the procedure regardless of prior biliary drainage.

3. In patients undergoing a simple right hepatectomy, embolization of segments 5 to 8 is sufficient. In those undergoing an extended right hepatectomy, which includes removal of segment 4, the segment 4 veins should be included in the embolization. The rationale for this is that segment 2 and 3 hypertrophy is greater when segment 4 is embolized than when it is not, and that isolated right PVE may produce hypertrophy of segment 4 in addition to segments 2 and 3 which increases the length of the transection plane and thus potentially complicates the surgery.

4. PVE can be performed from either an ipsilateral or a contralateral transhepatic approach. The ipsilateral approach avoids puncturing and thus potentially damaging the FLR and provides easier access to segment 4, but may otherwise be more technically challenging. It usually requires the use of reverse curve catheters, and the retrograde embolization increases the likelihood of inadvertent disruption of embolic material which both reduces efficacy and risks nontarget embolization. The contralateral approach is technically simpler but in rare cases may cause damage to the FLR, precluding curative resection. Furthermore, catheterization of segment 4 portal veins can be challenging, which may result in prolonged catheter dwell times and formation of thrombus within the left portal system. Notably, there is currently no evidence to suggest the superiority of either approach, and as such the choice is usually one of operator preference. Use of a trans-splenic approach is described elsewhere.

→ *Ipsilateral Approach*

For transhepatic right portal vein puncture, see Figure 39.1.

1. The accessed portal vein branch should be both peripheral and oriented to facilitate selection of the other veins to be treated. A segment 5/6 branch is generally well suited for this purpose. After confirming patency using Doppler imaging, a 22-gauge Chiba needle (Cook Medical, Bloomington, Indiana) is advanced into the target right portal branch under real-time guidance. The stylet is then removed and a 0.18-in guidewire is inserted through the needle centrally.

2. The needle is exchanged for a coaxial dilator system, either a Jeffrey set (Cook Medical) or an AccuStick system (Boston Scientific, Marlborough, Massachusetts), through which a stiff 0.035-in guidewire is introduced.

3. The outer portion of the dilator system is then exchanged over the wire for a 5-Fr vascular sheath, which is positioned with tip in the central aspect of the accessed vein.

4. A 5-Fr flush catheter is then introduced and positioned with tip in the main portal vein, after which digital subtraction portography is performed in multiple obliquities for anatomic delineation. Selective portograms are then obtained as needed.

5. The flush catheter is exchanged for 5-Fr end-hole catheter, which is used to select the first vein to be embolized. When segment 4 embolization is planned, it should be performed first so as to minimize catheter manipulation and potential embolic material dislodgement. Selection of segment 5 to 8 veins often necessitates use of a reverse curve catheter given their acute angulation relative to the sheath.

6. A microcatheter is introduced through the 5-Fr catheter and embolization performed. The authors prefer spherical particles, such as tris-acryl microspheres (Embosphere Microspheres, Merit Medical, South Jordan, Utah), with smaller sizes (100 to 500 μm) administered first followed by larger ones (500 to 900 μm). Once stasis is achieved, fibered microcoils or plugs are deposited centrally. The central 2 cm of right portal vein should be spared to facilitate subsequent surgical ligation.

7. Many other embolic materials have been used for PVE. Although a comprehensive discussion is beyond the scope of this text, the following points are worth noting:

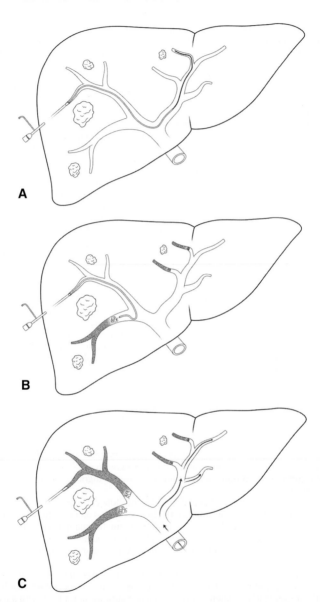

FIGURE 39.1 • Diagrams illustrate the technique of transhepatic ipsilateral right PVE extended to segment 4 using particulate embolic agent and coils. **A:** A vascular sheath is introduced into a right portal vein branch, after which a catheter is used to select segment 4. A microcatheter is then placed through the base catheter and embolization is performed. **B:** After embolization of segment 4, a reverse-curve catheter is used to sequentially select and embolized all right portal vein branches. **C:** After completion of embolization, blood flow is redistributed into the nonembolized liver (FLR), stimulating hypertrophy.

a. Spherical particles produce greater hypertrophy than do nonspherical particles.

b. The addition of coils to particles improves hypertrophy over particles alone.

c. In a small retrospective study, *n*-butyl cyanoacrylate (NBCA) mixed with iodized oil produced greater hypertrophy than the combination of spherical particles and coils (2).

The decision to use a particular agent ultimately depends on the operator's preference and his or her familiarity with the agent in question.

8. Once stasis has been achieved within a given portal vein branch, the catheter should be repositioned into another until all branches supplying segments 5–8 ± 4 have been treated. It is important to be familiar with variant portal vein branching as the "typical" anatomy is found in only 65% of cases. If the anatomy is atypical or unclear, 3D rotational cone-beam CT can be performed.

9. Embolization of the accessed branch should be performed last, followed by completion portography. The catheter and sheath can then be removed and the access tract embolized in standard fashion. Of note, extreme care should be taken as the catheter is retracted through the embolized access vessel as dislodgement of embolic material can occur.

→ *Contralateral Approach*

For transhepatic left portal vein puncture, see Figure 39.2.

1. This approach uses the same access system and technique as described above. A peripheral portal vein branch in the left, rather than right, hepatic lobe is targeted (the FLR). A vessel within segment 3 is generally preferred given its ready accessibility via a subxiphoid approach. Of note, extreme care must be taken during the puncture because injury to the FLR may preclude subsequent resection.

2. The access is upsized, a sheath placed, and portograms performed as described above. In contrast to the ipsilateral approach, use of a reverse curve catheter is generally not necessary for appropriate vessel selection. Rather, a short selective catheter is preferred because it provides less "dead space." Catheterization

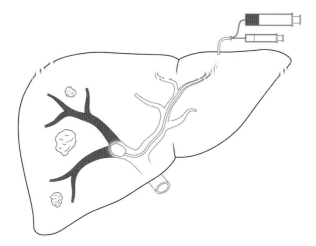

FIGURE 39.2 • Diagram illustrates the technique of transhepatic contralateral right PVE. A vascular sheath is introduced into a left portal vein branch and a balloon-occlusion catheter is positioned in the right portal vein. The balloon is inflated so as to prevent reflux and liquid embolic agent is delivered into the right portal vein.

of segment 4 portal veins may be challenging because of the proximity of the branches to the puncture site. In contrast to the ipsilateral approach, they are generally embolized last.

3. Choice and delivery of embolic agents follow the same principles used for the ipsilateral approach. Because the embolization is performed with the catheter positioned in the direction of portal venous flow, it is often technically easier. This may be particularly advantageous when liquid embolic agents are employed. If there is concern that embolic material may reflux into the left or main portal veins, a balloon occlusion catheter can be used.

Variations

Although PVE is generally effective for producing adequate FLR hypertrophy, patients with underlying liver disease may experience a less robust response which is ultimately insufficient to allow for safe hepatic resection. Attempts to further augment liver hypertrophy have focused on the observation that the DH correlates with the extent of ischemia, leading to treatment strategies in which PVE is combined with embolization of either the hepatic arteries or veins.

→ *Combination transarterial embolization (TAE) and PVE*

1. This involves sequential embolization of the hepatic arteries and portal veins supplying the liver parenchyma which will be removed.

2. The greater degree of ischemia results from (1) occlusion of arterial inflow, (2) attenuation of the hepatic arterial buffer response which occurs following PVE, and (3) obliteration of arterioportal shunts which are common in cirrhotic and tumor-bearing liver. An auxiliary benefit is the antitumor effect which accompanies TAE and may help to limit the degree of tumor growth between embolization and resection.

3. The major limitation to this approach is the potential for ischemic necrosis of hepatic parenchyma. Because of this concern, the procedures should be temporally separated by a minimum of three weeks, TAE should not be carried out to complete stasis, and use of particulate embolic agents should be avoided or limited. Although cases of hepatic abscess formation and sepsis have been reported, the risk appears highest in patients who underwent prior biliary intervention.

4. The procedures can be performed in either order, with most studies performing TAE prior to PVE. The benefit to performing PVE first is that the second procedure can potentially be avoided in patients who experience adequate hypertrophy following PVE alone.

→ *LVD*

1. This involves concurrent embolization of the portal and hepatic veins supplying the liver parenchyma which will be removed.

2. Because hepatic venous outflow is obstructed, the parenchyma becomes congested and inflow from both the hepatic artery and portal vein is reduced. When combined with PVE, this technique produces a degree of ischemia which is greater than that induced by PVE alone but less than that which results from combination of TAE and PVE. In theory this results in augmented hypertrophy without the risk of ischemic necrosis, and additionally allows performance of both procedures in the same session.

3. The PVE portion of the procedure is performed as described above. HVE can be performed via either a transjugular or a transhepatic approach.

   a. In the transjugular approach, access is obtained in the right internal jugular vein, the right hepatic vein is selected, and embolization is performed using vascular plugs and/or coils.

   b. In the transhepatic approach, direct transhepatic access is obtained into the right hepatic vein in a manner analogous to that for the portal vein and a vascular plug is deployed centrally in the vein. With this protection in place, further embolic material can then be administered such as NBCA glue.

4. Standard LVD involves embolizing the right hepatic vein alone. By contrast, extended liver venous deprivation (eLVD) refers to embolization of both the right and middle hepatic veins. In theory, the latter technique produces more complete obstruction to right hepatic venous outflow, which results in greater FLR hypertrophy.

Postprocedure Management

1. Because PVE predominantly induces apoptosis rather than necrosis, patients do not experience a postembolization syndrome and thus typically have limited postprocedure pain, nausea, or fever. Abdominal pain is reported in 20% to 30% but is easily managed via oral analgesia (3). In most cases patients are discharged the same or next day, and prescriptions for analgesics, antiemetics, and/or antibiotics are generally unnecessary.

2. Cross-sectional imaging, ideally of the same modality as that which was used for initial assessment, is performed 3 to 4 weeks following treatment to evaluate the extent of hypertrophy.

3. Patients with underlying hepatic dysfunction or certain systemic diseases such as diabetes mellitus may experience delayed hypertrophy. Consequently, if on initial postprocedure imaging the sLFR remains inadequate, repeating imaging in 3 to 4 weeks may be useful as further hypertrophy may occur.

4. Of note, prior PVE does not preclude chemotherapy administration, as one study demonstrated a clear survival benefit in those who underwent PVE and then received chemotherapy compared to those who did not (4).

Results

1. Reported rates of technical success are consistently greater than 95%. Published systematic reviews and metanalyses describe mean post-PVE FLR hypertrophy rates of 37.9% to 49.4% with subsequent successful hepatectomy rates of 75.9% to 96.1% (5,6).

   a. Guidelines from both the Society for Interventional Radiology (SIR) and Cardiovascular and Interventional Radiology Society of Europe (CIRSE) suggest thresholds of 95% to 100% for technical success and 85% for postembolization resection rate, although the CIRSE guidelines allow a lower threshold of 70% in patients with cirrhosis (3,7).

2. In addition to sFLR, the DH and kinetic growth rate (KGR) are predictive of postoperative outcomes (8).

   a. $DH = sFLR_{Post\ PVE} - sFLR_{Pre\ PVE}$
   b. $KGR = DH\ /\ (time\ since\ PVE\ in\ weeks)$
      Patients with DH <7.5% or KGR <2.0% per week have been reported to have higher postoperative complication rates with KGR the most strongly predictive of the three measures (8).

3. Preliminary data suggest combination TAE and PVE produces greater FLR hypertrophy than does PVE alone, and that this translates into improved postoperative outcomes (9). Importantly, pathologic analysis has shown preferential tumor necrosis with relative preservation of embolized hepatic parenchyma (10), suggesting that this may act as sufficient treatment should inadequate hypertrophy preclude surgery.

4. LVD and eLVD both appear to produce more significant FLR hypertrophy than does PVE, and the response to eLVD in turn is more robust than it is to LVD. In fact, the hypertrophy seen in eLVD is comparable to the dramatic proliferation which occurs following performance of surgical ALPPS but, unlike in that procedure, is accompanied by a proportionate increase in function.

Complications

1. The reported complication rate is 2.2% to 3.9% with an associated mortality rate of 0.1% or less (5,6). Specific complications include thrombosis of the main or left portal veins, nontarget embolization, transient liver failure, hepatic abscesses, cholangitis, subcapsular hematoma, hemoperitoneum, hemobilia, arterioportal fistulae, and pneumothorax. In cases where portal vein thrombosis involves the left or main branches, chemical and/or mechanical thrombolysis may be attempted.

2. A potentially unavoidable consequence of PVE is tumor progression in the time between PVE and resection. It is thought that tumor growth does not simply continue as before but rather is stimulated by PVE-induced trophic factor release. Combination TAE and PVE may help to mitigate this effect through direct treatment of the tumor, whereas the rapid hypertrophy induced by eLVD may allow for shortening of the interval to surgery and thereby limit time for tumor progression. Further study will be needed to see if these hypotheses are borne out.

References

1. Ribero D, Abdalla EK, Madoff DC, et al. Portal vein embolization before major hepatectomy and its effects on regeneration, resectability and outcome. *Br J Surg.* 2007;94(11):1386–1394.
2. Guiu B, Bize P, Gunthern D, et al. Portal vein embolization before right hepatectomy: improved results using n-butyl-cyanoacrylate compared to microparticles plus coils. *Cardiovasc Intervent Radiol.* 2013;36(5):1306–1312.
3. Denys A, Bize P, Demartines N, et al. Quality improvement for portal vein embolization. *Cardiovasc Intervent Radiol.* 2010;33(3):452–456.
4. Fischer C, Melstrom LG, Arnaoutakis D, et al. Chemotherapy after portal vein embolization to protect against tumor growth during liver hypertrophy before hepatectomy. *JAMA Surg.* 2013;148(12):1103–1108.
5. van Lienden KP, van den Esschert JW, de Graaf W, et al. Portal vein embolization before liver resection: a systematic review. *Cardiovasc Intervent Radiol.* 2013;36(1):25–34.
6. Wajswol E, Jazmati T, Contractor S, et al. Portal vein embolization utilizing n-butyl cyanoacrylate for contralateral lobe hypertrophy prior to liver resection: a systematic review and meta-analysis. *Cardiovasc Intervent Radiol.* 2018;41(9):1302–1312.
7. Angle JF, Siddiqi NH, Wallace MJ, et al. Quality improvement guidelines for percutaneous transcatheter embolization: Society of Interventional Radiology Standards of Practice Committee. *J Vasc Interv Radiol.* 2010;21(10):1479–1486.
8. Shindoh J, Truty MJ, Aloia TA, et al. Kinetic growth rate after portal vein embolization predicts posthepatectomy outcomes: toward zero liver-related mortality in patients with colorectal liver metastases and small future liver remnant. *J Am Coll Surg.* 2013;216(2):201–209.
9. Ogata S, Belghiti J, Farges O, et al. Sequential arterial and portal vein embolizations before right hepatectomy in patients with cirrhosis and hepatocellular carcinoma. *Br J Surg.* 2006;93(9):1091–1098.
10. Aoki T, Imamura H, Hasegawa K, et al. Sequential preoperative arterial and portal venous embolizations in patients with hepatocellular carcinoma. *Arch Surg.* 2004;139(7):766–774.

40 Transjugular Intrahepatic Portosystemic Shunts

Ziv J. Haskal, MD, FSIR, FAHA, FACR, FCIRSE and John T. Matson, MD

Introduction

A transjugular intrahepatic portosystemic shunt (TIPS) is a percutaneously created bypass that reduces portal vein pressure for treatment of complications of portal hypertension. Most typically, the decompressive channel is created between a hepatic vein and an intrahepatic branch of the portal vein. A similar procedure known as a direct intrahepatic portocaval shunt (DIPS) involves the creation of a shunt from the portal vein to the inferior vena cava (IVC). Creating a TIPS involves several key steps:

1. Catheterization of the hepatic veins and hepatic venography.
2. Passage of a long, curved transjugular needle from the chosen hepatic vein through the liver parenchyma into an intrahepatic branch of the portal vein.
3. Direct measurement of the systemic and portal vein pressures through the transjugular access.
4. Balloon dilatation of the tract between the hepatic and portal veins.
5. Deployment of an expanded polytetrafluorethylene-lined stent-graft or metallic stent spanning the parenchymal tract and outflow hepatic vein to maintain it against the recoil of the surrounding liver parenchyma and tissue ingrowth.
6. Angiographic and hemodynamic assessment of resultant portal and right atrial pressure changes.
7. Serial dilatation of the stent until satisfactory pressure levels has been reached.
8. Variceal embolization, when indicated (typically for bleeding indications).

Indications (1–5)

1. Efficacy determined by controlled trials:
   a. Secondary prevention of variceal bleeding
   b. Refractory cirrhotic ascites
2. Efficacy assessed in uncontrolled series:
   a. Hemorrhagic acutely bleeding varices
   b. Portal hypertensive gastropathy
   c. Bleeding gastric varices
   d. Refractory hepatic hydrothorax
   e. Hepatorenal syndrome (type 1 or 2)
   f. Budd–Chiari syndrome
   g. Restoration of portal vein patency prior to transplantation or during catheter-directed therapy of splenomesenteric thromboses
3. Unclear, variable efficacy described in small series or case reports
   a. Veno-occlusive disease (VOD)
   b. Hepatopulmonary syndrome
   c. Prophylactic preoperative decompression

Contraindications

Absolute
1. Severe or rapidly progressive liver failure
2. Severe or uncontrolled encephalopathy

3. Heart failure
4. Severe pulmonary hypertension

These contraindications hold for surgical and percutaneous portosystemic diversion procedures. Patients with very advanced stages of liver disease will not tolerate deprivation of nutrient portal flow that occurs after total or partially decompressive shunts. In these cases, shunts may accelerate liver failure and should be considered only as last measures, ideally as bridges to imminent transplantation.

Relative

1. Contraindications to angiographic procedures
   a. Recent myocardial infarction, serious arrhythmia, or substantial electrolyte imbalance
   b. Past serious documented contrast reaction—prophylaxis is required, or TIPS creation using carbon dioxide
   c. Uncorrectable coagulopathies
   d. Inability to lie flat on angiographic table due to congestive heart failure or compromised respiratory status—intubation may be required
   e. Pregnancy because of risk of exposure of fetus to ionizing radiation
2. Conditions that may increase the technical difficulty of creating a TIPS:
   a. Biliary obstruction
   b. Hepatic or pancreatic malignancy
   c. Polycystic liver disease
   d. Inferior vena caval or hepatic vein thrombosis
   e. Portal system thromboses (portal, splenic, or mesenteric). In cases of caval, hepatic vein, or portal system thromboses, modified procedures using transcaval, transhepatic, or trans-splenic approaches have been described. Targeting can be further aided by use of intravascular ultrasound (IVUS) for creation of TIPS in routine approaches, DIPS, or complex anatomy.

Preprocedure Preparation

1. Obtain informed consent. Table 40.1 lists procedural complications that should be discussed with the patient (6).
2. Preprocedural sonography, computed tomography (CT), or magnetic resonance (MR) imaging to assess portal vein patency and hepatic parenchyma because the incidence of hepatocellular carcinoma is increased in patients with cirrhosis.
3. Provide standard hemodynamic monitoring, including electrocardiogram (ECG), oxygen saturation, blood pressure, and possibly capnography, as appropriate for administration of sedation per hospital protocols.
4. In acutely bleeding patients, ensure that satisfactory resuscitation efforts are being undertaken prior to starting. These may include blood or plasma transfusions, vasopressor support, and placement of balloon tamponade catheters. In general, platelet counts are corrected to >50,000 per μL and international normalized ratio to $\leq$1.5 (though INR correction is optional in patients with advanced liver disease).
5. Intravenous antibiotic prophylaxis should be provided. Many medications may provide satisfactory coverage of skin and enteric flora (related to hepatic and biliary organisms), including cefoxitin or piperacillin/tazobactam or moxifloxacin in penicillin-allergic patients.
6. TIPS can be created under conscious sedation with intravenous fentanyl and midazolam, monitored anesthesia care, or general anesthesia.
7. Assemble required components:
   a. TIPS set. Several kits exist, including the Haskal (now retired), Rösch–Uchida, Ring sets (Cook Medical, Bloomington, IN), W.L. Gore needle set

Table 40.1 **Procedural Complications of Transjugular Intrahepatic Portosystemic Shunts (6)**	
	Reported Rate (%)
Major complications	3.00
Hemoperitoneum	0.50
Stent malposition	1.00
Hemobilia	2.00
Radiation skin burn	0.10
Hepatic infarction	0.50
Renal failure requiring dialysis	0.25
Death	1.00
Minor complications	4.00
Transient contrast-induced renal failure	2.00
Hepatic artery puncture causing clinically apparent injury	1.00
Fever	2.00
Entry site hematoma	2.00
Encephalopathy controlled by medical therapy	15.00–25.00

Dariushnia SR, Haskal ZJ, Midia M, et al. Quality improvement guidelines for transjugular intrahepatic portosystemic shunts. *J Vasc Interv Radiol.* 2016;27(1).

(W.L. Gore & Associates, Flagstaff, AZ), Scorpion (Argon Medical Devices, Plano TX), and Liverty set (Becton Dickinson, Franklin Lakes NJ). The factor most governing kit choice is operator preference. A TIPS set is suitable for VIATORR endoprosthesis delivery (W. L. Gore & Associates, Flagstaff, AZ), by virtue of the inclusion of a 10-Fr vascular sheath.

b. Metallic stents. Nearly every available metal stent has been used to support the parenchymal tract of a TIPS, including balloon expandable, self-expanding braided and laser-cut nitinol stents, and polytetrafluoroethylene (PTFE) stent-grafts. However, only two devices are FDA approved specifically for use in TIPS creation: the WALLSTENT (bare stent) and the VIATORR (expanded polytetrafluoroethylene [ePTFE]-lined stent-graft) (2,3,7). Other ePTFE endografts are under active development. With rare exception, stents must be lined with an ePTFE-covered stent-graft because of its far superior patency as compared to bare-metal stents (7).

c. Guidewires for portal entry are a matter of operator preference. A long-taper stiff shaft hydrophilic wire is useful, for example, Roadrunner (Cook Medical, Bloomington, IN) or Glidewire (Terumo Corporation, Tokyo, Japan).

d. Balloon angioplasty catheters, 8 to 10 mm diameter for tract dilation and subsequent stent expansion. With rare exception, stents should be dilated to no greater than 8 mm at the outset.

e. Pressure transducer (optional balloon occlusion catheter).

f. Optional adjunctive portal vein targeting equipment such as a directional IVUS catheter (intracardiac echocardiography [ICE] catheter commonly known as an "ICE" catheter).

8. Preprocedural echocardiography, in elective cases, is obtained at the discretion of the operator, especially if elevated right-sided heart pressures and pulmonary hypertension are suspected.

Procedure

The procedural steps for the creation of a TIPS are described below and in detail in virtual reality/ 360 Video with Dr. Haskal in YouTube channel (https://www.youtube.com/watch?v=ngFRoI6NivM).

1. The most common access is through the right internal jugular vein; however, shunts can be easily created using a left jugular approach. External jugular, femoral, transhepatic, and transcaval approaches have all been described. Sonographic-guided puncture of the internal jugular vein is performed. Once a guidewire is advanced toward the right atrium (RA), alert personnel to pay particular attention to the ECG. Arrhythmias may be induced during attempts to cross the Eustachian valve into the IVC. The author ensures that the ECG signal is audible to provide prompt indication of possible arrhythmias.

2. The vascular sheath is advanced into RA. Initial atrial pressures are recorded. If the mean RA pressure exceeds 10 mm Hg, consider reducing all unnecessary fluids. If the pressure is exceedingly high, consider whether unrecognized pulmonary hypertension or cardiac or valvular insufficiency may be present. As a general rule, TIPS patients should be "dry" with respect to intravenous fluids. TIPS increases cardiac preload by diverting higher-pressure portal blood to the RA. Purposefully minimize intravenous fluids during TIPS and in the postprocedure time period.

3. When using IVUS guidance for the hepatic vein to portal vein needle throw, femoral vein access is obtained. Right femoral or greater saphenous vein access is preferred but left can be used as well. ICE catheters are 8- or 10-Fr requiring appropriate sheath access. The IVUS probe is advanced over a wire into the intrahepatic IVC and rotated until the portal and hepatic venous anatomy can be assessed. The IVUS catheter may also be used to assist in selecting the correct hepatic vein in challenging cases. This approach can reduce fluoroscopy use in experienced hands (8).

4. A curved multipurpose (MPA/B) catheter is used to catheterize a suitable hepatic vein. The right hepatic vein ostium is typically one interspace higher than "expected" by fluoroscopy. The vascular sheath is advanced into the selected vein. Hand-injected free and wedged hepatic venography is performed. Rotational angiography may be helpful to confirm the selected hepatic vein. Wedged catheter or balloon occlusion carbon dioxide (due to the low viscosity of the gas) venography may be useful in opacifying the portal system for improved portal vein targeting. Alternatively, carbon dioxide portography can be performed by gas injection directly through the TIPS needle into the hepatic parenchyma. Caveat: Excessively forceful injection of iodinated contrast or carbon dioxide during wedged venography has led to serious or lethal hepatic lacerations and bleeding. If using IVUS portal vein targeting, do not to use carbon dioxide as residual gas within the parenchyma will obscure sonographic visualization.

5. An Amplatz guidewire is placed through the catheter into the selected hepatic vein, the diagnostic catheter removed, and the transjugular puncture needle, and its surrounding sheaths are advanced into the hepatic vein. Advancing the needle system over a "reversed" wire, that is, back-end of the Amplatz wire in the hepatic vein, can be helpful. The guidewire is removed, and gentle forward pressure is applied to the needle to prevent its retraction due to patient respiration. A partly filled syringe with contrast is attached to the needle hub.

6. In difficult cases (e.g., transcaval TIPS, Budd–Chiari, portal vein thromboses), a 60-cm coaxial fine needle can be used through the Colapinto needle. If using a coaxial fine needle, a 180-cm long, 0.018-in nitinol wire is used when a suitable portal branch is entered.

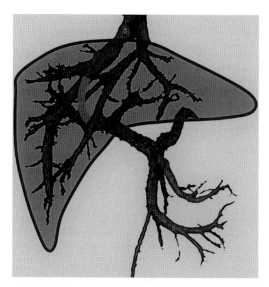

FIGURE 40.1 • Diagram of the typical intrahepatic course of a TIPS, extending from the right hepatic vein through the liver parenchyma into the right portal vein.

7. When using the right hepatic vein approach, the needle is rotated anteriorly and moved centrally within the vein to approximately 2 cm of the hepatic vein ostium. It is advanced parallel to the spine to the anticipated location of the intrahepatic portal vein (Fig. 40.1). The length of the needle pass is variable; it depends on the size of the actual liver and the relative positions of the portal and hepatic veins. Operators can modify the curve of the needle by bending it prior to insertion. This can be useful in cases of shrunken cirrhotic livers. These can often be estimated by fluoroscopic assessment of the liver or with wedged portographic images. Employ caution to avoid capsular transgression.

8. Aspirate the contrast syringe during slow needle and sheath withdrawal. When fluid is aspirated, inject contrast to identify the structure entered (portal vein, hepatic vein, hepatic artery, bile duct, lymphatic).

9. If a suitable portal branch has been punctured, the portal entry wire is manipulated through the main portal vein into the splenic or mesenteric veins. This is a critical step in TIPS creation—converting nearly any portal vein entry into one through which subsequently a stiff guidewire, sheath, angioplasty balloon and stent can be advanced. Due to respiratory motion, the liver is moving in a cephalocaudal direction (with needle in place), so it is important to maintain the rotatory orientation of the needle within the portal vein branch and advance the guidewire into the needle as quickly as possible to prevent loss of access to the portal vein. In cases performed under general anesthesia, some operators ask for brief respiratory cessation during these maneuvers.

10. Prior to needle removal, the needle guide and outer vascular sheaths are advanced forward into the parenchyma to the portal vein entry site, and occasionally into the portal vein. This step eases subsequent catheter and balloon passage across fibrotic periportal tissue. The needle is removed, and a 5-Fr diagnostic catheter is advanced into the parent vessel supplying the varices (splenic vein for esophageal and gastric varices, superior mesenteric vein [SMV] for

intestinal varices). For patients with ascites and hydrothorax, imaging of varices is not relevant because no embolization should be undertaken.

11. Portography is performed, and portal pressures are recorded.
12. The parenchymal tract is dilated with an 8-mm balloon (Fig. 40.2). Thereafter, a marker catheter (often a marker pigtail used previously for portography) is positioned within the parenchymal tract. Contrast venography is performed through the side arm of the vascular sheath ("tractogram"), positioned within

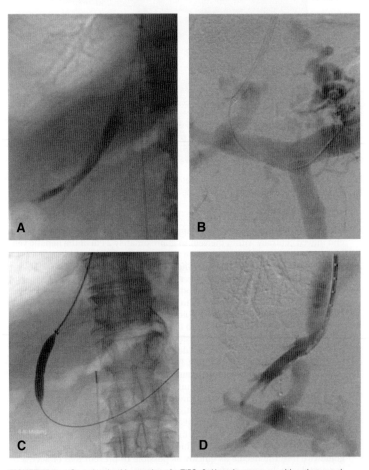

FIGURE 40.2 • Steps involved in creation of a TIPS. **A:** Hepatic venogram with catheter positioned in the right hepatic vein. **B:** Catheter advanced through the parenchymal tract to produce a contrast portogram. Note the gastroesophageal varices seen arising from the splenic vein. **C:** The liver tract is dilated with an angioplasty balloon. Note the presence of an "ICE" intravascular ultrasound catheter within the intrahepatic IVC oriented anteriorly toward the hepatic vein to portal vein intraparenchymal track. **D:** Simultaneous hepatic venogram with injection through the sheath and portogram with injection through a marker pig-tail catheter advanced into the main portal vein. The marker pig tail catheter is used to allow for accurate length measurement for stent selection.

the tract or cephalad portion of the main portal vein. Stent length measurements are obtained from these images.

13. The entirety of the TIPS tract is paved with an ePTFE-covered endoprosthesis, WALLSTENTS, or other bare stents, extending from the portal entry site to several millimeters into the IVC. The bare leading end of the endograft should just reach the main portal vein. For adults, as a general rule, 10-mm diameter bare stents or adjustable caliber VIATORR devices are used. In Asian countries, 8-mm Fluency (Benton Dickinson, Franklin Lakes, NJ) stent-grafts combined with a coaxial, leading bare-metal stent have been widely used. The specific technical aspects of VIATORR measurement (using a radio-opaque marker catheter) and deployment should be encompassed in specific device training.

End Points

   a. Primary objective: Create the smallest diameter shunt that achieves the desired clinical end point (9).
   b. Esophageal variceal bleeding—reduction of the portosystemic (porto-right atrial) gradient to ≤12 mm Hg. If there are large spontaneous splenorenal shunts in a patient with gastric varices, a lower gradient may be needed to divert flow from the varices into the TIPS, followed or preceded by ablative variceal embolization using coils, sclerosants, or other liquid embolics.
   c. Refractory ascites (or hepatic hydrothorax)—pressure-gradient end points are less clear. Some argue that the gradient needs to be lower than for esophageal varices; this must be offset against the often greater baseline encephalopathy seen in patients with longstanding refractory ascites. Because TIPS is palliative, the ascites effect should be balanced against risk of causing excessive portosystemic encephalopathy (or worsened liver function). For ascites patients, the shunt can always be enlarged at a second outpatient setting, once the clinical effect is measured after 2 to 3 weeks. For Budd–Chiari patients, there is evidence that higher initial gradient end points may be sufficient for the treatment of acute or subacute Budd–Chiari syndrome. In these patients, the gradients often rapidly drop with subsequent autodiuresis.

14. The VIATORR CX (Controlled eXpansion) is a self-expanding stent specifically designed with a higher radial expansile force than the WALLSTENT. It is specifically designed to expand to a minimum diameter of 8 mm unless balloon-dilated further and to maintain the set diameter over time, allowing for operator to select the desired diameter during implantation for the creation of the smallest shunt diameter that achieves desired pressure gradient. VIATORR CX endoprostheses are deployed over a 0.035-in wire and have a diameter range of 8 to 10 mm with a covered length of 4 to 8 cm and an uncovered portion of 2 cm.

15. If the patient is actively bleeding at the time of TIPS and a balloon tamponade catheter is present, deflate all balloons and repeat splenic venography and pressure measurements after shunt creation as demonstrated in Figure 40.3. If notable variceal flow remains, further expand the shunt and/or supplement with variceal embolization. Overdilatation of WALLSTENTS with balloons 1 to 2 mm larger than their nominal diameters will offset their relatively low radial expansile force and aid in achieving full stent expansion. Overdilatation is not performed with nitinol bare stents, VIATORRs, or other ePTFE endografts.

16. Remove all access catheters. It is preferred to not leave access site catheters in place, given prior reports of higher risks of site-related infection and fever.

Postprocedure Management

1. Postprocedure instructions and observation are governed by the patient's clinical status, that is, intensive care or floor recovery.
2. The right atrial pressure is routinely increased by TIPS formation. When the mean RA pressure is >10 mm Hg after TIPS, the author prescribes overnight

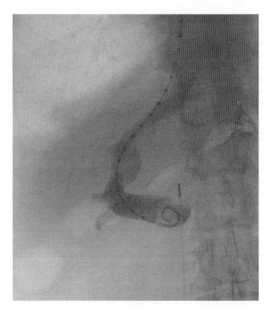

FIGURE 40.3 • Post-TIPS creation portogram demonstrating flow through the portosystemic shunt. Note the lack of opacification of the previously seen gastroesophageal varices.

diuresis of >1 L. The cardiac output, cardiac index, and right atrial pressure may remain elevated for more than 1 month after TIPS. Excessively high final right atrial pressures, particularly in acutely bleeding patients receiving fluid resuscitation, may both limit the decompressive effects of the shunt and lead to preventable secondary pulmonary edema (which may be confused with adult respiratory distress syndrome).

3. The majority of shunts are lined with ePTFE endografts. If the TIPS was created with bare-metal stents, postprocedural baseline TIPS sonography should be performed prior to discharge. This will serve as a baseline for comparison during outpatient shunt follow-up and detect any acute shunt thromboses or stenoses, such as those due to biliary-TIPS fistulae or hypercoagulability (e.g., in Budd–Chiari patients). If a VIATORR was used, avoid the immediate in-hospital post-TIPS sonogram; in the acute phase, the airspaces within the graft material will reflect sound, mimicking shunt occlusion. Within 1 to 2 weeks, the graft typically "wets out" by capillary action, becoming sonographically transparent. Perform the baseline post-VIATORR TIPS sonogram at the time of the first outpatient TIPS clinic visit.

4. If bare-metal stents are used, sonography should be performed at 3, 6, and 12 months in the first year and every 3 to 6 months after that depending on clinical status. Given the predilection for bare-metal shunts to develop stenoses, plans to line them with ePTFE endografts should be considered at each point. Sonographic follow-up may be less frequent in patients with VIATORR devices given expectations for long-term patency. If performed for recurrent ascites/hydrothorax, clinical follow-up should supplement TIPS ultrasonography. Recurrent ascites should prompt TIPS evaluation with venography and in rare cases could require shunt dilation or additional shunt creation, see Figure 40.4.

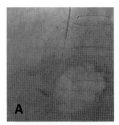
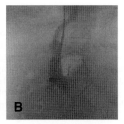
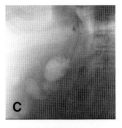

A **B** **C**

FIGURE 40.4 • A 45-year-old male with a history of TIPS creation in 2011 for refractory ascites. He is requiring large-volume paracentesis every 2 weeks. He presents for TIPS check and possible creation of parallel TIPS. TIPS check demonstrates elevated portal pressures to 32 mm Hg with a portosystemic gradient of 22 mm Hg. This did not improve with balloon angioplasty of the existing TIPS. **A:** Colapinto needle passed from intrahepatic IVC through the liver parenchyma. **B:** Portogram through the new transhepatic tract. **C:** Placement of VIATORR stent within the liver parenchymal track completing creation of DIPS in parallel to existing TIPS.

Results

1. Technical success: Creation of a TIPS between the hepatic vein and intrahepatic branch of the portal vein: 95% (6).
2. Hemodynamic success: Successful post-TIPS reduction of the portosystemic gradient below a threshold chosen for that indication: 95% (6).
3. Clinical success: Many randomized trials have compared TIPS to endoscopic treatment of esophageal variceal bleeding. The mean rates of rebleeding following TIPS and endoscopic treatment were 19% (range 9.8% to 24%) and 47% (range 24% to 57%), respectively (2,3,6). Increasing prospective controlled trials and large-scale registry data have emphasized the value to "early TIPS," that is TIPS created within days of an esophageal variceal hemorrhage have been shown to reduce rebleeding compared with endoscopic management, mortality, and morbidity (2,4).

Complications

1. Procedural complications are listed in Table 40.1.
2. Hepatic encephalopathy. Symptomatic or increased hepatic encephalopathy can occur after all forms of portosystemic diversion. The strongest prognostic factor is preexisting encephalopathy. In general, the risk is greater in patients with refractory ascites because of more severe underlying liver disease.
3. TIPS created with uncovered stents are prone to shunt stenoses resulting in portal hypertension in 25% to 50% of cases within 6 to 12 months. This emphasizes the mandatory need for routine TIPS follow-up and prophylactic revision. TIPS stenosis is vastly reduced with ePTFE-lined endografts (7). Establishing routine clinical follow-up of TIPS patients is a required aspect of interventional radiology care. Coordination with hepatologists, gastroenterologists, and when appropriate, liver transplant physicians is important.
4. Recurrent bleeding, and recurrent ascites to a lesser degree, is almost always associated with recurrent portal hypertension due to shunt stenosis or thrombosis. In the setting of recurrent bleeding or fluid accumulation, "negative" TIPS sonograms should not dissuade operators from direct shunt catheterization and hemodynamic assessment.

Management of Complications

1. Hepatic encephalopathy: First-line therapies include oral rifaximin, 550 mg twice daily in conjunction with oral lactulose. Lactulose is often started at 30 mL two or three times a day. Patients should be instructed to self-titrate their doses to an average of two to three bowel movements per day. If these measures prove inadequate (or liver function notably deteriorates after TIPS), shunt size reduction may be needed. This can be accomplished by deployment of a stenotic stent within the original TIPS. In cases of uncontrolled encephalopathy and progressive liver failure, intentional shunt occlusion can be performed using a balloon occlusion catheter or intravascular plug. This should be reserved for extreme cases because it may precipitate recurrent variceal bleeding or hepatorenal failure (10).

2. Shunt stenosis or thrombosis. Stent thrombosis usually is secondary to an underlying stenosis or occlusion. Shunt thrombus can be cleared by balloon dilation; chemical thrombolysis is rarely required. Stenoses occurring at the junction of the portal vein may be treated by angioplasty, although stents have a lower recurrence rate and may prevent restenosis in the future. The most common site of shunt stenosis is an unstented segment of native hepatic vein, emphasizing the need for extending endografts to the caval ostium. Stenosis within the intrahepatic portion of the bare stent-TIPS tracts may indicate a communication with bile ducts. If the occluded TIPS tract cannot be recanalized, a new TIPS can be created, usually from another hepatic vein.

3. Hyperbilirubinemia after TIPS. A partial differential diagnosis is provided: excessive (over)shunting, ischemic hepatopathy (due to hypotension related to acute bleeding or resuscitation—marked transaminitis), bile duct compression by the TIPS stents (elevated alkaline phosphatase without transaminase elevations), hemolysis (change in reticulocyte count, haptoglobin, low hemoglobin), ischemic liver due to hepatic artery injury (transaminitis), hemobilia (lower gastrointestinal bleeding or melena).

R e f e r e n c e s

1. He F, Zhao H, Dai S, et al. Transjugular intrahepatic portosystemic shunt for Budd-Chiari syndrome with diffuse occlusion of hepatic veins. *Sci Rep.* 2016;6:36380. doi:10.1038/srep36380

2. García-Pagán JC, Caca K, Bureau C, et al. Early use of TIPS in patients with cirrhosis and variceal bleeding. *N Engl J Med.* 2010;362(25):2370–2379. doi:10.1056/nejmoa0910102

3. Boyer TD, Haskal ZJ. AASLD practice guidelines the role of transjugular intrahepatic portosystemic shunt (TIPS) in the management of portal hypertension update 2009. *Hepatology.* 2010;51(1):306. Published online 2009. doi:10.1002/hep.23392

4. Lv Y, Yang Z, Liu L, et al. Early TIPS with covered stents versus standard treatment for acute variceal bleeding in patients with advanced cirrhosis: a randomised controlled trial. *Lancet Gastroenterol Hepatol.* 2019;4(8):587–598. doi:10.1016/S2468-1253(19)30090-1

5. Bureau C, Thabut D, Oberti F, et al. Transjugular intrahepatic portosystemic shunts with covered stents increase transplant-free survival of patients with cirrhosis and recurrent ascites. *Gastroenterology.* 2017;152(1):157–163. doi:10.1053/j.gastro.2016.09.016

6. Dariushnia SR, Haskal ZJ, Midia M, et al. Quality improvement guidelines for transjugular intrahepatic portosystemic shunts. *J Vasc Interv Radiol.* 2016;27(1):1–7. doi:10.1016/j.jvir.2015.09.018

7. Perarnau JM, Le Gouge A, Nicolas C, et al. Covered vs. uncovered stents for transjugular intrahepatic portosystemic shunt: a randomized controlled trial. *J Hepatol.* 2014;60(5):962–968. doi:10.1016/j.jhep.2014.01.015

8. Gipson MG, Smith MT, Durham JD, et al. Intravascular US–guided portal vein access: improved procedural metrics during TIPS creation. *J Vasc Interv Radiol.* 2016;27(8):1140–1147. doi:10.1016/j.jvir.2015.12.002

9. Trebicka J, Bastgen D, Byrtus J, et al. Smaller-diameter covered transjugular intrahepatic portosystemic shunt stents are associated with increased survival. *Clin Gastroenterol Hepatol.* 2019;17(13):2793–2799.e1. doi:10.1016/j.cgh.2019.03.042

10. Madoff DC, Wallace MJ, Ahrar K, et al. TIPS-related hepatic encephalopathy: management options with novel endovascular techniques. *Radiographics.* 2004;24(1):21–36. doi:10.1148/rg.241035028

41 Retrograde Transvenous Obliteration of Varices

John T. Matson, MD and
Ziv J. Haskal, MD, FSIR, FAHA, FACR, FCIRSE

Introduction

Gastric variceal bleeding is a life-threatening complication of portal hypertension. Retrograde transvenous obliteration (RTO) of varices is a procedure by which upstream occlusion of a pathologic portosystemic shunt is achieved using sclerosants and/or embolic solutions and mechanical occlusive devices. RTO of gastric varices using sclerosants such as ethanolamine has been used in Asia for over 20 years. It has become widely propagated in the West, and the techniques, device, and agents used have evolved. Variations of this procedure include the original balloon occluded (BRTO), plug-assisted (PARTO) and coil-assisted (CARTO) techniques using Gelfoam instead of sclerosant agents, which have shown to be quite effective (1).

Indications

1. Secondary prevention of recurrent gastric variceal hemorrhage. In most cases, BRTO (and variants) are not performed during acute variceal hemorrhage, although procedural evolution may allow its increasing use in this setting (2,3).
2. Primary prophylaxis of gastric varices. This is a common indication in Asia. Comparing published results of respective series must take into account the comparison of different cohorts, that is patients who have bled (secondary prevention) versus those who have never bled (primary prophylaxis).
3. Treatment of excess portosystemic encephalopathy (shunting-type) aggravated portal hypertension or secondary development of ascites or increased esophageal varices. Improved liver function can occur after such shunt obliteration (4,5).
4. Bleeding ectopic varices (e.g., duodenal) (6). Anatomically, all target varices (gastric or ectopic) must have a catheter-accessible efferent drainage (e.g., gastrorenal or gastrocaval shunt). See Figure 41.1 as an example of an anatomically amenable shunt

Contraindications

Absolute
1. Uncorrected coagulopathy
2. Patient is too unstable to tolerate time required for procedure. These patients may be more suitable for transjugular intrahepatic portosystemic shunt (TIPS).

Relative
1. Refractory ascites
2. Associated high-risk esophageal varices (RTO procedures increase absolute portal pressures and can lead to new or worsened ascites and esophageal varices)
3. Severe liver dysfunction

Preprocedure Preparation

1. Informed consent
2. Preprocedure imaging with either triple phase contrast computed tomography (CT) or magnetic resonance angiography (MRA)/magnetic resonance

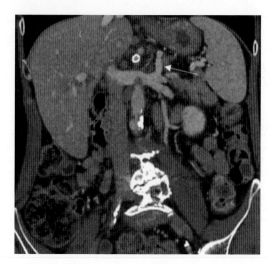

FIGURE 41.1 • A 62-year-old cirrhotic patient with submucosal gastric fundal varices and prominent gastrorenal shunt drainage (*arrow*) into the left renal vein which would be amenable to transvenous obliteration of varices.

venography (MRV) to evaluate the portal vein and the extent of portosystemic shunts, for example, Figure 41.1. Multiplanar imaging is essential for procedure planning, CT is often used due to its accessibility and ability for multiplanar reconstructions. It is important to evaluate the size of the gastrorenal shunt for suitability of the procedure and device selection. It is also important to understand the portal inflow to the shunt. This can be difficult because some shunts have multiple small inflow veins. Imaging can also be used to identify collateral veins that may require embolization prior to instillation of sclerosants (e.g., phrenic or pericardiophrenic veins).

3. Laboratory evaluation to include basic metabolic and electrolyte panels, complete blood counts, coagulation parameters, and liver function tests. Platelet counts above 40 to 50,000 are adequate to perform this procedure.

4. Hemodynamic monitoring with electrocardiography, blood pressure, and oxygen saturation.

5. Aggressive resuscitation should be implemented in acutely bleeding patients with hemodynamic instability. This may require packed red blood cells, fresh-frozen plasma, platelets, cryoglobulin, pressor support, and intravenous (IV) fluids.

6. Conscious sedation using IV fentanyl and midazolam is suitable for most patients.

7. Accumulate the required components:
   Embolic and/or sclerosing agent (7)
   a. Sodium tetradecyl sulfate (STS) (Sotradecol, AngioDynamics, Queensbury, NY)
   b. Ethanolamine oleate (Oldamin, Grelan Pharmaceutical, Tokyo, Japan). Haptoglobin is often required as part of its use.
   c. Polidocanol foam (Polidocasklerol, ZERIA Pharmaceutical, Tokyo, Japan)
   d. *n*-Butyl cyanoacrylate. Glues have been reported used in some RTO procedures.
   e. Gelfoam (Pharmacia & Upjohn, New York, NY). This is the primary embolic used during plug-assisted retrograde transvenous obliteration (PARTO) or CARTO procedures.

f. Ethiodol (occasionally mixed with other sclerosants per operator preference to enhance radio-opacity or increase foam stability)

g. Balloon-occlusion catheters (only required for BRTO; others may be equally suitable)

(1) Coda (Cook Medical, Bloomington, IN)

(2) Python occlusion balloon (Applied Medical, Rancho Santa Margarita, CA)

(3) Equalizer (Boston Scientific Corporation, Natick, MA)

h. Plugs (needed for PARTO technique)

(1) Amplatzer plug (St. Jude Medical, St. Paul, MN). Typically minimum sizes are 14 mm diameter or larger are required; these are oversized to the distal adrenal (juxtarenal) end of the shunt where a narrowed segment is typically present.

i. Coils (for coil-assisted techniques, CARTO)

(1) Pushable versus detachable, metallic, or polymer embolization coils

Procedure

Balloon-Occluded Retrograde Transvenous Obliteration (Fig. 41.2)

1. Access is through the femoral or internal jugular veins. An appropriate sheath is then placed based on estimated size of the shunt ostium and occlusion balloon required. Typically, 7- to 9 Fr, 50- to 70-cm long vascular sheaths are suitable.

2. Catheterization of gastrorenal shunt arising from the left renal vein

   a. A 4-Fr or 5-Fr catheter (Cobra, reverse curve, Simmons 1, or Headhunter) is used to select the left renal vein; a deflecting wire or hand curved back end of a guidewire (kept within the catheter lumen) can be useful. The outer sheath is advanced over the catheter into the central renal vein. The catheter is gently rotated while being drawn back, directed at the cephalic wall of the left renal vein. The gastrorenal vein empties into the left renal vein through the enlarged adrenal vein along its central cephalic aspect.

   b. A soft Teflon-coated metallic or hydrophilic guidewire is advanced into the gastrorenal shunt after which the long sheath advanced over the diagnostic catheter and guidewire beyond the junction of the shunt and renal vein. A parallel, "buddy wire" or catheter may be placed alongside the original guidewire. After shunt venography, the catheter is exchanged for the plug (an appropriately sized occlusion balloon. The balloon is positioned in a secure caudal location within the shunt, gently inflated and retrograde contrast venography performed, to begin to map the shunt. Iodinated contrast and carbon dioxide can be used as well as cone-beam CT.

   c. Reverse curve single and double balloon BRTO occlusion catheters are available in Asia; these can potentially reduce the number of steps in gastrorenal vein catheterization.

3. Balloon occlusion venography evaluation of shunt anatomy can reveal collateral veins, for example, paravertebral, pericardial, pericardiophrenic, or inferior phrenic veins, that may warrant coil embolization before instillation of the sclerosant. When using liquid sclerosants, these large veins may otherwise thwart contrast filling the entirety of varix, hence the need to skeletonize the shunt. The "inflow" of the shunt should be identified (i.e., its path toward the splenic vein) so that the proper amount of embolic solution is instilled, both sufficient to occlude the majority of the varix but not spill into the splenic vein.

4. Advance a microcatheter through the balloon lumen into the varix as far as feasible. The intent is to expose the majority of the varix to the occlusive agent or sclerosant, without reflux into the splenic vein.

5. The sclerosant agent of choice is mixed with gas and contrast agent. The following preparation of Sotradecol can be used: 2 mL of STS 3%, 1 mL of lipiodol, and 3 mL of air (8). Carbon dioxide can be used and may be preferable.

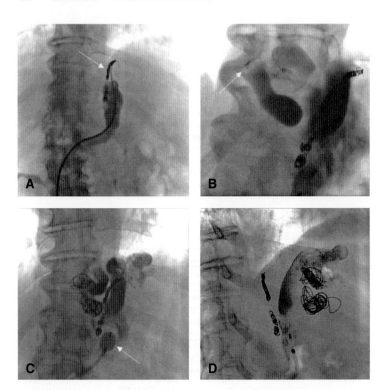

FIGURE 41.2 • A 68-year-old woman with history of nonalcoholic steatohepatitis, recanalized paraumbilical vein, and large gastric varices seen on cross-sectional imaging and endoscopy. **A:** Venography of the shunt revealed prominent competing outflow vein (phrenic in this case) which was embolized with coils (*arrow*). Following embolization, no additional collaterals were seen. **B:** Injection of Sotradecol foam sclerosant through a microcatheter (*arrow*) advanced coaxially through a Python occlusion balloon. **C:** Complete filling of the varix with coils and sclerosant. The occlusion balloon (*arrow*) was left inflated for 7 hours. At recheck, some movement of the sclerosant was seen upon balloon deflation and the balloon was reinflated and left inflated overnight. **D:** Stagnant contrast column with balloon deflation at recheck the next morning.

6. The sclerosant is injected under fluoroscopic guidance, and the occlusion balloon is left inflated.
7. The balloon is typically deflated ~4 or more hours later, although shorter protocols have been reported. Should flow persist, reinflation and resclerosis can be performed.

Plug/Coil-Assisted Retrograde Transvenous Obliteration (PARTO/CARTO) (Fig. 41.3)

1. Access into the shunt as described earlier. Use a long vascular sheath of sufficient caliber to allow delivery of a suitable plug (or coil mass) and parallel (para-axial) catheter for delivering the embolic solution.
2. Perform shunt venography.
3. Advance a microcatheter or 4/5-Fr diagnostic catheter deep into the shunt.
4. For plug-assisted retrograde occlusion, an oversized AMPLATZER Vascular Plug II (AVP-II) (available in sizes up to 22 mm diameter) is extruded into the shunt *but not detached from its delivery mandril.* For CARTO approaches, embolization

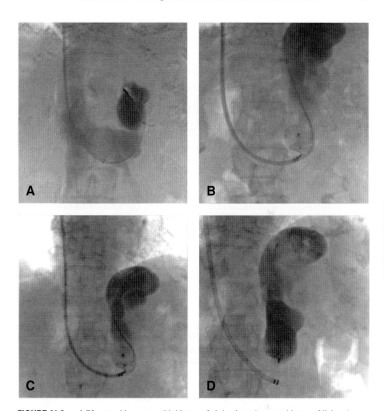

FIGURE 41.3 • A 76-year-old woman with history of cirrhosis and remote history of living donor liver transplant who presented with large gastric varices, recurrent episodes of hyperammonemia and encephalopathy with a large splenorenal shunt. **A:** The shunt is catheterized using a 7-Fr sheath coaxially within a 10-Fr sheath and headhunter catheter and venography of the shunt is performed. **B:** An Amplatzer II plug is positioned within the outflow of the draining vein with catheter advanced paraxially to the vascular plug with tip positioned deep within the varix. Venography confirms outflow occlusion. **C:** Embolization was then performed using thick Gelfoam slurry, care should be taken to avoid nontarget embolization of the renal or splenic veins. Imaging in multiple obliquities while filling the varix is helpful in determining the end point of filling the varix without reflux into the splenic vein. **D:** Once complete embolization/filling of the varix is achieved, the vascular plug is deployed.

coils are used, these are deployed alongside the microcatheter or 0.035-in catheter which has been placed deep into the varix.
5. A thick slurry of Gelfoam and iodinated contrast is injected into the varix via the catheter within the cephalic portion of the shunt. The occlusive plug prevents egress of this solution. Relatively large volumes of this solution may be required. The static column can be readily visualized as the varix is progressively filled. Oblique images are valuable to discern when the Gelfoam column begins to "turn" downward toward the splenic vein and/or sufficiently fills the fundal varices. Once a sufficient extent of varix stasis has been achieved, the plug is released at the central "base" of the varix and the procedure is concluded. Some operators have chosen to mix sclerosant agents into the Gelfoam solution.

6. The advantages of this approach include single-session only, absent need for collateral embolization, and lesser risk of sclerosis of nontarget vessels.

Postprocedure Management

1. Elective BRTO patients are often admitted for overnight observation; this is optional.
2. Laboratory evaluation in the first 48 hours may demonstrate a mild increase in total bilirubin and liver function tests, usually self-limited, perhaps related to increase portal flow and pressure. Persistent deterioration in liver function should prompt a liver Doppler ultrasound to exclude portal vein thrombosis.
3. The patient's fluid status and renal function should be monitored.
   a. Ascites, hepatic hydrothorax, and lower extremity edema may develop or increase after varix obliteration.
   b. Renal function can be affected by hemoglobinuria (particularly with the use of ethanolamine oleate), contrast, renal vein thrombosis, or the development of hepatorenal syndrome.
4. Upper endoscopy in combination with endoscopic ultrasound can be used in the postoperative period to verify obliteration of the gastric varices.
5. Cross-sectional imaging (computed tomography venography [CTV] or MRV) should be performed at least once during outpatient clinic follow-up at 3 to 6 months and then as clinically indicated.

Results (8–10)

1. Technical success reported between 80% and 100%.
2. Complete gastric varix thrombosis 75% to 100%. The majority of reports suggest greater than 95% complete thrombosis.
3. Recurrent GV bleeding between 0% and 9%.

Complications

1. Increased ascites and hepatic hydrothorax
2. Hemoglobinuria when using ethanolamine oleate-iopamidol sclerosing agent, which causes hemolysis. Haptoglobin 2,000 to 4,000 units can be given to prevent onset of renal failure.
3. Balloon rupture with leak of sclerosant or embolic agent can cause pulmonary embolus or renal vein thrombosis.
4. Worsening esophageal varices (9,10)
5. Portal vein thrombosis rate of 1% (10)
6. Abdominal pain
7. Fever

References

1. Kim DJ, Darcy MD, Mani NB, et al. Modified balloon-occluded retrograde transvenous obliteration (BRTO) techniques for the treatment of gastric varices: vascular plug-assisted retrograde transvenous obliteration (PARTO)/coil-assisted retrograde transvenous obliteration (CARTO)/balloon-occluded antegrade transvenous obliteration (BATO). *Cardiovasc Intervent Radiol.* 2018;41(6): doi:10.1007/s00270-018-1896-1.
2. Wang ZW, Liu JC, Zhao F, et al. Comparison of the effects of TIPS versus BRTO on bleeding gastric varices: a meta-analysis. *Can J Gastroenterol Hepatol.* 2020;2020:5143013. doi:10.1155/2020/5143013
3. Paleti S, Nutalapati V, Fathallah J, et al. Balloon-occluded retrograde transvenous obliteration (BRTO) versus transjugular intrahepatic portosystemic shunt (TIPS) for treatment of gastric varices because of portal hypertension: a systematic review and meta-analysis. *J Clin Gastroenterol.* 2020;54(7):655–660. doi:10.1097/MCG.0000000000001275

4. Kumamoto M, Toyonaga A, Inoue H, et al. Long-term results of balloon-occluded retrograde transvenous obliteration for gastric fundal varices: hepatic deterioration links to portosystemic shunt syndrome. *J Gastroenterol Hepatol.* 2010;25(6):1129–1135. doi:10.1111/j.1440-1746.2010.06262.x

5. Mukund A, Chalamarla LK, Singla N, et al. Intractable hepatic encephalopathy in cirrhotic patients: mid-term efficacy of balloon-occluded retrograde portosystemic shunt obliteration. *Eur Radiol.* 2020;30(6):3462–3472. doi:10.1007/s00330-019-06644-4

6. Minami S, Okada K, Matsuo M, et al. Treatment of bleeding stomal varices by balloon-occluded retrograde transvenous obliteration. *J Gastroenterol.* 2007;42(1):91–95. doi:10.1007/s00535-006-1960-5

7. Kim YH, Kim YH, Kim CS, et al. Comparison of balloon-occluded retrograde transvenous obliteration (BRTO) using ethanolamine oleate (EO), BRTO using sodium tetradecyl sulfate (STS) foam and vascular plug-assisted retrograde transvenous obliteration (PARTO). *Cardiovasc Intervent Radiol.* 2016;39(6):840–846. doi:10.1007/s00270-015-1288-8

8. Sabri SS, Swee W, Turba UC, et al. Bleeding gastric varices obliteration with balloon-occluded retrograde transvenous obliteration using sodium tetradecyl sulfate foam. *J Vasc Interv Radiol.* 2011;22(3):309–316. doi:10.1016/j.jvir.2010.11.022

9. Akahoshi T, Hashizume M, Tomikawa M, et al. Long-term results of balloon-occluded retrograde transvenous obliteration for gastric variceal bleeding and risky gastric varices: a 10-year experience. *J Gastroenterol Hepatol.* 2008;23(11):1702–1709. doi:10.1111/j.1440-1746.2008.05549.x

10. Park JK, Saab S, Kee ST, et al. Balloon-occluded retrograde transvenous obliteration (BRTO) for treatment of gastric varices: review and meta-analysis. *Dig Dis Sci.* 2015;60(6):1543–1553. doi:10.1007/s10620-014-3485-8

42 Varicocele Embolization

Lindsay Machan, MD

Introduction (1,2)

A varicocele is a collection of varicose veins within the pampiniform (spermatic venous) plexus secondary to reflux in the internal spermatic vein (ISV). The condition affects 10% to 15% of the general population; however, they are detected in as many as 30% to 40% of men undergoing infertility workup. Depending on the method used for diagnosis, they are reported as being bilateral in 17% to 77% of men. Isolated right varicoceles are uncommon; the traditional recommendation is to initiate cross-sectional imaging to exclude renal or retroperitoneal tumor, however recent data suggest this association is rare (3). Diagnosis was traditionally made by clinical examination; however, as for other venous reflux disorders, ultrasound has become the mainstay of diagnosis (4).

The proof that varicocele repair improves infertility remains elusive; however, there is general acceptance that treatment does improve abnormalities of semen production: by the traditional measures of decreased sperm motility, abnormal morphology, and decreased sperm count and by newer means of assessment such as the DNA fragmentation index. Although the connection between varicoceles and infertility remains controversial, associations with chronic groin pain and testicular atrophy in adolescent varicoceles are not.

Indications (5,6)

1. Chronic groin pain (other etiologies excluded)
2. Infertility and appropriate semen abnormalities
3. Recurrent varicocele after surgical repair
4. Testicular atrophy in a pediatric patient

Contraindications
1. Severe anaphylactoid reactions to contrast media
2. Uncorrectable coagulopathy
3. Severe renal insufficiency

Preprocedure Preparation
1. Scrotal ultrasound (4). There are published diagnostic criteria but they are not universally applied. Abnormal reflux with Valsalva maneuver rather than rigid size criteria are increasingly used as venous diameter varies significantly with hydration, anxiety, and inspiratory effort.
2. Laboratory workup (may be omitted in young patients with no pertinent medical history): hemoglobin (Hgb), platelet count, international normalized ratio (INR), creatinine (Cr) or estimated glomerular filtration rate (eGFR).
3. Oral intake restrictions per institutional protocol for IV sedation. The author's are no solids for 6 hours preprocedure, clear fluids only until 2 hours before.
4. Obtain informed consent. This is an outpatient procedure so ensure someone can accompany the patient home.
5. Establish a peripheral intravenous (IV) and appropriate monitoring.
6. Sedate with IV midazolam (Versed) and fentanyl.

Procedure (2,5)

1. Direct fluoroscopic imaging of the scrotum should be avoided. As far as possible imaging should be with low-dose fluoroscopy only, avoiding DSA, and archived using stored fluoro images. Testicular shielding is seldom used.
2. Ultrasound-guided insertion of 5- or 6-Fr sheath for right internal jugular vein, antecubital vein or common femoral vein access. The right internal jugular vein allows the most direct route to the right spermatic vein.
3. Catheters
   a. Right internal jugular or axillary vein: 5- or 6-Fr multipurpose-shaped catheters can be used to select the left and right spermatic veins, usually without the need for coaxial catheters or catheter exchange.
   b. Femoral approach
      (1) Left varicocele: A 5-Fr Cobra catheter allows access to the left renal vein. Some will pass this coaxially through a 6-Fr renal double curve–shaped sheath. A microcatheter may be used to manipulate across difficult valves and/or tortuous collateral vessels.
      (2) Right varicocele: A reverse curve catheter such as a Simmons 1 is helpful for selecting the right ISV. Invariably a coaxial microcatheter will be required for embolization.
4. The catheter should be advanced well into the left renal vein. Hand injection of contrast forceful enough to allow visualization of potential collateral veins should be performed during Valsalva maneuver. The origin of the left spermatic vein is noted.
5. To select the ostium of the left ISV (Fig. 42.1), during Valsalva maneuver the catheter is withdrawn along the inferior margin of the left renal vein while gently injecting contrast.
6. Once stable ISV catheter position is achieved, usually with the assistance of an angle-tipped glidewire, selective venography is performed. If there are incompetent valves, contrast should flow in a retrograde fashion toward the testis, especially during a Valsalva maneuver. Collaterals that originate from the renal hilum or paralumbar region may be noted. A tilt table may be of additional benefit.
7. The goal of embolization is occlusion of the ISV and collaterals (Fig. 42.1) from immediately above the spermatic cord to approximately 2 cm from its origin. The most reliable means of achieving this involves advancing the catheter or

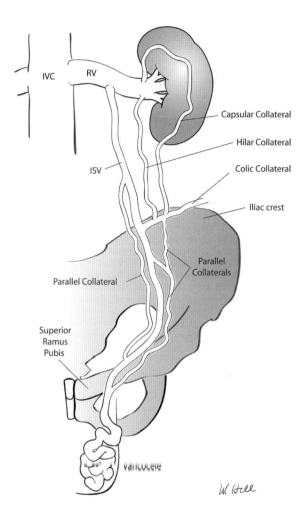

IVC

RV

Capsular Collateral

Hilar Collateral

ISV

Colic Collateral

Iliac crest

Parallel
Collaterals

Parallel Collateral

Superior
Ramus
Pubis

Varicocele

W. Hill

FIGURE 42.1 • Anatomy of the left ISV and collateral venous pathways.

coaxial microcatheter to the level of the inguinal ring (opposite the roof of the acetabulum). Particular care should be taken to avoid vessel spasm, which hinders the ability to proceed with the procedure and obscures collaterals—predisposing to a false impression of successful occlusion.

8. *Methods of embolization* (2,5). Several have been described, each with its own merits. The use of liquid embolics with or without metallic coils has become the most common practice. Embolization with coils alone should be avoided even for "straight forward" cases, due to a high rate of recurrence.

   a. **Glue**: Cyanoacrylate, particularly in countries where it is inexpensive, is increasingly used for varicocele occlusion as reported rates of late recanalization are lower than for other methods (7).

(1) Glue:lipiodol ratios (reported ratios range from 1:1 to 1:6), type of cyano-acrylate, or balloon occlusion versus injection from standard catheter are matters of individual choice.

(2) There are two modes of injection:

(a) When the catheter can be advanced into the distal ISV, the easiest method is to dribble a trail of glue as the catheter is withdrawn, with the patient performing a Valsalva maneuver. If the injection is stopped when the upper end of the glue column is at the level of the iliac crest the glue will typically migrate slightly cranially on its own to an optimal level of proximal occlusion. Continuing to inject until the column is within 2 to 3 cm of the renal vein usually results in overinjection.

(b) If the catheter cannot be advanced distally, glue can be refluxed from a secure proximal position. This is done with the patient performing a Valsalva maneuver and may be improved by a tilt table. Having an assistant poised to apply external compression as the glue flows into the distal ISV, and considerable dexterity with glue injection are required.

(3) Essential points

(a) The bolus of glue is introduced into the catheter after it has been flushed with 5% dextrose solution (D5W) and is pushed out of the catheter by another (carefully controlled!) bolus of D5W. Remove the catheter quickly as soon as the endpoint of glue injection is reached.

(b) Optimally, at the end of the procedure glue will fill the vein and collaterals from immediately above the roof of the acetabulum to approximately 2 cm from the ISV origin (Fig. 42.2). Coils in the proximal ISV are not necessary.

(c) Ideally injection of glue into the scrotum is avoided, either by previously placed distal coils or external compression. The author routinely uses both.

(d) Overinjection of glue will result in extension into the renal vein or embolization into the pulmonary artery. Delayed or slow removal of the catheter after glue injection may result in an adherent, and subsequently detached, trail of glue on the tip of the catheter with the same consequence.

b. **Metallic coils and sclerosants:**

(1) Coils (see below) are deployed at the level of the roof of the acetabulum. Occlusion of the lumen can usually be achieved with two or three coils.

(2) A venogram during Valsalva maneuver should again be performed. Sluggish flow or nonfilling of the pampiniform plexus should be seen.

(a) **Collateral veins**: Contrast injection after distal spermatic vein occlusion will often reveal new collaterals that have become visible with the higher pressure now present in the occluded spermatic vein (Fig. 42.2A). These may cause technical failure or recurrence and therefore must be occluded. If large enough or the operator is unsure of liquid embolic refluxing into the collateral, they can be entered directly and embolized with an appropriately sized coil placed as distally as possible. Alternatively, they can be occluded with sclerosant or glue infusion.

(3) **Sclerosants:** Sodium tetradecyl sulfate (STS) is most commonly used. Other sclerosing agents such as polidocanol have been reported.

(a) STS liquid

i. Can be opacified by mixing 2 mL of 1 or 3% STS with 0.5 to 1 mL of contrast.

ii. The vein is occluded at the inguinal ring by applying external pressure with a compression device or the patient's hand. Static contrast in the ISV is aspirated or displaced by saline injection.

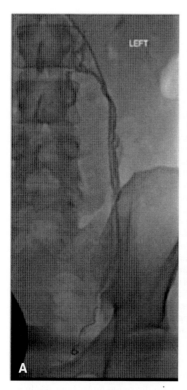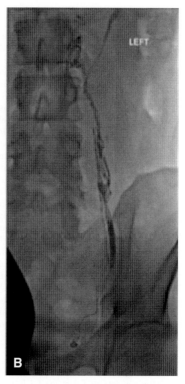

FIGURE 42.2 • Left varicocele embolization using glue. **A:** Venogram after coils placed in lower vein, during Valsalva maneuver with external compression. Multiple collateral channels are demonstrated, which were not apparent on initial venogram. **B:** Filling of collateral channels with glue/lipiodol injected under similar conditions as catheter was withdrawn.

    iii While the patient is performing a Valsalva maneuver, the STS is injected along the course of the vein from immediately above the coils at the inguinal ring to above the iliac crest (colic collateral) if a proximal coil is to be used. Otherwise, STS is injected to within 1 cm of the ISV origin. A volume of 2.5 to 5 mL is typically adequate.

(b) STS foam
    i. Can be injected to displace preexisting contrast, or opacified with contrast while the patient performs a Valsalva maneuver. This maneuver should be repeated as needed.
    ii. The STS foam is mixed in the following manner. A 2:1 mixture of 3% STS to sterile saline is aggressively agitated with an equal volume of air, thereby resulting in a 2% STS foam. This foam is injected into the catheter then the dead space of the catheter is flushed with saline to clear it. When a microcatheter is used, a similar technique may be used after 0.018-in coils are deployed.
    iii. The catheter should be retracted from the mid to upper ISV, and a repeat venogram is performed, paying particular attention to

the presence of any previously unidentified collateral channels. Further coils can be placed, or further displacement of the contrast with additional injections of the foam, taking care not to reflux proximally into the renal vein. If coils are used, additional foam is still injected.

iv. Some interventionists use STS foam alone without coils (8). In this instance, the vein is externally occluded distally, as above.

(4) **Metallic coils**: 0.035- or 0.038-in coils may be delivered through a 4- to 6-Fr catheter. If distal access is difficult, then 0.014- or 0.018-in coils are delivered via any appropriately sized coaxial microcatheter. The coils should be sized at least 20% larger than the diameter of the spermatic vein at the desired level of occlusion. Pushable (e.g., Nester or MReye coils) (Cook Medical, Bloomington, IN) are adequate in most cases, some physicians perceive additional safety using retrievable coils on 0.014- or 0.035-in platforms (see Chapter 95). Place the uppermost coil with care to occlude the cephalad portion of the spermatic vein (within 2 cm of the junction with left renal vein is usually adequate) without protruding into the left renal vein. Poorly deployed coils may migrate, eventually lodging in the pulmonary circulation. Occlusive plugs have been utilized; however, there are no data justifying the extra cost.

9. The right spermatic vein is cannulated and imaged in the same manner as the left. In 1% to 6% of patients the right ISV drains into the right renal vein. If the right ISV does not fill from the renal vein, it is usually located immediately anterior and inferior to the right renal vein ostium. If using femoral access, once the ISV orifice is engaged a coaxial 3-Fr microcatheter should be advanced into the upper right ISV. If using the jugular approach, an angled glidewire and multipurpose catheter will suffice in most cases. Right spermatic venography and if positive, embolization, are performed as on the left.

Postprocedure Management

1. Remove all catheters and the sheath; attain hemostasis at the puncture site.
2. Monitor patient for at least 1 hour prior to discharge (outpatient discharge evaluation criteria must be met).
3. Ten percent of patients will have back or scrotal pain that lasts for 24 to 48 hours. Nonnarcotic analgesic and nonsteroidal antiinflammatory drugs (NSAIDs) and avoidance of any activity more vigorous than walking for 3 days will usually suffice.
4. With the coil and STS foam method, up to 10% of patients may have mild scrotal swelling and discomfort, relieved easily with NSAIDs and a heating pad for 24 to 48 hours.
5. Follow-up scrotal ultrasound in 3 months. It should be performed in precisely the same manner as the preembolization examination.

Results (2,7)

1. Clinical outcomes of surgical or endovascular techniques are almost identical (9,10). Embolization offers a shorter recovery time and there is no possibility of hydrocele.
2. Technical success of embolization for previously untreated varicoceles and postsurgical recurrences is 93% to 100%.
3. Thirty to 35% of infertile couples will have a normal pregnancy if there are no female infertility factors. In the literature, pregnancy rates from 11% to 60% have been reported.
4. Patients usually return to work the next day, compared with an average of 6 days following microsurgical techniques. Patients who have surgery initially and then embolization for recurrence express a strong preference for embolization.

Complications

1. Coil misplacement or migration into the central venous circulation. Retrieval typically is possible (see Chapter 83), but not always essential.
2. Venous perforation, usually self-limiting and clinically inconsequential, may occur when an angled glidewire is allowed too far into a tiny parallel branch vein or venospasm is present and one perseveres with catheter manipulation. The best option is to wait 5 minutes for the spasm to abate spontaneously. If there is concern distribution of embolic agent will be limited by spasm, abandoning the procedure and rebooking in at least 6 weeks may be necessary.
3. Phlebitis, clinically manifesting as scrotal or flank pain typically resolves within 3 days postprocedure. In less than 1% of patients it can persist for weeks or months. Treatment with antiinflammatory agents to maximal tolerable dose, limitation of activity to nothing more strenuous than walking until resolution, and patience are recommended.

References

1. Su JS, Farber NJ, Vij SC. Pathophysiology and treatment options of varicocele: an overview. *Andrologia*. 2021;53(1):e13576.
2. Baigorri BF, Dixon RG. Varicocele: a review. *Semin Intervent Radiol*. 2016;33(3):170–176.
3. Gleason A, Bishop K, Xi Y, et al. Isolated right-sided varicocele: is further workup necessary? *AJR Am J Roentgenol*. 2019;212(4):802–807.
4. Freeman S, Bertolotto M, Richenberg J, et al. Ultrasound evaluation of varicoceles: guidelines and recommendations of the European Society of Urogenital Radiology Scrotal and Penile Imaging Working Group (ESUR-SPIWG) for detection, classification, and grading. *Eur Radiol*. 2020;30(1):11–25.
5. Wadhwa V, Kashanian JA, Schiffman M, et al. Varicocele embolization: patient selection: preprocedure workup, and technical considerations. *Semin Intervent Radiol* 2021; 38(2):176–181.
6. Silay MS, Hoen L, Quadackaers J, et al. Treatment of varicocele in children and adolescents: a systematic review and meta-analysis from the European Association of Urology/European Society for Paediatric Urology Guidelines Panel. *Eur Urol*. 2019;75(3):448–461.
7. Makris G, Efthymiou E, Little M, et al. Safety and effectiveness of the different types of embolic materials for the treatment of testicular varicoceles: a systematic review. *Br J Radiol*. 2018;91(1088):20170445.
8. Gandini R, Konda D, Reale CA, et al. Male varicocele: transcatheter foam sclerotherapy with sodium tetradecyl sulfate—outcome in 244 patients. *Radiology*. 2008;246(2):612–618.
9. Persad E, O'Loughlin CA, Kaur S, et al. Surgical or radiological treatment for varicoceles in subfertile men. *Cochrane Database Syst Rev*. 2021;4(4):CD000479.
10. Jing Y, Wang R, Liu Z, et al. Analysis of internal spermatic vein embolization through catheter versus laparoscopic high ligation in treatment of left varicocele. *Vascular* 2020; 28(5):583–590.

Ovarian and Pelvic Vein Embolization

Lindsay Machan, MD and
Maureen P. Kohi, MD, FSIR, FCIRSE, FAHA

Introduction (1–3)

The three most common ways pelvic venous varicosities come to clinical attention are:

1. Chronic pelvic pain. Dilated veins can be the only cause, or (importantly!) part of a multifactorial etiology. The classical presentation is a multiparous woman with pain worse at the end of the day or with long periods of standing. Dyspareunia, especially after intercourse, vulvar/perineal varicosities, and buttock pain are not uncommon.
2. Lower extremity varicose veins in an unusual distribution (e.g., labia or buttock), or leg varicosities which are resistant or recurrent after appropriate treatment.
3. Incidental finding on imaging studies in asymptomatic women. Reported incidence is 10% to 63% and if asymptomatic requires no treatment.

Assessment of the patient can be complex; on cross-sectional imaging or laparoscopy there can be dilated pelvic veins in parous women who don't have symptoms and transiently nondilated veins (especially on supine imaging) in patients who do. In addition, there can be an obstructive component, principally of the left common iliac vein (3) (see Chapter 37), or from renal vein nutcracker syndrome.

Indications

1. Chronic pelvic pain with varicosities seen on cross-sectional imaging, laparoscopy, venography, or open operation
2. Lower extremity varicose veins recurrent immediately after adequate surgical treatment, or of an atypical distribution
3. Symptomatic labial/perineal varicosities

Contraindications

1. Ovarian or pelvic veins without demonstrated reflux
2. Coexisting cause of pelvic pain not adequately treated (relative)
3. Contraindications to angiography
   a. Severe anaphylactoid reactions to contrast media
   b. Uncorrectable coagulopathy
   c. Severe renal insufficiency
4. Phobia to medical implants

Preprocedure Preparation

Pretreatment Assessment (4,5)

1. If the patient suffers from pelvic pain
   a. Detailed clinical assessment by gynecologist or pelvic pain specialist ± laparoscopy.
   b. Pelvic duplex ultrasound or magnetic resonance venography (MRV) (6). Multiple published criteria including tortuous parauterine veins ≥ 4 mm diameter with slow flow (<3 cm per second) on ultrasound; and ≥4 dilated ipsilateral parauterine veins at least 1 measuring ≥4 mm in diameter, or ovarian vein diameter ≥8 mm on MR. Ultrasound in particular is a nuanced examination and familiarity with performing it, or with the sonographer, is essential.

    c. Patient education: Before diagnostic venography, the patient should be informed that pelvic venous insufficiency is not accepted as a cause of pelvic pain by many physicians (or insurers), and that ovarian or pelvic venous reflux can be an incidental finding and not responsible for the patient's symptoms.

2. If the patient suffers from lower extremity varicosities
    a. Detailed clinical assessment by physician expert in venous disease
    b. Pelvic and lower extremity duplex ultrasound

Patient Preparation

1. Timing of the procedure in relation to menstrual or pain cycle is unimportant.
2. Oral intake restrictions per institutional protocol for IV sedation. The author's are no solids for 6 hours preprocedure, clear fluids only until 2 hours before.
3. Obtain informed consent. Ensure someone can accompany the patient home.
4. Establish a peripheral intravenous (IV).
5. Sedate with IV midazolam (Versed) and fentanyl. These patients may be anxious and require a lot of sedation, sometimes even general anesthetic.

Procedure (6–8)

1. Transjugular route
    a. Position the patient supine on the table with head turned to the left.
    b. Sterile skin preparation and draping.
    c. Puncture the jugular vein under ultrasound guidance.
    d. Using Seldinger technique, introduce a 5- to 7-Fr sheath into the jugular vein.
    e. Advance multipurpose shape (MPA) catheter through sheath into the peripheral left renal vein.
    f. Perform a left renal venogram by forceful injection of 20 mL of contrast with the patient performing a Valsalva maneuver to identify all collateral channels.
    g. If there is no reflux into the ovarian vein, and it clearly arises from the renal vein, this is considered a negative study.
    h. If there is ovarian vein reflux, direct the catheter into the main trunk of the ovarian vein and repeat injection of 20 mL of contrast with the patient performing a Valsalva maneuver to identify all varicosities and collateral channels. Include bottom of pubic bones at inferior aspect of image and obtain delayed images because varicosities may fill and drain slowly. There are multiple published venographic criteria for pelvic venous insufficiency including ovarian or utero-ovarian arcade veins >5 mm diameter, gonadal vein reflux, contrast stagnation, opacification of pelvic, labial or thigh varicosities (undulating dilated veins with delayed contrast clearance). Considering the capriciously dynamic nature of veins, the authors consider the venogram abnormal if there is reflux resulting in static flow in varicosities regardless of briskness of reflux or ovarian vein diameter.
    i. Advance the diagnostic catheter (some exchange for a balloon occlusion catheter) into the main trunk just above the major branches, or into each of the major branches of the ovarian vein. Embolize varicosities in continuity back to the main ovarian vein, and all visible collateral channels to within 2 to 5 cm of the ovarian vein origin. Methods described (without a clear "best" agent or concentration include sclerosant (liquid or foam), glue, onyx, and/or coils. One preferred method is infusing a slurry from the main ovarian vein immediately above the major bifurcation while the patient does a Valsalva maneuver, to fill all varicosities and until stasis at the end of the catheter (usually 7 to 20 mL). The basic ratio is 2 mL 3% tetradecyl sulfate (TDS), 5-mL lipiodol and at least one brick of gelfoam (enough to make consistency of oatmeal, "runniness" depending on rate of flow in the varicosities). The main ovarian vein is occluded with coils, principally to prevent reflux of the embolic liquid/slurry. As undersized coils will migrate centrally it is important to oversize. Consider a detachable coil the closer you get to the upper end of the vein.

j. Perform a left renal venogram with the catheter in the peripheral renal vein to confirm left ovarian vein occlusion and that there are no patent collaterals.

k. Direct the catheter into the right renal vein and perform a right renal venogram to ensure that the right ovarian vein does not arise from it (1% to 4% incidence).

l. If not, direct the catheter immediately anterior and inferior to the right renal vein orifice. Gentle probing along inferior vena cava wall in an up-and-down motion extending from the right renal vein orifice to the iliac confluence is performed, beginning laterally, and rotating anteriorly slightly between each sweep. It may arise anteriorly to the left of the midline.

m. A right ovarian venogram and, if needed, embolization are performed in the same fashion as described for the left.

n. Select each internal iliac vein sequentially and inject 20 mL of contrast with the patient performing a Valsalva maneuver. Some physicians perform internal iliac venography and embolization using a balloon occlusion catheter. The authors use the same MPA catheter in the fashion described earlier for selective embolization if there is reflux and varicosities.

o. To assess left common iliac vein compression select the left common femoral vein and inject 20 mL of contrast in quiet respiration and with the patient performing a Valsalva maneuver. Narrowing of the left common iliac vein is common and not always pathologic. IVUS is a more sensitive and accurate method of assessing left common iliac vein compression. Decision to treat with a venous stent (see Chapter 37) should be based on the patient's symptoms, venographic evidence of obstruction such as stasis, retrograde filling of the left internal iliac vein and well-established collateral venous pathways and/or luminal narrowing >50% on IVUS. Some treat outflow occlusion at the same time as embolization, others at a separate session if there is inadequate symptom improvement months after embolization.

p. Note: Some authors use coils alone without sclerosant, or don't routinely assess and treat internal iliac vein reflux or left common iliac vein obstruction. While there isn't level I evidence confirming improved patient outcomes, most experts in the field recommend all three.

2. Transfemoral route

   a. Sterile skin preparation as for femoral angiography.

   b. Insert a 5- to 7-Fr sheath into the right femoral vein and direct a Cobra catheter into the peripheral left renal vein, each internal iliac vein, and left common femoral vein. Selective venography and embolization are performed using the same diagnostic criteria and methods as described for the transjugular route.

   c. The catheter is exchanged for a Simmons I catheter or equivalent and directed into the right ovarian vein. A coaxial microcatheter is frequently necessary.

3. Labial varicosities

   a. Very difficult to eradicate; often multiple sclerotherapy sessions are needed.

   b. Some physicians exclude and treat ovarian and pelvic vein reflux first, others do this if there is persistence or recurrence after multiple injections.

   c. Direct puncture with 25- or 27-gauge butterfly needle under direct vision or ultrasound. Tilt table may help. Venography is not necessary in most cases.

   d. Inject sclerosant of choice (usually 0.25% to 0.5% TDS) until vein blanches (direct vision) or there is stasis of sclerosant (ultrasound).

   e. Patient to wear compression shorts ± pad for at least 2 days after. Avoid workouts for 48 hours and hot baths for 7 days.

Postprocedure Management

1. Observe the patient on bed rest for 60 minutes, and if stable and alert, discharge to a responsible adult who can drive her home.

2. Analgesic requirements vary greatly. Nonsteroidal antiinflammatory drugs (NSAIDs) or acetaminophen/codeine for 3 days is usually adequate. Consider steroids which help alleviate the pain and swelling, for example Medrol pack.
3. Patient to avoid activities more strenuous than walking for 3 days postprocedure.
4. Chronic pain syndromes are complex and improvement may be gradual. Reassuring the patient of this is an essential part of postprocedure management.
5. Follow-up pelvic ultrasound and consultation in 3 months.

Complications

1. Postembolization syndrome in 80% to 90% of patients, consisting of pain, fever, and nausea varying from minor ache to agony. It can last from a few hours to several days. Treatment is analgesia, possible addition of steroids, and avoidance of activity more strenuous than walking until the pain resolves.
2. Other significant complications are rare (9).
3. Recurrent symptoms after treatment. Exact incidence not reported but as with all venous therapies are frequent and expected. Development of reflux in a previously normal vascular bed or previously unrecognized May–Thurner syndrome are frequent causes. Repeat pelvic ultrasound and venography in the same manner as previously described. It is essential to consider that symptoms may have been only partially or not at caused by varices and may need gynecologic reassessment.

Results (9,10)

1. Technical success ranges from 96.7% to 100%.
2. Reported improvement in pain occurs in 68.3% to 100%, most commonly approximately 75%. Pain resolution reported as complete in 0% to 57.9% of studies.
3. This compares to bilateral oophorectomy and hysterectomy with subsequent hormone replacement (symptom improvement in 66% of women) and surgical ligation of the left ovarian vein (improvement in 73%).

References

1. Knuttinen MG, Xie K, Jani A, et al. Pelvic venous insufficiency: imaging diagnosis, treatment approaches, and therapeutic issues. *AJR Am J Roentgenol.* 2015;204(2):448–458.
2. Bendek B, Afuape N, Banks E, et al. Comprehensive review of pelvic congestion syndrome: causes, symptoms, treatment options. *Curr Opin Obstet Gynecol.* 2020;32(4):237–242.
3. Santoshi RKN, Lakhanpal S, Satwah V, et al. Iliac vein stenosis is an underdiagnosed cause of pelvic venous insufficiency. *J Vasc Surg Venous Lymphat Disord.* 2018;6(2):202–211.
4. Maratto S, Khilnani NM, Winokur RS. Clinical presentation, patient assessment, anatomy, pathophysiology, and imaging of pelvic venous disease. *Semin Intervent Radiol.* 2021;38(2):233–238.
5. Weston M, Soyer P, Barral M, et al. Role of interventional procedures in obstetrics and gynecology. *Radiol Clin N Am* 2020;58(2):445–462.
6. Bookwalter CA, VanBuren WM, Neisen MJ, et al. Imaging appearance and nonsurgical management of pelvic venous congestion syndrome. *Radiographics.* 2019;39(2):596–608.
7. Durham JD, Machan L. Pelvic congestion syndrome. *Semin Intervent Radiol.* 2013;30(712): 372–380.
8. Joh M, Grewal S, Gupta R. Ovarian vein embolization: how and when should it be done? *Tech Vasc Interv Radiol.* 2021;24(1):100732
9. Brown CL, Rizer M, Alexander R, et al. Pelvic congestion syndrome: systematic review of treatment success. *Semin Intervent Radiol.* 2018;35(1):35-40.
10. Daniels JP, Champaneria R, Shah L, et al. Effectiveness of embolization or sclerotherapy of pelvic veins for reducing chronic pelvic pain: a systematic review. *JVIR* 2016; 27(10): 1478–1486.

44 Thermal and Nonthermal Saphenous Vein Ablation

Ronald S. Winokur, MD, FSIR, RPVI, Kimberly L. Scherer, DO, Robert J. Min, MD, MBA, FSIR, FACR, and Neil M. Khilnani, MD, FSIR, FAVLS

Introduction

Chronic venous disease (CVD) of the lower extremity results from venous hypertension. Most commonly, this is caused by incompetent valves in the saphenous veins and their primary tributaries and less frequently by chronic deep venous obstruction and reflux after prior deep vein thrombosis (DVT). In patients with saphenous vein reflux, treatment often begins with ablation of these veins.

Thermal versus Nonthermal Ablation

Thermal ablation is the induction of nonthrombotic vein occlusion by delivery of thermal energy directly to the vein walls. Thermal ablation procedures require tumescent anesthesia (TA) for compressing and insulating the treated veins as well as for local anesthesia. Endovenous laser ablation (ELA) (also called endovenous laser treatment [EVLT]) and radiofrequency ablation (RFA) are the most commonly used thermal ablation techniques. Nonthermal, nontumescent (NTNT) techniques developed for closure of the saphenous vein include cyanoacrylate (CA) glue (VenaSeal, Medtronic, Santa Rosa, CA), mechanochemical ablation (MOCA) (ClariVein, Merit Medical, South Jordan, UT), and polidocanol endovenous microfoam (Varithena, Boston Scientific, Marlborough, MA).

The underlying mechanism of thermal and nonthermal ablative procedures is to produce irreversible occlusion and fibrosis of the vein by thermal injury, mechanical-assisted chemical injury for MOCA, early vein wall coaptation and a secondary giant cell inflammatory response for VenaSeal or protein theft endothelial denaturation for Varithena (1,2).

Thermal ablative modalities have proven track records as safe, effective, and durable treatments to eliminate varicose veins. Nonthermal techniques have also produced effective closure with decreased postprocedure discomfort and decreased risk of adjacent thermal nerve injury. In addition, VenaSeal obviates the need for use of postprocedure graduated compression stockings. The nonthermal modalities have been promoted as alternatives to thermal ablation with the potential for less intra- and postprocedure pain as well as eliminating the low incidence of injury to adjacent nerves found with lower calf thermal ablation.

Anatomy of Superficial Veins of the Leg

Successful outcomes require a thorough understanding of the disease process and the anatomy of the superficial venous system and a thorough examination utilizing duplex ultrasound (DUS). The superficial venous system of the lower extremity is composed of innumerable subcutaneous collecting veins and the saphenous trunks and their tributaries. The most recognized components of the superficial venous system are the great saphenous vein (GSV) and small saphenous vein (SSV). The saphenous veins are located between the superficial and muscular fascia in a compartment known as the saphenous space.

The GSV begins on the dorsum of the foot and ascends the medial calf and thigh to join the common femoral vein (CFV) at the fossa ovale (Fig. 44.1). Important tributaries include the anterior and posterior circumflex veins of the calf, the very common anterior accessory great saphenous vein (AA-GSV), less common posterior accessory GSV, and the superficial accessory saphenous vein (SA-SV, a

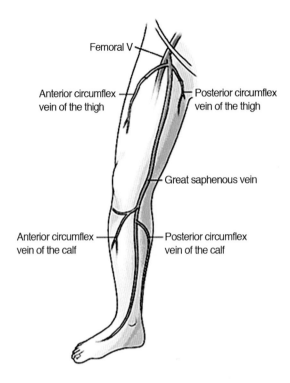

FIGURE 44.1 • Diagram of the GSV and its named tributaries.

vein running parallel to the GSV course but outside the superficial fascia). These tributary veins are often found segmentally in the calf and/or thigh but may serve as the primary flow channel when the true GSV is either congenitally very small or absent in segments. The saphenous nerve runs close to the GSV in the mid-calf and more so in the lower third of the calf.

The SSV begins on the lateral aspect of the foot, passes posterior to the lateral malleolus, and then ascends up the midline of the calf (Fig. 44.2). The cephalad termination of the SSV is variable. The classic anatomy is for the SSV to drain into the popliteal vein just above the level at which the two heads of the gastrocnemius diverge. However, a dominant popliteal termination is present in up to 60% of cases. In the remainder of cases, the SSV will also or only extend more cephalad in a space between the deep muscular and superficial fascia. These cephalad terminations of this vein are variable and include termination into a perforating vein in the posterior thigh as well as a vein that communicates with the GSV (also known as Giacomini or intersaphenous vein). Practically, combinations of the described SSV termination patterns are common in many patients. The sural nerve runs close to the SSV in the mid-calf and more closely in the lower third of the calf.

Thermal ablation has been successfully performed in the GSV, SSV, the AA-GSV, the anterior and posterior circumflex veins of the thigh, as well as the thigh extension of the SSV.

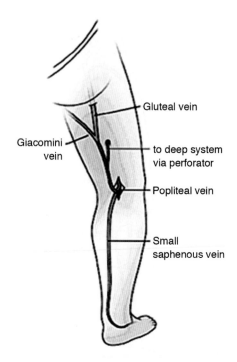

FIGURE 44.2 • Diagram of the veins of the posterior calf and thigh. The SSV begins posterior to the lateral malleolus and ascends the midline of the calf. In about two-thirds of cases, its primary termination is into the popliteal vein about 2 cm about the knee crease. In the remainder of cases, its primary termination extends more cephalad.

Indications

1. Clinical
   a. Symptoms: heaviness, aching, swelling, throbbing, itching (the so-called "HASTI" symptoms) when affecting quality of life.
   b. Signs: healed or active venous ulceration and recurrent superficial venous thrombophlebitis or spontaneous bleeding. Skin changes associated with chronic venous hypertension such as lipodermatosclerosis and atrophie blanche may also be indications.
   c. Cosmetic (restorative) concerns.
2. Clinical tools
   a. CEAP (Clinical, Etiology, Anatomy, Pathophysiology) is useful to classify the stage of CVD.
   b. The Venous Clinical Severity Score (VCSS) and the disease-specific patient-reported quality-of-life instruments including the Aberdeen Varicose Veins Score, VV-SymQ, SQOR-V, CIVIQ, and VEINS-QOL/Sym are often utilized to assess patients before and following treatment.
3. Anatomic
   a. Clinically significant saphenous vein reflux documented on DUS examination classically defined as reflux >0.5 second, although nearly all patients with clinically relevant reflux have durations >1 second.

    b. Straight vein segment for catheter-based ablation techniques.

    c. Reflux seems responsible for the clinical indication.

Contraindications

Absolute

1. Nonrefluxing saphenous vein
2. Patients in whom the saphenous vein being considered for ablation is responsible for significant antegrade collateral flow around a deep vein occlusion

Relative

1. Related to the clinical condition of the patient
   a. DVT or SVT in the prior 3 months (patients remain hypercoagulable for up to 3-months postthrombosis)
   b. Large diameter saphenous vein. Thermal ablation is successful in larger diameter veins (>12 mm diameter proximal) in small retrospective series. VenaSeal of >12 mm diameter veins may also be effective with procedural modifications. Varithena and MOCA are not recommended above 12 mm diameter given lack of data to support success
   c. Inability to adequately ambulate postprocedure
   d. Pregnancy or nursing female patients (concerns related to anesthetic use, heated blood effluent which may pass through the placenta to the fetus or exposure to drugs associated with sclerosis or adhesives). "Pump and dump" of breast milk would mitigate this contraindication in the postpartum period
   e. For thermal tumescent procedures: Liver dysfunction or allergy making it impossible to use a local anesthetic (cold saline may be useful as an alternative)
   f. Severe hypercoagulability syndromes (where risk of treatment outweighs potential benefits, despite prophylactic anticoagulants)
   g. Severe uncorrectable coagulopathy. Ablation can be performed safely and successfully on patients receiving therapeutic anticoagulation or antiplatelet agents
   h. Inability to wear compression stockings secondary to inadequate arterial circulation, hypersensitivity to the compressive materials, or musculoskeletal or neurologic limitations to donning the stocking itself for all except VenaSeal
   i. COVID-19 infection (hypercoagulability associated with cases may persist for 3 months as well)
2. Related to anatomy
   a. SA-SV less than 5 mm from the skin or GSV segments in very thin patients. With all forms of ablation this may lead to postprocedure prolonged induration and pain, hyperpigmentation and skin puckering (puckering usually in looser thigh skin) or increased rate of type IV delayed hypersensitivity to CA.
   b. Tortuous vein segments may preclude the ability to use catheter thermal ablation devices. In those cases, Varithena or ultrasound (US) guide foam sclerotherapy may be a treatment option.
   c. Postthrombotic intraluminal changes or similar changes related to prior endovenous ablation in saphenous veins with catheter-based approaches, as the catheter may not be able to traverse the relevant segments. Multiple punctures may allow application of catheter-based techniques. Varithena can also be useful in these situations since catheterization of the entire segment is not necessary. MOCA should not be used secondary to risk of device being ensnared on a web after activation.
   d. Sciatic vein reflux with thermal devices because of proximity to sciatic and common peroneal nerves. Risk of NTNT approaches for sciatic nerve vein is unknown but likely lower.

Preprocedural Evaluation

1. Complete medical history including symptoms of venous insufficiency, family history, pregnancy history, prior treatment for varicose veins, and personal or family history of DVT, SVT, and/or hypercoagulable states.
2. Directed physical examination of the lower extremity including the lower abdomen.
3. Use of the clinical tools described above.
4. Complete DUS examination of the entire deep and superficial venous system should be performed. The superficial venous examination should be performed while the patient is upright or in a steep reverse Trendelenburg position to avoid both false-negative and false-positive evaluations for the presence of significant reflux. This examination should identify all incompetent venous segments and should explain all abnormal visible veins.

Preprocedure Preparation

1. No dietary restrictions. Procedure usually is performed with only local anesthetics.
2. Obtain informed consent.
3. Use a procedure table that allows a supine patient to be tilted into both Trendelenburg position as well as elevation of the patient's head and torso.
4. Perform DUS in the upright position to mark the location and extent of the vein or veins to be ablated and the locations of important anatomic landmarks including the deep vein junctions; aneurysmal, tortuous, hypoplastic, and aplastic segments; and large vein tributaries or communication with incompetent perforating veins. The US unit should have a linear 7.5- to 13-MHz probe.
5. If performing thermal ablation, prepare TA fluid. This is often prepared by mixing 440 mL 0.9% normal saline, 50 mL 1% lidocaine (with or without epinephrine 1:100,000)), and 10 mL 8.4% sodium bicarbonate. (Note: we do not use epinephrine.)

Procedure

Thermal Ablation

1. The patient is placed on the procedure table in the reverse Trendelenburg position and prepared in standard sterile fashion. The GSV and its tributaries are treated in a supine position with the knee turned outward. The SSV and the thigh extension are treated in the prone position.
2. Using US guidance, access is obtained at the most peripheral point of the incompetent vein segment to be treated. Occasionally, more than one access point may be necessary to allow treatment of the entire incompetent segment for aplastic, hypoplastic, tortuous vein segments; previously treated veins, webs, or vein spasm preventing advancement of the ablation device; or sheath. It is recommended that when venous access for ablation is required directly into a tributary vein or into the AA-GSV that these veins are accessed first and efficiently because they are most likely to undergo spasm or empty first.
3. Insert a vascular sheath (if needed) and position the thermal ablation device typically just peripheral to the superficial epigastric vein (SEV) confluence (or 2 cm peripheral to the saphenofemoral junction [SFJ]) for the GSV. For the SSV, the catheter tip/ablation tool is positioned peripheral to the thigh extension of the SSV or just below the point that the vein angles deep to join the popliteal vein. Some laser and radiofrequency (RF) tools can be inserted without the need for a guidewire and positioned as above.
4. Place the patient in 10 to 15 degrees of Trendelenburg position.
5. Using US guidance, inject TA solution around the veins to be treated, from the entry point to the most central location to be ablated at about 5 to 10 mL per cm of vein.

a. The purpose of the tumescent fluid is to empty the vein by extrinsic compression to improve heat transfer to the vein wall, to separate the vein from surrounding structures, and provide a protective halo of fluid to prevent extravenous thermal injury to them (Fig. 44.3A,B) as well as for its anesthetic effect.

b. Tumescent delivery can be accomplished using a syringe and needles, a syringe connected to a reservoir with a one-way valve, or a needle connected to a mechanically driven foot-accentuated TA pump. A standard 25-gauge, 1.5-in-long needle is well tolerated by unsedated patients. Others use 21- to 23-gauge needles such as micropuncture or spinal needles which allow faster delivery although attention is needed to limit the TA dose to that required.

6. The thermal energy is then delivered.

a. For ELA, the laser fiber is withdrawn at a rate allowing for adequate heat transfer to the vein wall and varies depending on the wavelength and power settings of each system. Data suggest that for 810- to 980-nm laser ablation,

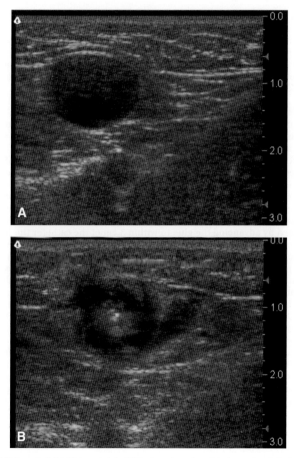

FIGURE 44.3 • **A:** Axial US image of the GSV prior to insertion of the laser sheath. **B:** Axial US image at the same level as **A** with the ELA fiber and sheath in place and surrounding TA fluid.

at least 80 J per cm is needed to accomplish successful ablation judged by occlusion and resorption at 12 months. Larger vein segment diameters and the proximal part of the vein may require larger amounts of energy. For longer wavelength lasers (1,320, 1,470, and 1,510 nm), successful vein closure can be achieved with linear energy deposition (LEED) of 72.4 to 83 J per cm (3).

   b. For RFA with the ClosureFAST system (Medtronic), withdrawal is performed in 6.5-cm segments after each 7-cm section has been treated with a standard "cycle." A double cycle of the first 7 cm is recommended in the instructions for use (IFU) but is used by many with larger diameter veins in subsequent cycles as well.

7. Aspirating the sheath if close to the tip of a laser or external compression of the skin over the tip of a thermal ablation catheter is used by some in an attempt to empty the vein and to contain any heated blood from entering the deep vein beyond the junction.

8. Upon completion of ablation and sheath removal, manual compression is applied to the vein puncture site to gain hemostasis and a sterile dressing is applied.

9. After the procedure, the treated leg is placed in a graduated compression stocking (30 to 40 mm Hg, usually thigh high) for 10 to 14 days with continuous use during the first 18 to 24 hours including overnight wear (an additional dressing and compression is often used for the first 48 hours if microphlebectomy is performed concurrently). There is no evidence to support the need for compression after simple thermal ablation but pain and bruising are less if it is used for at least a week after combined thermal ablation and microphlebectomy.

VenaSeal Cyanoacrylate Closure

1. VenaSeal is approved for use for the GSVs, accessory saphenous veins, and SSVs. Patient preparation, positioning, and target vein access are the same as for thermal ablation.

2. After venous access at the lowest level of GSV reflux, an 80-cm long 7-Fr introducer sheath provided by the manufacturer in the kit is then advanced to near the SFJ over a 0.035-in guidewire.

3. A syringe with a proprietary CA is connected to a dispensing gun, connected to a specially designed hydrophobic delivery catheter that is highly visible on DUS and designed not to induce polymerization of the adhesive and primed by advancing the glue to within 3 cm of the catheter tip. It is very important to avoid injecting saline into this catheter as the saline will initiate polymerization.

4. The delivery catheter is placed into the sheath and positioned approximately 5 cm below the SFJ. Compression with the US probe about 2 to 3 cm above the point of initial injection is initiated to block cephalad migration of CA.

5. The initial delivery of CA is performed in two injections of 0.09 mL (one 3-second trigger pull at 5 cm and then immediately afterward, a second 3-second trigger pull at 6 cm below the SFJ). The catheter is then withdrawn another 3 cm while maintaining external compression, both with the US probe as above as well as with a hand over the injection site, to coapt the vein segment containing CA for 3 minutes. Additional CA is subsequently repetitively delivered at 3-cm intervals followed by 30 seconds of US probe and hand compression. The last injection site is 4 to 6 cm from the access site. After allowing the last drop of glue to polymerize, the outer sheath is advanced back into the vein over the delivery catheter which is then removed to prevent any CA in the catheter from being left in the subcutaneous tissue. If any is left extending to the skin, it is removed as much as possible and trimmed with a scissor if still adherent.

6. Graduated compression stockings are not recommended in the IFU following VenaSeal.

Mechanicochemical Ablation

1. The ClariVein (MOCA) catheter is approved for infusion of drugs into peripheral vessels. Patient preparation, positioning, and target vein access are the same as for thermal ablation.

2. The MOCA catheter, with its dispersion wire protected within is inserted into a short sheath at the puncture site. The device will fit through the outer catheter of a micropuncture set. It is advanced to just below the SFJ; the dispersion wire can be deployed earlier and used to steer the catheter upward if any difficulty is encountered. The dispersion wire is unsheathed from the catheter and positioned 1 to 2 cm from the SFJ under US guidance.

3. The patient position is changed from reverse Trendelenburg to flat.

4. The catheter wire rotation is activated at approximately 3,500 rpm for 2 to 10 seconds to induce venospasm and prevent central flow of sclerosant.

5. The catheter is withdrawn at a maximum rate of 1.5 mm per second (7 seconds per cm) with simultaneous instillation of 1.5% sodium tetradecyl sulfate. The delivery of the drug is titrated to spread out over the full length of the vein, generally 6 to 10 mL in the GSV and 2 to 4 mL in the SSV based on the vein diameter as recommended by the manufacturer. After ablation of the first 10 cm, if the treated segment still has flow, readvance the catheter and retreat the segment a second time. The tip of the device is then resheathed and removed and manual compression applied to the puncture site.

6. The patient is placed in a graduated compression stocking postprocedure, which is worn during the day for 10 to 14 days.

Polidocanol Endovenous Microfoam (Varithena)

1. Varithena is approved for use for the GSV, accessory saphenous veins, and their varicose tributaries. In addition to marking the course of the incompetent GSV, the SFJ, any mid-thigh perforating vein, and high calf paratibial perforating veins should be marked. The skin 5 cm below the SFJ is also marked for ease of identification. Finally, the varicose tributaries that are to be treated at the same time are also marked including the reentry perforating veins.

2. The patient is prepped in a similar fashion to thermal ablation.

3. The target vein is accessed with an angiocatheter or micropuncture set. The optimal initial access is in the mid-thigh, unless a mid-thigh perforating vein is found in which case the access needs to be at a higher or more central level. Multiple access sites may allow more targeted delivery of the drug with less dispersion of drug to nontarget tributaries and perforating veins in longer target vein segments. Do not to access too close to the SFJ. The catheter is then connected to a saline-filled connecting tube and confirmed intraluminal by aspiration of blood flushed with saline and secured to the skin with tape.

4. The Varithena canister is charged according to the IFU and allowed to sit for 1 minute.

5. A specifically designed syringe is connected to the canister and 3 mL of Varithena is purged to eliminate air in the syringe and canister top. Then 5 mL of Varithena is withdrawn into the syringe and left on the canister for an additional 3 seconds.

6. The leg is then elevated to at least 45 degrees, which can be accomplished with Trendelenburg bed positioning. The syringe is then removed and an initial aliquot of the drug is injected into the connecting tube under US guidance and while manually compressing the vein below the IV access. When the injection reaches approximately 3 to 5 cm below the SFJ, the injection is stopped temporarily and pressure is placed on the GSV just above this level (to prevent foam progression to the CFV) until venous spasm occurs, which generally takes up to 3 minutes. Additional drug is then injected distally after releasing pressure in that location to fill any distal GSV and visible varicose vein tributaries that the physician wishes to treat (2). Additional needle or IV access for injections into

the tributary varices can then be performed with pressure placed over important perforating veins to minimize filling of the deep venous system. A maximum of 5 mL per injection, for a total of 15 mL per session, are the maximum amounts recommended in the IFU.

7. A 30 to 40 mm Hg, thigh high graduated compression stocking is placed, with or without additional compression rolls, over the treated veins. The patient's leg is lowered and the patient allowed to ambulate. The compression is worn for 2 days without taking it off. At that point, the pads are removed and the compression is continued for 2 weeks, except to sleep or shower, similar to thermal ablation.

8. The patient may need a second treatment in approximately 40% of cases. In general, they return after about 1 to 2 weeks for assessment and possible retreatment. An opened Varithena canister may be reused with a new sterile dispensing cap each time for 30 days for several patients, so coordination of future treatments is recommended.

Postprocedure Management

1. Ambulation is initiated immediately and encouraged following all of the aforementioned procedures. We recommend 2 hours of walking per day for 2 weeks and at least a 1-hour walk immediately following the procedure, although no scientific data exist for this recommendation.

2. Vigorous exercise is generally discouraged for the first 1 to 2 weeks following treatment. Long periods of immobility such as those that occur with long air flights or car rides soon after endovenous ablation should likely be discouraged to minimize venous stasis that could increase the risk of DVT. These practices are not based on data.

3. Patients should return for clinical and DUS evaluation to confirm vein closure and exclude complications.
   a. If a physician is attempting to identify thrombus extension across the saphenopopliteal junction (SPJ) or SFJ, a DUS in the first 72 hours postprocedure seems to be necessary. However, given the transient and benign clinical course of endothermal heat-induced thrombus (EHIT) extension in the deep veins at the junctions as well as the seemingly low rate of thrombosis in the deep veins of the calf, the necessity of evaluating all patients at 72 hours for thrombus cannot be substantiated.
   b. Clinical evaluation and DUS at 1-month postablation allow one to assess the early outcome of the ablation and plan further treatment as needed.

4. The value of periodic postprocedure DUS is controversial. However, follow-up DUS of a treated vein is not needed once it is no longer visible. Periodic follow-up DUS may be needed to evaluate the etiology of any symptom or varicose vein recurrences.
   a. The natural history of a successfully thermally treated truncal vein includes acute vein wall thickening without significant intraluminal thrombus in the first few weeks after treatment. This is followed over the next few months by progressive vein shrinkage and eventual disappearance on US examination (4).
   b. The disappearance of the treated vein apparently occurs more slowly after ClariVein and Varithena, with skip segments and recanalization more common. Patients with recanalizations found on DUS after Varithena and MOCA ablation have similar clinical improvement to those with successful closure with thermal devices as measured by generic and disease specific QOL tools.
   c. After VenaSeal ablation, the vein lumen appears more echogenic immediately after the ablation and will remain echogenic and not completely shrink when followed over the first year, with few recanalizations beyond 6 months.

Results

1. Thermal ablation
   a. ELA and RFA result in durable obliteration of the GSV in 88% to 100% of cases and 88% to 96% of cases in the SSV with up to 5-year follow-up.
   b. Successfully treated veins occlude and shrink with time and become difficult to detect. The average period for a treated GSV to shrink to a fibrous cord of <2.5 mm diameter is 6 months. At 1 year following ELA of the GSV, 95% of the treated segments were not visualized, 2% were occluded but visible, and 2% were still patent.
   c. There is no clear difference in outcomes between RFA and ELA; however, four trials have suggested decreased immediate postprocedure pain with RFA and higher long-term venous closure rates with ELA although this difference is very small (5).
2. VenaSeal
   a. The VeClose trial demonstrated GSV closure rates of 100% at 1 month, 99% at 3 months, 97.2% at 12 months, 95.3% at 24 months, and 94.4% at 36 months following CA closure (6).
3. MOCA
   a. In a clinical trial of 30 veins treated with MOCA, the primary closure rate at 260 days was 96.7% with no adverse events (AEs) up to 6 months following treatment.
   b. This study also noted no complaints of pain during the procedure, which only required 1 mL of local anesthesia at the cannulation site and no postprocedure bruising.
   c. A systematic review of 1,521 vein (1,267 GSV and 254 SSV) showed pooled anatomical success of 92% at short-term follow-up (less than 8 weeks), 92% at 6 months, 91% at 12 months, 91% at 2 years, and 87% at 3 years (7).
   d. A recent RCT comparing MOCA to RF and laser demonstrated a 1-year occlusion rate of 100% for thermal and 82% for MOCA with similar improvements in QOL and a lower postprocedure sensory disturbance rate with MOCA (0% MOCA vs. 8% with thermal ablation) (8).
4. Varithena
   a. The VANISH II trial reported the outcomes of 232 patients randomized to receive ablation with polidocanol endovenous foam or placebo with 8-week follow-up. Treatment with Varithena showed a statistically significant improvement in patient-reported outcomes Varicose Vein Symptom Questionnaire (VVSymQ), appearance from the patient perspective and by a blinded physician, and DUS response (63% and 86% closure rate with 0.5% and 1% polidocanol foam, respectively) at 3 months (2).
   b. Pooled data showed a 77.7% moderate to much improved symptoms relief following treatment with Varithena (0.5%, 1%, and 2%).
   c. 56 patients out of the original 230 enrolled in the VANISH II trial were assessed at 1 year for follow-up demonstrating 85% of patients demonstrating VVSymQ score reduction (2).

Complications

1. Thermal ablation
   a. Most AEs following endovenous ablation are minor (9).
      (1) Soreness, bruising, tenderness, and induration over the treated segment frequently occur and normally resolve by 7 to 14 days. Following GSV ablation, patients may develop a feeling of tightness similar to that after a strained muscle in the medial thigh, which is self-limited and usually improves with stretching, the use of nonsteroidal antiinflammatory drugs and graduated compression stockings.

(2) Superficial phlebitis of the varicose tributaries is reported in about 5% of cases and can occasionally be avoided with the concurrent use of ambulatory phlebectomy if ablation isolates the inflow and outflow from a varicose vein tributary (9).

b. Significant AEs include sensory nerve injuries, skin burns, and DVT. The overall rate of these complications is higher at low case–volume centers. Dysesthesia and skin burns have been reported in a small number of cases, and DVT in less than 1% of patients after ELA and RFA. The risk of saphenous and sural injury when treating in the lower third of the calf is higher with thermal ablation. Recent data suggest this risk is small with adequate TA and avoiding treating vein segments adjacent to nerves. For most patients, treatment of the lower GSV and SSV is felt not needed, even when it is refluxing, except in C5 and C6 patients.

2. VenaSeal

a. Reddening and tenderness to palpation over the treated vein was seen in 11.4% in a multicenter trial of 70 patients (1).

b. In the initial feasibility trial in 38 patients, there were 8 (21.1%) incidences of threadlike thrombus extension across the SFJ; however, in the follow-up multicenter trial using a greater starting point distance from the SFJ, there was only 1 case (1.4%) of thrombus extension across the SFJ (1).

c. Mild AEs such as phlebitis, paresthesia, access site infection, and superficial thrombophlebitis were similar for RFA and CA closure in the first 3 months postprocedure.

d. In a cohort of 379 limbs in 286 patients treated with VenaSeal CA closure, 18 patients (5.8% of treatments, 6.3% of limbs) developed redness and itching over the treated vein (likely a hypersensitivity reaction) with 4.2% representing mild reactions, (responding in 24 to 48 hours to oral antihistamines, topical steroids and NSAID) 1.3% moderate (not responding in 24 to 48 hours but responding to a Medrol dose pack). More severe allergies have been reported with recurrent generalized hives in one patient in this series requiring vein and CA removal (0.3%). The incidence anecdotally is reduced by not using VenaSeal in patients with or at risk to CA sensitivity (chronic occupational exposure or a history of Krazy Glue [Elmer, Westerville, OH]), Histoacryl (B Braun, Melsungen, Germany), DermaBond (Ethicon, Raritan, NJ), artificial nail or eyelash sensitivity or patients with an extensive allergy history, avoiding glue deposition in the subcutaneous tissue and avoiding treatment of veins <5 to 10 mm from the skin. Cases of glue being extruded several days to weeks later are described but can be avoidable as mentioned. More concerning granuloma formation with extrusion through the skin required local excision or vein and glue removal along the treatment zone have been reported (10). The manufacturer estimates this to occur in about 1 in 10,000 cases based on post market data collected.

e. No DVT or pulmonary emboli were identified in patients up to 36 months postprocedure (6).

3. MOCA

a. In 1,464 veins treated in the systematic review that reported complications, 3 cases of DVT were reported (0.2%) and 2 cases of PE (0.1%). Transient paresthesia occurred in 1 patient (<0.1%) (7).

4. Varithena

a. Polidocanol endovenous microfoam (PEM) has a low risk of AE with 95% of them classified as mild or moderate and no cerebrovascular events or migraines.

b. At the approved formulation (1% PEM), the most commonly reported AE was retained coagulum (27.6%), which can be expected with chemical sclerosis.

c. The incidences of DVT (with average volume of thrombus about the size of a peanut M&M and mostly in calf veins), CFV thrombus extension, and superficial thrombophlebitis were 8.6%, 6.9%, and 3.4%, respectively. None of the cases of CFV thrombus extension were occlusive. There was no difference in the outcome of the patients who received anticoagulation to treat a thrombotic complication, which was used in about half of the patients with such complications.

References

1. Proebstle TM, Alm J, Dimitri S, et al. The European multicenter cohort study on cyanoacrylate embolization of refluxing great saphenous veins. *J Vasc Surg Venous Lymphat Disord.* 2014;2(2):1–6.
2. Todd KL III, Wright DI, Group V-I. The VANISH-2 study: a randomized, blinded, multicenter study to evaluate the efficacy and safety of polidocanol endovenous microfoam 0.5% and 1.0% compared with placebo for the treatment of saphenofemoral junction incompetence. *Phlebology.* 2014;29(9):608–618.
3. Cowpland CA, Cleese AL, Whiteley MS. Factors affecting optimal linear endovenous energy density for endovenous laser ablation in incompetent lower limb truncal veins – A review of the clinical evidence. *Phlebology.* 2017;32(5):299–306.
4. Pichot O, Kabnick LS, Creton D, et al. Duplex ultrasound scan findings two years after great saphenous vein radiofrequency endovenous obliteration. *J Vasc Surg.* 2004;39(1) 189–195.
5. Gloviczki P, Comerota AJ, Dalsing MC, et al. The care of patients with varicose veins and associated chronic venous diseases: clinical practice guidelines of the Society for Vascular Surgery and the American Venous Forum. *J Vasc Surg.* 2011;53:2S–48S.
6. Morrison N, Kolluri R, Vasquez M, et al. Comparison of cyanoacrylate closure and radiofrequency ablation for the treatment of incompetent great saphenous veins: 36-month outcomes of the VeClose randomized controlled trial. *Phlebology.* 2019;34(6): 380–390.
7. Witte ME, Zeebregts CJ, de Borst GJ, et al. Mechanochemical endovenous ablation of saphenous veins using the ClariVein: a systematic review. *Phlebology.* 2017;32(10): 649–657.
8. Vahaaho S, Mahmoud O, Halmesmaki K, et al. Randomized clinical trial of mechanochemical and endovenous thermal ablation of great saphenous varicose veins. *Br J Surg.* 2019;106(5):548–554.
9. Khilnani NM, Grassi CJ, Kundu S et al. Multi-society consensus quality improvement guidelines for the treatment of lower-extremity superficial venous insufficiency with endovenous thermal ablation from the Society of Interventional Radiology, Cardiovascular Interventional Radiological Society of Europe, American College of Phlebology and Canadian Interventional Radiology Association. *J Vasc Interv Radiol.* 2010;21(1): 14–31.
10. Gibson K, Minjarez R, Rinehardt E, et al. Frequency and severity of hyperpigmentation in patients after VenaSeal cyanoacrylate treatment of superficial venous insufficiency. *Phlebology.* 2020;35(5):337–344.

45 Varicose, Perforator, and Spider Veins: Liquid Ablation and Microphlebectomy

Kimberly L. Scherer, DO, Neil M. Khilnani, MD, FSIR, FAVLS, and Ronald S. Winokur, MD, FSIR, RPVI

Introduction (1,2)

Distention and dysfunction of the small veins which ultimately feed into the axial superficial venous system can occur alone or in association with truncal vein reflux. Abnormal small veins include telangiectasias, reticular veins and varicose veins. Telangiectasias, also known as spider veins are intradermal, flat red vessels smaller than 1 mm in diameter. Telangiectasias are present in up to 28.9% of men and 40.9% of women. Reticular veins are subdermal veins with a cyanotic hue and measure 1 to 3 mm in diameter. Varicose veins are larger, ropy veins which measure >3 mm in diameter. Risk factors for these abnormal veins include heredity, pregnancy, female hormones, weight gain, and prolonged sitting or standing.

Perforator veins connect the superficial and deep venous systems. When incompetent, venous hypertension can result in skin ulceration, which can benefit from perforator vein closure.

Sclerotherapy is the primary treatment for telangiectasias and reticular veins. Ambulatory Phlebectomy (aka Microphlebectomy) and Sclerotherapy are the primary treatments for varicose veins in cases where they arise from axial vein reflux or alone. When managing patients with lower extremity varicose veins, it is important to assess for the cause of varicosities and begin treatment with incompetent truncal or axial veins prior to treating the resultant tributaries and varicosities.

Sclerotherapy

Indications (1,3)
1. Spider and reticular veins
   a. Cosmesis
2. Varicose veins
   a. Cosmesis
   b. Symptom relief
   c. Remnant disease after surgical or endovenous treatment of truncal reflux
3. Incompetent perforator veins
   a. All treatments of coexisting superficial reflux have been exhausted
   b. Diameter >3.5 mm
   c. Reflux >0.5 seconds
   d. Close proximity to an active or recently healed venous ulceration

Contraindications
1. Absolute
   a. Allergy to sclerosing agent
   b. Acute thrombophlebitis/deep vein thrombosis (DVT)
2. Relative
   a. Pregnancy/breastfeeding
   b. Needle phobia
   c. Hypercoagulable state
   d. Inability to tolerate compression
   e. Peripheral vascular disease with ABI <0.6
   f. Systemic or infectious skin disease
   g. Known patent foramen ovale (for physician compounded foam)

Table 45.1 Common Agents Used for Sclerotherapy

Detergents—disrupt endothelial cell membrane
  Sodium tetradecyl sulfate (Sotradecol)
  Polidocanol (Aethoxysclerol)
  Sodium morrhuate (Scleromate)
  Ethanolamine oleate (Ethamolin)

Osmotic agents—endothelial cell dehydration and cell membrane denaturation
  Hypertonic saline
  Saline solution with dextrose (Sclerodex)

Chemical irritants—caustic endothelial destruction
  Chromated glycerin (Sclermo)
  Polyiodinated iodine

---

h. Inability to ambulate/impending immobilization (e.g., surgery or prolonged travel)
i. Deep venous obstructive disease and/or postthrombotic changes

Preprocedure Preparation

1. Detailed history and physical examination should be performed. The patient's expectations should be clearly defined and, if necessary, realistically modified.
2. Duplex ultrasound. If reflux is demonstrated in the saphenous or other superficial truncal veins, this must be treated first. Some practitioners will perform sclerotherapy in the same session after truncal vein ablation; we prefer to wait >2 to 12 weeks (tributary improvement may occur up to 12 weeks following ablation).
3. Consider taking pretreatment photographs for documentation and comparison with the postoperative results.
4. Informed consent should include discussion that multiple treatment sessions are typically necessary and that new vessels may develop over time.

Procedure (2,4)

A list of injectable agents used for sclerotherapy is shown in Table 45.1. Only the detergent sclerosants sodium tetradecyl sulfate and polidocanol are U.S. Food and Drug Administration (FDA) approved for intravenous injections.

Spider and Reticular Veins

1. The guiding principle is to ablate the desired vessels while avoiding damage to normal collaterals and surrounding tissue by using the lowest effective volume and concentration of sclerosant. Suggested concentrations of commonly used sclerosing agents are listed in Table 45.2.
2. There is no evidence to demonstrate advantage of foam over liquid sclerotherapy of reticular and spider veins. Adverse reactions may be more common with foam.

Table 45.2 Suggested Concentrations for Small Vessel Sclerotherapy

	Reticular Veins and Venulectasias (%)	Telangiectasias (Spider Veins, %)
Hypertonic saline	23.4	11.7
Sodium tetradecyl sulfate	0.25–0.4	0.1–0.2
Polidocanol	0.5–1.0	0.25–0.75

3. Larger veins are treated before smaller vessels and injections should begin at the most central point of reflux progressing peripherally (i.e., Varicose and reticular veins before spider veins).
4. *First*, clean the skin with sterile solution or alcohol. No sedation or anesthesia is generally required.
5. Puncture a straight segment of the spider or reticular vein with a small needle, usually 27- to 30-gauge, bevel up.
6. Ensure there is blood return with aspiration (may not be possible with spider veins).
7. Slowly and gently inject 0.1 to 0.4 mL of sclerosant with no smaller than a 3-mL syringe. The injected area will change color. Avoid blanching skin to minimize risk of adverse events. Remove needle and compress. Massaging may enhance sclerosant distribution.

Varicose Veins

1. Larger veins are treated before smaller vessels and injections should begin at the most central point of reflux progressing peripherally.
2. The concentration of drug and volume will increase with larger-diameter veins. Multiple injections result in more effective sclerosis and less nontarget vein occlusions compared with single injections when a long vein or plexus of veins are treated.
3. *First*, clean the skin with sterile solution or alcohol. No sedation or anesthesia is generally required.
4. Using sterile technique, cannulate the vessel with a 25-gauge or larger needle (if using foam, a smaller needle disrupts the bubbles).
5. Ultrasound or transillumination guidance can be used to guide the puncture and to monitor dissemination of the sclerosant during injection.
6. If using a liquid sclerosant inject until the target vein is thought to be filled. *When using foam*, target and nontarget vein filling can be monitored by ultrasound.
7. Foam sclerotherapy (injection of a detergent sclerosing agent mixed with air or CO_2, or CO_2/O_2 mixtures) requires a smaller volume of sclerosing agent, results in a lesser dilution with blood, achieves a homogeneous effect in the injected veins, and is visible on ultrasound.
   a. Foam is at least twice as strong as the liquid drug from which it is prepared.
   b. 0.5% to 3% sodium tetradecyl sulfate or 1% polidocanol are mixed 1:4 with room air (or other more physiologic gas) using two syringes connected by a three-way stopcock, alternatively moving the syringe pistons up and down with 10 to 20 movements to create physician compounded foam.
   c. The syringe containing foam is then connected to a needle in the vein and depending on the vein size, total volumes of 3 to 5 mL are typically injected (until foam is distributed throughout the desired vein).
   d. Commercial 1% polidocanol CO_2/O_2 foam is also available (Varithena, Boston Scientific, Marlborough, MA).
   e. Guidelines suggest that adverse reactions are felt more common when >10 mL of foam are injected per session.
   f. Anecdotal evidence suggests ultrasound-guided foam injection of the periulcer venous plexus facilitates the rate of ulcer healing.

Perforator Veins

1. Sclerotherapy is typically performed with foam under ultrasound guidance.
2. With patient supine cannulate the vein, or preferably a related tributary close to the perforating vein, with a 21- to 27-gauge needle.
3. Foam is injected until just before it extends into the deep vein, usually with a volume of 0.5 to 1 mL injected at each point. Ask the patient to contract the calf several times after the injection is completed to dilute the foam that invariably passes into the deep venous system.

4. Other treatment methods include surgery, thermal ablation with laser or radiofrequency, and occlusion with cyanoacrylate. These techniques are not discussed in this chapter (Table 45.2).

Postprocedure Management

1. Compression after sclerotherapy improves clinical outcomes, but there is no consensus on duration or intensity. Although 3 days of compression results in greater improvement than no compression, 3 weeks of continuous compression with 20 to 30 mm Hg or 30 to 40 mm Hg graded compression stockings yielded the best results in a single study.
   a. Patient compliance can be an issue; if a patient does not tolerate compression well, graded compression stockings should at the least be worn the first night and then daily for 1 week.
2. The patient should begin walking immediately after treatment but avoid aggressive exercise for 1 week.
3. Nonsteroidal antiinflammatory drugs (NSAIDs) may be taken as needed after sclerotherapy.
4. Arrange further small vessel treatment session at 2- to 8-week intervals for further injections.
5. Expression of intravascular coagulum (trapped blood) with an 18- to 25-gauge needle at the same intervals has been demonstrated to reduce the intensity, duration, and likelihood of permanent skin staining post sclerotherapy.

Results

1. Small vein sclerotherapy—there are no publications of evidence-based treatment results. Published reports indicate 60% to 80% patient satisfaction and statistically significant reduction of detectable telangiectasias compared with untreated regions (5).
2. Nontruncal varicosities—limited published data are available (3).
3. Veins >5 mm diameter—81% technical success (occlusion seen by Duplex ultrasound)
4. Veins <5 mm diameter—92% technical success
5. Persistence of occlusion at 2-year follow-up
   a. 53% after foam injection
   b. 12% after liquid sclerotherapy
6. Perforator sclerotherapy—with perforator incompetence alone, sclerotherapy can result in rapid ulcer healing in 86.5% of patients with a mean time of healing of 36 days (6).

Complications (7)

1. Allergic reactions—0.3% including anaphylaxis. Having appropriate resuscitation medications and equipment available and knowledge of their use is required.
2. Bruising—common and self-limited
3. Hyperpigmentation—10% to 30%
4. Telangiectatic matting (development of fine red telangiectasias in the area of treatment)—15% to 20%. This can occur spontaneously but may be due to rapid injection, too high concentration of sclerosant or injection of veins without correction of axial or perforator reflux to the area. In many cases, it resolves spontaneously or after injection of refluxing inflow veins, but in others it may persist permanently.
5. Superficial thrombophlebitis—thrombosis (not sclerosis) of nontarget veins.
6. Tissue necrosis (cutaneous ulceration)—most common with hypertonic saline but may be seen with any sclerosant. The cause may be extravasation, excessive pressure resulting in arterial filling across the capillary network, or direct injection into an arterial branch.
7. DVT—rare, but more common with larger doses (concentration and volume) foam and underlying coagulopathy. The natural history of these may be different

than typical DVT as they are likely secondary to direct chemical injury rather than a systemic activation of the coagulation system.

8. Foam sclerotherapy-specific adverse effects—especially in patients with a patent foramen ovale.
   a. Visual (scotoma or amaurosis)
   b. Neurologic (transient ischemic attack [TIA], stroke, migraine)
   c. Pulmonary symptoms (cough, pain)

Management of Complications (8)

1. Extravasation—if there is extravasation of a large volume or high concentration of sclerosant, immediate dilution by regional injection of hyaluronidase (75 units in 3 mL), normal saline, lidocaine, or a mixture of the latter two should be performed.
2. Hyperpigmentation—reassurance is usually adequate as spontaneous resolution occurs in 70% of patients at 6 months and 99% at 1 year. Removal of intravascular coagulum beginning 3 weeks after each treatment helps mitigate the duration and intensity of pigmentation and reduce the risk of permanent pigmentation.
3. Telangiectatic matting
   a. May resolve spontaneously in 3 to 12 months.
   b. Gentle sclerotherapy and treatment of feeding veins can provide resolution.
   c. Can be permanent.
4. Superficial thrombophlebitis—treatment is with compression stockings, NSAIDs, evacuation of the liquefied thrombus.
5. Tissue necrosis—may be secondary to extravasation or injection into an arterial branch. If blanching of the skin is encountered while injecting sclerosant, massage, topical 2% nitroglycerin ointment, or both may lessen or prevent necrosis. If the patient develops skin necrosis after sclerotherapy, standard wound care with debridement of any necrotic tissue and dressings is necessary. Consultation with a dermatologic or plastic surgeon would be of value with larger or deep ulcers in the absence of local expertise with wound care.

Microphlebectomy

Indications

1. Varicose veins
   a. Cosmesis
   b. Symptom relief
   c. Remnant disease after surgical or endovenous treatment of truncal reflux

Contraindications (9)

1. Absolute
   a. Infectious dermatitis/cellulitis in surrounding areas
   b. Severe peripheral edema
   c. Severe arterial insufficiency with ABI <0.6
   d. Seriously ill patients
2. Relative
   a. Therapeutic anticoagulation
   b. Hypercoagulable states
   c. Pregnancy

Preprocedure Preparation

1. Detailed history and physical examination should be performed. The patient's expectations should be clearly defined and, if necessary, realistically modified.
2. Duplex ultrasound. If reflux is demonstrated in the saphenous or other superficial truncal veins, this should be treated first or in the same treatment session as microphlebectomy.

3. Clear mapping of varicose tributaries to be treated and discussion of patient expectations.

Procedure (9)

1. Varicose veins marked on the skin prior to the procedure with surgical marker. Transillumination is often used to clearly define the location of the varicosities. Ultrasound can be of value as well. Marking in the position the procedure will be performed is recommended.
2. Skin cleaned with sterile solution and sterile field draped in a Trendelenburg position.
3. Tumescent anesthesia administered in the perivenous tissues using a 25-gauge needle.
4. Two to 3 mm incisions or needle punctures can be made with a no. 15 or 11 blade, or 18- or 16-gauge needle. Incisions/punctures should be made along Langer's lines to minimize scarring.
5. Phlebectomy hook is inserted through the puncture site and used to grasp the vein, which is brought to the skin and through the opening using a "windshield wiper" motion. Care is used not to hook nerves or lymphatics.
   a. The most commonly used phlebectomy hooks are Müller, Oesch, Tretbar, Ramelet, Varady, and Dortu-Martimbeau.
6. The vein is grasped with fine-tipped, serrated clamps and removed with gentle traction. As the vein is removed it is regrasped at the skin level with clamps. Very often, the vein will tear; compression over the vein tunnel for a few minutes will control any bleeding. Compression may be applied while the next segment is hooked and removed.
7. Another incision is made and the segments are removed sequentially along the course of the marked pathway.
8. If the vein does not tear but requires too much tension to remove or is painful secondary to branches, you can ligate the vein with a suture, transect above the suture and release the vein back into the soft tissues.
9. The procedure is completed when the desired vein segments are completely addressed.

Postprocedure Management

1. Steri-Strips may be used at incisions to assist in healing although our preference is to leave them open to drain any blood and tumescent anesthetic.
2. Absorbent pads for eccentric compression and 30 to 40 mm Hg compression stockings or bandages are applied immediately after the procedure.
3. Patients are instructed to use the bandages or graduated compression stockings for 48 hours without taking them off. Thereafter, they should use the graduated compression stockings for 1 to 2 weeks postprocedure, except to sleep and shower.
4. Ambulation of at least 1 to 2 hours per day is encouraged postprocedure and vigorous activity or exercise is discouraged for 7 to 10 days.
5. Bruising and mild tenderness is to be expected and can be managed with NSAIDs.

Results

1. Overall effective treatment option for varicose veins, however no large studies have been performed directly comparing microphlebectomy to sclerotherapy.

Complications (8,10)

1. Skin blistering (1.3% to 20%)—usually related to tight bandages or movement of the dressings under the compression, especially over bony prominences such as the knee and ankle.
2. Bleeding/hematoma (0.1%).
3. Superficial phlebitis (1.1% to 2.8%)—often the result of segments of the vein that are retained between segments that are removed. Usually resolves on its own over a few weeks.

4. Wound infection (0.07%).
5. Nerve damage (dysesthesia or hypoesthesia, temporary or permanent)
   a. Paresthesias for small nerve injuries occur in 0.2% to 4.6%.
   b. Common peroneal nerve injury <1%—use extreme care or avoid treatment when the veins pass over the superficial course of this nerve between the lateral popliteal fossa and the fibular head. Injury to this motor and sensory nerve may include foot drop.
6. Telangiectatic matting (0.5% to 9.5%)—relatively unusual in our experience.
7. Hyperpigmentation of scars (0.01% to 4.6%).

Management of Complications
1. Blisters can be managed conservatively and usually resolve on their own.
2. Pigmentation, telangiectatic matting, superficial phlebitis—see above in Sclerotherapy section.
3. Temporary dysesthesia—no treatment required, it may resolve spontaneously.

References

1. Winokur RS, Khilnani NM. Superficial veins: treatment options and techniques for saphenous veins, perforators, and tributary veins. *Tech Vasc Interv Radiol*. 2014;17(2):82–89.
2. Sadick N, Khilnani N, Morrison N, eds. *Practical Approach to the Management and Treatment of Venous Disorders*. Springer-Verlag; 2013.
3. Leopardi D, Hoggan BL, Fitridge RA, et al. Systematic review of treatments for varicose veins. *Ann Vasc Surg*. 2009;23(2):264–276.
4. Coleridge Smith P. Foam and liquid sclerotherapy for varicose veins. *Phlebology*. 2009;24(Suppl 1):62–72.
5. Hamel-Desnos C, Allaert FA. Liquid versus foam sclerotherapy. *Phlebology*. 2009;24(6):240–246.
6. Masuda EM, Kessler DM, Lurie F, et al. The effect of ultrasound-guided sclerotherapy of incompetent perforator veins on venous clinical severity and disability scores. *J Vasc Surg*. 2006;43(3):551–556.
7. Guex JJ, Allaert FA, Gillet JL, et al. Immediate and midterm complications of sclerotherapy: report of a prospective multicenter registry of 12,173 sclerotherapy sessions. *Dermatol Surg*. 2005;31(2):123–128.
8. Weiss MA, Hsu JT, Neuhaus I, et al. Consensus for sclerotherapy. *Dermatol Surg*. 2014;40(12):1309–1318.
9. Kabnick LS, Ombrellino M. Ambulatory phlebectomy. *Semin Intervent Radiol*. 2005;22(3):218–224.
10. Olivencia JA. Complications of ambulatory phlebectomy. Review of 1000 consecutive cases. *Dermatol Surg*. 1997;23(1):51–54.

SECTION IV
NONVASCULAR PROCEDURES

46 Biopsy Procedures of the Lung, Mediastinum, and Chest Wall

Matthew D. Cham, MD, Claudia I. Henschke, PhD, MD, and David F. Yankelevitz, MD

Indications

1. Evaluation of a solitary pulmonary nodule (solid, part-solid, and nonsolid nodules) with features suspicious for primary lung cancer and lacking benign features such as fat composition or calcification in a benign pattern (1,2)
2. Evaluation of pulmonary nodules with documented growth at a malignant rate
3. Evaluation of positron emission tomography (PET)-positive pulmonary lesions that are suspicious for malignancy
4. Evaluation of pulmonary nodules as part of a staging strategy in patients with known malignancies (lung cancer and extrathoracic malignancies)
5. Obtaining tissue for molecular and genetic characterization to guide therapy
6. Evaluation of focal pulmonary infections that are refractory to standard therapy
7. Evaluation of pleural masses, pleural thickening, or pleural fluid collections
8. Evaluation of mediastinal masses, hilar masses, and lymphadenopathy
9. Evaluation of chest wall masses and lytic rib lesions

Contraindications

1. An uncooperative patient (considered by some as the sole absolute contraindication)
2. Bleeding diathesis (international normalized ratio [INR] ≥ 1.5, platelet count <50,000 per μL)
3. Medications associated with increased risk of bleeding (relative risk, some or all can be discontinued prior to procedure; also depends on the location of the lesion)
4. Severe bullous emphysema
5. Contralateral pneumonectomy or severely limited function in the contralateral lung
6. Intractable cough
7. Suspected hydatid cyst (due to risk of an anaphylactic reaction)
8. Possible pulmonary arteriovenous malformation (AVM), vascular aneurysm, or vessel supplying a pulmonary sequestration (intralobar or extralobar)
9. Pulmonary hypertension (especially when biopsy of a central lesion is considered)
10. Patients on positive pressure ventilation

Preprocedure Preparation

1. Explain or provide information regarding the procedure and its possible complications to the patient 1 week prior to the biopsy if performed in the outpatient setting. Referring clinicians can also provide suitable information about the

Table 46.1 **Needles Used for Transthoracic Needle Biopsy**

Type of Needle	Brand and Manufacturer	Commonly Used Gauge
Aspiration needle	Chiba (Cook Medical, Bloomington, IN)	20–25
Aspiration needle that also yields tissue fragments	Westcott (BD Medical, Franklin Lakes, NJ)	20–22
	Turner (Cook Medical)	18–22
Coaxial needle system	Greene (Cook Medical)	Outer needle: 19 Inner needle: 22
Cutting needle with spring-activated handle	Biopty (BD Bard, Tempe, AZ) Temno (Merit Medical, South Jordan, UT)	18–20

procedure at that time which can be reviewed prior to the procedure when obtaining consent.

2. Discontinue aspirin 5 days before biopsy when possible. Discontinue other nonsteroidal antiinflammatory drugs (NSAIDs) 2 days prior to the procedure. Patients on oral anticoagulants should be switched to heparin for 2 to 3 days, which in turn should be discontinued several hours before the procedure. Discontinue low–molecular-weight heparin 24 hours before biopsy.

3. Obtain INR, prothrombin time, partial thromboplastin time, and platelet count 1 day prior to biopsy.

4. Correct any bleeding disorders with fresh-frozen plasma, platelets, protamine, or vitamin K.

5. Patient instructed to have only a light meal 4 hours prior to the biopsy.

6. Choose the appropriate image guidance for the procedure.

   a. **Computed tomography (CT) guidance** is used for most transthoracic needle biopsies (TNBs). CT may allow planning of a trajectory that avoids traversing aerated lung, interlobar fissures, bullae, vascular structures, and bone. In addition, CT may help to differentiate necrotic from viable areas within tumor.

   b. **CT fluoroscopy** offers the advantages of CT combined with real-time imaging but is not as widely available as CT. There is also the potential risk of increased radiation exposure for radiologists performing this procedure frequently.

   c. **Fluoroscopic guidance** offers real-time imaging for lesions visualized in two projections. Although previously the standard of care, currently this modality is less useful for smaller pulmonary nodules and has been largely replaced by CT guidance.

   d. **Ultrasound guidance** is useful for biopsy of chest wall, pleural, anterior mediastinal, and peripheral lung lesions.

7. Choose the appropriate needle for the procedure (Table 46.1).

   a. There are two main types of biopsy needles: **Aspirating needles** provide a cellular aspirate for cytologic examination. **Core biopsy needles** provide a core of tissue for histologic examination. Some needles, such as Turner needles and Westcott needles, yield small fragments as well as a cellular aspirate. Most biopsy needles are available in diameters ranging from 16 to 25 gauge.

   b. When a **single-needle technique** is used, multiple pleural punctures are required to obtain multiple samples. Alternatively, a **coaxial needle system** can be used to obtain multiple samples using a single pleural puncture. In this type of needle system, a thinner inner needle is inserted through a larger outer needle called an introducer. Therefore, the pleura will be punctured by a needle that is larger than the one used to obtain the sample. Many core biopsy needles are powered by spring-activated handles that can be used to obtain a large core of tissue. These are particularly effective for sampling benign lesions (e.g., hamartomas, granulomas) and anterior mediastinal lesions (e.g., thymomas, lymphomas).

c. The single-shaft aspiration needles have up to a 70% lower complication rate due to its smaller needle gauge (3). However there has been a gradual shift toward using both aspiration and core needles during each biopsy procedure to improve the diagnostic efficacy of molecular analysis compared to either aspiration or core needle alone (4).

8. Review the procedure, possible complications, and alternatives with the patient. Obtain signed informed consent minutes prior to the biopsy.

Procedure

1. Position the patient on the biopsy table so that the skin entry site is placed upright. When ease of performance and risk of complications are not substantially affected by the patient's position, prone position is preferred to minimize chest wall motion and patient anxiety from seeing the needle. Biopsy side down post-procedure is also facilitated which reduces pneumothorax rates.

2. Perform preliminary examination.
   a. For CT-guided biopsies, a scout view is obtained followed by localizing trans-axial images through the lesion. Upper lobe lesions generally do not require any special breathing instructions. When nodule motion is observed near the diaphragm, breath-holding instructions are given. A small inspiration is requested so that there will be minimal amount of motion once the needle has passed through the pleura and less chance of a pneumothorax, as with deeper breath holds there will be greater motion and more chance of tearing the pleural surface. Patients are requested to maintain the same degree of inspiration each time they are asked to breath-hold (whenever the lesion is scanned or the biopsy needle is advanced). It is useful to practice breath-holding with patients before beginning the procedure.
   b. When ultrasound guidance is used, a preliminary examination is performed to confirm visibility of the lesion.

3. When CT is used for guidance the dose should be reduced to the minimal amount necessary for monitoring of the procedure as it is not being performed for diagnostic purposes. Both kV and mA should be lowered to achieve an estimated dose of less than 1.0 mSv for the entire procedure.

4. Plan the desirable needle path and mark the skin entry site.
   a. Whenever possible, a needle path that avoids aerated lung should be chosen to reduce the likelihood of developing a pneumothorax. If aerated lung must be traversed, structures such as interlobar fissures, bullae, cysts, and large vascular structures should be avoided. Lesions that lie directly underneath an obstructing rib can be accessed using an oblique approach, with or without angling of the gantry.
   b. A convenient way to localize the skin entry site is to place a row of metallic objects (e.g., injection needles) on the skin at the desired level and scan them. Commercial skin markers are also available for this purpose. The skin directly underneath or in between these objects can be marked with a felt-tipped pen. It is useful to trace and plan the desired needle trajectory on the CT console.

5. Cleanse the skin entry site using a povidone-iodine or chlorhexidine disinfectant. Cover the skin with sterile drapes. Anesthetize the skin and subcutaneous tissue by infiltrating 5 to 10 mL of 1% lidocaine down to, but not crossing, the pleura. The pleural surface can be very sensitive, and adequate anesthesia is needed to minimize discomfort and motion. The patient should also be informed of the normal pressure sensations during needle manipulation. Patients who do not anticipate

these sensations may become anxious with the false notion that the local anesthesia was insufficient. Sedation is not necessary for this procedure except for rare situations such as severe claustrophobia in the CT scanner. Patient reassurance and cooperation are paramount to a successful lung biopsy.

6. Use the anesthetic needle as a guide for placement of the biopsy needle. Advance the biopsy needle along the planned trajectory until the needle tip is within the target lesion. When the procedure is performed with CT guidance, at least one image superior and inferior to the needle tip must be obtained to document that the needle tip is actually within the lesion. This avoids sampling error caused by partial volume-averaging.

7. Sample the lesion. The actual sampling process varies depending on the needle design and biopsy technique used (core biopsy or fine-needle aspiration). For aspiration needles, the needle's central stylet is removed and a syringe is attached to the needle's hub. The plunger is then pulled back to generate suction, and the needle is carefully shaken up and down to cut away cells from the lesion and draw them into the syringe. The suction is then relieved as the needle and the attached syringe are withdrawn. For spring-loaded core biopsy needles, the spring mechanism is cocked, and the needle is advanced into the introducer until the tip is in the lesion. The core needle's sliding mechanism is then advanced fully (but not fired) while keeping the needle's collecting receptable within the lesion. After confirming that the collecting receptacle is within the lesion, the firing mechanism is activated. Using this technique, firing the needle will slice and load tissue into the receptacle without changing the needle tip position, thus preventing unanticipated injury.

8. Ideally, the needle and attached syringe are then given to an on-site cytopathologist for immediate cytologic evaluation. As the evaluation of small samples of material has become far more sophisticated in recent years, the need to have a well-developed protocol with the cytologist is increasingly important. The specimens may need to be divided and allocated to the various necessary tests (5). In the absence of an on-site pathologist, the aspirate is smeared on slides and fixed in 95% alcohol for cytologic evaluation, while larger fragments are placed in a formalin solution for histopathologic evaluation. Additional analyses for molecular markers such as epidermal growth factor receptor (eGFR) and Kirsten Rat Sarcoma Viral Oncogene Homolog (K-RAS) are also performed for newly diagnosed lung cancers to determine their susceptibility to targeted drug therapies. If an infectious cause is suspected, part of the obtained sample should be placed in a sterile test tube or sterile saline solution for further microbiologic evaluation.

9. If a coaxial needle system is used, the blood patch technique can be applied to reduce the pneumothorax rate. The blood patch technique involves the injection of 4 mL of autologous blood into the most peripheral 2 cm of the pulmonary needle tract. This requires the use of a coaxial needle, with the inner needle used to perform the biopsy and the outer needle used to inject the autologous blood. The success of the blood patch technique depends on the injection of autologous blood into nonemphysematous lung parenchyma. Other materials such as chemical sealants and normal saline have also been used with some success (6).

Postprocedure Management

1. If the biopsy was performed using CT guidance, obtain an immediate postbiopsy scan at approximately the level of the biopsy site to detect a possible pneumothorax. Alternatively, an expiratory portable chest radiograph can be obtained with the patient sitting upright (Fig. 46.1).

2. If no significant pneumothorax is noted and the patient is asymptomatic, then the patient is transported on a gurney to the recovery area for observation.

3. Observe the patient for 1 to 2 hours following the procedure. The patient should remain recumbent throughout the observation period. Vital signs should be

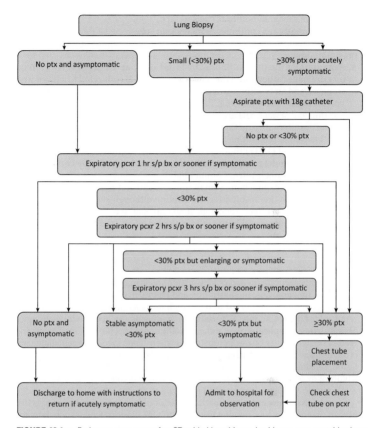

FIGURE 46.1 • Patient management after CT-guided lung biopsy. bx, biopsy; pcxr, portable chest x-ray; ptx, pneumothorax; s/p, status post.

monitored at least twice an hour. Measures that can reduce pneumothorax rates and facilitate the resorption of an existing small pneumothorax include placing the patient in a "puncture site down" position and administration of supplemental nasal oxygen. Stable inpatients can be monitored from their patient rooms.

4. If a significant (>30%) pneumothorax is clinically suspected during the observation period (e.g., increasing pleuritic pain, dyspnea, or hypoxia), an expiratory chest radiograph should be obtained immediately.

5. If there is no pneumothorax and there is no symptom attributable to a pneumothorax, then the patient can be discharged after 1 hour of observation. The vast majority of pneumothoraces requiring chest tube placement occur within 1 hour of biopsy. Instruct patients to abstain from strenuous activities for 3 days and to visit the nearest emergency room promptly if dyspnea or pleuritic chest pain develops. A contact number for the physician who performed the procedure should also be provided.

6. Pneumothoraces that are small (<30%), asymptomatic, and stable do not require treatment. A postbiopsy pneumothorax must be treated if:

   a. The patient is dyspneic or has an acute onset of chest pain that may be attributable to pneumothorax.

   b. The size of the pneumothorax exceeds 30%.

   c. The pneumothorax continues to increase in size.

7. Two general approaches can be undertaken in the treatment of a postbiopsy pneumothorax:

   a. Aspiration of the pneumothorax by insertion of an 18-gauge Angiocath or 6-Fr drainage catheter into the pleural space. This is connected to a three-way stopcock and air is withdrawn using a 60-mL syringe. The catheter is removed upon reexpansion of the lung. The patient is placed in the "biopsy side down" position and serial CXRs are obtained to observe for recurrence of pneumothorax. An alternative method is to place the patient in the "biopsy side down" position prior to aspirating the pneumothorax.

   b. Placing a small (11-Fr) thoracic catheter at the second or third intercostal space at the midclavicular line. The thoracic catheter may be connected to a one-way Heimlich valve. Commercial thoracic vents are available for this purpose. Patients in whom a small thoracic catheter has been inserted may be admitted to the hospital for observation although successful outpatient management has been reported. If the air leak has ceased, the catheter can be removed several hours following placement, and the patient can be discharged.

Results

1. TNB is highly accurate for diagnosing intrathoracic malignancy, including malignancies of the lung, hila, mediastinum, and pleura. In general, the sensitivity for malignant nodules is reported to be as high as 95% (7), whereas the sensitivity reported for benign nodules is variable depending on the needle and technique. This is further complicated by whether specific or nonspecific diagnosis is considered as benign. Under those circumstances where a nonspecific benign diagnosis is made based on multiple samples and documentation of the needle tip within the lesion, sensitivity of 90% has been reported (8). However, because there is a possibility of missing a malignant lesion, a plan for further follow-up must be made.

2. A false-positive diagnosis is rare and is estimated at about 2% (9).

3. Although TNB is accurate for the diagnosis of malignancy, the rate of specific benign diagnoses is low, ranging from 16% to 68% in series where such data are available. A negative cytologic or histopathologic diagnosis should be interpreted with caution, as it may not represent a truly benign diagnosis but merely failure to reach a malignant one.

4. Factors that improve the diagnostic yield of TNB include (8):

   a. Careful positioning of the patient and documentation of the needle tip in the lesion.

   b. When necessary, sampling different areas within the lesion. Guidance by analysis of PET images, when available, to areas of increased activity may be helpful.

   c. Larger size and favorable site of the lesion.

   d. Experience of the performing radiologist and of the cytopathologist.

   e. Use of a cutting needle is particularly beneficial in improving the likelihood of obtaining a specific diagnosis in noninfectious benign lesions.

5. The presence of an on-site cytopathologist is ideal. Prospective studies have consistently found that immediate cytologic evaluation significantly improves the diagnostic accuracy of CT-guided TNB (10).

Complications

Common

1. Pneumothorax: The reported incidence of pneumothorax related to TNB ranges from 5% to 60%. The typically reported frequency of developing a postbiopsy pneumothorax is 20% to 25%, whereas the reported frequency of pneumothoraces requiring thoracic vent or chest drain placement is 2% to 15%. Risk factors that increase the occurrence of pneumothorax include:

a. Underlying emphysema or chronic obstructive lung disease
b. The use of cutting or core biopsy needles (vs. aspirating needles)
c. Large-gauge needles (especially 18-gauge needles or introducers)
d. Traversing more than one visceral pleural surface (e.g., crossing an interlobar fissure)
e. Decreased needle-to-skin angle
f. Inability to place the patient in a "biopsy side down" position after biopsy
g. Increased length of needle path (controversial)

2. Hemorrhage
a. The occurrence of hemorrhagic complications depends on the presence of a bleeding diathesis, vascularity of the lesion, and use of medications that induce a bleeding tendency. Pulmonary hemorrhage, manifesting as hemoptysis, occurs in 5% to 10% of biopsies and is usually self-limited. Patients should be alerted about the possibility of hemoptysis as part of the informed consent.
b. If hemoptysis occurs, the patient should be reassured and placed biopsy site down to prevent transbronchial aspiration of blood. Although massive pulmonary hemorrhage is rare, hemorrhage is the most frequent cause of death following needle biopsy of the lung. Death results from massive tracheobronchial aspiration and asphyxia.
c. To decrease the risk of serious hemorrhage, a small-caliber aspiration needle can be used.

Infrequent
1. Hemothorax and chest wall hematoma
2. Vasovagal reaction

Rare
1. Air embolism
2. Massive hemoptysis
3. Cardiac tamponade
4. Malignant seeding of the needle tract
5. Lung torsion
6. Fatal hemorrhage

References

1. MacMahon H, Naidich DP, Goo JM, et al. Guidelines for management of incidental pulmonary nodules detected on CT images: from the Fleischner society 2017. *Radiology.* 2017;284(1):228–243.
2. Henschke CI, Salvatore M, Cham M, et al. Baseline and annual repeat rounds of screening: implications for optimal regimens of screening. International early lung cancer action program investigators. *Eur Radiol.* 2018;28(3):1085–1094.
3. Heerink WJ, de Bock GH, de Jonge GJ, et al. Complication rates of CT-guided transthoracic lung biopsy: meta-analysis. *Eur Radiol.* 2017;27(1):138–148.
4. Chen L, Jing H, Gong Y, et al. Diagnostic efficacy and molecular testing by combined fine-needle aspiration and core needle biopsy in patients with a lung nodule. *Cancer Cytopathol.* 2020;128(3):201–206.
5. Crapanzano JP, Saqi A. Adequacy and tissue preservation of small biopsy and cytology specimen. In: Moreira AL, Saqi A, eds. *Diagnosing Non-small Cell Carcinoma in Small Biopsy and Cytology.* Springer; 2015:39–59.
6. Huo YR, Chan MV, Habib AR, et al. Post-biopsy manoeuvres to reduce pneumothorax incidence in CT-guided transthoracic lung biopsies: a systematic review and meta-analysis. *Cardiovasc Intervent Radiol.* 2019;42(8):1062–1072.

7. Yankelevitz DF, Bulman W. Advances in nonsurgical sampling techniques for the diagnosis and staging of lung cancer. In: Moreira AL, Saqi A, eds. *Diagnosing Non-small Cell Carcinoma in Small Biopsy and Cytology*. Springer; 2015:15–38.
8. Gelbman BD, Cham MD, Kim W, et al. Radiographic and clinical characterization of false negative results from CT-guided needle biopsies of lung nodules. *J Thorac Oncol*. 2012; 7(5):815–820.
9. Khorsandi M, Shaikhrezai K, Wallace W, et al. Is fine-needle aspiration diagnosis of malignancy adequate prior to major lung resections including pneumonectomy? *Interact Cardiovasc Thorac Surg*. 2012;15(2):253–257.
10. Tachibana K, Nakazato Y, Tsuchida S, et al. Immediate cytology improves accuracy and decreases complication rate in real-time computed tomography-guided needle lung biopsy. *Diagn Cytopathol*. 2013;41(12):1063–1068.

47 Catheter Drainage of Intrathoracic Collections

Jared D. Christensen, MD, Edward F. Patz Jr, MD and Jeremy J. Erasmus, MD

Introduction

Numerous disease processes result in the accumulation of pleural fluid or intraparenchymal pulmonary collections. Effective diagnosis and management typically require intervention. This chapter reviews common indications, procedural considerations, and techniques for the drainage of intrathoracic collections including malignant pleural effusion (MPE), parapneumonic effusion, empyema, and lung abscess.

Indications

1. Malignant pleural effusion (MPE) (1–5)
   a. Tumor invasion into the pleural space may lead to lymphatic obstruction resulting in increased pleural fluid production and reduced fluid absorption. Removal of fluid in this setting can be performed for both diagnostic and therapeutic purposes. MPE is an indicator of a poor prognosis with a mean survival of only 4 to 7 months from diagnosis.
   b. Indications for intervention
      (1) Therapeutic drainage in patients with dyspnea, cough, and/or chest pain; intervention is not recommended in asymptomatic patients.
      (2) Large effusions prior to chemotherapy to prevent accumulation of therapeutic agents in the pleural space.
      (3) Symptomatic refractory/recurrent effusions.
      (4) Diagnosis and/or tumor staging information. Predictors of need for definitive therapy (indwelling catheter and/or pleurodesis) at diagnosis are low pH (<7.2), large size, and advanced patient age.
   c. Diagnosis and staging
      (1) Initial tumor diagnosis may be obtained from cytologic evaluation of pleural fluid with yield rates reported between 40% and 87%.
      (2) In addition, cytologic evaluation of pleural fluid may provide important clinical staging information, with MPE indicative of stage IV disease for most cancers.
      (3) Although analysis of pleural fluid is often helpful for diagnostic and staging purposes, MPE may not be sufficient for genetic mutational analysis;

however, with technical advances some studies have reported improved molecular analysis of MPE for patients with lung cancer and malignant pleural mesothelioma.

2. Parapneumonic effusion/empyema (2,5,6)

   a. Pneumonia can be complicated by complex pleural collections resulting in a parapneumonic effusion or empyema. The evolutionary process and classification with associated treatment recommendations are as follows:

   (1) *Uncomplicated:* Interstitial parenchymal fluid accumulates adjacent to a site of infection and flows across the visceral pleura into the pleural space resulting in a sterile, exudative collection with pH >7.2, glucose >60 mg/dL, and elevated protein. Gram stain and culture are negative. Antibiotic therapy is generally effective in treating both the underlying pneumonia and effusion.

   (2) *Complicated:* Bacteria, polymorphonuclear leukocytes, and cellular debris collect within the pleural space resulting in a fibropurulent collection. In addition, fibrin barriers can create loculated components that complicate treatment. Percutaneous drainage is recommended when the fluid analysis shows a pleural glucose <60 mg/dL or a pH <7.2. Cultures are negative.

   (3) *Empyema:* Frank pus in the pleural space or evidence of bacterial infection by Gram stain or culture constitutes an empyema. Fibroblasts produce an extensive organized collection with a thickened pleural peel, creating resistance to respiratory motion. Percutaneous drainage is of limited value; definitive management requires surgical washout and debridement.

   b. Parapneumonic effusions occur in 20% to 57% of patients with pneumonia and approximately 10% require drainage. The American College of Chest Physicians classifies and recommends management of parapneumonic effusions on the basis of size, chemistry, and bacteriology.

   (1) *Category 1:* Free-flowing pleural effusion <1 cm in thickness on decubitus radiograph does not require treatment.

   (2) *Category 2:* Small to moderate (>1 cm, <50% of hemithorax) free-flowing effusions with pleural pH >7.2, glucose >60 mg per dL, lactate dehydrogenase (LDH) less than three times the upper limit of serum, and Gram stain and culture negative do not usually require drainage as most patients respond to antibiotic therapy.

   (3) *Category 3:* Large (>50% of hemithorax) free-flowing effusions, loculated effusions, or effusions with thickened parietal pleura and/or pleural pH <7.2, and/or pleural glucose <60 mg per dL, and/or Gram stain and culture positive require drainage.

   (4) *Category 4:* Frank pus in the pleural space requires drainage.

3. Lung abscess (2,6,7)

   a. Pulmonary abscess occurs in the setting of microbial infection-induced liquefactive necrosis of lung tissue resulting in cavitation. Abscess formation may be bronchogenic (aspiration or inhalation) or hematogenous (spread from another site, such as with septic emboli). A total of 10% to 20% of patients with a pyogenic abscess will fail to respond to medical therapy (systemic antibiotics, postural drainage). Percutaneous drainage is recommended for:

   (1) Persistent sepsis 5 to 7 days after initiation of antibiotic therapy

   (2) Abscess size >4 cm with an air fluid level

   (3) Increase in abscess size during medical therapy

   (4) Children <7 years of age, as abscesses in this population often do not drain spontaneously and are less likely to respond to medical management

   b. Surgical management should be considered for an abscess >6 cm in size, that has not responded to medical treatment beyond 12 weeks, or has failed percutaneous treatment.

Contraindications

1. Relative
   a. Clotting deficiency
      (1) International normalized ratio (INR) >1.5
      (2) Thrombocytopenia (<50,000 platelets per µL)
      (3) Anticoagulation therapy
   b. Extensive fibrothorax: prevents lung reexpansion and limits the value of percutaneous drainage
2. Absolute: There are no absolute contraindications to tube thoracostomy

Choice of Drainage Catheter (1–3,5–8)

1. Malignant pleural effusion
   a. Inpatient drainage: 14-Fr all-purpose drainage (APD) catheter (Flexima APD, Boston Scientific Inc, Natick, MA)
   b. Outpatient (ambulatory) drainage: 10-Fr APD catheter
   c. Treatment of refractory/recurrent malignant effusions and symptomatic MPE with underlying trapped lung: indwelling 15.5-Fr drainage catheter (PleurX catheter, Denver Biomaterials Inc, Golden, CO)
2. Parapneumonic effusion/empyema
   a. Inpatient drainage: 12- to 14-Fr APD catheter or 10- to 14-Fr Malecot catheter
   b. Outpatient (ambulatory) drainage: 10-Fr APD catheter
3. Lung abscess
   a. Tube selection depends on the size of the cavity, although an 8- to 14-Fr APD catheter is usually sufficient. In children, tube size may also depend on the age of the patient.

Preprocedure Preparation

1. Stop oral intake, preferably 8 hours prior to procedure.
2. Obtain informed consent.
3. Lab work: Clotting indices (prothrombin time [PT]/INR) and platelets. If the patient is on anticoagulation therapy, the procedure should be timed to coincide after the cessation of therapy per manufacturer pharmacologic recommendations to minimize bleeding risk.
4. Establish IV access.
5. Monitor vital signs: electrocardiogram (ECG), blood pressure, and pulse oximetry.
6. Imaging/guidance selection: fluoroscopy, ultrasound (US), or computed tomography (CT). Most malignant effusions can be drained with fluoroscopic or US guidance, although complicated fluid collections in the pleural space (parapneumonic effusion, empyema) and lung abscesses may require CT guidance.
7. Administer sedation/analgesia. Although a local anesthetic may be sufficient in some circumstances, pleural drain placement is well tolerated with minimal (light) conscious sedation; commonly achieved by a combination of IV midazolam and fentanyl administration.
8. Choose a drainage system based on the underlying pathology and clinical considerations as previously detailed.
9. Prepare and drape skin entry site.

Technique

Malignant Pleural Effusion (1–3,5,8)
1. Common in cancer patients (15%) with more than 75% due to lung malignancy, breast malignancy, and lymphoma.
2. Aim of treatment is palliation by symptomatic relief and prevention of recurrence.

Contraindications

1. Thick pleural peel of malignant tissue encasing the visceral pleura prevents complete lung reexpansion after drainage of effusion (trapped lung syndrome); pleurodesis is rarely successful
2. Central mass obstructing the airway that prevents reexpansion of the lung
3. Multiple loculated, complex fluid collections
4. Karnofsky index <40

Procedure

1. Patient position and imaging guidance
   a. Usually performed with patient in supine position using US or fluoroscopy
2. Percutaneous drainage approach
   a. Typically, the sixth or seventh intercostal space in the midaxillary line is selected. Enter at mid–two-thirds of intercostal space to avoid subcostal neurovascular structures and irritation of the periosteum.
3. Placement of APD catheter
   a. Small-bore APD catheters (12 to 14 Fr) are the treatment of choice as they are easy to insert, well tolerated, and have response rates similar to large-bore catheters.
   b. Inject local anesthesia (1% to 2% lidocaine) into the soft tissues to the level of the pleura. Always aspirate after advancing the needle tip prior to injection to avoid intravascular injection of lidocaine.
   c. Cut skin with a small blade to facilitate needle and catheter entry.
   d. Insert an 18-gauge trocar needle into the pleural space; entry into the pleural space is indicated by an abrupt decrease in resistance to forward movement of the needle. Accurate placement is facilitated by image guidance.
   e. Remove the inner stylet. Confirm needle position by aspirating a small quantity of pleural fluid. If the tip is in the pleural space, fluid will usually flow back freely.
   f. Introduce a 0.038-in 100-cm floppy-tip guidewire (Cook Medical Inc, Bloomington, IN) through the trocar into the pleural space. Remove the trocar, leaving the wire in place. The wire position can be confirmed by imaging.
   g. Serially dilate the track up to the required catheter French size. Some advocate slightly under dilating to minimize potential air or fluid leaking around the catheter.
   h. Set up the previously selected catheter assembly with the metal stiffener and introduce over the guidewire. The metal stiffener is used to facilitate passage of the APD catheter through the subcutaneous tissues. Once the catheter tip enters the pleural space, disconnect the stiffener from the catheter; while the stiffener is held fixed, advance the catheter into the pleural space.
   i. The metal stiffener is slowly removed when the catheter is in satisfactory position, followed by guidewire removal, leaving the catheter in place. Confirm desired positioning with imaging.
   j. The pigtail catheter is formed, locked, and anchored externally with a suture an adhesive skin disc (Hollister Inc, Libertyville, IL) or Molnar external retention disc (Cook Medical Inc, Bloomington, IN).
   k. Up to 1 L of fluid may be aspirated. If the patient begins to cough before 1 L is removed, active aspiration is discontinued to avoid reexpansion edema.

Postprocedure Management

1. A postprocedure radiograph is obtained to ensure proper tube placement and establish a baseline for follow-up.
2. Bed rest for 2 to 4 hours.
3. Check vital signs every 15 minutes for 1 hour, every 30 minutes for 1 hour, and then every 60 minutes for 2 hours.
4. Inpatient tubes are connected to a Pleur-Evac system (Teleflex, Wayne, PA) with continuous suction at 20-cm H_2O.

5. Outpatient tubes are connected to a Tru-Close 600-mL bag (UreSil, Skokie, IL) or Dover urine leg bag (Cardinal Health, Dublin, OH) for gravity drainage.

6. Tubes are flushed with 5- to 15-mL bacteriostatic saline every 8 hours.

7. Daily fluid output is recorded, and while drainage remains high, *daily chest radiographs are not required.* When drainage decreases to approximately 100 to 200 mL over a 24-hour period, a chest radiograph is obtained to exclude loculated fluid and ensure complete lung reexpansion. If pleural fluid and air have been completely evacuated (usually 2 to 5 days), pleurodesis with a sclerosing agent may be performed.

8. Several sclerosing agents have been used to treat MPEs. Talc is currently the agent of choice for pleurodesis (poudrage, slurry 5-g talc, 50-mL saline, 10-mL 1% Xylocaine). Doxycycline (500-mg, 30-mL saline, 30-mL 1% Xylocaine), bleomycin (60 units in 50-mL saline), and silver nitrate (20 mL 0.5%) have been used as alternatives to talc for pleurodesis, but effectiveness is lower, availability is inconsistent, and pain on instillation is common.

   a. The selected sclerosing agent is introduced into the pleural space through the drainage catheter.

   b. Patient changes position every 15 minutes for 2 hours in an effort to distribute the sclerosing agent completely throughout the pleural space.

   c. The APD catheter is then reopened to suction for 24 hours.

   d. The APD catheter is removed if drainage remains less than 200 mL over 24 hours over the same period. A second dose of the sclerosing agent can be administered if the fluid drainage level is higher than 200 mL.

9. APD catheter removal is performed by cutting across the distal aspect of the catheter. This allows the locking suture to be freed and the pigtail loop to uncoil as the catheter is withdrawn. The skin site is covered with a Vaseline gauze dressing.

10. In patients with long-term drainage catheters, fluid is drained periodically into 600-mL vacuum bottles by placing the preconnected tube with a firm dilator into the valve at the distal end of the PleurX catheter.

Results

1. Response, as measured by improvement of symptoms and prevention of fluid reaccumulation, depends on complete drainage of fluid and lung reexpansion.

2. A total of 70% to 90% of patients will respond; however, without sclerosis, drainage will fail in more than 90% of patients and reaccumulation of fluid can occur as early as 3 days after APD catheter removal.

3. In patients with long-term/indwelling catheters, the degree of symptomatic improvement in dyspnea is comparable to pleurodesis. Late recurrence of effusions is uncommon (<15%), and about 50% of patients will have spontaneous pleurodesis usually within a month.

4. Even in patients with trapped lung (inability of the lung to reexpand following drainage), most patients still have symptomatic improvement (decreased dyspnea, improved exercise tolerance).

Complications

1. Tube malfunction (e.g., clotting, kinking, malposition). In patients with a long-term catheter, tube malfunction is uncommon, and the catheter usually remains in place until the patient's demise (mean, 115 days).

2. Infection

3. Hemorrhage

4. Pneumothorax: Up to 30% of patients following chest tube placement will have air in the pleural space. This is most likely due to an *ex vacuo* phenomenon, as the lung is relatively stiff and cannot rapidly reexpand. In most cases, the air resolves completely over a few days.

5. Loculation: This is an unusual complication, and multiple drainage catheters may be required for effective treatment. Alternatively, fibrinolytic agents such as streptokinase and urokinase can be used to successfully drain complex/

loculated MPEs with a low complication rate (see "Parapneumonic Effusions and Empyema").

6. Reexpansion pulmonary edema: uncommon; the incidence can be decreased by judicious removal of fluid (i.e., <500 mL per hour).

Parapneumonic Effusions and Empyema (2,5–7,9,10)

1. Parapneumonic effusions occur in up to 57% of patients with pneumonia.
2. Early diagnosis and intervention are important to decrease morbidity associated with complicated pleural effusions and empyema.

Contraindications

1. Thick pleural rind/fibrothorax, which prevents lung reexpansion and limits the value of percutaneous drainage.

Procedure

1. Placement of APD catheter (see "Malignant Pleural Effusion" procedure section).

Postprocedure Management

1. A postprocedure radiograph is obtained to ensure proper tube placement and establish a baseline for follow-up.
2. Bed rest for 2 to 4 hours.
3. Check vital signs every 15 minutes for 1 hour, every 30 minutes for 1 hour, and every 60 minutes for 2 hours.
4. Record daily drainage output.
5. If the pleural fluid is loculated, multiple drainage catheters or fibrinolytic agents can be useful.
6. APD catheters are typically left in place until the patient demonstrates clinical improvement, drainage is minimal (<50 mL per 24 hours), and antibiotics are changed from intravenous (IV) to oral (PO) administration.
7. Catheter removal (see prior description).

Results

1. Catheter drainage is usually successful or complete within 5 to 10 days of insertion, and resolution of fluid collection is reported in 70% to 90% of cases.

Complications

1. Tube malfunction (e.g., clotting, kinking, malposition)
2. Hemorrhage
3. Pneumothorax
4. Loculation: not uncommon due to fibrin content within the pleural exudate. Multiple drainage catheters or fibrinolytic agents can be used. Fibrinolytic agents decrease fluid drainage time and hospitalization.
   a. Recombinant-tissue plasminogen activator (r-tPA) (2 to 6 mg in a volume of between 50 mL and 250 mL depending on the size of the effusion, infused daily for 1 to 3 days), streptokinase (250,000 units in 100-mL normal saline daily for 1 to 3 days), or urokinase (80,000 units every 8 hours for 1 to 3 days) instilled into the pleural space may be used to mobilize viscous purulent fluid.
   b. r-tPA and urokinase have the advantage of being nonantigenic and are not associated with fever that occurs in approximately 25% of patients after streptokinase instillation.
   c. After instillation, the APD catheter is closed for 2 hours to allow the fibrinolytic agent to distribute through the pleural space and is then reopened to continuous suction.
   d. Although fibrinolytics may be useful in patients with parapneumonic effusions, they should not be used in patients with an empyema or in the setting of a suspected or confirmed bronchopleural fistula.

Lung Abscess (2,5,6,7,10)
1. Usually caused by anaerobic bacteria and typically occurs after aspiration.
2. Medical therapy (systemic antibiotics, postural drainage) is the initial treatment of choice and is curative in most patients.
3. Percutaneous drainage may be considered when medical therapy fails or complications develop (see "Indications" section).

Contraindications
1. None
2. It is important in children to differentiate a lung abscess from necrotizing pneumonia as percutaneous aspiration of necrotizing pneumonia is associated with a high complication rate (i.e., bronchopleural fistula and persistent pneumothoraces).

Procedure
1. Patient position and imaging guidance
   a. Proper positioning is important for safe and successful drainage. Although percutaneous drainage can be performed with the patient supine, prone, or in decubitus position, the abscess should be in a gravity-dependent position to avoid aspiration of pus into the normal lung.
   b. Due to the need for precise localization, drainage is most easily facilitated by CT imaging guidance.
2. Percutaneous drainage approach
   a. Optimal approach ensures that the needle catheter traverses the minimal number of pleural surfaces.
   b. Avoidance of normal lung may reduce development of a bronchopleural fistula or pyopneumothorax.
3. Placement of drainage catheter
   a. Drainage can be performed either using a trocar or Seldinger technique. Although direct puncture of the abscess cavity with a single-puncture trocar drainage system saves time, Seldinger technique with placement of the drainage catheter over a guidewire allows greater control and may decrease the complication rate.
   b. With Seldinger technique, an 18-gauge trocar needle is placed through the chest wall into the abscess. Transthoracic needle aspiration of pus is performed and may completely drain the abscess. Aspiration of pus can be used as both a diagnostic and therapeutic measure and may be all that is required for effective treatment. If drainage is incomplete, a catheter is placed.
   c. First, a 0.038-in guidewire with a floppy distal segment (Cook Medical Inc, Bloomington, IN) is inserted through the needle into the collection, followed by sequential dilators until the diameter of the drainage catheter is reached.
   d. A 12- to 14-Fr APD catheter (Flexima APD, Boston Scientific, Natick, MA) is inserted into the collection. Pus is aspirated and the pigtail loop is formed and locked in place.
   e. The catheter is maintained in place by an adhesive skin disc (Hollister Inc, Libertyville, IL) or Molnar external retention disc (Cook Medical Inc, Bloomington, IN).
   f. Repeat CT scan is performed to confirm correct catheter placement. If the abscess is loculated, additional catheters can be inserted.
   g. Catheters are connected to an underwater drainage system, such as a Pleur-Evac (Teleflex, Wayne, PA), with continuous suction at 20- to 30-cm water. Periodic irrigation of the catheter with 5 to 15 mL of saline is performed to facilitate the drainage of viscous purulent fluid.

Postprocedure Management
1. A postprocedure radiograph is obtained to ensure proper tube placement and establish a baseline for follow-up.
2. Bed rest for 2 to 4 hours.
3. Check vital signs every 15 minutes for 1 hour, every 30 minutes for 1 hour, and every 60 minutes for 2 hours.
4. Record daily drainage.
5. When clinical parameters (e.g., temperature, white cell count) and chest radiographs indicate resolution of the abscess, the catheter(s) can be removed.

Results
1. Placement of a drainage catheter is usually curative, and in most cases, surgery is avoided. Clinical and radiologic improvement usually occurs rapidly after catheter drainage. Mean time to resolution is 10 to 15 days although marked improvement of sepsis (i.e., fever, leukocytosis) usually occurs within 48 hours.
2. Drainage failure may occur when the abscess:
    a. Contains viscous, organized material
    b. Is multiloculated
    c. Has a thick, noncollapsible wall

Complications
1. Potential complications include bleeding, bronchopleural fistula, and empyema.
2. Mortality rate for percutaneous pulmonary abscess drainage is <5%. The morbidity and mortality of patients treated with percutaneous catheter drainage is lower than surgical resection even though these patients are typically more ill than those undergoing surgery.

References

1. Feller-Kopman DJ, Reddy CB, DeCamp MM, et al. Management of malignant pleural effusions. An official ATS/STS/STR clinical practice guideline. *Am J Respir Crit Care Med.* 2018;198(7):839–849.
2. Bhatnagar R, Corcoran JP, Maldonando F, et al. Advanced medical interventions in pleural disease. *Eur Respir Rev.* 2016;25(140):199–213.
3. Al-Tariq QZ. Percutaneous strategies for the management of pulmonary parenchymal, chest wall, and pleural metastases. *AJR Am J Roentgenol.* 2014;203(4):709–716.
4. Pleural diseases. Light RW. 6th ed. Lippincott Williams & Wilkins; 2013.
5. Maskell N. British thoracic society pleural disease guidelines—2010 update. *Thorax.* 2010; 65(U)|ii6/ hh9
6. Hyeon Y. Management of pleural effusion, empyema, and lung abscess. *Semin Interven Radiol.* 2011;28(1):75–86.
7. Owali S. An update on the drainage of pyogenic lung abscesses. *Ann Thorac Med.* 2012; 7(1):3–7.
8. Walker S, Mercer R, Maskell N, et al. Malignant pleural effusion: keeping the flood gates shut. *Lancet Respir Med.* 2020;8(6):609–618.
9. Rahman NM, Maskell NA, West A, et al. Intrapleural use of tissue plasminogen activator and DNase in pleural infection. *N Engl J Med.* 2011;365(6):518–526.
10. Janda S, Swiston J. Intrapleural fibrinolytic therapy for treatment of adult parapneumonic effusions and empyemas: a systematic review and meta-analysis. *Chest.* 2012;142(2): 401–411.

48 Lymphatic Interventions

Alexey Gurevich, MD and Maxim Itkin, MD

Introduction

The lymphatic system is designed to remove proteins and fluid from interstitial tissues and return them back to systemic circulation. Each organ in the body generates slightly different types of lymph which can clinically be differentiated into three types: liver lymph, intestinal lymph, and soft tissue lymph. Liver lymph is characterized by a high concentration of albumin (90% of plasma level), intestinal lymph (chyle) has a high concentration of triglycerides and relatively high concentration of proteins, and soft tissue lymph is characterized by a low concentration of albumin. Lymphatic leaks can present clinically as a surface leakage or accumulation of the fluid in body cavities. It is very important to differentiate the leaks based on the source of the lymph (Fig. 48.1).

Chylous leaks are the leakage of intestinal lymph from the lymphatic system. They may occur at any point along the course of chyle transit, beginning in the intestinal lymphatic ducts, through the cisterna chyli (CC) and the thoracic duct (TD) (Fig. 48.2). The manifestation of chylous leaks depends on the location of the leakage (Fig. 48.1). Chylous leaks may be traumatic or, less commonly, nontraumatic in etiology. Traumatic causes include iatrogenic injury of the TD or its branches during thoracic, cardiac, or neck surgery and secondary to blunt or penetrating chest trauma. Nontraumatic causes include idiopathic, malignancy (e.g., lymphoma), congenital, lymphatic vessel disease (lymphatic malformation), systemic diseases (e.g., sarcoidosis, systemic lupus erythematosus, and Behçet diseases) and associated with genetic syndromes (Noonan disease) (1). In nontraumatic chylothorax, chylous leaks can originate from abnormal pulmonary lymphatic flow from the TD into the lung parenchyma, from retroperitoneal lymphatic masses into lung parenchyma, and from chylous ascites (2). In chylous ascites, chylothorax is a result of migration of lymphatic fluid through diaphragmatic fenestrations due to negative pressure within the chest cavity.

Thoracic duct embolization (TDE) is a percutaneous, image-guided, minimally invasive alternative to surgical interventions for treating chylous leaks. This technique comprises of three steps: first, an intranodal lymphangiogram in order to opacify the lymphatic system followed by transabdominal access of the TD and embolization of the TD. Compared to the "blind" surgical method, visualization of the leak and lymphatics significantly improves the outcomes (3).

Recently a technique of interstitial lymphatic embolization was developed, allowing the embolization of lymphatic leaks through the lymphatic vessel–rich tissues (lymph nodes, lymphatic malformations). This technique is especially useful to treat chylous ascites and nonchylous lymphatic leaks, such as lymphocele and protein losing enteropathy (4).

Indications for TDE

1. Chylothorax
2. Chylopericardium
3. Plastic bronchitis
4. Chyle leaks post neck surgery

Initial conservative management includes treatment of the underlying disease (e.g., lymphoma), repeated thoracentesis, octreotide infusion, and dietary modification such as low-fat diets or keeping the patient NPO. Conservative therapy fails in up to 70% of cases and intervention is then performed.

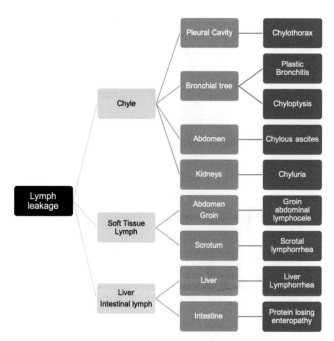

FIGURE 48.1 • Different types of lymph are associated with different leak locations which can manifest with unique pathologies. Knowing the origin of the leak can greatly impact approach to treatment.

Contraindications

Absolute
1. Uncorrectable coagulopathy

Relative
1. Pregnancy
2. Prior severe anaphylactic reaction to iodinated contrast media

Preprocedure Preparation

1. History and physical examination should be conducted with an emphasis on the lymphatic system and assessment for prior thoracic trauma or intervention.
   a. An assessment using the American Society of Anesthesiologists' (ASA) classification for conscious sedation should be performed.
   b. Contrast allergy and reaction should be carefully documented with appropriate preprocedural treatment prescribed.
2. Laboratory analysis of the fluid is performed.
   a. Chylothorax is assessed for a significantly elevated triglyceride level (>200 mg per dL) in the pleural fluid in patients on a regular diet.
   b. In addition, the lymphatic fluid is assessed for a significant proportion of lymphocytes in the cell differential (more than 60%) (5).
   c. Presence of chylomicrons is diagnostic for chyle unless the fluid contains blood.

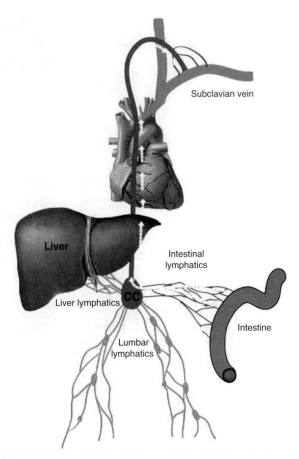

FIGURE 48.2 • Schematic representation of the chyle path *(arrows).* Chylous fluid originates in the intestinal lymphatics and then it passes through intestinal lymphatic vessels into the CC and then in the TD. Interruption of this flow can result in chylous effusions (chylous ascites, chylothorax, chylopericardium, etc.). In rare cases, this path can be altered (lymphatic malformations) and the chyle can be redirected outside the usual path, for example, into the perineum or lower extremities.

3. Obtain informed consent with comprehensive discussion of possible complications.
4. Magnetic resonance (MR) imaging
   In cases of nontraumatic chylothorax, heavily T2-weighted MR imaging of the chest and abdomen is initially performed. The goal is to exclude ascites and lymphatic malformations. This is followed by dynamic contrast-enhanced MR lymphangiography (DCMRL) using intranodal injections of a gadolinium-based agent followed by sequential imaging using a 4D MRA protocol (6).
   a. If MR demonstrates free fluid in the abdomen, chylous ascites with chyle transmigration into the chest through diaphragmatic fenestrations should be suspected. Abdominal fluid sampling and analysis for chyle is advised and TDE should be avoided in order to reduce backflow pressure.

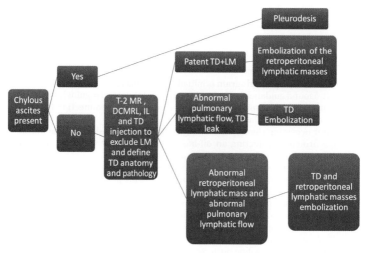

FIGURE 48.3 • Treatment algorithm for nontraumatic chylothorax. LM, lymphatic malformation.

   b. If a retroperitoneal lymphatic malformation that extends into lung parenchyma is identified on the MRI, and TD is found to be patent on conventional lymphangiogram, TDE should not be attempted. Instead, interstitial embolization of the lymphatic masses should be performed (see below).

   c. If DCMRL visualizes a lymphatic leak, or abnormal pulmonary lymphatic flow from TD into lung parenchyma is identified, TDE should be performed.

5. Coagulation profile should be within acceptable limits—international normalized ratio (INR) <1.5. In case of coagulopathy, blood products are administered to correct coagulopathy.

6. The procedure can be performed under general anesthesia or conscious sedation managed by nursing staff with incremental administration of midazolam and fentanyl.

   a. Oral intake should be appropriately restricted for at least 6 hours preprocedure with the exception of normal medications taken with a sip of water.

   b. For insulin-dependent diabetics, fasting preprocedure, morning insulin doses should be halved.

7. Prophylactic periprocedural antibiotics (e.g., cefazolin 1 g intravenously [IV]) are administered at the beginning of the procedure.

8. The patient should be equipped with sequential pneumatic compression devices on lower extremities in order to increase the speed of lymphatic contrast propagation.

9. For nontraumatic chylothorax (Fig. 48.3) this treatment algorithm is a good route of management.

   a. Exclude chylous ascites. If fluid in abdomen is present, we assume that the source of the leak is in the abdomen, and in this case, there are several management options. TDE must be avoided in order to prevent an increase in ascites due to lymphatic backflow.

   b. Next, perform contrast- and noncontrast-enhanced MRI to exclude lymphatic malformation and define anatomy. T2-MRI is followed by DCMRL to visualize potential leaks. MRI is followed by conventional intranodal lymphangiogram. If TD is occluded proximally or leak is identified, embolization of the TD is indicated.

c. In case of patent TD with no abnormal collaterals and presence of retro-peritoneal lymphatic masses, attempt to embolize the masses via interstitial embolization.

Procedure

1. **Intranodal lymphangiogram** is initially performed (7).
   a. Ultrasound guidance is used to directly access bilateral inguinal lymph nodes using a 25-gauge spinal needle connected to a small connection tubing (BD Medical, Franklin Lakes, New Jersey, NJ).
   b. After accessing the hilum of the lymph node, the position of the needle is confirmed by injecting an oil-based contrast agent (Lipiodol, Guerbet, Villepinte, France) using fluoroscopic guidance.
   c. The contrast is injected by hand using either a 3-mL polycarbonate syringe or a balloon inflator at a rate of approximately 1 to 2 mL per 5 minutes. Up to 6 mL of contrast should be injected into each lymph node to achieve appropriate opacification of abdominal and pelvic lymphatics in an average-sized adult patient.
   d. If opacification of the target vessels is not achieved at the completion of the contrast injection, 20 mL of saline is injected through the same needles ("saline push"). Less viscous saline propels the contrast further into the lymphatic system. A saline push results in faster and better opacification of the TD and CC which significantly reduces the procedure and fluoroscopy time, and improves the success of embolization.
2. **Thoracic duct access.**
   a. When the target duct is confirmed, a 21- or 22-gauge, 15- to 20-cm Chiba needle (Cook Inc, Bloomington, IN) is used for access of the lymphatic system. Access is performed transabdominally regardless of the abdominal structures which could be in the needle trajectory. A gentle 5- to 10-degree bend of the distal 2 cm of the needle is made manually to augment directionality.
   b. Under fluoroscopic guidance, swift staccato-like thrusts with the Chiba needle are made. This latter technique helps minimize needle deflection by bowel and other intervening structures.
   c. The safest access to the lymphatic system is below the CC through one of the lumbar feeders. Although technically more challenging due to the smaller size of these feeders, this approach prevents one of the potential complications from TDE—leak from the CC.
   d. As double wall penetration of the duct is achieved, a stiff 0.018-in guidewire (V18 Control, Boston Scientific, Natick, MA) is engaged to probe for the TD. Successful access of the TD is confirmed by easy advancement of the wire into the upper thorax.
   e. A 3-Fr 65-cm microcatheter (e.g., Renegade, Boston Scientific, Marlborough, MA) is advanced over the wire into the TD.
   f. Using a 3-mL syringe, water-soluble iodinated contrast is injected into TD through the catheter to assess for the source of the chylous leak and TD anatomy. This may be characterized by contrast extravasation and/or abnormal pulmonary lymphatic flow.
   g. Specifically, in instances of *plastic bronchitis*, it is suggested to inject blue dye within the approximate area of leak and look for it with concurrent bronchoscopy. Visualization of the dye within the bronchi confirms location of the leak and proper catheter positioning.
3. Thoracic duct embolization
   a. The TD and/or its branches are embolized proximal (upstream) to the leak or lymphatic abnormality with a combination of embolization coils and glue (e.g., *n*-butyl cyanoacrylate [*n*-BCA]) (Trufill, Codman Neuro, Raynam, MA).
   b. Coils are placed proximal (upstream) to the leak/abnormality which may be identified in the TD or within one of its lymphatic branches. The coils

provide a scaffold for polymerization of the glue. Optimal coil deployment is promoted by controlled gentle to-and-fro maneuvers of the catheter. Of note, if visualized leak is suspected to arise from multiple diminutive collaterals, embolization with glue alone can be performed.

c. Prior to glue injection, 0.2 mL of 5% dextrose solution (D_5W) is used to flush the catheter to avoid intracatheter polymerization of the glue. The use of greater volumes of D_5W tends to result in retarding of the glue polymerization in the TD, which often results in recanalization of the glue cast.

d. n-BCA diluted 1:1 in lipiodol is prepared for embolization. The rate at which the n-BCA polymerizes is determined by the speed at which the glue is exposed to the ionic compounds. Experience suggests that 1:1 glue/lipiodol dilution provides sufficient time for injection for embolization of the TD. The glue mixture is injected immediately proximal (upstream) to the site of leak or occlusion. In cases of access to the TD via lumbar lymphatics, it is possible to administer a small amount of glue at the site of lymphatic ductal access. The microcatheter is removed immediately following glue embolization.

4. **TD needle disruption.**
   a. May be performed when TD catheterization fails.
   b. A "twiddling" motion with the needle is used to disrupt the retroperitoneal lymphatics. This controlled trauma to the lymphatic vessels produces local venous thrombosis and an inflammatory cascade which seals the leak.

5. Interstitial lymphatic embolization technique. Some body regions such as groin, axilla, and retroperitoneum are rich in lymphatic lymph nodes and vessels. They are arranged into tight networks of lymphatic interconnections and can act as an array of lymphatic leakage origins. Typical conditions are postsurgical lymphocele and chylous ascites. These areas cannot be directly accessed with a catheter; however, they can be accessed directly with a needle and embolization material such as n-BCA glue mixed with lipiodol can be injected directly into these structures resulting in distal propagation of the glue mixture into leaking lymphatic vessels.
   a. After the needle is placed into the lymphatic rich area, iodinated contrast is injected to confirm needle position.
   b. The needle is then flushed with a significant amount of 5% dextrose solution to allow more distal propagation of the glue mixture.
   c. A ratio of 1:3 to 1:4 of n-BCA to lipiodol allows sufficient penetration within the lymphatic networks leading to an interstitial embolization. n-BCA injections are painful and should be preceded by infusion of a local anesthetic.

Postprocedure Management

1. General care of the patient
   a. Patients need not be routinely admitted overnight; however, a decision to admit a patient for postprocedural monitoring may be made on clinical grounds.
   b. Postembolization pain is usually minimal. Adequate pain management should align with the care of the patient's underlying disease state in conjunction with referring clinicians.
2. Chylous output management
   a. Monitor output from pleural drainage tubes following embolization.
      (1) If output has decreased significantly shortly after the procedure, a food challenge test consisting of administration of ice cream or cream is prescribed.
      (2) If food challenge test is negative (no increase in chest tube output), the patient's diet may be advanced and chest drains removed.
   b. In patients without a chest tube, serial follow-up chest radiographs may be used to monitor the success of the treatment.

c. In cases of technically successful catheterization and embolization of the TD but a failed clinical response marked by persistent chylous effusions, repeat embolization should be considered. The causes of the failed first embolization attempt include second parallel duct and leakage from the CC access point.

Results

1. Traumatic chylothorax: Overall intent-to-treat success rate in largest series of 109 patients was 71% (3). Success rate directly relates to technical ability to catheterize the CC and/or the TD. If TDE was technically successful, the clinical success was 90%. TDE with coils alone demonstrates a lower clinical success rate than embolization with coils and glue (84% vs. 91%) (3). Coils not only serve as a matrix for glue polymerization but also provide a dual source of embolization when the liquid embolic fails.
2. Nontraumatic chylothorax: Overall intent-to-treat clinical success rate in largest series of 52 patients was 86%. This compares favorably to the 27% success rate reported by Maldonado et al. (8) who employed combined conservative and surgical management for nontraumatic chylothoraces. In a study by Gurevich et al., three lymphangiographic patterns were observed with varying clinical success rates (9):
   a. Originating from TD only (60%): 97% clinical success rate.
   b. Originating from TD and retroperitoneal masses (19%): 90% clinical success rate.
   c. Chylous ascites presenting as chylothorax (21%): 55% clinical success, 75% of those that chose to undergo treatment.
3. Plastic bronchitis: In early reports, six of seven patients demonstrated abnormal pulmonary lymphatic flow based on DCMRL imaging, which was confirmed with TD cannulation. Of the six patients identified, embolization leads to complete resolution in five and partial improvement in one (10).

Complications

1. Immediate complications
   a. Nontarget embolization: Two reported cases of embolization of the pulmonary artery from isolated embolization with *n*-BCA.
      (1) First case (asymptomatic) involved retrograde spilling of glue into the inferior vena cava and then into the pulmonary circulation.
      (2) Second case (symptomatic) likely involved over injection of glue into the TD, with antegrade spillage of glue through the TD into the subclavian vein and into the pulmonary circulation (1).
2. Long-term complications
   a. Protein-losing enteropathy, lymphedema, and chylous ascites manifesting as chronic diarrhea (12%), lower extremity edema (7%), bilateral breast swelling (2%), and abdominal swelling (5%) after pedal lymphangiography (11).
   b. Recent update from inguinal lymphangiography followed by TDE, with an average follow-up time of 40.2 months, showcased complications in just 4 of 65 (6.2%) patients surveyed. These complications manifested as one lower extremity swelling and three instances of abdominal swelling. There were no reports of diarrhea, shortness of breath, or weight loss.

Management of Complications

1. Nontarget embolization: Given that 1 to 4 mL of glue is used for TDE, escape of a fraction of this volume into the pulmonary circulation is not deemed enough to cause symptoms in patients with adequate lung reserve. To preempt this complication, embolize the TD with coils just upstream to the leak to construct a scaffold on which the glue may polymerize.
2. Chronic sequelae: Treatment is expectant and often conservative.

References

1. Nadolski GJ, Itkin M. Thoracic duct embolization for nontraumatic chylous effusion: experience in 34 patients. *Chest.* 2013;143(1):158–163.
2. Goity LD, Itkin M, Nadolski G. An algorithmic approach to minimally invasive management of nontraumatic chylothorax. *Semin Intervent Radiol.* 2020;37(3):269–273.
3. Itkin M, Kucharczuk JC, Kwak A, et al. Nonoperative thoracic duct embolization for traumatic thoracic duct leak: experience in 109 patients. *J Thorac Cardiovasc Surg.* 2010; 139(3):584–590.
4. Itkin M, Nadolski GJ. Modern techniques of lymphangiography and interventions: current status and future development. *Cardiovasc Intervent Radiol Springer US.* 2018;41(3):366–376.
5. Agrawal V, Doelken P, Sahn SA. Pleural fluid analysis in chylous pleural effusion. *Chest.* 2008;133(6):1436–1441.
6. Dori Y, Keller MS, Rome JJ, et al. Percutaneous lymphatic embolization of abnormal pulmonary lymphatic flow as treatment of plastic bronchitis in patients with congenital heart disease. *Circulation.* 2016;133(12):1160–1170.
7. Nadolski GJ, Itkin M. Feasibility of ultrasound-guided intranodal lymphangiogram for thoracic duct embolization. *J Vasc Interv Radiol.* 2012;23(5):613–616.
8. Maldonado F, Cartin-Ceba R, Hawkins FJ, et al. Medical and surgical management of chylothorax and associated outcomes. *Am J Med Sci. 2010;339(4):314–318.*
9. Gurevich A, Hur S, Singhal S, et al. Nontraumatic chylothorax and chylopericardium: diagnosis and treatment using an algorithmic approach based on novel lymphatic imaging. *Ann Am Thorac Soc.* 2022;19(5):756–762.
10. Itkin MG, McCormack FX, Dori Y. Diagnosis and treatment of lymphatic plastic bronchitis in adults using advanced lymphatic imaging and percutaneous embolization. *Ann Am Thorac Soc.* 2016;13(10):1689–1696.
11. Laslett D, Trerotola SO, Itkin M. Delayed complications following technically successful thoracic duct embolization. *J Vasc Interv Radiol.* 2012;23(1):76–79.

49 Percutaneous Abdominal Biopsy

Daniel I. Glazer, MD and Stuart G. Silverman, MD, FACR

Introduction

Image-guided percutaneous abdominal biopsy is a commonly utilized technique which has largely replaced surgical biopsy for almost all disease processes in the abdomen. This chapter describes established and emerging indications and techniques for common biopsy procedures performed in the abdomen and pelvis (1).

Indications

Including, but not limited to (1)
1. Diagnosis of primary malignancy
2. Confirmation of suspected metastasis
3. Staging of malignancy
4. Confirmation of a benign diagnosis (benign tumor, cyst, infection, inflammation)
5. Molecular analysis for treatment planning
6. Monitoring treatment

Contraindications (1)

1. Uncorrectable bleeding diathesis
2. Hemodynamic instability
3. Lesion inaccessible percutaneously (e.g., surrounded by bone, no safe path)
4. Uncooperative or unwilling patient

Preprocedure Assessment and Patient Preparation

1. Consultation—Is a percutaneous biopsy indicated? Are special preparation steps needed? Evaluate medical record; review pertinent imaging examinations to establish indication and determine feasibility. Establish if patient is able to consent, determine need for appropriate sedation or anesthesiology support; assess need for preprocedure laboratory tests.
   a. Consider inpatient biopsies when
      (1) Patient is in hospital for other reasons.
      (2) Risk of biopsy is increased (e.g., medical comorbidities, lesion type, and location).
      (3) Patient lives alone or far away.
2. Preprocedure patient preparation (2,3): deliver preparation instructions to patient. Withhold solid food (except medications) for 6 hours and clear liquids for 2 hours when minimal or moderate sedation (formerly known as conscious sedation) is planned. Withhold solid food for 8 hours when deep sedation or general anesthesia is planned; both require presence of an anesthesiologist.
   a. Instruct patient to arrive 1 to 1.5 hours prior to procedure.
   b. Ask patient to arrange for a responsible adult companion to provide transport to home (if sedation is being administered), and, if possible, someone to accompany them overnight.
   c. Advise patient of possible signs and symptoms of adverse events and provide contact information.
   d. Determine if patient is on anticoagulation medication.
   e. Discontinue medications that affect hemostasis (e.g., heparin, warfarin, aspirin, clopidogrel) if procedure has high risk of bleeding (SIR category II).
   f. Discuss risks of discontinuing anticoagulant medications with care providers if patient has a high thrombotic risk before considering for biopsy.
   g. May forego discontinuing medications if procedure is urgent.
   h. Warfarin should be discontinued for procedures with high risk of bleeding (typically 5 days); low–molecular-weight heparin (LMWH) bridge can be considered if patient is high risk for thrombosis, for example, heart valve surgery, recent pulmonary embolism, and deep vein thrombosis.
   i. Discontinue full-dose aspirin or clopidogrel for at least 5 days for procedures with high risk of bleeding. Stopping other nonsteroidal antiinflammatory drugs (NSAIDs) is optional. Restart aspirin, clopidogrel, or NSAIDs >12 hours after the procedure when low risk for bleeding and >24 hours when high risk for bleeding.
   j. Heparin (unfractionated, intravenous [IV] or subcutaneous [SQ]): if prophylactic dose, discontinue for 4 to 6 hours, no need to recheck partial thromboplastin time (PTT); restart >12 hours when low risk for bleeding and >24 hours when high risk for bleeding. If therapeutic dose, discontinue for 4 to 6 hours, recheck PTT; restart >12 hours when low risk for bleeding and >24 hours when high risk for bleeding. For patients on LMWH, prophylactic dose (5,000 IU once per day) stop 12 hours before and therapeutic dose (≥5,000 IU once per day) stop 24 hours before the procedure. Restart prophylactic and therapeutic dose >12 hours after the procedure when low risk of bleeding >24 hours when high risk for bleeding.

3. Day of procedure: obtain written informed consent. Detail indications as they relate to the patient's medical problem, the benefits, risks (including specific potential complications, their probability of occurrence, and steps to minimize their risk), alternative procedures, and other relevant aspects of the procedure (e.g., the planned approach and how long the procedure will take). Give patient specific instructions on how to cooperate during the biopsy (e.g., breath holding).

4. Laboratory tests (3)
   a. Obtain serum prothrombin time (PT) (international normalized ratio [INR]) and complete blood count (CBC) if normal values have not been documented in the medical record in the prior 30 days for procedures with high risk of bleeding. If normal values have been documented, these tests do not need to be repeated unless there are risk factors for bleeding such as medications that could alter coagulation, diseases known to alter hemostasis (e.g., liver disease), or other reasons to suspect a bleeding diathesis. Obtain serum PTT only for procedures with high risk of bleeding, and only if a normal value has not been documented in the past. PTT does not need to be remeasured unless there are new risk factors such as medications, diseases, or other reasons to suspect an alteration in PTT. General guidelines for hemostatic parameters include PT <15 seconds, INR <1.5, PTT <1.5 × control, and platelet count >50,000 per μL; however, deviation from these guidelines can be considered if clinically indicated.
   b. Adrenal mass biopsy: if pheochromocytoma is a consideration, measure plasma-free fractionated metanephrines (high sensitivity especially in patients with hereditary predisposition to pheochromocytoma, but false positives possible especially in sporadic cases), and if positive, the specificity can be increased by 24-hour measurement of urine-fractionated metanephrines and catecholamines.
   c. Liver cyst aspiration: consider echinococcal serology in suspected cases.

5. Consider "on-site" cytopathologist for preliminary reading of fine-needle samples if target is difficult to visualize or procedure is technically challenging.

6. Advantages of real-time cytopathology review:
   a. Offers immediate assessment of adequacy of specimen.
   b. Allows for altering approach or technique if preliminary tissue specimen is insufficient.
   c. Allows selective processing of specimen for special studies (e.g., culture if material suggests infection, marker studies for lymphoma, electron microscopy, cytogenetics for some tumors, and measurement of tumor-specific markers).
   d. Limits the number of passes to no more than what is necessary, particularly in high-risk procedures.

7. Choose an image-guidance system (1).
   a. Fluoroscopy—Not typically used for percutaneous biopsy procedures.
   b. Ultrasound (US)
      (1) Advantages: rapid localization, real-time and multiplanar, flexible patient positioning, no ionizing radiation, Doppler can reveal vascularity.
      (2) Disadvantages: suboptimal imaging in large patients. Target may be obscured by overlying structures (e.g., bone, lung, bowel).
   c. Computed tomography (CT)
      (1) Advantages: helps visualize deep lesions, depicts tissue components, vascularity, precise anatomic relationships (e.g., bowel and pleural space), precise needle localization possible, multiplanar guidance possible with reconstructions. CT fluoroscopy with either intermittent "quick check" scans or continuous, near real-time scans can shorten needle placement time.
      (2) Disadvantages: ionizing radiation. More costly and time-consuming compared to US

d. Magnetic resonance imaging (MRI)
   (1) Advantages: useful for lesions seen on MRI alone, multiplanar, no ionizing radiation
   (2) Disadvantages: expensive, limited availability, MRI-compatible equipment required, time consuming
e. PET/CT
   (1) Advantages: developed recently to guide biopsy of lesions only visible on PET imaging or to target PET avid portions of a lesion.
   (2) Disadvantages: expensive, limited availability, PET/CT scanner needed

Procedure

Intraprocedure Preparation

1. Patient preparation
   a. Establish IV access if needed. Procedures with a lower risk of bleeding (SIR category I) may not require placement of an IV.
   b. Sedation and analgesia: minimal or moderate sedation using parenteral narcotics and benzodiazepines is typically satisfactory. Deep sedation and general anesthesia are rarely needed.
   c. Position the patient comfortably without compromising access to needle entry site.
   d. Sterilize the overlying skin (field) with iodinated scrub and alcohol, or chlorhexidine.
   e. Place sterile drapes and towels surrounding the field of intervention.
2. Physician preparation
   a. Thorough hand washing
   b. Wear impermeable gowns, caps, masks, and facial shields. Double gloving has been showing to reduce hand contact with patient's blood and/or body fluids.
   c. Protective equipment, such as needle receptacles, and specially designed biopsy trays can be used.

Procedure (1)

1. Anesthetize the skin and subcutaneous tissues with local 1% or 2% lidocaine. Make a 3- to 5-mm superficial skin incision with scalpel blade.
2. Biopsy needle selection
   a. Needle size
      (1) Fine needles (20 to 25 gauge): ideal for cytology, can transgress bowel to access solid structure if necessary, minimal hemorrhagic potential
      (2) Large needles (14 to 19 gauge): samples can be analyzed for cytology or histology, increases yield, helps subtype tissue particularly in lymphoma, may have increased hemorrhagic potential. Large-needle samples may be needed for molecular testing and genomic analysis.
   b. Cutting edge
      (1) End-cutting needle types
         (a) Acute bevel
         (b) 90-degree bevel
      (2) Side-cutting needle types
         (a) Cannula gap
         (b) Stylet gap
   c. Spring-loaded/automated (side cutting)
   d. Choose a biopsy needle based on the following:
      (1) Lesion size and depth: small, deep lesions may require a 20-gauge needle (or larger) that is stiff enough to be directed accurately, as 22- and 25-gauge needles tend to "bow" out of intended track.
      (2) Access route: in the rare instance that bowel needs to be traversed, a fine needle (20 to 25 gauge) is recommended.

(3) Suspected diagnosis
 (a) *Known primary malignancy:* requires less tissue, fine-needle biopsy may be sufficient.
 (b) *Unknown primary malignancy:* larger needle samples (14 to 19 gauge) may be needed.
 (c) *Suspected lymphoma:* fine needles (20 to 25 gauge) may be adequate to diagnose lymphoma versus other solid malignancies, but larger needles (14 to 19 gauge) typically needed for subtyping lymphomas.
 (d) *Increased hemorrhagic potential* (bleeding diathesis, hypervascular lesion): fine needles (20 to 25 gauge) probably have less hemorrhagic potential. Larger needles (14 to 19 gauge) may have increased hemorrhagic potential but may be needed in some cases.
(4) Cytopathologist preference: a preliminary "cell-layer thick" specimen for slide preparation is often preferred; hence, the first pass should be with a fine needle, but large samples may be subsequently needed.
(5) General principle: use the thinnest needle that can be used successfully to target the lesion and obtain sufficient material. Needles as thin as 25 gauge have been shown to be diagnostic.
(6) Large-needle samples needed for histology are commonly obtained using side-cutting needles as these are thought to be provide better specimens.
3. Image-guidance technique (1)
 a. US-guided biopsy
  (1) Perform full US examination of lesion and surrounding region to confirm lesion and plan biopsy. This should be done by the radiologist who will be performing the biopsy.
  (2) Localize the lesion, assess path, distance, and angle.
  (3) Free-hand technique: prepare transducer by placing sterile cover. Monitor needle placement with real-time US using a sterile, covered transducer.
  (4) Biopsy transducer guide: consider use of biopsy transducer guide with built-in needle slots to direct the needle at a predetermined angle within the plane of view of the transducer (particularly useful for novice operators).
  (5) Demonstrate needle tip in target lesion, preferably on two tangential images. Some prefer scanning with the transducer perpendicular to the target, whereas others prefer scanning close proximity to the entry site. Regardless of where the transducer is placed, the US beam should parallel the needle shaft. Needle "jiggling" or "bobbing" (in and out motion) may help. Biopsy needles with echogenic tips can be used. These ensure a strong echo reflection and may improve needle tip visibility during scanning.
 b. CT-guided biopsy
  (1) Review prior imaging examinations to determine approximate site of skin entry site. Commercially available radiopaque grids are typically used to mark the exact skin entry site.
  (2) Perform preprocedure CT scan of lesion and surrounding region with patient in the biopsy position to confirm lesion and plan approach. Consider IV contrast material to assess lesion vascularity and surrounding vessels if needed.
  (3) The angle, distance, and potential structures in the path of the needle are identified by drawing a line connecting the skin entry site determined by the grid marker and the lesion.
  (4) Plan and then place needle. Maintaining trajectory in axial plane allows subsequent scans to visualize entire needle length. Angled approach (out of the axial plane) may be necessary and may require multiple scans to visualize needle path and tip.
  (5) CT fluoroscopy can be used to directly monitor needle placement either in real time or intermittently after partial insertions or to quickly scan the position of an already placed needle.

4. Biopsy technique (1)
   a. General principles
      (1) When biopsying masses that move with respiration, a breath hold is generally desired for all needle placements and CT scans. Breath holds at end expiration, half-breaths, or simply stopping breathing can be used. Regardless of which is used, it is helpful to have the patient practice before the procedure, and with an explanation to the patient that the goal is consistency.
      (2) Choose shortest path possible (unless adjacent critical structures need to be avoided).
      (3) Tandem technique (in which the biopsy needle is placed alongside a reference needle) can be used when wider regions of a mass need to be sampled. A coaxial technique (in which a biopsy needle is placed within an introducer needle) is often preferred to minimize needle passes and reduce the potential for tumor seeding along the biopsy track.
      (4) Use the least number of needle placements to obtain diagnostic tissue.
      (5) Critical structures to avoid during needle placement
         (a) Lung: be sure that the position of the lung is known in the biopsy position, and at the breath hold used at the time of the needle insertion.
         (b) Gallbladder
         (c) Pancreas
         (d) Dilated duct (biliary, pancreatic)
         (e) Small and large bowel: the colon and small intestines should not be transgressed if a fluid-containing structure is targeted so as not to contaminate the patient or the specimen with flora; however, the colon and small intestines can be transgressed with a fine needle, if absolutely necessary, to biopsy a solid lesion.
         (f) Major blood vessels
   b. Needle placement techniques: this requires precise placement of one needle, which serves as a reference (tandem technique) or a conduit (coaxial technique) guide for all subsequent needle placements.
      (1) Tandem technique
         (a) Mandatory short (3 to 5 mm) superficial incision
         (b) Place initial 20- or 22-gauge reference needle.
         (c) Image and confirm reference needle-tip in or adjacent to lesion.
         (d) Place a second biopsy needle via same incision site parallel to reference needle (tandem) (20- to 25-gauge needles if fine needles desired; larger needles may be used).
         (e) Biopsy with the second needle for cytology smear.
         (f) Obtain additional (typically two or three) tandem passes, using larger gauge needles if necessary.
         (g) Obtain images that document appropriate position of biopsy needles within the targeted lesion.
         (h) Complete procedure using reference needle as the final specimen.
      (2) Coaxial technique is useful for small and deep lesions requiring greater precision (i.e., narrow "window" between two or more critical structures along the path to target) or when multiple biopsy samples are required.
         (a) Determine appropriate skin entry point and advance introducer needle into position just proximal to lesion.
         (b) Coaxially place biopsy needle (fine or large needle) through introducer needle.
         (c) Obtain images that document appropriate position of biopsy needle within the targeted lesion.

(d) A 17-gauge introducer is needed for biopsy specimens obtained with 18-gauge needles, 19-gauge introducer is needed for 20-gauge needles, 22-gauge needles can be placed coaxially through 19-gauge (or larger introducers or needles), 25-gauge needles can be placed coaxially through a 20-gauge needle, and multiple biopsy specimens can be acquired.

(e) Remove introducer needle at conclusion of procedure.

c. Technical maneuvers that may be helpful (1,4)

(1) Alternative patient positioning: the patient may be placed in a different position, such as oblique or lateral decubitus, to remote critical structures from the planned needle path.

(2) Hydrodissection: sterile saline, dilute contrast material, or dextrose water injection may help displace intervening bowel loops.

(3) Compression device: abdominal compression may facilitate displacement of bowel.

(4) Utilization of a blunt needle: slow advancement of an introducer needle with blunt stylet in place may help avoid inadvertent puncture of bowel or blood vessel.

(5) Curved needle: use of a manually curved needle (typically 22 gauge) advanced coaxially through a larger gauge reference needle may help target a mass that is not in direct line with the reference needle.

(6) Administer IV contrast material: isodense lesions not visible on preprocedure unenhanced CT can be targeted after IV contrast material is administered. Typically a reference needle is placed in the area of the target prior to contrast material administration.

(7) Triangulation method may be used to determine optimal angle and calculate distance to lesion.

(8) Gantry tilt technique (maintains needle in imaging plane while facilitating an angled approach)

(9) Dual-modality image fusion can be used to guide the biopsy of lesions which are inconspicuous on one modality, for example, fusing positron emission tomography (PET) images to unenhanced CT for lesions visible only on PET and fusing contrast-enhanced CT or MR images to US for lesions visible only with CT or MRI.

(10) Electromagnetic tracking using skin fiducials and needles with internal sensors allows spatial tracking of the needle tip and can facilitate US- or CT-guided needle placement. Multiplanar image displays and multimodality image coregistration can be used with real-time feedback.

5. Sampling technique

a. Fine-needle biopsy—use rotatory corkscrew drilling motion, maintaining continuous suction on a small volume syringe. Transgress the most optimal portion of the lesion with each insertion and retraction. Release suction before withdrawing needle.

b. Automatic spring-loaded devices may be used to obtain a core of tissue.

c. Cytology smears are obtained dry.

d. Specimen processing:

(1) Fine-needle biopsy specimen can be handed to cytotechnologist for smears and cell block. Alternatively, smears can be prepared using sterile slides; the remaining material in the needle and syringe can be submitted in sterile solution for cell block, and the needle reused.

(2) Large-needle specimens should be submitted in formalin for histology examination. If lymphoma is suspected, a specimen can also be submitted in saline for flow cytometry.

(3) Gram stains and cultures are obtained as necessary and typically submitted in saline.

6. Fine-needle specimens may be sufficient for diagnosis of epithelial malignancies, however, the greater demand for specimen processing (e.g., molecular and genetic testing) has changed clinical practice to use large needles in most patients.
7. Organ-specific approaches to focal masses (5-7)
   a. Liver (under US, CT, or MRI guidance): use a transparenchymal route by interposing normal "cuff" of liver tissue to decrease the risk of hemorrhage into the peritoneal space, particularly when sampling a hypervascular lesion. A direct approach into a mass is also acceptable if needed.
   b. Adrenal gland: CT and MRI approaches are given (consider using US for large lesions).
      (1) Lateral decubitus (affected side down) offers a posterior approach with a path that is caudal to posterior sulcus and typically avoids transgressing the lung and compresses/pushes the ipsilateral lung out of the posterior sulcus.
      (2) Right (lateral) transhepatic
      (3) Left (anterior) transhepatic
      (4) Transrenal (only if necessary)
      (5) Alternative approaches (all designed to avoid or minimize pleural space transgression)
      (6) Prone position, skin entry site caudal to the posterior sulcus with needle angled superiorly
      (7) Triangulation method and gantry tilt techniques
   c. Kidney mass (under US, CT, or MRI guidance)
      (1) Lateral or prone posterior approach
      (2) Historical indications include the following:
         (a) Patients with a renal mass and known extrarenal primary malignancy
         (b) Patients with a renal mass and imaging findings that suggest unresectable renal cancer
         (c) Patients with a renal mass and surgical comorbidity
         (d) Patients with a renal mass that may have been caused by an infection
      (3) More recently established indications include the following:
         (a) Patients with a renal mass considered for percutaneous ablation or radiotherapy
         (b) Patients with renal masses that are multiple or bilateral
         (c) Patients with a renal mass in solitary or transplant kidney
         (d) Patients with a renal mass that could be clinical T1a (4 cm or smaller) renal cell carcinoma
   d. Retroperitoneum (typically under CT or MRI guidance; US rarely used): although anterior and posterior approaches can be used, the latter is generally preferred employing needles 19 gauge or larger (e.g., suspected lymphoma). Also, an anterior approach may necessitate transgressing the bowel.
   e. Presacral/pelvic mass (typically under CT or MRI guidance; US rarely used)
      (1) Transgluteal: posterior half of greater sciatic notch, close to sacrum posteriorly, to avoid the sciatic nerve anteriorly, and below the level of piriformis muscle, to avoid the gluteal vessels anterior to piriformis
      (2) Alternative approaches include transvaginal and transrectal biopsy (only using US guidance) if no other safe access route is possible.
   f. Spleen (typically under US, CT, or MRI guidance)
      (1) Traversing the least amount of parenchyma en route to the lesion may reduce bleeding risk.
   g. Pancreas: because of the close anatomic relationship of the pancreas to the stomach and duodenum, many pancreatic lesions are biopsied with endoscopic US. However, tissue sampling is generally limited to fine needles. When tissue is needed for histologic evaluation, a percutaneous approach may be needed.

(1) Anterior approach can be attempted. If a transgastric or transduodenal route is necessary, cystic masses could be contaminated if gastric pH is not normal.

(2) When an anterior approach is not feasible, posterior approach may be possible in some cases for lesions in body and tail of pancreas.

(3) The risk of pancreatitis can be reduced by not traversing normal pancreas and not including pancreatic tissue in the sample.

8. Nonfocal organ biopsy
   a. Liver parenchyma (8)
      (1) US is adequate in most cases. CT may be required in large patients.
      (2) Left lobe approach: epigastric subxiphoid approach to the left hepatic lobe avoids pleural space transgression. This technique is performed near the midline away from major vessels, in the region of the linea alba.
      (3) Right lobe approach: subcostal or low intercostal approach is preferred.
      (4) Two or three, 18-gauge specimens are often sufficient.
      (5) The patient typically recovers for 3 to 5 hours after the procedure.
   b. Kidney parenchyma (9)
      (1) US typically used for guidance. CT may be required in large patients.
      (2) Target the lower pole cortex. Sample should be obtained from the most peripheral portion of the kidney as possible.
      (3) Two or three, 18-gauge specimens are often sufficient.
      (4) Patient typically recovers for 6 to 24 hours after procedure although shorter recovery times may be considered, particularly for transplant kidneys.

9. Reduction of bleeding risk: optional intraprocedural steps (1)
   a. Compress skin entry site
   b. Tamponade site by positioning ipsilateral side down
   c. Plugging the track with autologous clot or foam: when postprocedure bleeding is suspected or risk is high and a coaxial technique is used, the stylet can be inserted half way and left for 1 to 2 minutes to allow the subsequent clot to be injected by advancing the stylet before removing the stylet-introducer assembly. Alternatively, absorbable compressed gelatin sponge (Gelfoam, Pfizer Inc, New York, NY) or polyvinyl alcohol foam (e.g., Contour, Boston Scientific, Natick, MA) can be injected along the track as the introducer is withdrawn.

Postprocedure Management

1. Monitor vital signs in recovery area every 15 minutes for 1 hour, every 30 minutes for 2 hours, and then every hour.
2. Limit activity in the recovery room; bathroom use with assistance.
3. Clear liquid diet for the first hour; regular diet thereafter as tolerated.
4. If vital signs are stable and no adverse events are noted, the patient may be discharged, usually after 1 to 3 hours.
5. Advise patient of possible signs and symptoms of adverse events and provide contact information. Give instructions to outpatients regarding follow-up.

Pathology Results

1. Diagnostic tissue should be recovered in at least 80% to 95% of cases.
2. False negatives are most often due to inaccurate targeting of small lesions or sampling necrotic portions of large lesions. Diagnostic yield is improved by assuring that the needle tip is within the lesion at the time of the procedure.
3. Biopsy of the periphery of a large lesion may avoid a necrotic center.

Adverse Events

1. Overall, variable, and estimated: <2%
2. Bleeding: most common adverse event but clinically significant bleeding occurs in less than 2% of biopsies overall; death due to bleeding is extremely rare.
3. Infection: extremely rare
4. Organ injury needing surgery or other intervention (primary organ or adjacent organ [e.g., viscous or duct perforation], often depends on route): <2%
5. Pneumothorax: variable, depends on access route, probably <1%
6. Pancreatitis (depends on access route): 2% to 3% if normal pancreas is biopsied; less if normal pancreas not transgressed
7. Needle-tract tumor seeding. Reported with most tumors but overall extremely rare; approximate frequency: 0.003% to 0.009%
8. Mortality rate: 0.006% to 0.031%

Genomics (10)

In the era of personalized medicine and targeted therapy, a molecular pathology test (e.g., immunohistochemistry, polymerase chain reaction, fluorescence in situ hybridization, sequencing, messenger RNA arrays, methylation) may be often performed on the biopsy specimen. Previously, tissue was used to establish a benign or malignant nature of a lesion at the time of initial diagnosis. However, molecular analysis is more frequently being used to guide therapy at multiple timepoints to help guide targeted therapy or establish prognosis. Common malignancies that frequently can be treated with precision therapy include: lung, colon, pancreas, liver, and kidney. Uses for molecular testing include assessing for:

1. Molecular biomarkers that predict the natural course of disease and prognosis
2. Expressed receptors (e.g., vascular endothelial growth factor [VEGF]) and genetic variability that has been linked to differing therapeutic response and toxicity
3. Hallmarks of cancer signaling pathways and targets for specific drug interventions
4. Heterogeneity that is inherent to many cancers and affects success of therapies

More tissue may be needed for genomic testing compared to standard histopathology as up to 20% of biopsies performed for molecular testing may be nondiagnostic.

References

1. Carberry GA, Lubner MG, Wells SA, et al. Percutaneous biopsy in the abdomen and pelvis: a step-by-step approach. *Abdom Radiol (NY)*. 2016;41(4):720–742.
2. Davidson JC, Rahim S, Hanks SE, et al. Society of Interventional Radiology Consensus Guidelines for the Periprocedural Management of Thrombotic and Bleeding Risk in Patients Undergoing Percutaneous Image-Guided Interventions-Part I: Review of Anticoagulation Agents and Clinical Considerations: Endorsed by the Canadian Association For Interventional Radiology and the Cardiovascular and Interventional Radiological Society of Europe. *J Vasc Interv Radiol*. 2019;30(8):1155–1167.
3. Patel IJ, Rahim S, Davidson JC, et al. Society of Interventional Radiology Consensus Guidelines for the Periprocedural Management of Thrombotic and Bleeding Risk in Patients Undergoing Percutaneous Image-Guided Interventions-Part II: Recommendations: Endorsed by the Canadian Association for Interventional Radiology and the Cardiovascular and Interventional Radiological Society of Europe. *J Vasc Interv Radiol*. 2019;30(8): 1168–1184.e1.
4. Epelboym Y, Shyn PB, Hosny A, et al. Use of a 3D-printed abdominal compression device to facilitate CT fluoroscopy-guided percutaneous interventions. *AJR Am J Roentgenol*. 2017;209(2):435–441.
5. Potretzke TA, Saling LJ, Middleton WD, et al. Bleeding complications after percutaneous liver biopsy: do subcapsular lesions pose a higher risk? *AJR Am J Roentgenol*. 2018; 211(1):204–210.

6. Zhang CD, Delivanis DA, Eiken PW, et al. Adrenal biopsy: performance and use. *Minerva Endocrinol.* 2019;44(3):288–300.
7. Lim CS, Schieda N, Silverman SG. Update on indications for percutaneous renal mass biopsy in the era of advanced CT and MRI. *AJR Am J Roentgenol.* 2019;37:1–10.
8. Patel NJ, Bowman AW. Assessment of appropriate recovery time after liver biopsy. *J Am Coll Radiol.* 2018;15(9):1266–1268.
9. Patel A, Kriegshauser J, Young S, et al. Detection of bleeding complications following renal transplant biopsy. *AJR Am J Roentgenol.* 2020;216(2):428–435.
10. Dalag L, Fergus JK, Zangan SM. Lung and abdominal biopsies in the age of precision medicine. *Semin Intervent Radiol.* 2019;36(3):255–263.

50 Drainage of Abdominal Abscesses and Fluid Collections

Ashraf Thabet, MD and Ronald S. Arellano, MD, FSIR

Introduction

Percutaneous drainage of abdominal and pelvic collections is one of the most commonly performed interventional procedures and is a well-established management option in patients who do not have another indication for immediate surgery.

Indications

1. Fluid characterization (1,2)
   a. Distinguish purulent fluid, blood, bile, urine, lymph, and pancreatic secretions.
   b. Determine if collection is infected or sterile.
2. Treatment of sepsis (3)
   a. Curative in patients with simple abscesses.
   b. Curative or temporizing in patients with complex or pancreatic abscesses (4,5).
3. Relief of symptoms
   a. Alleviate pressure and pain due to size or location of collection (e.g., pancreatic pseudocyst).
   b. Obliterate recurring cysts or collections with sclerosing agents (6).

Contraindications

Absolute (1,2)
1. Lack of a safe pathway to the collection due to interposed vessels or viscera.
2. Uncooperative patient.

Relative (1,2)
1. Coagulopathy: Requires correction with appropriate blood products before proceeding.
2. Sterile collections (e.g., hematoma): prolonged catheter drainage may increase the risk of secondary infection.
3. Procedure requires transgression of pleura: risk of pneumothorax, pleural effusion, and empyema.
4. Echinococcal cyst: leakage of contents may elicit anaphylactic reaction.
5. Tumor abscess: may require lifelong catheter drainage.

6. Lack of a safe pathway to the collection due to interposed viscera.
7. Hemodynamic instability or cardiopulmonary compromise.

Preprocedure Preparation

1. NPO for 8 hours before procedure. (Note: If oral contrast use is anticipated for CT guidance, time for NPO requirement.)
2. Written informed consent.
3. Intravenous access: 20 gauge or larger.
4. Recent coagulation studies: Stop anticoagulation and antiplatelet medications such as coumadin and aspirin. Laboratory studies: PT <15 seconds, INR <1.5, platelets >50,000 per mm^3.
5. Prophylactic antibiotics required when draining abscess or potentially infected collection; preprocedure antibiotics generally do not affect cultures.
6. Conscious sedation with monitoring of physiologic parameters, including blood pressure, pulse, and oxygen saturation.
7. General anesthesia in young children, uncooperative patients or patients with significant medical comorbidities.

Imaging Guidance

1. Ultrasound (US)
   a. Enables real-time visualization of anatomy and needle/catheter during the procedure.
   b. Produces no radiation.
   c. May be used to guide primary needle access into the collection. For drainages performed using Seldinger technique, can then transition guidance to fluoroscopy for wire manipulation and tract dilation.
   d. Provides ability to perform portable procedures.
   e. Visualization is degraded by body habitus, bowel gas, and bone. This may make drainage of retroperitoneal and pelvic collections more difficult, particularly in obese patients.
2. CT
   a. Provides excellent tomographic visualization of anatomy and fluid collections irrespective of the overlying structures.
   b. Lack of real-time imaging guidance; this is mitigated with the use of CT fluoroscopy although radiation dose to patient and operator may be of concern.
3. Fluoroscopy
   a. Used in combination with other modalities, most often US, particularly when using Seldinger technique.
   b. Used to guide catheter exchanges and upsizing.

Procedure

1. **Preliminary imaging**
   a. Review prior imaging to (1) visualize the abnormality, (2) decide on the appropriate guidance method to be used, and (3) select route for drainage.
   b. Immediately prior to the procedure, confirm that the collection is clearly seen with the imaging-guidance method selected and verify safe route to the collection.
   c. Preliminary CT
      (1) Place the patient in the optimal position for drainage (supine, prone, lateral decubitus) and attach a radiopaque grid over the area of collection.
         (a) The lateral decubitus position may help reduce the risk of pleural transgression as it splints the ipsilateral hemithorax.

(b) If possible, both of the patient's arms are placed above the head to optimize image quality for drainage of upper quadrant collections.

(2) 5- to 10-mm thick contiguous slices are obtained through the region of interest. If there is concern, bowel (oral, rectal) and/or intravenous contrast medium may be given and imaging repeated to distinguish collection from surrounding normal structures. Timing of administration of oral contrast should take into account need for NPO status for sedation.

(3) From these preliminary images and with the aid of grid markings, a safe route for drainage is identified and the site of skin puncture, angle of needle entry, and distance to the collection are determined. Occasionally, when there is no safe route for puncture, angling the gantry or changing patient position may reveal a safe path for drainage.

2. **Determination of catheter route**

a. The optimal path for catheter drainage should consider the size and shape of the abscess and the safest route from skin to collection that does not transgress vital structures. If possible, an extraperitoneal approach is preferable as this reduces the risk of peritoneal contamination.

(1) When performing fine-needle aspiration alone, it is safe to traverse certain viscera such as liver, kidney, and small bowel. However, these structures should be avoided as much as possible when using catheter drainage.

(2) Traversing colon and normal pancreas should be avoided as this may risk superinfection of collections or pancreatitis, respectively.

(3) Aspiration and drainage of splenic abscesses can be done safely, as long as coagulation parameters are normal and vascular tumors are excluded.

(4) Interloop abscesses in inflammatory bowel disease may not be drainable due to surrounding small bowel loops, although fine-needle aspiration may be performed.

b. The usual anterior approach may not be possible in the pelvis due to overlying structures. In such cases, alternative routes such as the transgluteal, transvaginal, or transrectal approaches may be considered (7).

c. Organ displacement techniques may help displace nonvascular vital structures to create a window for percutaneous needle aspiration or drainage (8).

3. **Diagnostic needle aspiration**

a. Prior to drainage, preliminary fine-needle (22- to 20-gauge) aspiration of the collection is helpful to determine the nature of the collection. No more than 5 mL of fluid should be aspirated to prevent the cavity from collapsing should catheter drainage become necessary. If fluid is not obtained on initial aspiration and needle tip is optimally placed, then aspiration using a larger needle (18 gauge) may be attempted, with subsequent needles placed parallel and in tandem to the first needle. If no fluid is obtained on reaspiration, then, depending on the clinical suspicion, either a biopsy of the area or a trial with catheter drainage may be performed.

b. When fluid is aspirated, it can be inspected macroscopically, assessing for color, viscosity, turbidity, and smell. Fluid may be sent for laboratory testing to determine its origin. If the question of infection is important, as in the case of a sterile hematoma where catheter insertion may not be desirable, a rapid Gram stain analysis of the aspirate will determine the presence of bacteria and neutrophils. Thus, information from the preliminary needle aspiration can determine if no further action is to be taken, complete needle aspiration alone is sufficient, or catheter drainage is required.

c. If after aspiration the needle is found to be in a good position, it can be left in place and used as a parallel guide to place a catheter into the collection when using the trocar technique (i.e., tandem trocar technique), or it can be used for introduction of an 0.018-in guidewire as the first step in drainage using the Seldinger technique.

4. **Seldinger versus trocar technique**
   a. Percutaneous catheters are placed using the modified Seldinger or trocar techniques. The particular technique used is determined by the size of the collection, its location, operator preference/experience, and imaging guidance employed.
      (1) In general, large superficial collections are drained using the trocar technique because it is a one-stick procedure that is quick, simple, and safe to perform.
      (2) The Seldinger technique is preferred in potentially difficult drainages where the collection is small, is remotely situated, or has limited access. With this technique, multiple passes can be made using a thin needle such as a 20-gauge Chiba needle or a Ring needle. Once safe access is obtained, the tract can be serially dilated using coaxial exchanges of guidewires and dilators until insertion of a large catheter is possible. However, in inexperienced hands, particularly when not using real-time guidance, a number of complications, including guidewire kinking, loss of access, and catheter malposition, can occur.
   b. The catheters used commonly range in size from 7 to 14 Fr and can be either single lumen or double lumen (sump).
      (1) Larger catheters are traditionally used in the bigger and more complex collections. However, smaller bore catheters may be just as effective.
      (2) Similarly, the 12- to 14-Fr double-lumen sump catheters should theoretically allow more free drainage.
      (3) The use of a multi–side-hole catheter, such as a Cope-type loop biliary catheter, placed over the length of the collection may provide better drainage of spread-out collections, such as a subphrenic collection.
   c. CT-guided drainages performed using the trocar technique.
      (1) The optimal path for drainage between the abscess and skin is determined from the preliminary CT. The skin puncture site is marked on the patient using combined information from CT slice position and radiopaque markers. The skin is cleaned and draped using sterile technique.
      (2) Approximately 10 to 20 mL of 1% lidocaine is given as local anesthesia. A small skin incision is made and the subcutaneous tissue stretched using clamps or hemostats.
      (3) The angle of needle entry and distance to the collection are calculated from the preliminary CT images. Using these measurements, a 20-gauge needle is advanced into the collection. Repeat imaging is performed to confirm needle position. If the position is not optimal, the same needle is repositioned correctly or a second needle advanced in tandem.
      (4) Once the needle is optimally positioned, up to 5 mL of fluid is aspirated. The catheter is then loaded on a trocar delivery system (stiffening cannula and sharp inner stylet) and its tip placed in the skin wound while holding the shaft parallel to the diagnostic needle. The catheter is then advanced in tandem to the needle to the predetermined depth to enter the cavity.
      (5) As the catheter pierces the proximal wall of the abscess, there is usually a palpable "give" suggesting cavity puncture. This is confirmed by removal of the inner stylet and aspiration of fluid through the metal stiffener. Once fluid is aspirated, the catheter is unlocked from the stiffening cannula and slid forward to coil within the collection while holding the cannula steady. The cannula is removed and, if applicable, pigtail locked.
5. **Aspiration and irrigation**
   a. The catheter is attached to a drainage bag through a three-way stopcock. The use of a three-way stopcock provides a convenient, clean, and closed system through which the contents of the cavity can be aspirated and subsequently irrigated.
   b. The cavity should be aspirated until there is no more return. The cavity should then be irrigated with small volumes of saline (5 to 20 mL) no larger

in volume than the total volume of fluid initially aspirated from the cavity as overdistention may elicit bacteremia. Irrigation should be continued until the aspirate becomes clear or is merely blood-tinged.

c. Following this, a completion CT is performed through the drainage area to (a) ensure that the cavity is completely emptied, (b) detect any undrained separate collections, (c) form a baseline for future evaluation, and (d) screen for complications such as bleeding. If the cavity is incompletely drained due to loculation or there are additional separate collections, then additional needle aspiration or catheter drainage may be required.

6. **Catheter fixation:** Most catheters have some form of intrinsic locking device such as a string that can be tightened to coil and fix the catheter tip within the cavity. Additional security can be obtained by externally fixing the catheter to the skin. This can be achieved by attaching a tape around the catheter near the skin and suturing this tape to a skin adhesive (disk-type) device.

7. **Visceral collections**
   a. Liver (10)
      (1) When draining hepatic collections, avoid transgression of large vessels, dilated bile ducts, and the gallbladder.
      (2) Care should be exercised to avoid transgression of the pleura, although this is not always possible. Employ a subcostal and as anterior an approach when possible; such access may be more obtainable when using a combination of US and fluoroscopy rather than CT as the needle can be angled and advanced cranially.
      (3) Pyogenic abscesses are the most common hepatic collections amenable to percutaneous drainage.
      (4) Medical therapy is considered first-line therapy for hydatid cysts. Drainage can be performed in refractory disease in patients who have undergone at least 2 weeks of medical therapy. Small aspirates can be replaced with hypertonic saline prior to placing catheter to help reduce the risk of intraperitoneal spillage.
      (5) Medical therapy is also considered first-line therapy for amebic disease, although drainage can be performed for refractory disease or peripheral hepatic collections that may be more prone to rupture.
      (6) Bilomas, particularly if superinfected, are also amenable to percutaneous drainage.
   b. Spleen (1,9): Abscesses may also be aspirated or drained as long as coagulation parameters are normalized. Traverse as little splenic parenchyma as possible.
   c. Pancreas: symptomatic pseudocysts and abscesses are amenable to drainage. Persistent output from catheters suggests pancreatic fistula, which may be confirmed by contrast injection of the catheter; adjunctive octreotide therapy may be helpful to close the fistula.
   d. Urinomas: can be treated with catheter drainage, but may need an adjunctive nephroureteral catheter or percutaneous nephrostomy catheter with ureteral stent if there is persistent output.

8. **Subphrenic collections**
   a. Given their location, there is a risk of pleural transgression that may lead to pleural effusion, empyema, or pneumothorax.
   b. Combination of US and fluoroscopy may allow a subcostal approach to be used, where cranially located collections can be accessed by angling the needle superiorly.
   c. CT guidance may also be utilized and pleura traversed if no other access available; however, lung parenchyma generally should not be transgressed. Assess for pneumothorax and hemothorax on postprocedure images.

9. **Transgluteal drainage** (7): Catheter insertion should be as close to the sacrococcygeal margin as possible and below the piriformis muscle, generally at the

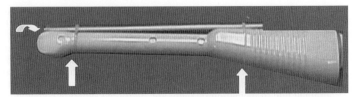

FIGURE 50.1 • Probe-guide assembly. The modified guide (fashioned from catheter protector tubing from packaging) is securely attached to the probe along the guide-groove with two sterile rubber bands (*straight arrows*). It should not project past the transducer head (*curved arrow*). The guide needs to be cut to the right length to allow at least 5 cm of catheter advancement through the vaginal vault. This stiff plastic tube is large enough to accept up to a 14-Fr trocar catheter. It needs to be preslit along its length so that it can be removed from the catheter after deployment. (Reprinted with permission from O'Neill MJ, Rafferty EA, Lee SI, et al. Transvaginal interventional procedures: aspiration, biopsy, and catheter drainage. *Radiographics.* 2001;21:657–672.)

level of the sacrospinous ligament. This helps avoid neurovascular structures that are located more laterally and superiorly; inadvertent traversal of the sacral plexus or inferior gluteal vessels may lead to transient buttock pain or bleeding, respectively. Angling the gantry may help achieve optimal access. The transgluteal approach is suitable in children as well.

10. **Transrectal and transvaginal drainage (7)**
    a. Transrectal: Suitable for collections anterior or posterior to rectum as well as prostatic abscess. For this approach, the patient is placed in the left lateral decubitus position.
    b. Transvaginal: Given the concern for seeding in certain pelvic malignancies, the transvaginal approach is used in specific circumstances, including recurrent endometriotic cysts, symptomatic hemorrhagic cysts, postoperative collections, poor surgical candidates, and pregnant patients. But it is not suitable for presacral collections. For the transvaginal approach, the patient is placed in the dorsal lithotomy position, a speculum inserted, and vaginal vault sterilized with povidone–iodine solution.
    c. A Foley catheter is helpful to decompress the bladder.
    d. Seldinger technique may be used. Once the wire is placed into the collection under US, further exchanges are performed using fluoroscopy. However, the Seldinger technique may be difficult due to wire kinking and distance of hand to point of wire entry. In transvaginal approaches, the muscular wall of the vagina is tough and may make wire exchanges challenging.
    e. In general, trocar technique is preferred as it is quicker to perform and can be done using only US. A peel-away sheath may be attached to the biopsy guide of the US probe. However, this occasionally may not be adequately stiff to maintain catheter position during manipulations. Alternatively, the plastic connector that comes with the catheter can be used as a guide (Fig. 50.1).
       (1) A longitudinal slit is cut along the length of the catheter. The protector is then shortened such that approximately 5 cm of catheter protrudes from its distal tip.
       (2) A sterile condom is placed over the probe and secured with rubber bands. The protector is then attached to the guide and secured with a distal and proximal rubber band. A second sterile condom is placed over the assembly.
       (3) A needle may be placed initially through the protector for diagnostic aspiration.
       (4) Subsequently, the catheter with stiffening cannula and sharp inner stylet are advanced into the protector (Fig. 50.2A).

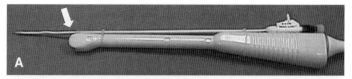

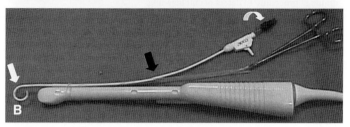

FIGURE 50.2 • Catheter delivery and probe-guide removal. **A:** Photograph shows the trocar catheter advanced through the guide and projecting approximately 5 cm past the end of the probe *(arrow).* **B:** Photograph shows that the catheter has been advanced and the pigtail has been formed *(straight white arrow).* The inner needle of the trocar has been removed for safety, but the outer metal cannula stiffener *(curved arrow)* is left in the straight portion of the catheter to stiffen it and ease the peeling away of the guide (attached to hemostat) from the catheter *(black arrow).* (Reprinted with permission from O'Neill MJ, Rafferty EA, Lee SI, et al. Transvaginal interventional procedures: aspiration, biopsy, and catheter drainage. *Radiographics.* 2001;21:657–672.)

(5) The catheter is advanced at least 2.5 cm into the collection to allow the pigtail to form. Doppler US may be helpful to avoid vessels. The stylet is removed, distal rubber band cut, and outer condom peeled away. The probe is carefully removed, the proximal rubber band cut, and protector guide removed (Fig. 50.2B).

(6) The inner stiffener is removed from the catheter and catheter secured to the medial thigh.

11. **Percutaneous abscess drainage in children (4)**
   a. The most common indication for percutaneous drainage in children is peri-appendiceal abscess.
   b. Technique and success rates are similar to adults
   c. As with other interventional procedures, consideration should be made of potential body heat losses in children. Special attention is given to the use of blankets, heat lamps, and warm US gel.
   d. Radiation dose should be minimized. This can be achieved by the use of pulsed fluoroscopy, low CT dose, use of gonadal shields, minimizing the distance between the patient and the image intensifier, acquiring fluoro stores rather than spot images, judicious use of magnification, and collimation.
   e. The transrectal approach may be used for periappendiceal abscesses. However, if the patient is too young that an endorectal probe is not suitable, a transrectal catheter can be placed with sonography performed from an anterior transabdominal view; the bladder should be distended to provide an acoustic window.

Complications

Overall, complication rates are reported to be less than 15% (1) and 30-day mortality approximately 1% to 6%. Complications may be categorized as major or minor (2).

Major (1)

1. Major complications include hemorrhage, septic shock, enteric fistula, peritonitis, and hemopneumothorax.
2. Puncture of a blood vessel can cause brisk and severe bleeding that may require blood transfusion, angiography with embolization, or even laparotomy for treatment. Therefore, all patients require close monitoring of their vital signs after a drainage procedure to detect occult bleeding.
3. Underlying viscera such as bowel can be punctured during catheter insertion. If there are signs of peritonitis, bowel obstruction, or enteric fluid draining from the catheter, catheter injection should be performed to check for catheter position, detect any fistula, and identify free peritoneal spill. If bowel communication, with or without free peritoneal leak, is found, immediate surgical consultation is required. This allows a combined decision to be made as to whether to remove the catheter immediately, remove it during laparotomy if peritonitis is present, or leave it in position for 3 to 4 weeks for a mature tract to develop.

Minor (1)

1. Minor complications include pain, bleeding, infection, and pericatheter leak.
2. The reasons for catheter nonfunction and pericatheter leak include kinking, blockage, or dislodgment. If simple bedside measures such as aspiration or flushing are not effective, then catheter injection and manipulation, or replacement under fluoroscopy may be required. If the catheter falls out inadvertently, then, depending on the duration and volume of drainage, nature of drainage, imaging findings, and patient clinical condition, a trial without catheter may be undertaken or a new catheter inserted using a new tract.
3. If infection is suspected at the catheter insertion site, swabs may be sent for culture and appropriate antibiotics started.
4. Bleeding from the catheter insertion site is usually self-limiting but occasionally may require angiographic investigation.

Catheter Care

Catheter care is best undertaken by the radiologists who have intimate knowledge of the procedure and catheter complications. This is best achieved by daily interventional ward rounds where a member of the interventional team sees the patient and deals with any problems related to the procedure. The catheter should be inspected to make sure that the stopcock is open to the drainage bag, the catheter has not been externally retracted, there is no pericatheter leak, and there are no local skin complications such as cellulitis. Orders should be written to flush the catheter with 10 mL of saline every 8 hours, 5 mL toward the collection and 5 mL toward the bag, for catheter occlusion prophylaxis. It is not necessary to attach catheters to suction, as gravity drainage to a bag is just as effective. This visit also provides an opportunity to review recordings of the patient's catheter outputs and vital signs, assess clinical progress, and make progress note report.

Catheter Removal

1. Catheter drainage is required until the patient's vital signs return to normal and the body can promote complete healing of the abscess cavity. Early removal will result in recurrence of the collection, while prolonged drainage will increase morbidity.
2. Usually, the catheter is removed when there is drainage of less than 20 mL per day from the catheter coupled with return of vital signs to normal. Repeat imaging is only required if (a) the patient's condition is not improving, (b) there is less than expected drainage, or (c) there is sudden reduction in drainage from the catheter.
3. If there is high output from the catheter (>50 mL per day) after the fourth day of catheter insertion, the possibility of a fistula to the bowel, pancreatic duct, or

biliary system should be considered and a catheter injection performed to identify any communication. If a fistula is found, prolonged (4 to 6 weeks) percutaneous catheter drainage or primary treatment of the fistula is required before the catheter can be removed. Adjunctive treatment of pancreatic fistulas with octreotide may be helpful.

4. If there is a persistent collection and poor outputs from the catheter, adjunctive use of tissue plasminogen activator (tPA) can be very helpful (4). In general, 4 to 6 mg of tPA is diluted in 50-mL normal saline. Up to 50 mL is injected into the catheter twice daily for 3 days (care should be taken not to inject a volume larger than the collection size), with the catheter clamped for 30 minutes after injection. This can be successful up to nearly 90% of the time, with failure more likely in patients with pancreatic collections, fungal infection, or enteric fistula.

Results

1. The success of percutaneous drainage of uncomplicated collections can exceed 90% (1). However, this decreases significantly with complex collections such as those with loculation or inflammation (e.g., pancreatic abscess).

2. The recurrence rate of a collection after drainage is between 8% and 20% and is commonly due to early removal of catheter, undetected fistula, or drainage of tumor abscess.

R e f e r e n c e s

1. Dariushnia SR, Mitchell JW, Chaudry G, et al. Society of Interventional Radiology Quality Improvement Guidelines for image-guided percutaneous drainage and aspiration of abscesses and fluid collections. *J Vasc Interv Radiol.* 2020;31(4): 662–666.

2. Charles HW. Abscess drainage. *Seim Intervent Radiol.* 2012;29: 325–336.

3. Dissanayake B, Burstow MJ, Jeyakumar A, et al. Operative surgery is rarely required in the acute management of diverticulitis in the modern era. *Am Surg.* 2020; 84(4):308–312

4. Shawyer AC, Amaral JGPV, Langer JC. The role of tissue plasminogen activator in the management of complex intra-abdominal abscesses in children. *J Pediatr Surg.* 2012 47(7): 1380–1384.

5. Cronin CG, Gervais DA, Fernandez-del Castillo C, et al. Interventional radiology in the management of abdominal collections after distal pancreatectomy: a retrospective review. *AJR Am J Roentgenol.* 2011;197(1):241–245.

6. Ballard DH, Mokkarala M, D'Agostino HB. Percutaneous drainage and management of fluid collections associated with necrosis or cystic tumors in the abdomen and pelvis. *Abdom Radiol.* 2019;44(4) 1562–1566.

7. Maher MM, Gervais DA, Kalra MK, et al. The inaccessible or undrainable abscess: how to drain it. *Radiographics.* 2004;24(3):717–735.

8. Arellano RS, Gervais DA, Mueller PR. CT-guided drainage of abdominal abscesses: hydrodissection to create access routes for percutaneous drainage. *AJR Am J Roentgenol.* 2011;196(1):189–191.

9. Li G, Gao L, Zhou J, et al. Management of splenic abscess after splenic arterial embolization in severe acute pancreatitis: a 5-year single-center experience. *Gastroenterol Res Pract.* 2019: 2019:60669179.

10. Zu S, Shi BQ, Chao LM, et al. Prognostic nomogram for the combination therapy of percutaneous catheter drainage and antibiotic in pyogenic liver abscess patients. *Abdom Radiol (NY).* 2020;45(2):393–402.

51 Percutaneous Gastrostomy, Percutaneous Gastrojejunostomy, Jejunostomy, and Cecostomy

Ji Hoon Shin, MD and Ho-Young Song, MD, PhD

Percutaneous Enteral Tubes

Although temporary enteral tubes (e.g., nasogastric [NG] and nasojejunal) may be placed through natural orifices, percutaneously placed feeding tubes offer the best options for patients who require long-term nutrition. Percutaneous radiologic gastrostomy (PRG) is associated with low morbidity and mortality rates. These minimally invasive procedures are generally simpler, associated with higher technical success rates, and have lower complication rates than percutaneous endoscopic gastrostomy (PEG) or surgical placement techniques.

Types of Tubes

1. Dedicated single function (feeding or decompression alone)
   a. Gastrostomy (G-tube)
      (1) Simplest technically, requiring the least manipulation
      (2) Shortest tube, providing for less clogging over time
      (3) Preserves gastric function, allowing for high diet variety and simplicity in maintenance
      (4) Can be converted into gastrojejunostomy (GJ) tube after percutaneous tract matures (10 to 21 days)
   b. Jejunostomy (J-tube)
      (1) Bypasses stomach, requires elemental diet and slow pump infusion to prevent dumping syndrome
      (2) A higher level of tube care is required
      (3) Single-lumen GJ
         (a) Catheter placed via the stomach with tip at or beyond the ligament of Treitz
         (b) Simpler to place under fluoroscopy than direct J-tube
         (c) Longer catheter than direct J-tube, making it more prone to clogging
2. Split function: Double-lumen gastrojejunostomy (DLGJ)
   a. Requires elemental diet and slow jejunal infusion using a pump
   b. Gastric lumen required for either of the following:
      (1) Decompression in patients with gastroparesis or gastric outlet obstruction
      (2) Medications that are only absorbed by the stomach

Percutaneous Gastrostomy

Indications (1–5)
1. Nutritional support for patients with inadequate oral intake due to dysphagia, risk of aspiration, or obstruction secondary to
   a. Stroke and neuromuscular disorders
   b. Esophageal mass/neoplasm
   c. Lesions of the head, neck, and mediastinum (including recent surgery or radiation)
2. Diversion of feedings from esophageal leaks caused by recent surgery or trauma

3. Decompression of gastroenteric contents and/or need for jejunal feeding
   a. Gastric outlet or proximal small bowel obstruction
   b. Patients with gastroparesis (e.g., diabetic gastropathy, scleroderma)
4. Intestinal access for biliary procedures (e.g., patients with Roux-en-Y anastomosis)

Contraindications (1–5)

Absolute
1. Unsatisfactory anatomy (e.g., no safe percutaneous access to stomach secondary to interposed colon or liver)
2. Uncorrectable coagulopathy

Relative
1. Prior gastric surgery with anatomic distortion (e.g., subtotal gastrectomy or gastric bypass). Access to the stomach may be extremely difficult and require advanced techniques and/or CT guidance
2. Massive ascites. Preprocedural paracentesis and gastropexy can help reduce the incidence of peritoneal leakage
3. Gastric or abdominal wall varices due to portal hypertension
4. Inflammatory, neoplastic, or infectious involvement of the gastric wall (may result in poor wound healing and tract formation)
5. Severe gastroesophageal reflux. Feedings should be delivered into the jejunum via PGJ or percutaneous jejunostomy (PJ) tube
6. Ventriculoperitoneal shunt

Preprocedure Preparation
1. Review surgical history and prior imaging for evidence of altered gastric anatomy, safe percutaneous access route, and ascites.
2. Review and correct as necessary any coagulopathy.
3. Approximately 200 mL of dilute barium suspension is given 12 hours before the procedure to outline the colon. Alternatively, colonic gas is typically sufficient to outline the colon, or when not present, a small amount of air or contrast can be instilled retrograde per rectum at the time of the procedure.
4. Maintain nil per os (NPO) status for 8 hours prior to procedure.
5. An NG tube (preferably placed bedside the evening before the procedure) is necessary for insufflating air to bring the stomach into apposition with the anterior abdominal wall, displacing adjacent viscera, and facilitating safe gastrostomy tube placement. If there is difficulty placing the NG tube at bedside, an angiographic catheter placed under fluoroscopic guidance immediately prior to the procedure may be used for insufflation.
6. Conscious sedation should be given judiciously in patients with head and neck malignancies or respiratory compromise in neuromuscular disorders such as amyotrophic lateral sclerosis (ALS). In fact, the ability to safely and comfortably place radiologic gastrostomy tubes with minimal sedation is a particular advantage in this patient population.

Procedure
1. Prepare the left subcostal area and epigastrium in a sterile manner.
2. Glucagon (0.5 to 1.0 mg) or butylscopolamine (20 mg) intravenously (IV) may be administered to diminish gastric peristalsis.
3. Insufflate air into the stomach via NG tube until adequate gastric distention is achieved fluoroscopically.
4. Although the need for routine gastropexy remains debated, clinical scenarios suggesting an impaired ability to form a mature tract (e.g., patients on chronic steroids) or at high risk for peritoneal leakage (patients with ascites) mandate secure gastropexy (1,2,6).

5. If gastropexy is not employed, it may be necessary to continue air insufflation during the procedure to keep the stomach distended—so it is wise to limit the volume of air used initially. In patients with partial gastrectomy or other surgeries involving a vagotomy, it will be more challenging to maintain gastric distension during tube placement. Conversely, the presence of adhesions often simulates a gastropexy.

6. After air insufflation, frontal and oblique views of the upper abdomen are helpful to determine the depth to the anterior gastric wall and location of the transverse colon. Rarely, lateral imaging may be needed.

7. Choose the puncture site—distal body of the stomach, equidistant from the lesser and greater curvatures to minimize the risk of arterial injury (Fig. 51.1). Avoid punctures that transgress the colon or left lobe of the liver. The risk of hemorrhage is minimized by avoiding the inferior epigastric artery as it courses the junction of the medial two-thirds and lateral one-third of the rectus muscle (Fig. 51.1).

8. Infiltrate local anesthesia (1% lidocaine) down to the peritoneal surface; a small skin incision is made.

9. Many operators routinely use gastropexy devices (Saf-T-Pexy T-Fasteners [Avanos, Alpharetta, GA] or 18-gauge needle preloaded with a T-fastener [Cook Inc, Bloomington, IN]). Two to four T-fasteners are deployed to fix the anterior gastric wall to the abdominal wall (1,2). Gastric puncture is performed with the kit needle preloaded with an anchor system. An intragastric position is confirmed both by aspiration of air into a syringe and injection of contrast with visualization of gastric rugae. A stylet is introduced through the needle, advancing the anchor into the stomach. The stylet and needle are subsequently removed and the stomach is gently approximated to the anterior abdominal wall by gentle traction on the anchor suture. Alternatively, the needle is removed over a safety guidewire (GW) to retain original access. If gastropexy is not employed, a Seldinger needle is used for a new gastric puncture.

10. Whatever the choice, the puncture should be made with a brief, deliberate thrust so as not to push the anterior gastric wall away from the anterior abdominal wall. Usually, the puncture needle is directed slightly toward the pylorus, to facilitate future conversion to a PGJ if needed (Fig. 51.2). When placing a pull-type gastrostomy tube under fluoroscopy, access can be directed slightly toward the gastroesophageal junction to facilitate cannulation of the esophagus.

11. Once the gastric lumen is entered, the needle position is confirmed by injection of contrast, outlining gastric rugal folds. With the Seldinger needle tip within the stomach, a stiff 0.035-in GW is inserted and looped in the stomach.

12. Fascial dilators, of adequate diameter to accommodate the feeding tube, are introduced over the 0.035-in GW to make a tract (Fig. 51.2). Because of the thick muscular wall of the stomach, the dilator can easily push the stomach wall forward rather than dilating the puncture hole within the wall. If this happens, the GW may prolapse outside the stomach into the peritoneum. A GW with the proper stiffness and fluoroscopic visualization during manipulation helps avoid this problem.

13. Place the selected gastrostomy tube over the wire, through an appropriately sized peel-away sheath if placing a balloon retention gastrostomy tube (e.g., Entuit gastrostomy catheter, Cook, Bloomington, IN) (typically 2 Fr larger than the gastrostomy tube to accommodate the balloon). A 12-Fr or larger locking loop multipurpose drainage catheter can also be used (Fig. 51.2).

14. Following tube placement, contrast is injected and fluoroscopic images of the upper abdomen are obtained to confirm proper position.

15. The feeding tube is secured to the skin with sutures or commercially available retaining devices.

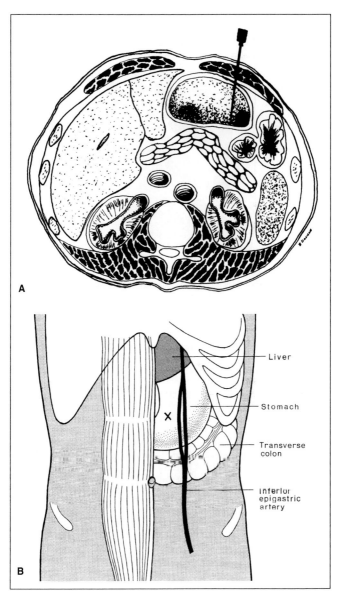

FIGURE 51.1 • **A:** Axial cross-section of abdomen at the level of the body of the stomach with patient supine. No liver or colon noted anteriorly. **B:** Frontal cutaway view shows window to body of the stomach (*X*), avoiding the inferior epigastric artery, left lobe of the liver, and transverse colon. (*continued*)

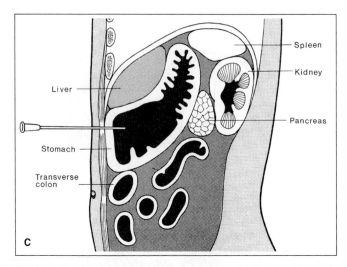

FIGURE 51.1 • (*Continued*) **C:** Sagittal view demonstrating superficial location of the anterior wall of a distended stomach. Liver is cephalad to, and lumen of transverse colon is caudal to, the stomach.

Postprocedure Management

1. Vital signs and serial abdominal examination must be closely followed, looking for signs of peritonitis that may indicate leakage of gastric contents. Pneumoperitoneum on routine imaging is not unexpected and slowly resolves over 24 to 72 hours.

2. The PG tube should remain connected to a gravity drainage bag or to low, intermittent suction for the first 24 hours following placement, before attempting feedings. If documented overnight output is not excessive, and if the abdominal exam is benign, feedings may begin the next morning.

3. For a PG tube, the initial infusion rate is usually 10 mL per hour, increased as tolerated by 10 mL per shift to goal rate as determined by the nutritional support team. J-tubes require a slower infusion rate. Although gastric residuals are commonly checked and recorded by the nursing staff, what more accurately predicts a well-functioning feeding tube is the absence of symptoms such as reflux, aspiration, nausea, and bloating.

4. If these symptoms persist over several days after initiating feeding, the patient should be assessed for presence of ileus; if absent, agents to increase gastric motility may be initiated. If motility agents are not successful in decreasing tube residuals, the G-tube may be converted to a G–J tube to allow more distal feeding while providing the option for proximal decompression.

5. If the PG tube is placed for decompression of small bowel obstruction, low, intermittent suction should begin early and continued as needed.

6. Long-term management: Routine G-tube changes are not usually performed; commonly, the clinical team, patient, or outside caretaker calls if there are problems—this usually results in a tube change in 4 to 6 months. However, a proactive involvement by the interventional radiology (IR) service with patients is preferable. Most problems are resolved by asking the right questions of the person (caregiver or the patient) accessing the tube most frequently. Common scenarios and their management are as follows:

   a. The retention device failed, causing the tube to partially back out.

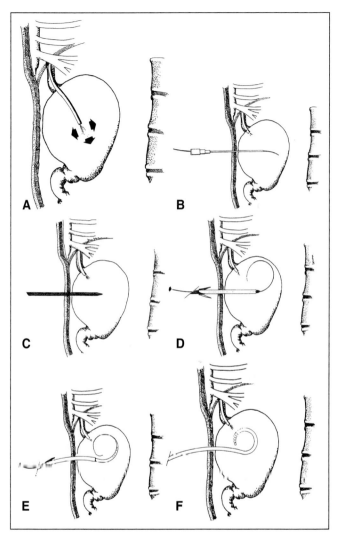

FIGURE 51.2 • Alternative method for placement of a percutaneous gastrostomy tube. **A:** The stomach is inflated with air through the nasogastric tube to bring the gastric wall close to the abdominal wall. **B:** The puncture is made with a 16-gauge needle/catheter pointing vertically down, and a 0.035-in J-tipped guidewire is advanced through it. **C,D:** Before inserting the peel-away introducer sheath, fascial dilators are advanced over the guidewire until an adequate diameter is reached. **E:** The catheter is advanced over the guidewire through the peel-away sheath. **F:** After the catheter is in place, the guidewire is removed and the sheath is peeled away. (Reprinted with permission from Castaneda-Zuniga WR, Tadavarthy SM. *Interventional Radiology.* 2nd ed. Wolters Kluwer; 1992:1218–1219.)

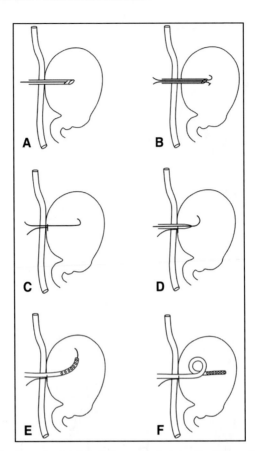

FIGURE 51.3 • One-anchor technique. **A:** The puncture is made with a 17-gauge needle pre-loaded with a single anchor. **B:** After confirming its location within the stomach, the anchor is released by pushing with a guidewire. **C:** After removing the 17-gauge needle, the anchor is pulled firmly toward the anterior abdominal wall. **D:** Fascial dilators are advanced over the guidewire until an adequate diameter is reached. **E,F:** A gastrostomy tube (10 to 16 Fr) is introduced over the guidewire into the stomach. *Note:* A similar technique is employed for percutaneous jejunostomy tube placement.

     (1) If the catheter is functioning normally, it should be refixed in place.

     (2) If malfunction of the catheter is suspected, it is appropriate to check under fluoroscopy and possibly replace the catheter.

  b. The tube fell out/was pulled out completely: In the setting of a mature tract, the tube can be replaced at the bedside. If the tract has constricted, there is difficulty with bedside replacement, or concern about tube malposition, fluoroscopy can be used to recannulate the existing tract with an angled catheter and wire, facilitating placement of a new tube.

  c. The tube is leaking around the skin insertion site.

     (1) If the patient has a balloon retention catheter, the balloon is likely ruptured. Instruct the patient to fix the catheter to the skin until arriving in IR for tube replacement.

(2) If the patient has a multi–side-hole catheter, either the side holes have backed into the tract or the patient is developing gastric outlet obstruction. Rarely, this occurs from the catheter loop migrating to, and obstructing, the pylorus.

d. The tube is clogged.

(1) This is typically from inadequately crushed pills or suboptimal flushing after use. The catheter should be vigorously flushed with a 3-mL syringe.

(2) If the above is unsuccessful, the catheter should be exchanged. In the setting of a mature tract, if the tube is too obstructed to allow GW passage, it may be removed completely and the tract recanalized. Alternatively, the external hub is cut and a properly sized peel-away sheath is coaxially introduced over the old tube to retain original access.

e. The patient is not tolerating feeds or has diarrhea: This history is classic for a gastrostomy tube that has migrated to the duodenum. Bolus feeds no longer slowly drain through the pylorus and the patient develops dumping syndrome. The tube should be repositioned into the stomach with fluoroscopy.

f. The patient has abdominal pain: Physical examination is important to determine the cause: skin infection, tube migration, gastric outlet obstruction, or other causes.

g. The patient is complaining of skin irritation/breakdown at the insertion site.

(1) A liquid antacid may be applied topically to the area.

(2) Evaluate for infection and treat with antibiotics as appropriate.

Modifications of PG Placement

1. One-anchor technique

a. Controversy exists as to the number of anchors that is sufficient—one placed through the gastrostomy tract (i.e., one-anchor technique) to four placed in the form of a square around the tract (2).

b. With this technique, a single anchor is inserted through the preloaded 17-gauge puncture needle (Cope gastrointestinal suture anchor sets, Cook, Bloomington, IN) (Fig. 51.3). After confirming its location within the stomach, the anchor is released by pushing with the GW. The anchor is pulled firmly toward the anterior abdominal wall; serial dilators are introduced over the GW through the same tract. Finally, a gastrostomy tube (10 to 16 Fr) is introduced over the GW into the stomach (Fig. 51.3).

c. Although the one anchor technique is a simple procedure, there is an increased risk of anchor dislodgment and related peritonitis

2. Pull-type gastrostomy tube placement: The problem associated with the retention of radiologically inserted gastrostomy tubes led to the development of peroral *endoscopic* placement of pull-type gastrostomy tubes (7). However, these tubes may also be placed percutaneously using fluoroscopic guidance:

a. The pull-type gastrostomy tube is pulled down through the oropharynx. Because this may transport oral bacteria to the gastrostomy site, prophylactic antibiotics are advised (generally penicillin-based prophylaxis).

b. Percutaneous gastric access is similar to that of PG tube placement, but the use of gastropexy is debated.

c. Following successful access, a 5- to 7-Fr angiographic catheter and GW are used to cross the gastroesophageal junction from the stomach to the esophagus. The catheter and GW are advanced in a retrograde direction and pulled out of the patient's mouth.

d. After exchanging the GW for a "traction wire" or preferably an exchange-length GW, a pull-type gastrostomy tube is introduced coaxially, passing in an antegrade direction down the mouth into the esophagus and out the anterior abdominal wall. The tapered tip of the gastrostomy tube is then cut to the desired length. A 20-Fr mushroom-retained catheter (Flow 20, Cook, Inc, Bloomington, IN) is commonly used.

e. The tube is affixed externally at the skin.

Results
Technical success of PRG and PGJ placement approaches 100% (1–5).

Complications
1. 30-day mortality from all causes ranges from around 4% (1) to 8% (3) depending on the severity of the underlying illness, according to one meta-analysis of the literature (3). Procedure-related 30-day mortality is under 0.5%.
2. Major complications (hemorrhage, peritonitis, wound infection, gastrointestinal perforation, aspiration, displacement of the tube requiring a repeat procedure, and sepsis) are under 8% (3). Surgical and endoscopic gastrostomies carry higher mortality and complication rates (3); PRG is often the preferred approach.
3. Peritonitis associated with PRG is a rare but most serious major complication (8). This devastating complication is caused by extravasation of gastric contents into the peritoneum, either from intraperitoneal leakage around an enteral puncture site or from tube migration and erosion causing frank perforation of the stomach (or small bowel in the case of direct jejunostomy). Tube feeding should be held; clinical evaluation should dictate surgical consultation and exploratory laparotomy, if necessary.
4. Aspiration pneumonia occurs less frequently with PRG (0.8% to 5%) than with PEG (6% to 20%, related to profound sedation and the technique used during the endoscopic procedure).
5. Minor complications (superficial wound infection, minor peritubal leakage, tube dislodgment) are reported in 5% to 10% of cases (3).
6. Gastrointestinal complications such as hemorrhage and perforation following PRG or PGJ tube placement occur in less than 2% of cases (3). Transarterial embolotherapy is useful for controlling massive hemorrhage (2).
7. Other potential complications—laceration of the liver, pancreas, or spleen, and gastroenteric fistula—are very rare.

Percutaneous Gastrojejunostomy

In patients with a history or risk of gastroesophageal reflux or aspiration, percutaneous gastrojejunostomy (PGJ) is considered. PGJ can be performed as an initial feeding tube placement (primary PGJ) or by converting a prior gastrostomy tube to a GJ (conversion PGJ) tube. Conversion may be performed any time after successful placement of a PG if gastropexy is used, or if not, after the tract matures (usually in 1 to 3 weeks). A successfully placed or converted PGJ tube may be used within hours of insertion. Multiple types of GJ tubes are available, with gastric and jejunal ports. Typical size ranges are 16 to 22 Fr and lengths 15 to 45 cm (e.g., MIC Gastric-jejunal Feeding Tube, Avanos, Alpharetta, GA).

Conversion of a Mature PG Tube to PGJ Tube
1. Conversion PGJ can be difficult if the initial angle of entry of the PG tube is directed toward the fundus. An angled 5-Fr vascular catheter (usually C-1), 7-Fr seeking catheter, and a rigid sheath or vascular dilator have all been described to facilitate the redirection of the tract. Redirection can avoid proximal migration and recoil of a PGJ tube after it has been successfully placed.
2. If the original tract is unfavorable for redirection, a new puncture directed toward the pylorus is needed.

3. Regardless of the type of tube deployed (coaxial configuration or a single tube with dual ports), the tip of PGJ tubes should be placed well beyond the ligament of Treitz and the gastric port should be located within the stomach lumen.

Primary Placement of a PGJ Tube

1. For primary PGJ tube placement, follow all steps as described for PG placement but direct the initial needle puncture toward the pylorus.
2. Using an angled catheter–GW combination, maneuver the catheter into the jejunum.
3. Replace the initial GW for a stiffer exchange GW, with the tip well into the jejunum.
4. Dilate the entry site and place a peel-away sheath.
5. Introduce the PGJ tube with jejunal and gastric ports optimally positioned as described above.
6. Inject a small amount of contrast through each port to confirm satisfactory position.
7. Secure the catheter at the skin.
8. The jejunal port (not the gastric, if a fresh introduction) may be used immediately for feeding.
9. Irrigate copiously with fresh tap water after each use to prevent clogging.

Percutaneous Jejunostomy

Primary PJ tube placement is indicated for patients with a history of chronic aspiration, gastric surgery (i.e., gastrectomy), or abnormal gastric position. Percutaneous puncture of the jejunum is more difficult than that of stomach because of the high mobility and easy collapsibility of the jejunum. The technical success of the PJ placement ranges between 85% and 95% (8,9). A 12-Fr or larger pigtail multipurpose catheter, or balloon retention single lumen jejunostomy tube (e.g., MIC Key jejunostomy tube, Avanos, Alpharetta, GA) of size ranges 12 to 22 Fr, up to 51 cm long, are used.

1. A 5-Fr angled catheter (cobra or head-hunter) and a 0.035-in GW (hydrophilic, if needed—these wires may be stiffer than necessary) are introduced through the nostril and directed through the esophagus into the jejunum under fluoroscopic guidance.
2. Dilatation of jejunal loops is achieved by slow saline injection. Upon frontal and lateral fluoroscopy, the catheter tip is located in an air-filled proximal jejunal loop, as a target, in a position that is sufficiently close to the anterior abdominal wall.
3. Puncture of the distended jejunum is performed under fluoroscopic and/or ultrasound guidance (8). A 17-gauge needle preloaded with a Cope suture anchor is commonly used (8)—Note: The technique is similar to that illustrated in Figure 51.3 for gastrostomy tube placement. A 21-gauge Chiba needle (Cook) can alternatively be used for puncture (9). After confirming the intraluminal positioning of the needle, a 0.018-in GW is advanced as far as possible into the jejunum to allow insertion of the sheath from a 6-Fr Neff introduction set (Cook). A single Cope suture anchor is then deployed into the jejunum through the Neff sheath. Following serial dilation of the entry site, the tube is inserted.
4. Postprocedure feeding and tube management are similar to PGJ tubes.

Percutaneous Cecostomy

Cecostomy is indicated for decompression and/or diversion in the setting of fecal incontinence, colonic pseudo-obstruction (Ogilvie syndrome), or cecal volvulus (10). Cecostomy tubes can also be used to deliver laxatives for antegrade irrigation for patients who have chronic constipation caused by a neurogenic colon, avoiding the need for multiple retrograde enemas (10). The posterolateral extension of the peritoneum around the cecum along with the overlying posterolateral iliac bone is the rationale for using an anterior intraperitoneal approach rather than a retroperitoneal approach.

1. When needed, the cecum is distended using air introduced through a Foley catheter placed through the rectum.
2. A single-wall puncture is made under fluoroscopic guidance with a 18-gauge, 7-cm, single-wall needle with a Seldinger shield (e.g., MajeSTIK, Merit Medical, South Jordan, UT). The needle is preloaded with two metallic retention sutures (Cook). After confirming intraluminal location of the needle tip with contrast injection, a 0.035-in Amplatz GW is used to deploy the retention sutures, and the needle is removed leaving the GW in place.
3. Although the retention sutures are pulled tight for the cecum to be drawn close to the abdominal wall, the tract is dilated (using a Coons Dilator, Cook) over the GW so that an 8.5- to 10-Fr cecostomy tube (Dawson-Mueller Catheter, Cook) can be accommodated. Conversions to a cecostomy button (Chait Trapdoor Cecostomy Catheter, Cook) with a coil-shaped distal tip may be needed for long-term use.
4. The tube is attached to external drainage for decompression or used for antegrade irrigation/enemas as needed.
5. Technical success is high in patients with fecal incontinence (~100%); 89% of them have improvement of fecal incontinence (10).
6. Complications are rare. Granulation tissue formation around the tube insertion site or tube dislodgment can occur.

References

1. Brown AS, Mueller PR, Ferrucci JT Jr. Controlled percutaneous gastrostomy: nylon T-fastener for fixation of the anterior gastric wall. *Radiology*. 1986;158:543–545.
2. Kim JW, Song HY, Kim KR, et al. The one-anchor technique of gastropexy for percutaneous radiologic gastrostomy: results of 248 consecutive procedures. *J Vasc Interv Radiol*. 2008;19(7):1048–1053.
3. Wollman B, D'Agostino HB, Walus-Wigle JR, et al. Radiologic, endoscopic, and surgical gastrostomy: an institutional evaluation and meta-analysis of the literature. *Radiology*. 1995;197(3):699–704.
4. Kuo YC, Shlansky-Goldberg RD, Mondschein JI, et al. Large or small bore, push or pull: a comparison of three classes of percutaneous fluoroscopic gastrostomy catheters. *J Vasc Interv Radiol*. 2008;19(4):557–563.
5. Park JH, Shin JH, Ko HK, et al. Percutaneous radiologic gastrostomy using the one-anchor technique in patients after partial gastrectomy. *Korean J Radiol*. 2014;15(4):488–493.
6. Dewald CL, Hiette PO, Sewall LE, et al. Percutaneous gastrostomy and gastrojejunostomy with gastropexy: experience in 701 procedures. *Radiology*. 1999;211(3):651–656.
7. Clark JA, Pugash RA, Pantalone RR. Radiologic peroral gastrostomy. *J Vasc Interv Radiol*. 1999;10(7):927–932.
8. van Overhagen H, Ludviksson MA, Laméris JS, et al. US and fluoroscopic-guided percutaneous jejunostomy: experience in 49 patients. *J Vasc Interv Radiol*. 2000;11(1):101–106.
9. Yang ZQ, Shin JH, Song HY, et al. Fluoroscopically guided percutaneous jejunostomy: outcomes in 25 consecutive patients. *Clin Radiol*. 2007;62(11):1060–1068.
10. Chait PG, Shlomovitz E, Connolly BL, et al. Percutaneous cecostomy: updates in technique and patient care. *Radiology*. 2003;227(1):246–250.

52 Percutaneous Biliary Interventions

Pouya Entezari, MD and Ahsun Riaz, MD

Introduction

Peroral endoscopic procedures by Interventional Gastroenterology (GI) are considered the standard of care in management of biliary disease. However, there have been many advances in percutaneous approaches, including endoscopy, by interventional radiology (IR) which offer a safe and effective alternative in cases of failed or difficult endoscopic intervention.

A meta-analysis on patients with malignant obstructive jaundice revealed a similar rate of therapeutic success and overall complication rates between peroral endoscopic and percutaneous approaches. Percutaneous interventions demonstrate a lower risk of pancreatitis and cholangitis with a higher risk of bleeding when compared to peroral endoscopic procedures (1).

Frequently, multiple underlying conditions in patients undergoing percutaneous interventions render these procedures technically challenging. Precise planning of the procedure, close collaboration of interventional radiologists and gastroenterologists, and close follow-up provide effective care to these patients. This chapter will focus on IR management of benign/malignant biliary ductal diseases and will touch on the gallbladder.

Preprocedural Preparation

Precise evaluation of the patient prior to the biliary intervention is a crucial step. Multidisciplinary discussions with gastroenterologists, surgeons, and oncologists can help achieve the best treatment option (including rendezvous treatment plans).

1. Clinical status evaluation
   a. Scrutinizing of patient's history and clinical examination provides valuable information to assure that the appropriate procedure is performed.
   b. Examination of cardiopulmonary functional status is important to make sure patient tolerates anesthesia and procedure.
   c. Personal review of surgical procedure notes relating to biliary anatomy is integral.
2. Laboratory investigations
   a. Complete blood count (CBC)
      (1) Drop in hemoglobin postprocedure indicates bleeding.
      (2) Leukocytosis can indicate infection (e.g., cholangitis).
      (3) Platelet levels should be ≥50,000 per mL (2).
   b. Liver function tests (LFTs) including alkaline phosphatase, gamma-glutamyl transferase (pediatric population), and bilirubin levels should be obtained at baseline and postprocedure to assess intervention efficacy.
   c. International normalized ratio (INR)
      (1) Aim for INR ≤1.5 (2).
      (2) Consider fresh-frozen plasma to correct INR in emergent procedures.
3. Imaging
   a. Ultrasound (US) and computerized tomography (CT) can provide adequate information regarding biliary pathology and ductal anatomy variations.
   b. Magnetic resonance (MR) and MR cholangiopancreaticography (MRCP) are of great value in diagnosis of biliary pathologies and understanding the anatomical structure of biliary tree.
   c. Review of reports/images from prior ERCP/endoscopic US (EUS) should also be performed.

4. Antiplatelets and anticoagulation
   a. Hold antiplatelet agents 5 days prior to the procedure, if clinically possible.
   b. Hold warfarin for 5 days until INR ≤1.8. For patients with high risk of thrombosis, consider bridging anticoagulation. Withhold heparin 4 to 6 hours before the procedure (2).
5. Antibiotics (3)
   a. Biliary interventions are classified as clean-contaminated/contaminated and administration of prophylactic antibiotics is recommended. The most common strains found in biliary secretions are Enterococcus, Candida species, and gram-negative aerobic bacilli. Prophylactic antibiotic should be administered within 1 hour before start of the procedure. In prolonged procedures (>2 hours), a supplemental dose of antibiotic should be considered.
   b. There is no consensus regarding first-choice antibiotic. Recommended antibiotic regimens:
      (1) 1-g ceftriaxone IV
      (2) 1.5 to 3 g ampicillin/sulbactam IV (Unasyn)
      (3) 1-g cefotetan IV plus 4-g mezlocillin IV
      (4) 2-g ampicillin IV plus 1.5-mg per kg gentamicin IV
      (5) In case of penicillin allergy, use a combination of aminoglycoside with vancomycin or clindamycin
6. Anesthesiology: Pain control is critical in patients undergoing biliary interventions. Epidural anesthesia provides significantly better pain control, compared to IV sedation. General anesthesia or monitored anesthesia care greatly improves the ease of the procedure.

Percutaneous Transhepatic Cholangiography (PTC)

Indications
1. Evaluation of ductal anatomy to reveal biliary pathology, potential etiologies, and proper planning of the intervention. Note that currently, PTC is not frequently used for sole diagnostic purposes as imaging modalities such as MRCP can provide essential information in many cases.
2. Used as an adjunct procedure to obtain appropriate access and guidance for therapeutic peroral endoscopic and percutaneous interventions to decompress central bile ducts.

Contraindications

Relative
1. Correctable coagulopathy
2. Large-volume ascites
   a. Use left-sided approach
   b. Consider paracentesis before the procedure
3. History of allergy to contrast agents
4. Hemodynamic instability

Absolute
1. Persistent coagulopathy not responding to treatment
2. Suspicion of hydatid cysts

Procedure
1. US to reconfirm hepatobiliary anatomy and expected pathologies and plan the point/trajectory of needle puncture.
2. Use local anesthesia to desensitize skin, muscles, and liver capsule.
3. Under US guidance, obtain access to a peripheral duct using a 21-gauge (G) needle.

a. For access to right intrahepatic ductal system, consider using right mid-axillary line in the 11th/12th intercostal space. Use a subcostal approach where possible.

b. Consider using left subxiphoid approach to access left intrahepatic ductal system.

c. Use lower part of intercostal space to avoid intercostal neurovascular bundle injury.

(1) Pulmonary complications, although rare following PTC, are more likely to occur with right-sided approach.

(2) Patients usually experience more discomfort with intercostal approach.

(3) Left-sided approach can lead to difficulty advancing the drain. Operator exposure to radiation is also increased with left-sided approach.

4. Observation of bile reflux or injection of contrast can verify appropriate access to the bile duct.

5. Use serial dilatation to upsize the access over a wire.

6. Traverse biliary stricture(s)

a. Advance wire through the biliary stricture to reach duodenum or jejunum (depending on biliary-enteric anatomy).

b. In cases of very tight strictures, use digital subtraction angiography to find outflow path. Do use microsystems, if needed.

7. Inject contrast to opacify biliary tree under fluoroscopy.

a. Always use minimal contrast to diminish risk of developing sepsis.

b. In patients with obstructed bile ducts (demonstrated as biliary dilatation), decompression of the biliary tree should be performed before injecting contrast. Failure to do so can increase the pressure within biliary tree, increasing the risk of bacteremia and sepsis. Consider keeping the side-arm of the sheath open for decompression.

c. Injection into bile duct should result in centrally directed slow flow with slow clearance of contrast. Hepatic vein, portal vein, hepatic artery, and lymphatics can all be opacified while attempting a PTC access.

8. Note that severe obstruction prevents passage of contrast into some biliary branches, making them unidentifiable on PTC. Hence, correlation of fluoroscopic findings with MRCP is crucial for proper interpretation of PTC.

9. Tips

a. In cases of multiple drains, do the easy side first. This allows for possible opacification of the other segmental ducts. This can serve as a fluoroscopic target for percutaneous puncture. In addition, it can help find way to the common hepatic duct.

b. Use 3D imaging such as MRIP-IIPAIII CT or conventional CT to see filling of other ductal systems. Consider using Lumason (ultrasound contrast; Bracco Diagnostics, Monroe Township, New Jersey, NJ) to help confirm filling of other ductal system on US.

c. Nondilated PTCs: A more central stick may be needed to opacify the biliary system. A fluoroscopy-guided stick of a more peripheral duct can be then performed. Alternatively, through a microsystem advanced into a peripheral (relatively superficial) duct, a microsnare can be advanced which can be targeted under fluoroscopy.

Postprocedure Management

1. For a clinically appropriate time (1 to 3 hours) following procedure, monitor for signs of hypotension or tachycardia.

2. Closely monitor patients with underlying cholangitis for 2 hours for signs and symptoms of sepsis.

3. Instruct patient to seek medical attention for any new or worsening dyspnea, chest pain, abdominal pain, signs of infection, or melena.

Success Rate

PTC success rates threshold for dilated and nondilated ducts are 95% and 65%, respectively (4).

Complications and Their Management

Reported rate of complications following PTC is 2%. Complication rate of greater than 4% necessitates reviewing institutional policies regarding preparation, technical aspects, and postprocedure monitoring to reduce the incidence of complications (4). Using smaller-gauge needles for initial access helps to lower the rate of complications.

1. Local infection, cholangitis, and sepsis
   a. Start a course of antibiotics for 7 to 10 days if cholangitis is suspected.
   b. If sepsis is suspected, continue administration of proper antibiotics. Use serum infusion to provide enough intravascular volume. Obtain blood and bile samples to identify the pathogen. Transfer patient to ICU.
2. Hemobilia (arterial/venous bleeding into the bile duct)
   a. Can present as upper/lower gastrointestinal hemorrhage.
   b. Hepatic angiography and selective embolization are curative.
3. Bilhemia (bile leak into a vein)
   a. Can demonstrate as significant postprocedural bilirubin increase.
   b. Can be difficult to diagnose and treat. Consider performing ERCP/PTC which may demonstrate filling of veins. Consider HIDA scan to see blood pooling. These usually resolve spontaneously.
   c. Bile thromboemboli can occur in severe cases and be catastrophic.
4. Bleeding
   a. Assess patient's stability. Closely monitor vital signs.
   b. Obtain necessary blood tests (CBC, coagulation panel, blood type and cross-matching).
   c. Correct present coagulopathies. Make sure appropriate IV access is present/obtained for volume repletion/blood transfusion.
   d. Obtain contrast-enhanced three-phase CT scan to identify bleeding source, if clinically possible.
   e. In unstable patients, perform urgent hepatic angiography and embolization.
5. Pneumothorax
   a. Obtain chest radiograph to assess pneumothorax.
   b. Place chest tube, if indicated.

Percutaneous Transhepatic Biliary Drainage (PTBD)

Indications

1. Biliary obstruction
   a. Patients with biliary-enteric anastomosis.
   b. When endoscopic approach fails to provide adequate drainage.
   c. In obstructions above the insertion of cystic duct (high-level obstructions)
   d. In order to decrease bilirubin to allow patients to get chemotherapy
2. Biliary leak
   a. Iatrogenic
   b. Posttraumatic
3. Cholangitis
   a. Intrasegmental cholangitis.
   b. Patients with altered anatomy (Roux-en-Y anatomy).
   c. Failure of ERCP to provide appropriate drainage.
   d. Cholangitis should be diagnosed using clinical presentation (RUQ pain and fever) and jaundice (hyperbilirubinemia). This is not very sensitive. To

overcome this limitation, the Tokyo Guidelines (TG) were developed and TG-13 should be used as standard diagnostic criteria in clinical practice (5).
   e. Recurrent cholangitis due to intrahepatic choledocholithiasis: PTBD can be utilized to facilitate transhepatic cholangioscopy and lithotripsy.
4. Biliary drainage in patients with hilar/perihilar malignancy: Bismuth Corlette classification can be used to help guide drainage.

Contraindications

Relative
1. Coagulopathy
2. Obligatory use of antiplatelet agents
3. Ascites: Diffuse ascites increases the risk of post-PTBD septic and hemorrhagic complications. There are limited data that suggest increased peritoneal tumor and tract seeding.

Absolute
None.

Procedure
1. Perform PTC (Fig. 52.1). Dilate the tract and ducts.
2. Insert a drainage catheter (either external [only in the biliary ducts] or internal–external [drain going through the bile duct to the duodenum/jejunum]) and fix the catheter to the skin. Consider cholangioplasty of the stricture to assist in drain placement. Consider using a peel-away sheath to decrease "accordion-ing" of the drain in the tract.
   a. Due to higher risk of dislodgment and fluid loss associated with external drains, it is preferred to use internal–external drainage catheters.
   b. If the stricture is so severe that does not allow wire/catheter to cross, use external drainage catheters to drain bile for a few days and reattempt drain internalization after the inflammation has resolved.

Postprocedure Management
1. Closely monitor vital signs and patient's condition (every 15 to 30 minutes for 2 hours and then every 4 hours) for 24 hours for any signs/symptoms of sepsis and hemorrhage.
2. Check wound dressing for evidence of bile leaks.
3. Skin around the catheter should be evaluated every 24 hours.
   a. Mild erythema can be normal finding.
   b. Presence of pus, blisters, or excoriated skin renders evaluation necessary to rule out infection and bile leak.
4. Flush catheter daily with 10-mL saline (operator dependent).
5. Catheter outputs should be recorded daily.
6. Schedule routine IR follow-ups to check and exchange catheters and obtain follow-up laboratory investigation.
7. Instruct patient to seek medical evaluation if experiencing any abdominal pain, fever, pain, or erythema of skin around the drain, or significant changes in bile output.

Success Rate
Cannulation should be successful in at least 95% and 70% of dilated and nondilated ducts, respectively. After appropriate cannulation, adequate internal drainage should be established in more than 90% of cases. Among patients who undergo PTBD for stone removal, greater than 90% of cases should be successful; otherwise a review of procedure technique should be conducted (4).

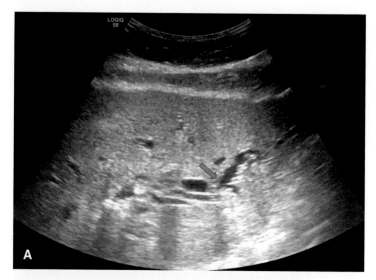

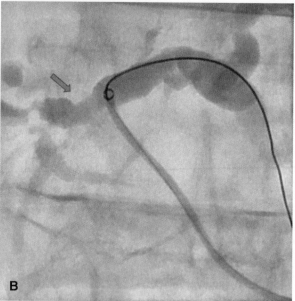

FIGURE 52.1 Multifocal structuring and choledocholithiasis due to Caroli disease. **A:** Ultrasound image demonstrating dilated left biliary ducts (*blue arrow*). **B:** Access of the duct with the wire going peripherally instead of centrally (*blue arrow*) toward the hilum. (*continued*)

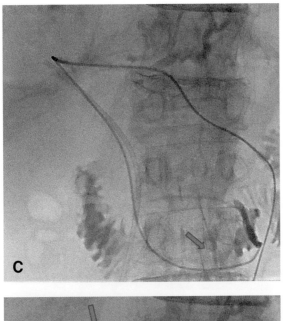

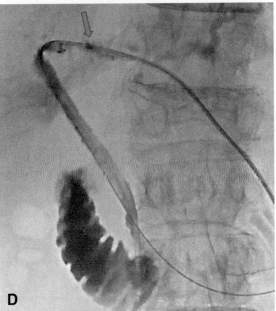

FIGURE 52.1 • (*Continued*) **C:** Five-French catheter advanced via the left hepatic/common hepatic/common bile duct into the duodenum (*blue arrow*). **D:** Sheath cholangiogram (*blue arrow*) confirming multifocal structuring with sludge/debris in the biliary system. (*continued*)

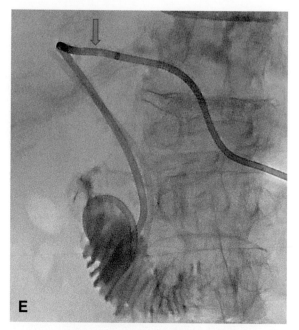

E

FIGURE 52.1 • (*Continued*) **E:** Left internal external biliary drain (*blue arrow*).

Complications and Management of Complications

Overall rate of complications after PTBD vary from 9% to 40%. However, major complications are reported in only approximately 4% of patients. Suggested threshold for most major complications following the procedure is 5% (4). There are higher rates of post-PTBD complications in patients with nondilated biliary ducts or underlying hepatobiliary malignancies. Extra care should be taken in these situations to minimize the risk.

1. Catheter-related complications
   a. Occlusion: If catheter stops drainage, instill 5 mL of normal saline with firm, yet gentle, push. If bile does not still drain, imaging evaluation and even replacement might be needed.
   b. Dislodgment: In immature tracts, attempts for reinsertion of the catheter should be performed as soon as possible since there is a risk of tract closure. If tract is mature, reinsertion of the catheter can be performed within 2 days.
   c. In obese patients, a left-sided approach decreases the risk of drain dislodgment. If right-sided approach is necessary, try a high (lower intercostal) and more anterior puncture site.
2. Skin irritation/leakage
   a. Clean skin gently. Use several gauzes in dressing to absorb bile discharges. Change dressing frequently. Use powdered absorbing agents to prevent further breakdown of the skin. Apply topical antibiotics if necessary.
   b. Catheter might need to be repositioned or replaced.
   c. Cholangiogram through existing drain to confirm that the drain is (a) in appropriate position and (b) patent.
   d. Consider upsizing the drain to help with drainage through the drain. This may be a very temporary solution.

   e. Sheath cholangiogram if the above fails to confirm that an additional biliary duct was not traversed to get to the duct with the drain. Consider wiring the "intermediate duct," if that is the case.

3. Pain: In addition to oral analgesia, consider long-acting local anesthetic (bupivacaine) to perform an intercostal nerve block.

4. Bleeding

   a. Hemobilia after catheter exchange is common and might be due to placement of a side hole into a vein. This can be confirmed by performing a tractogram through a sheath. Catheter repositioning can resolve the issue. If bleeding continues, upsizing the catheter (by 2-Fr sizes) can tamponade the vein and stop the bleeding.

   b. Persistent or severe hemobilia (in cases of external drainage) or profound melena (in cases of internal drainage) can indicate arterial bleeding. Hepatic arteriogram should be performed to identify source followed by selective embolization.

   c. If arteriography fails to identify offending artery, the biliary catheter should be taken out over a wire to remove the tamponade and repeat arteriography should be performed.

5. Cholangitis and biliary sepsis

   a. Management as described previously.

   b. External drainage carries a lower risk of post-PTBD infection.

6. Bilothorax

   a. Try to puncture bile ducts as low as possible to prevent iatrogenic leakage of bile into the pleural cavity.

   b. Thoracentesis to confirm high bilirubin content in pleural fluid. Chest tube may be needed.

   c. Use currently present drain to opacify the biliary system and place a new drain as inferior as possible to decrease risk of pleural transgression.

7. Quick internalization: The best thing to do is to remove or internalize drains when clinically appropriate and the tract has matured.

Percutaneous Transjejunal Cholangiography and Endoscopy

Indications

1. Performing cholangiography for evaluation of biliary tree in patients with prior Roux-en-Y hepaticojejunostomy (e.g., Whipple, liver transplantation).

2. To obtain biliary access when ERCP is not feasible in patients with biliary-enteric anastomoses.

3. To obtain access for therapeutic percutaneous interventions to address biliary complications related to Roux-en-Y anatomy (e.g., stricture, biliary leak, cholangitis, stone formation).

Contraindications

1. Cellulitis of percutaneous access area.

2. Coagulopathies.

3. Complicated surgical history or presence of peritoneal adhesions.

Procedure

1. Obtain MRCP prior to the procedure to scrutinize postsurgical biliary anatomical features. Review operative reports (including donor biliary anatomy in cases of liver transplantation and presence/absence of a Modified Hutson loop) (6).

2. Moderate sedation or general anesthesia should be considered.

3. Access patient's Roux limb with a 21-G needle under guidance of US/fluoroscopy (6). Inject dilute contrast to confirm appropriate intraluminal position of the needle (Fig. 52.2).

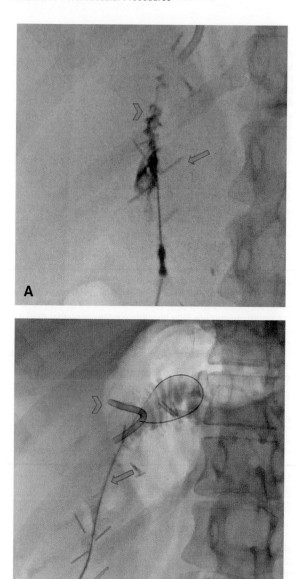

FIGURE 52.2 • Patient post-liver transplant with elevated alkaline phosphatase. **A:** Percutaneous access of the modified Hutson loop (*blue arrow*) with opacification of the biliary limb (*blue arrowhead*). **B:** Wire in the biliary limb (*blue arrow*) with a previously placed Cotton-Leung stent across the biliary-enteric anastomosis (*blue arrowhead*). (*continued*)

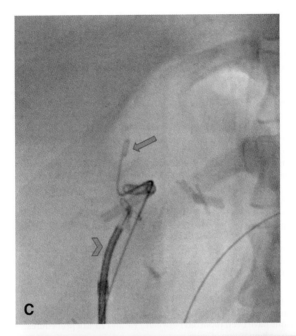

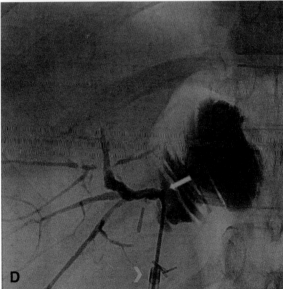

FIGURE 52.2 • (*Continued*) **C:** Cholangioscope in the biliary limb with the stent snared (*blue arrowhead*) and a safety wire placed across the anastomosis (*blue arrow*). **D:** Cholangiogram following stent removal demonstrating patent anastomosis (*blue arrow*) and the sheath in the biliary limb (*blue arrowhead*).

4. Direct the sheath in a retrograde fashion toward the liver.
5. Inject contrast to opacify the biliary-enteric anastomosis. Try these techniques, if contrast injection fails to opacify the anastomosis/biliary tree:
   a. Place patient in Trendelenburg position to benefit from assist of gravity.
   b. Inflate a Foley catheter to pressurize the limb and push contrast into the biliary system.
   c. Use a 5-Fr angled catheter to access the ostium under fluoroscopic guidance.
   d. Use an endoscope (Lithovue [Boston Scientific, Marlborough, Massachusetts] or SpyGlass Discover [Boston Scientific, Marlborough, Massachusetts]) to assist in visualization of the anastomosis and the bile ducts.
6. Correlate cholangiography findings with preprocedure imaging to ensure all biliary branches are evaluated.
7. If cholangiogram indicates need for additional biliary interventions, cholangioplasty and stenting can be performed (procedure details are explained below).

Postprocedure Management
1. If only cholangiography was performed, use PTC protocol.
2. Management of patients with therapeutic interventions is described below.

Success Rate
Percutaneous access to biliary tree through transjejunal approach was reported to be successful in 88% to 95% of cases.

Complications and Management of Complications
Major complications have been reported in approximately 4% of procedures. Minor complications have been reported between 11% and 23% of procedures.
1. Irritation or hematoma of skin:
   a. Apply local skin care for irritation.
   b. Apply manual pressure to prevent expansion.
2. LFT abnormalities
   a. Many LFT toxicities will resolve within 1 month of the procedure.
3. Cholangitis, perihepatic abscess and biliary sepsis
   a. Cholangitis and sepsis: Manage as described previously.
   b. Perihepatic abscess: Start empirical therapy with aminoglycoside plus ampicillin (treatment length depends on number of abscesses). Drain under guidance of US/CT. Obtain pathogen sensitivity and adjust antibiotic regimen accordingly.
4. Abdominal pain
   a. Monitor patient for any signs/symptoms of peritonitis. Obtain imaging if necessary.
   b. Conservatively manage cases of mild abdominal pain.
5. Duodenal/jejunal perforation/peritonitis
   a. To diminish the risk of bowel perforation in patients within 4 weeks of surgery, only perform diagnostic cholangiography using catheters smaller than 5 Fr.
   b. Request for urgent surgical consultation to repair the defect.

Biopsy

Brush Biopsy
Brush biopsy of the strictured region can be performed through the percutaneous biliary access. The sensitivity is less than 50%.

Endoscopic
The ability to advance a scope through a 10- or 12-Fr sheath, either via a percutaneous transhepatic or transjejunal access, significantly improves ability to visualize

the stricture/intraductal lesion and biopsy using small forceps that can go through the lumen of the scope. This increases the sensitivity of the biopsy.

Percutaneous Fluoroscopic/Ultrasound-Guided Biopsy
Patients with obstructive hilar lesions can be biopsied using a percutaneous US/fluoroscopic-guided approach following a cholangiogram to target the region of the stricture.

Percutaneous Cholangioplasty

Indications
Cholangioplasty should be considered for the following indications:
1. Postsurgical stricture (bile duct reconstruction, liver transplantation)
2. Ischemic stricture
3. Primary sclerosing cholangitis
4. Hepatobiliary malignancies to help advance drains/stents
5. Enterohepatic anastomotic stricture
6. Cholangioplasty of interstices in patients with previously existing biliary/duodenal stents

Contraindications
Relative: Identical to PTC.

Absolute: Identical to PTC. Early postsurgical cholangioplasty (within a month of surgery) should be discussed in detail with the surgical team due to risk of anastomotic disruption.

Procedure
1. Obtain access using PTC or PTJA, as previously described. Perform cholangiography to identify the level of the stricture.
2. Advance a guidewire through a catheter/sheath to traverse the stricture.
3. Pass a balloon over the guidewire. Conventional balloon cholangioplasty is most commonly performed. In severe cases not responsive to conventional cholangioplasty, consider cutting balloons or drug-coated balloons (minimal data to support their use).
4. Inflate balloon to dilate the stricture: Prolonged cholangioplasty should be considered.
5. Insert an internal–external catheter and obtain a cholangiogram to assess the success of the dilation.

Postprocedure Management
1. Most cases can be managed as outpatient procedures.
2. Apply general catheter postprocedure management protocols mentioned in PTBD.
3. Schedule a follow-up cholangiography to assess biliary patency.
4. Consider upsizing drain. A technique where an 8-Fr drain is placed through a 12-Fr drain and an 8 Fr drain exits one of the side holes to then have two drains (8 and 12 Fr) crossing the stricture. External leakage at the site of connection of the two drains externally remains an issue with this technique. Surgical revision should be considered in strictures not responding to cholangioplasty.
5. Clinical and laboratory assessment should be performed at 3 and 6 months after external catheter removal.

Success Rate
1. The majority of the studies have evaluated posttransplant patients. Success rates of 51% to 93% have been reported (7).
2. Long-term success of biliary dilation is not significantly different between anastomotic and nonanastomotic strictures (7).

3. Patients with multiple strictures and multiple dilation sessions are more prone to restenosis.

Complications and Management of Complications

Complication rate following cholangioplasty is reported between 5.6% and 14.7% (8).

1. Bile duct perforation
   a. Utilizing an appropriately sized balloon is crucial to prevent bile duct perforation.
   b. Place a drain in perforated area. Many cases will resolve with proper drainage.
   c. If perforation is accompanied by bleeding, consider balloon inflation for 15 minutes (and up to 30 minutes in persistent cases). If treatment fails, insert covered stent.
2. Drain complications: Manage as described in PTBD section.
3. Abscess and sepsis: Manage as described previously.
4. Hemobilia: Manage as described previously.
5. Stricture recurrence:
   a. Restenosis has been reported in 11.8% of cases (8).

Percutaneous Stent Placement

Indications

Plastic Stents

Median patency of plastic stents ranges from 1.5 to 3 months.

1. Benign strictures (postsurgical or secondary to inflammation): Multiple plastic stent placement is superior to uncovered self-expandable metal stents in patients with benign extrahepatic biliary strictures (9).
2. Choledocholithiasis where previous attempts of extraction have failed.
3. Bile leaks: Schedule stent removal and a repeat cholangiography at 4 to 8 weeks.
4. Hilar and nonhilar malignant strictures
   a. When GI can access biliary-enteric anastomosis/ampulla and can make exchanges.
   b. Consider plastic stents in hilar malignancies as well. Metal stents may not be the best way to "reconstruct" the hilar bile ducts as some patients with cholangiocarcinoma are living beyond the patency of the stents. The GI community now suggests placing plastic stents in such cases if exchanges are possible.

Self-Expanding Metal Stents (SEMS)

1. Malignant strictures: In patients with life expectancy less than a year.
2. Benign strictures: Single-covered self-expandable metallic stent can be considered in patients with benign biliary stricture who have bile duct diameter greater than 6 mm, if the stent does not cover the cystic duct.

Covered versus Uncovered Self-Expanding Metal Stents (10)

a. Stent occlusion: Significantly higher in the uncovered stent (48%) compared to covered stents (25%). The median patency of uncovered metal stents is approximately 6 months compared to 8 to 10 months for covered metal stents.
b. Migration: Before the advent of Viabil (Gore, Newark, Delaware), stent migration was much more of a problem with covered stents (41%), when compared to uncovered stents (0%).
c. Cholecystitis and pancreatitis: Cholecystitis and pancreatitis are slightly more commonly seen with covered metal stents.

Contraindications
Relative: Identical to PTC.
   Absolute: Identical to PTC.

Procedure
1. Using the same techniques described before for PTC or PTJA. Obtain cholangiogram and wire access.
2. The wire should cross the stricture. If initial attempt to cross the stricture failed, decompress the biliary tree for 2 to 3 days and reattempt traversal.
3. Place stent over the appropriate wire through an appropriate sheath. Deploy in the appropriate position under fluoroscopic guidance (Fig. 52.3). Consider injecting contrast in the gut and bile duct(s) prior to stent deployment to know where the stent's leading and trailing edges should be. In patients with biliary malignancy, consider overextending both proximal and distal ends of the stent to delay tumor overgrowth. This can be also considered in patients with benign stricture, due to soft tissue hyperplasia.
   a. Uncovered metal stents are more prone to occlusion due to tumor overgrowth. Consider using covered stents to overcome the risk. However, risk of stent migration and sludge formation is higher in covered stents.
   b. There is no significant difference of technical success and complication rate between bilateral and unilateral stenting. However, bilateral stenting carries a longer duration of patency for patients.
4. In instances with severe stricture, a high-pressure balloon can be used to fully expand the stent.
5. An external drain can be considered to maintain access and confirm stent patency in a week. In patients with evident biliary sepsis, place an internal/external drain and postpone stent insertion until the sepsis has resolved.

Postprocedure Management
1. Most cases can be managed as outpatient procedures.
2. Apply general catheter postprocedure management protocols mentioned in PTBD.
3. Monitor patients for any signs/symptoms of biliary sepsis.
4. Perform cholangiography after 3 to 7 days to check for stent patency and proper position. Remove external drain once appropriate position and drainage of the stent is approved.
5. A comprehensive follow-up including clinical evaluation, liver function investigation, and lab assessment should be performed 1 week after the procedure and regularly every 1 to 3 months after drain removal.

Success Rate
1. In patients with benign extrahepatic stricture (9):
   a. Technical success rates for uncovered SEMS, single plastic stents, and multiple plastic stents were 98.9%, 94.8%, and 94%, respectively.
   b. Multiple plastic stents had the best clinical success rate, followed by self-expanding stents and single plastic stents.
   c. Self-expanding stents are best choice for stricture due to chronic pancreatitis. Multiple plastic stents are most favorable for stricture secondary to surgical interventions.
2. For patients with malignant stricture: Technical success, clinical success, and overall complication rate of SEMS and plastic stents are comparable. However, SEMS carry a higher patency rate and lower risk of recurrent obstruction.

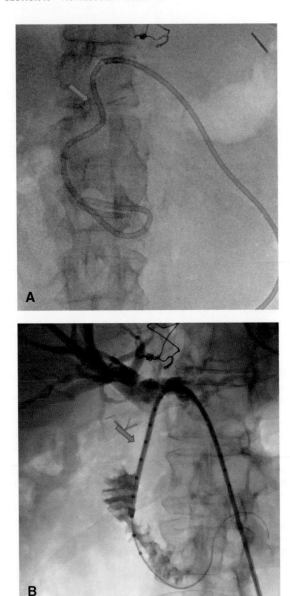

FIGURE 52.3 Common bile duct (CBD) stricture due to pancreatic cancer. **A:** Internal external biliary drain (*blue arrow*). **B:** Sheath cholangiogram demonstrating the long-segment CBD stricture (*blue arrow*). (*continued*)

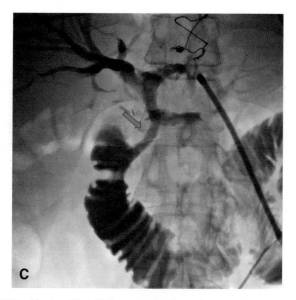

FIGURE 52.3 • (*Continued*) **C:** Viabil (Gore, covered self-expanding stent; blue arrow) was placed across the stricture and the drain was removed.

Complications and Management of Complications

In patients with benign biliary stricture, complications were reported in 39.5%, 36%, and 20.3% of patients with uncovered SEMS, single plastic stent, and multiple plastic stents, respectively (9).

In patients undergoing SEMS for malignant biliary obstruction, early (less than 30 days) stent occlusion, late stent occlusion, stent migration, and cholangitis occur in 3%, 27%, 0.8%, and 8%, respectively. The complications listed above are more frequent with plastic stents when compared to SEMS.

1. Hemorrhage
   a. Manage as described before
   b. In cases of significant hemobilia, inserting a drain catheter and regular irrigation is necessary
2. Cholangitis and sepsis development: Manage as described previously
3. Pancreatitis: Most cases resolve by conservative treatment
4. Stent occlusion/migration
   a. Insert a drain to enhance drainage
   b. Removal or exchange of the stent might be required

Pediatric Biliary Interventions

For the most cases, biliary interventions in the pediatric population are similar to the adult population. The Kasai procedure (Roux-en-Y hepaticojejunostomy) is performed in patients with biliary atresia. Pediatric liver transplants are also routinely performed for various indications. Peroral endoscopic access to the hepaticojejunostomy is difficult in infants, toddlers, and preschoolers (2 to 5 years) due to size of the endoscopes used by gastroenterology. Given these limitations, percutaneous transhepatic biliary interventions are performed frequently.

Combined Procedures

"Rendezvous" procedures where peroral endoscopic procedures are unsuccessful should be strongly considered. These may create scenarios where IR and GI can do a combined procedure to maximize success. This also increases patient comfort as no drains may be needed.

An example of such a procedure would be a patient with biliary obstruction (without cholangitis) and a failed ERCP intervention. A PTC can be performed and a wire or a small-diameter catheter (≤4 Fr) could be advanced through the stricture. This can help GI guide their devices to place stents via an endoscopic approach. No drains may be needed. This approach should be definitely considered before GI does procedures where they use EUS to puncture the distal CBD (high complication rate).

Another example would be of a patient where there is a severe benign stricture which cannot be traversed by IR or GI. A combined procedure where GI places a scope in the biliary limb of the Roux-en-Y and IR advances their catheter as close to the scope as possible. A radiofrequency wire can then be advanced to create a "neo-duct."

Percutaneous Cholecystostomy (PC)

Indications
1. Acute calculous cholecystitis: PC should be considered in critically ill patients when surgical intervention is not feasible. This should be a temporizing measure to get patient to surgery whenever possible.
2. Acute acalculous cholecystitis: This is usually definite treatment. Acalculous cholecystitis usually resolves when patient's clinical status improves.
3. Given communication of the gallbladder with the biliary tree, a PC can be considered for:
   a. Decompression in acute cholangitis/jaundice due to common bile duct obstruction.
   b. Providing an access to biliary tree, if transhepatic approach fails.
4. A diagnostic and potentially therapeutic procedure, in septic patients with unidentifiable source.

Contraindications
Relative: Coagulopathy.
   Absolute: None, as patients are usually critically ill.

Procedure
1. Use US to evaluate liver, gallbladder, and point/trajectory of needle entry.
2. The procedure is usually performed with moderate sedation.
3. A needle is used to puncture the gallbladder under US guidance.
   a. Transhepatic approach is preferred as there is a decreased risk of peritoneal bile leaks. Direct gallbladder sticks may be considered in some cases.
   b. Consider Seldinger (using a fine needle and serial dilation of the tract) or Trocar (direct insertion of a 6- to 8-Fr catheter) techniques. Seldinger is appropriate for nondistended gallbladders. It lowers the risk of bleeding and perforation but prolongs procedure time. Trocar technique should be used in extreme circumstances (e.g., ICU patient unable to come to an IR fluoroscopy suite with a distended gallbladder). It carries a higher risk of bleeding and perforation.
4. Confirm successful puncture.
   a. Bile aspiration indicates appropriate puncture.
   b. Appropriate puncture can also be approved by fluoroscopy. Contrast volume should be less than 5 mL to minimize the risk of sepsis exacerbation.

5. Place a wire through the needle into the gallbladder. Upsize/dilate.
6. Insert an 8- to 10-Fr locking pigtail catheter and use US or fluoroscopy to confirm placement of catheter loop inside gallbladder lumen.
7. Obtain bile sample for diagnostic purposes.
8. Secure the catheter to the skin.
9. Gravity drainage.

Postprocedure Management
1. Monitor patient following the procedure.
2. Apply general catheter care principles described in PTBD.
3. Consider flushing the catheter daily with 10 mL of sterile saline to prevent occlusion.
4. If catheter is to be removed (in cases of acalculous cholecystitis), ensure the tract is mature.
   a. Tract maturation takes at least 2 weeks in transhepatic and 3 weeks in transperitoneal approach.
   b. Advance a wire through the catheter and then remove the catheter.
   c. Inject 10 to 15 mL of contrast through a 6- to 8-Fr sheath to evaluate for any peritoneal leakage.
   d. If any leakage is found, place a catheter over the wire and repeat the maneuver after a suitable time to reassess tract maturity.
5. Once duct patency and tract maturity are confirmed and patient is stable, the catheter can be removed.
6. If decision is made to keep catheter inserted, it should be exchanged every 3 months (operator dependent).
7. Consider internalization:
   In patients with calculous cholecystitis who are not surgical candidates, do consider removing the drain using the following options.
   a. Percutaneous stent placement: This is in experimental stages. Consider placing plastic stents across the cystic duct, through the CBD, into the duodenum. Placement of two stents is better than one stent due to the space created between the stents in addition to the lumen of the stents.
   b. EUS-guided cholecystoduodenostomy/cholecystogastrostomy: GI can help place a stent between the gallbladder and the stomach/duodenum. There is a risk of bleeding/bile leak.
   c. Lithotripsy followed by drain removal: There are centers that are performing electrohydraulic or laser lithotripsy of calculi in the gallbladder followed by drain removal. The long-term data on this procedure are limited.

Success Rate
1. Clinical success threshold for acalculous, and calculous cholecystitis are 65% and 75%, respectively (4).
2. Technical success rate of using an 18- and 21-gauge needle for the procedure should be greater than 95% and 80%, respectively.
   a. The majority of technical failures in performing PC is related to high bile viscosity and not due to failure in accessing gallbladder (4).

Complications and Management of Complications
Most major complications of PC occur in less than 3% of patients. Suggested overall threshold for all major complications is 5% (4). Overall 30-day mortality of patients following PC is reported as 15.4%. However, only 0.36% of the mortality is attributed to the procedure itself.
1. Sepsis: Treat as described for PTBD.
2. Hemorrhage: Manage as described for PTBD.
3. Bile leak: If it is due to catheter dislodgment, reinsert catheter. If persistent, exchange the catheter. Immediate care should be taken to avoid bile peritonitis.

4. Perforation of adjacent organs.
  a. May demonstrate as septic shock.
  b. Obtain imaging and manage accordingly.
5. Pneumothorax. Manage as described previously.
6. Bradycardia and vasovagal reactions.
  a. Closely monitor blood pressure.
  b. Administer IV fluids.
  c. 0.4- to 1-mg atropine, IV, may be required.
7. Catheter-related problems: Manage as described in PTBD.

References

1. Duan F, Cui L, Bai Y, et al. Comparison of efficacy and complications of endoscopic and percutaneous biliary drainage in malignant obstructive jaundice: a systematic review and meta-analysis. *Cancer Imaging.* 2017;17(1):1–7.
2. Patel IJ, Rahim S, Davidson JC, et al. Society of Interventional Radiology Consensus Guidelines for the Periprocedural Management of Thrombotic and Bleeding Risk in Patients Undergoing Percutaneous Image-Guided Interventions—Part II: Recommendations: Endorsed by the Canadian Association for Interventional Radiology and the Cardiovascular and Interventional Radiological Society of Europe. *J Vasc Interv Radiol.* 2019; 30(8): 1168–1184.e1.
3. Venkatesan AM, Kundu S, Sacks D, et al. Practice guideline for adult antibiotic prophylaxis during vascular and interventional radiology procedures. *J Vasc Interv Radiol.* 2010;21(11):1611–1630.
4. Saad WE, Wallace MJ, Wojak JC, et al. Quality improvement guidelines for percutaneous transhepatic cholangiography, biliary drainage, and percutaneous cholecystostomy. *J Vasc Interv Radiol.* 2010;21(6):789–795.
5. Kiriyama S, Kozaka K, Takada T, et al. Tokyo Guidelines 2018: diagnostic criteria and severity grading of acute cholangitis (with videos). *J Hepatobiliary Pancreat Sci.* 2018;25(1): 17–30.
6. Riaz A, Entezari P, Ganger D, et al. Percutaneous access of the modified Hutson loop for retrograde cholangiography, endoscopy, and biliary interventions. *J Vasc Interv Radiol.* 2020; 31(12):2113–2120.e1.
7. Zajko AB, Sheng R, Zetti GM, et al. Transhepatic balloon dilation of biliary strictures in liver transplant patients: a 10-year experience. *J Vasc Interv Radiol.* 1995;6(1):79–83.
8. Janssen JJ, van Delden OM, van Lienden KP, et al. Percutaneous balloon dilatation and long-term drainage as treatment of anastomotic and nonanastomotic benign biliary strictures. *Cardiovasc Intervent Radiol.* 2014;37(6):1559–1567.
9. van Boeckel PG, Vleggaar FP, Siersema PD. Plastic or metal stents for benign extrahepatic biliary strictures: a systematic review. *BMC Gastroenterology.* 2009;9:96.
10. Isayama H, Nakai Y, Kawakubo K, et al. Covered metallic stenting for malignant distal biliary obstruction: clinical results according to stent type. *J Hepatobiliary Pancreat Sci.* 2011;18(5):673–677.

53 Percutaneous Nephrostomy and Antegrade Ureteral Stenting

Sirish A. Kishore, MD and Anne M. Covey, MD, FSIR

Introduction

There are four types of percutaneous urinary drainage catheters:

1. Percutaneous nephrostomy (PCN) refers to an external drainage catheter, placed via a flank approach, positioned in the renal pelvis (Fig. 53.1A).
2. A nephroureteral stent (NUS)/nephroureterostomy (NUT) enters the collecting system via a flank approach (like a PCN) with a locking loop in the renal pelvis, and extends down the ureter terminating in the bladder, allowing both internal and external drainage (Fig. 53.1B). These catheters are less prone to dislodgment than a PCN, especially in large patients.
3. A ureteral or "double-J" stent is an internal catheter that extends from the renal pelvis to the bladder and can be placed in patients who are able to fill and empty their bladder normally (Fig. 53.1C). Stents relieve patients of the lifestyle limitations associated with an exteriorized device.
4. Retrograde PCN catheters are placed through a urinary stoma (i.e., ileal conduit). The locking loop of the catheter is positioned in the renal pelvis and the hub exits the stoma draining directly into the ostomy bag (Fig. 53.1D).

Indications (1–4)

1. Obstructive uropathy including ureteral obstruction from iatrogenic, neoplastic, or inflammatory causes, particularly in setting of urosepsis/infection, acute renal failure, or intractable pain
2. Urinary diversion
   a. Urine leak
   b. Vesicovaginal or vesicocolic fistula
   c. Hemorrhagic cystitis
3. Access for percutaneous intervention
   a. Percutaneous nephrolithotomy
   b. Tumor biopsy, ablation/fulguration, or intracavitary delivery of medications
   c. Stricture dilation or rendezvous ureteral recanalization (4,5)
   d. Endopyelotomy
   e. Foreign-body retrieval (e.g., dysfunctional ureteral stent)
   f. Ureteral occlusion/embolization for refractory urinary fistula
4. Preoperative localization of the ureter
5. Before and after extracorporeal shock wave lithotripsy (ESWL)
6. Following a surgical procedure involving the ureter to maintain patency during healing
7. Whitaker test

Contraindications

Absolute

There are no absolute contraindications. Risk of procedural intervention for urinary obstruction should be weighed against the risk of untreated urinary obstruction (e.g., sepsis, renal injury, pain).

Relative

1. Uncorrectable coagulopathy—the risk of not performing drainage is weighed against the risk of bleeding and kidney loss. Patients with severe uremia/azotemia are at increased risk of bleeding.

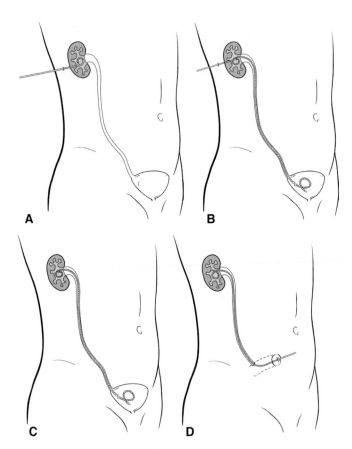

FIGURE 53.1 • Types of renal drainage: **(A)** Percutaneous nephrostomy is an obligate external drainage catheter; **(B)** nephroureteral catheter can drain both internally and externally; **(C)** ureteral stent is an internal device draining into the native bladder; and **(D)** retrograde nephrostomy, placed via an ileal conduit, drains the renal pelvis to the urostomy device on the anterior abdominal wall.

2. Severe hyperkalemia—higher risk of sedation-related complication.

Specific to Antegrade Ureteral Stents
1. Untreated bladder outlet obstruction
2. Untreated urinary tract infection
3. Spastic or noncompliant bladder; urinary incontinence
4. Bladder fistula
5. Non-native bladder (because of high risk of catheter occlusion)
6. Difficult future stent exchange (e.g., extensive bladder tumor, challenging urethral anatomy, etc.)[a]

---

[a]Multidisciplinary coordination with urology is recommended prior to ureteral stent placement to ensure possibility of future exchanges for patients who may require future cystoscopic stent exchanges.

Preprocedure Preparation

1. Prior to renal drainage, *cross-sectional imaging* is important to evaluate the presence of hydronephrosis, anatomic variants (duplication, malposition, horseshoe kidney), cysts, tumors, stones, and/or perinephric urinoma. On occasion, radionuclide renography can be useful in measuring differential renal function.

2. Patient education should include a description of the procedure, risks and complications, alternative therapies, catheter maintenance, and long-term plan, including need for routine exchanges, and whether the patient is a candidate for internalization.

3. Relevant labs include hematocrit (Hct), white blood cell (WBC), platelet count, international normalized ratio (INR), and creatinine (Cr).

4. Coagulopathy should be corrected to local guidelines. 2019 SIR guidelines recommend an INR of <1.5 to 1.8 and a platelet count >50,000 per µL for new catheter placements (high bleeding risk), and oral anticoagulation should be withheld, utilizing a bridging strategy with LMWH if anticoagulation cannot be stopped entirely. For routine exchange (low bleeding risk) INR <2 to 3 and platelet count >20,000 per µL are recommended (6).

5. Obtain urinalysis and urine culture and sensitivity, if relevant to the case.

6. Nil per os (NPO) according to hospital guidelines to allow safe sedation.

   a. Anesthesia consultation may be considered for patients who have difficulty with prone positioning or with respiratory compromise that may be exacerbated by prone position.

7. Establish intravenous (IV) access for sedation and *preprocedure antibiotic prophylaxis*, if needed:

   a. Risk-stratified appropriate prophylactic antibiotics reduce the rate of infectious complications, though choice of agent may vary based on local culture and sensitivity data (7,8). There is no consensus first-line antibiotic in current guidelines, though endorsed consensus regimens (including 2018 SIR guidelines) for new catheter placement include the following:

      (1) 1- to 2-g ceftriaxone IV once prior to tube placement

      (2) 1.5- to 3-g ampicillin/sulbactam IV +/− gentamycin 5 mg per kg IV

      (3) Vancomycin recommended in penicillin-allergic patients

      Patients with indwelling catheters and ileoureteral anastomoses may have atypical or multidrug resistant (MDR) for which review of cultures may guide prophylaxis.

      Antibiotics are not routinely given after the procedure but may be considered based on signs or risk of infection.

8. Catheter selection

   a. Options to consider when choosing catheters for urinary drainage include catheter material, locking mechanism, size, and shape. The most common materials include hydrophilic- or non–hydrophilic-coated silicone or polyurethane. Hydrophilic coating facilitates placement by reducing friction but may promote encrustation because it is permeable to inorganic salts. Silicone is softer and generally more comfortable for patients, but it is less strong, requiring a thicker wall to have the same tensile strength as polyurethane (8).

   b. The most common locking mechanism is the Cope or "locking loop" that is formed by pulling on a monofilament suture that runs through the body of the catheter (Fig. 53.2B). A Malecot- or tulip-type locking mechanism is designed so the distal sides of the catheter flare outward (Fig. 53.2A). This occupies less space than a loop catheter and is useful when there is a very small renal pelvis or when a staghorn calculus fills the renal pelvis.

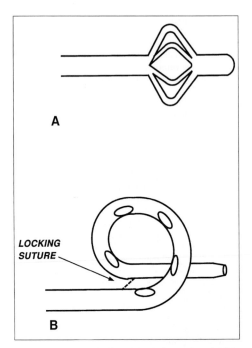

FIGURE 53.2 • The two basic shapes of self-retaining drainage tubes. **A:** Malecot or tulip type. **B:** Cope self-retaining loop.

    c. In most cases, an 8-Fr catheter is sufficient for drainage. In cases of pyonephrosis or hematuria with clots, 10- or 12-Fr catheters may decrease the incidence of catheter occlusion.

Procedure

Percutaneous Nephrostomy
1. Patient position: Prone or prone-oblique when possible. During pregnancy, the patient may only able to lie on her side.
2. Fluoroscopy and/or ultrasound are used to determine an appropriate access site which is then prepped and draped.
3. The *skin entry site* is along the ipsilateral posterior axillary line, preferably below the 11th rib to avoid entering the thorax. A subcostal approach is most comfortable for patients.
   a. To avoid bleeding complications, the needle *path to the kidney* should be along "Brodel bloodless line" (Fig. 53.3). This path, typically 30 to 45 degrees with respect to the table surface (when the patient is prone) should also avoid other interpositioned structures such as the liver and colon. Ideally, a posterior lower pole calyx should be targeted.
   b. If the PCN is being placed for treating stones, the choice of the calyx for entry is critical and should be selected for optimal access to the stone.
   c. A direct posterior entry is only useful for opacifying the collecting system; this approach should not be used to place a catheter as it is uncomfortable for the patient and leads to catheter kinking and poor function.
   d. Direct puncture into the renal pelvis for the purpose of catheter placement should be avoided due to the risk of bleeding.

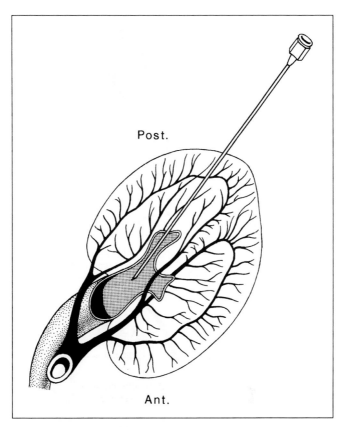

FIGURE 53.3 • Cross-section of kidney showing needle pathway through Brodel avascular line and the relationship of the anterior and posterior divisions of the renal artery to the renal pelvis and infundibula. Plane of arterial division is the least vascular area of the kidney and is usually the place where nephrostomy punctures are performed to avoid damage to large vascular structures. (Redrawn from Castaneda Zuniga WR, ladavarthy SM. *Interventional Radiology*. 2nd ed. Wolters Kluwer, 1992:707.)

4. Administer local anesthesia (1% lidocaine) at the chosen skin entry site.
5. Make a small skin incision through the dermis to facilitate catheter passage.
6. Commonly used introduction systems include the Cope, Jeff, or Neff (Cook, Bloomington, IN) and AccuStick (Boston Scientific, Marlborough, MA) sets that allow initial access with a skinny (21- or 22-gauge) needle and subsequent placement of 0.035- or 0.038-in guidewire through a coaxial 6-Fr introducer.
   a. During gentle respiration, advance the skinny needle toward the intended calyx using either fluoroscopic or ultrasound guidance (Fig. 53.4A).
      (1) Ultrasound guidance is preferred when there is hydronephrosis.
      (2) Fluoroscopic guidance is more appropriate when radiopaque landmarks (e.g., calcified stones, surgical clips, indwelling ureteral stent, contrast in the renal collecting system) are present.

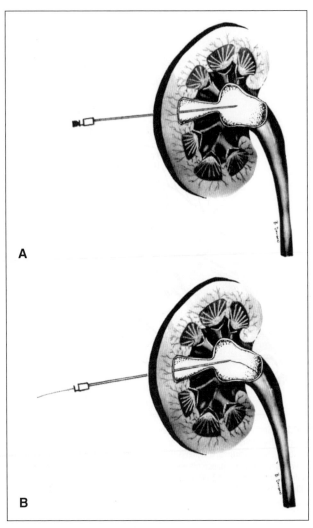

FIGURE 53.4 • Percutaneous nephrostomy using Cope introduction system. **A:** Skinny 22-gauge, 15-cm long puncture needle tip in pelvis through a posterior midpole calyx. **B:** A 0.018-in wire is introduced through the puncture needle after the stylet is removed. (*continued*)

  (3) For nondilated collecting systems in patients with normal or near-normal Cr, 50 to 100 mL IV contrast can be injected to opacify the renal collecting system.
  (4) Computed tomography (CT) guidance can also be used if there is challenging anatomy (e.g., morbid obesity, interposed bowel, nondilated system) (9)
  b. When the needle enters the renal parenchyma, the tip will move synchronously with the kidney. When the collecting system is entered, there is an abrupt decrease in resistance to forward movement of the needle.

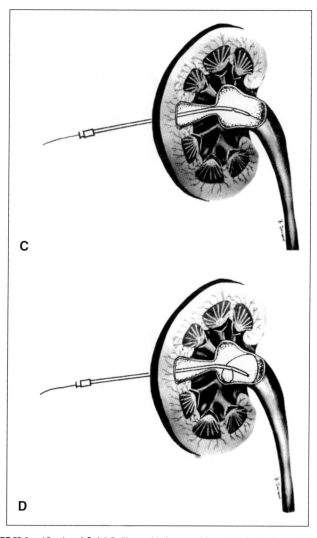

FIGURE 53.4 • *(Continued)* **C:** A 6-Fr dilator with tip tapered for a 0.018-in wire is introduced over the wire. The metal cannula is removed. **D:** The 0.018-in wire is removed, and a 0.038-in standard J-tipped guidewire is introduced through the dilator and exits through the distal side hole. *(continued)*

   c. Remove the stylet from the needle. In cases of hydronephrosis, urine will drain freely. Otherwise, slowly retract the needle while aspirating with a plastic syringe half filled with contrast on a connecting tube until urine emerges.

   d. Inject a small amount of dilute contrast to confirm needle position and, only if there is no suspicion of infection, to opacify the collecting system. In cases of suspected infection, the system should be partially decompressed prior

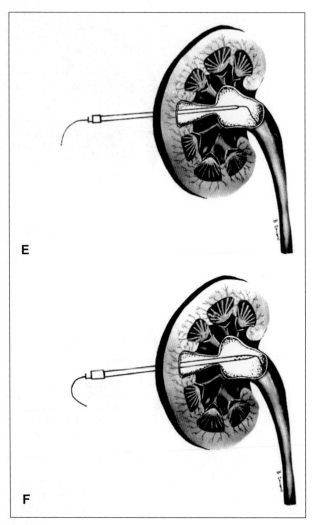

FIGURE 53.4 • (*Continued*) **E:** Optional tract dilation with fascial dilator over wire is performed. **F:** The nephrostomy catheter is introduced over wire with stiffening cannula providing support while crossing subcutaneous soft tissue. (*continued*)

to contrast injection to minimize bacterial translocation due to further distension of the collecting system (9). Complete decompression should be avoided as it will make subsequent entry difficult if access is inadvertently lost.

e. If a central puncture is made, the collecting system may be gently opacified to visualize an appropriate peripheral calyx for puncture with a second needle.

f. Once access into the target calyx is achieved, the needle is exchanged over a 0.018-in wire for the coaxial introducer (Fig. 53.4B,C). (Note: Internal

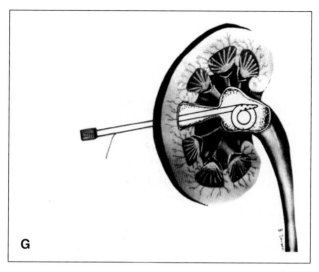

G

FIGURE 53.4 • (*Continued*) **G:** Cope PCN catheter with pigtail formed in renal pelvis.

metallic stiffeners should be advanced no further than the entry point of the collecting system in order to avoid inadvertent perforation of the renal pelvis.)

g. Urine is aspirated through the 6-Fr introducer for culture and/or cytology as indicated. Patients at high risk for positive urine culture include those with urinary diversion, cystectomy, recent catheter or stent placement, or clinical signs of infection (9).

h. Widen the skin nick with a hemostat to a depth of about 0.5 cm prior to introducing the catheter.

7. The coaxial introducer is exchanged over a 0.035-in or 0.038 in guidewire for a PCN catheter (Fig. 50.1D–G).

a. Introduction of an 8-Fr or larger PCN catheter may be facilitated by the passage of Teflon dilators.

b. The metal stiffener of the PCN is used only to facilitate passage through the extrarenal soft tissues and should not be advanced beyond the renal parenchyma. If it is difficult to pass the catheter through the soft tissues, a peel-away sheath may be used.

c. Once the catheter tip is well within the renal pelvis or proximal ureter, reform the pigtail tip within the renal pelvis. To do this, remove the metal stiffener, partially retract the guidewire, and lock the tip by applying slight tension on the external string (Fig. 53.4).

8. Remove the guidewire completely and inject contrast to confirm catheter position.

9. Open the catheter to external drainage and obtain an image to document decompression of the collecting system, confirming good function of the catheter.

10. Anchor the catheter to the skin with a retention disk and/or suture. In obese patients, consider both forms of catheter securement, as obesity is a risk factor for dislodgment of nephrostomy tubes likely due to movement of the tube with the pannus (10).

11. Attach a drainage bag to the external hub.

Nephroureterostomy (Nephroureteral Stent) Placement

1. After accessing the renal collecting system as discussed earlier, advance a straight or angled 5-Fr catheter, such as a multipurpose or Kumpe catheter, into the ureter over the guidewire. Advance the catheter over the wire to just above the level of obstruction. Use a small amount of dilute contrast to opacify the ureter and optimize the angle of approach to the obstruction using oblique angulation of the image intensifier.

2. An angled 0.035-in hydrophilic-coated guidewire can be used to probe for the narrowed orifice. A stiff hydrophilic-coated guidewire may be necessary to cross fibrotic obstructions. Use care, as these low–surface-friction wires may perforate the ureter. If the ureter is perforated it is very difficult to traverse the occlusion at the same sitting because the wire repeatedly exits the microperforation. A PCN should be placed and a second attempt to cross the obstruction after allowing 2 to 4 weeks for the perforation to heal.

3. If the guidewire cannot be passed across a redundant or S-shaped ureter, advance an angled catheter such as a Kumpe catheter to a level approximately 5 mm above the first bend and advance a floppy-tipped or angled-tipped hydrophilic-coated guidewire across the bend. Deep expiration may also partially straighten the redundant segment.

4. Once a guidewire is passed into the bladder, advance the NUT catheter over the wire until several centimeters are in the bladder. Once the wire is retracted the distal pigtail will form in the bladder. The wire is then pulled back to the kidney and the proximal pigtail is formed in the renal pelvis by slight tension applied to the external string.

Antegrade Ureteral Stent Placement

Antegrade ureteral stents are reserved for patients with functioning native bladders. It is common to wait at least 1 week following placement of a nephrostomy tube before stent placement to decrease the risk of clot or debris occluding the lumen of the stent. However, clinical judgment should be used, and stents may be placed sooner. If the patient has an NUT in place, a capping trial can be performed to assess whether the patient will tolerate internalization with a ureteral stent. If the Cr remains stable and there is no pericatheter leakage or fever with the catheter capped for several days, there is a high likelihood that a ureteral stent will provide adequate drainage.

1. If there is an NUT in place, pass a guidewire through the catheter into the bladder. Otherwise, obtain access to the bladder as described for NUT placement.

2. The length of the ureter can be measured by passing a Teflon-coated guidewire through the catheter into the bladder. When the tip of the guidewire is at the intended position of the distal J of the stent, place a clamp on the guidewire at the skin. Withdraw the guidewire tip to the intended position of the proximal loop of the stent and place a second clamp on the guidewire at the skin surface. The distance between clamps is the desired stent length. Stents are sized in centimeters (22 to 28 cm) by the distance between the pigtail or J curves (Fig. 53.5).

3. Coil an Amplatz Super Stiff (Boston Scientific/Medi-Tech Marlborough, MA) 0.035-in guidewire in the bladder. Prepare the catheter before placing the stiff wire in the bladder to minimize the time the wire is in the bladder because this can cause discomfort.

4. Mount the stent on the guidewire and advance over the wire down the ureter into the bladder. Depending on the type of stent being deployed, it may be premounted on a long delivery system or may need to be advanced by using a stiff "pusher" mounted on the guidewire behind the stent (Fig. 53.6A).

5. When the tip of the stent is beyond the ureteral orifice of the bladder (UVJ), retract the guidewire and the flexible stiffener, if one is used. The distal loop of the stent will then coil if free in the bladder. If the stent has been measured properly, the proximal loop will form within the renal pelvis when the guidewire and stiffener are removed (Fig. 53.6B,C).

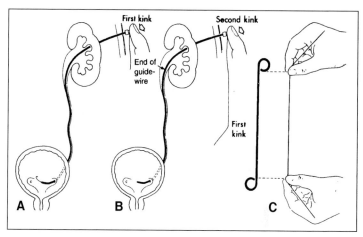

FIGURE 53.5 • Measuring the ureter to determine stent catheter length. **A:** The guidewire and catheter extend past the ureterovesical junction (UVJ). When the guidewire is positioned in the bladder 2 to 3 cm from the UVJ, the guidewire that extends from the flank is bent at the catheter hub. **B:** The guidewire is retracted until the tip is located in the renal pelvis approximately 1 cm above the ureteropelvic junction. A second kink is now made in the guidewire at the catheter hub. **C:** The distance between the two guidewire bends will determine the length of the catheter between the pigtail curves. (Reprinted with permission from Pollack HM. *Clinical Urography: An Atlas and Textbook of Urological Imaging.* Vol. 3. WB Saunders; 1990:2771.)

6. It may be desirable to leave a nephrostomy until stent patency is confirmed (Fig. 53.6D). In this situation, a nephrostomy catheter can be used as the "pusher" to advance the ureteral stent into place. The loop of the nephrostomy is formed adjacent to the proximal loop of the ureteral stent. The nephrostomy tube can be capped for a physiologic trial so that drainage is internal through the stent. The tube is fixed to the patient's skin in the usual manner and is left in place for at least 24 hours.

7. Very *tight or hard strictures* will not allow soft ureteral stents to pass easily. The stricture may be widened by passage of a Van Andel Teflon dilator (Cook, Inc, Bloomington, IN) over the wire, 0.5- to 1.0-Fr diameter larger than the stent to be placed (usually 8 or 10 Fr) into the ureter. Balloon ureteroplasty can also be performed to dilate the stricture prior to stent placement. Another option is to pass a guidewire into the bladder, snare the wire from transurethral access and externalize it through the urethra. With control of both ends of the guidewire, a stent may be passed in an antegrade manner. These *maneuvers* may be painful; adequate sedation and analgesia are necessary.

8. If a stent still cannot be passed, a nephrostomy may be placed. A second attempt to convert to ureteral stent may be successful after a period of external drainage. Short-segment occlusions may be candidates for rendezvous recanalization procedures, in collaboration with urology (4,5)

9. If the indication is treatment of a ureteral leak, a stent with holes only in the renal pelvis and bladder (rather than along the entire course of the catheter) should be used.

10. After stent placement, when the patient passes the physiologic trial of a capped nephrostomy (i.e., the Cr is stable, the patient is able to void, and remains asymptomatic without pain or fever), the nephrostomy can be removed over a wire to

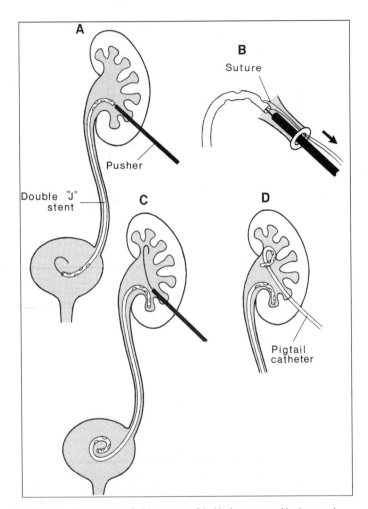

FIGURE 53.6 • Double-J stent. **A:** Advancement of double-J stent over guidewire passed beyond site of obstruction. **B:** Close-up view of proximal end of a Silastic double-J stent with suture passed through a side hole for repositioning purposes. **C:** With the proximal end of the stent held in place with the pusher, the suture is removed, thus releasing the proximal loop. **D:** Stent has doubled back into the lower pole infundibulum, and the pusher has been replaced by a pigtail catheter for temporary external drainage. (Redrawn from Castaneda-Zuniga WR, Tadavarthy SM. *Interventional Radiology*. 2nd ed. Wolters Kluwer; 1992:881.)

prevent inadvertent dislodgment of the ureteral stent, either with or without an antegrade contrast study to document stent patency. Because flow of urine through the stent is gravity dependent, using a tilting fluoroscopy table facilitates quick assessment of the stent:

a. If contrast is seen to traverse the stent and collect within the bladder, remove the nephrostomy tube over a guidewire under fluoroscopy to ensure that the proximal loop of the ureteral stent is not dislodged by removal of the PCN tube.

b. If contrast does not pass into the bladder, ask the patient to void completely, or, if this is not possible, place a Foley catheter and repeat the antegrade injection through the PCN tube. One cause of stent malfunction is elevated pressure in a bladder that cannot be emptied completely.

Retrograde Nephrostomy
When an ileal conduit is present following cystectomy, a retrograde nephrostomy is the preferred urinary drainage system (Fig. 53.1D).
1. Antegrade access to the kidney is achieved as for PCN placement.
2. An angled catheter and hydrophilic wire are advanced past the obstruction into the conduit.
3. With the patient semiprone, the urostomy site is prepped. The catheter and wire are directed out of the ostomy (this requires a second operator).
4. A stiff wire is then advanced retrograde from the end of the catheter (exiting the stoma) to the hub (at the flank) and the angled catheter is removed.
5. A retrograde nephrostomy catheter (40 to 50 cm in length) is advanced over the wire through the stoma until the locking loop is in the renal pelvis.
6. An antegrade "safety" catheter may be advanced over the floppy end of the wire (via the flank) into the kidney before the wire is removed to maintain antegrade access.
7. The wire is removed and the locking mechanisms of the catheter(s) are deployed.
8. Contrast is injected into either catheter to confirm adequate drainage through the retrograde catheter into the urostomy.
9. If an antegrade catheter has been left in place, it can be capped and removed at the first successful exchange of the retrograde catheter in 1 to 3 months. Because the conduits are of variable length and tortuosity, exchange of the retrograde catheter can be difficult and it may be necessary to revert to antegrade (PCN) access.

Removal or Exchange of PCN or Nephroureterostomy
1. A scout image is obtained with and without contrast injection. The hub and locking mechanism are cut from the tube with scissors. This allows the locking suture to be free when the loop is uncoiled. Some physicians grasp the suture with a mosquito forceps to prevent it from balling up inside the catheter.
2. A guidewire (with a firm distal body) is used to uncoil the fixation loop and to retain access to the renal pelvis or bladder, if a replacement is to be made. The replacement catheter can then be advanced over the wire into the renal pelvis or bladder.
3. Remove the nephrostomy tube over a guidewire.
   a. It is more comfortable for the patient.
   b. It helps prevent the PCN tube from catching and dragging a ureteral stent with it, if one is in place.
   c. It maintains access to the collecting system in situations where bleeding into the tract is suspected.

Exchange of Ureteral Stents
1. Routine exchange is usually performed cystoscopically, especially in men because access to the ureter may be lost when the stent is pulled through the penile urethra.
2. In women, a short sheath can be placed into the urethra and a snare (e.g., Gooseneck) advanced through the sheath and used to snare the distal pigtail of the ureteral stent.
   a. The stent is pulled through the sheath, taking care to make sure access to the ureter is maintained by the proximal portion of the stent.
   b. A stiff wire (e.g., Amplatz) is advanced through the stent into the renal collecting system.

c. The stent is removed and exchanged for a 5-Fr catheter. Dilute contrast is injected into the catheter to evaluate for hydronephrosis (that would suggest stent malfunction).

d. The catheter is exchanged over a stiff wire for a stent which is advanced to the renal pelvis. The wire is pulled back to allow the pigtail to form in the renal pelvis.

e. A "pusher" is used to advance the end of the stent through the urethra while the wire is pulled back, allowing the distal pigtail to form in the bladder. The sheath in the urethra can then be removed.

Postprocedure Management

1. For new catheter placement or catheter exchanges with sedation, bed rest and every 15- to 30-minute vital sign monitoring for 2 to 4 hours.

2. If drainage was performed to relieve obstruction, there may be a profuse postobstructive diuresis. Monitoring urine output permits IV replacement of volume.

3. If PCN is for decompression, continue external drainage until antegrade flow is restored. If PCN is to provide a tract for later stone removal and there is no obstruction, the catheter may be capped until the stone removal procedure.

4. Resume preprocedure diet.

5. Continue antibiotics only if signs of infection are present.

6. Treat pain and fever symptomatically.

7. If blood clot(s) obstruct the catheter and prevent good drainage, forward-flush 5 to 10 mL of bacteriostatic normal saline every 4 to 8 hours.

8. Blood-tinged urine may be seen for up to 48 hours:
   a. If gross hematuria persists, a tract study may be performed.
   b. If Hct falls without gross hematuria, check for retroperitoneal hemorrhage.
   c. Pericatheter bleeding may be a sign of arterial injury.

9. After NUT or antegrade stent placement, patients may experience bladder irritation and urinary frequency for a few days. It resolves in the majority, but if persistent and lifestyle limiting, may be an indication for PCN.

10. PCN catheters and NUT catheters are routinely changed every 3 months (or more commonly as needed) to prevent occlusion from encrustation and debris. Routine exchange generally requires little or no IV sedation. Antegrade ureteral stents are routinely changed every 3 to 6 months.

11. Patients with frequent catheter occlusions may benefit from routine forward flushing with normal saline (10 mL twice daily).

12. The use of antibiotic prophylaxis for routine catheter exchange is debatable.

Results

1. Placement of a PCN tube, especially into dilated collecting systems, is highly successful (95% to 100%).

2. Overall ureteral stent patency is 80%, with most failures occurring within 2 months of placement.
   a. Stent life can be optimized by
      (1) Increasing urine flow by encouraging patients to keep well hydrated
      (2) Administering prophylactic antibiotics at the time of stent placement
      (3) Avoiding placement of stents into bloody or infected collecting systems

Complications and Management (1–4)

Major: 4.0%

1. Massive hemorrhage requiring surgery or transcatheter embolization: 1% to 3.6%
   a. Angiography and embolization may, on rare occasion, be necessary.
   b. If a culprit vessel is not seen, the PCN should be retracted over a wire and repeat renal arteriogram performed to allow visualization of any bleeding or

abnormal vessels that are obscured or tamponaded by the catheter. Immediately after the angiogram, the PCN is quickly reinserted to tamponade the bleed.

2. Sepsis: 1% to 2%
3. Pneumothorax: <1%
4. Death due to hemorrhage: <0.2%
5. Peritonitis: rare

Minor: 15%, Usually Without Sequelae

1. Macroscopic hematuria: very common, clears within 12 to 24 hours
2. Pain: common; usually treated with acetaminophen but occasionally requires short-term opioids
3. Urine extravasation: <2.0%
4. Perirenal bleeding: rare
5. Urinary infection: 1.4% to 21% (45% of patients with struvite stones) will develop signs of infection following PCN tube placement.
   a. Postprocedure rigors may respond to meperidine (Demerol): 25 to 50 mg IV.
6. Catheter-related problems
   a. Dislodgment: 1% in early postprocedural period; 2% by end of the first month; and as high as 11% to 30% with longer follow-up.
      (1) If the catheter has been in for at least several weeks, the existing tract can usually be recatheterized after it is opacified using a 5-Fr dilator inserted into the skin entry site. Then, a 0.035-in angled Glidewire (Terumo Corp, Tokyo, Japan) may be manipulated through the dilator and into the renal collecting system.
      (2) When there is dislodgment before a tract can form, a new puncture may be required.
   b. Catheter occlusion occurs in 1% of patients; these tubes require replacement. PCN tubes placed to relieve hydronephrosis during pregnancy seem particularly susceptible to blockage by gritty material.
   c. Encrustation of the tube with the inability to uncoil the loop during attempted removal.
      (1) If the tube becomes encrusted from being bathed in infected urine or has been in situ for too long, the loop may not open when a guidewire is advanced within the lumen (Fig. 53.7).
      (2) The hub and locking mechanism are cut off from the end of the tube and a 2-0 silk suture is sewn through the cut end of the indwelling tube and secured.
      (3) The suture material is brought through the lumen of the outer portion of a peel-away sheath that is the same size or 1 Fr larger than the failed nephrostomy tube.
      (4) A 0.035-in guidewire is advanced through the indwelling nephrostomy tube and coiled in the renal collecting system. With traction placed on the suture material, the sheath is advanced over the indwelling tube until it is in the renal collecting system. The loop can then be straightened against the Teflon peel-away sheath and removed.
      (5) A new tube can be placed through the lumen of the peel-away sheath that has its tip within the renal collecting system. If the peel-away sheath should become dislodged in the removal process, the guidewire should remain in place to provide access for placement of a replacement nephrostomy tube.
      (6) An NUT or ureteral stent that cannot be withdrawn with reasonable traction, particularly if in situ for more than 6 months, may be encrusted. Use of excessive force can cause catheter fracture, or result in ureteral injury or avulsion.

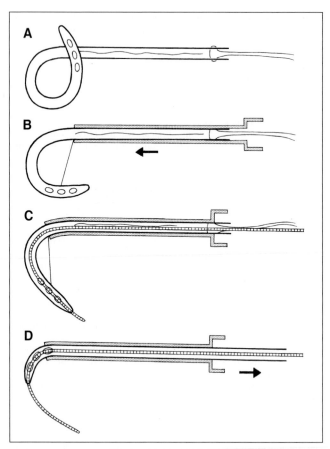

FIGURE 53.7 • Diagram illustrating removal of stuck Cope loop. **A:** Severe incrustation of urinary salts has produced binding of loop drawstring in Cope loop. Hub of catheter has been cut and a silk suture has been passed through the blunt end of catheter. **B:** The silk suture has been passed into the lumen of the peel-away sheath, which has then been advanced over the shaft of the Cope loop, forcing the leading edge of the introducer to release the drawstring and straighten the loop. **C:** Once the loop has been straightened, a 0.035-in guidewire is passed through the lumen of the loop into the collecting system. **D:** While the guidewire is kept in position, the Cope loop is pulled back through the peel-away sheath. (Redrawn from Castaneda-Zuniga WR, Tadavarthy SM. *Interventional Radiology.* 2nd ed. Wolters Kluwer; 1992:838.)

Complications Specific to Antegrade Ureteral Stent Placement

1. Stent migration due to improper positioning or length.
2. Stent occlusion, most commonly from an obstructing blood clot, but transient ureteral obstruction from severe mucosal edema has been described.
3. Bladder irritation and urinary frequency that usually resolve within days. Agents that decrease bladder muscle spasm may provide relief; however, occasionally severe irritation and discomfort persist, and stent removal and PCN placement are necessary.

References

1. ACR-SIR-SPR Practice parameter for the performance of percutaneous nephrostomy; 2016. www.sirweb.org/practice-resources/clinical-practice/guidelines-and-statements
2. Scheidt MJ, Hohenwalter EJ, Pinchot JW, et al. ACR appropriateness criteria radiologic management of urinary tract obstruction. *J Am Coll Radiol.* 2020;17(5S):S281–S292.
3. Thornton RH, Covey AM. Urinary drainage procedures in interventional radiology. *Tech Vasc Interv Radiol.* 2016;19(3):170–81.
4. Herr A, Malhotra A, White M, et al. *Ureteral Interventions. Tech Vasc Interv Radiol.* 2016; 19(3):182–93.
5. Lopez Zarraga F, Maynar FJ, Bastida R, et al. Percutaneous transrenal-ureteral connection: a new rendezvous modification. *J Vasc Interv Radiol.* 2018;29(9):1336–1338.
6. Patel IJ, Rahim S, Davidson JC, et al. Society of interventional radiology consensus guidelines for the periprocedural management of thrombotic and bleeding risk in patients undergoing percutaneous image-guided interventions—Part II: recommendations. *J Vasc Interv Radiol.* 2019;30(8):1168–1184.
7. Chebab MA, Thakor A, Tulin-Silver S, et al. Adult and Pediatric Antibiotic Prophylaxis during Vascular and IR Procedures: A Society of Interventional Radiology Practice Parameter Update Endorsed by the Cardiovascular and Interventional Radiological Society of Europe and the Canadian Association for Interventional Radiology. *J Vasc Interv Radiol.* 2018;29(11):1483–1501.
8. Batura D, Rao GG. A systematic review of the clinical significance of nephrostomy urine cultures. *World J Urol.* 2020;38(1):45–55.
9. Brandt MP, Lehnert T, Czilwik T, et al. CT-guided nephrostomy—an expedient tool for complex clinical scenarios. *Eur J Radiol.* 2019;110:142–147.
10. Bayne D, Taylor ER, Hampson L, et al. Determinants of nephrostomy tube dislodgement after percutaneous nephrolithotomy. *J Endourol.* 2015;29(3):289–92.

54 Lymphocele and Cyst Drainage and Sclerosis

Parag Amin, MD, Danny Cheng, MD, and Thuong G. Van Ha, MD

Introduction

In 1846 British physician-anatomist Sir Benjamin C. Brodie cautiously described palliative needle aspiration of "watery fluid" from cystic lesions he believed to be what are now known as hepatic cysts (1). Cystic lesions are commonly encountered on cross-sectional imaging and are either congenital or acquired in etiology. While congenital cysts can occur in virtually any solid organ (e.g., liver, pancreas, kidney, and ovary), acquired cystic lesions such as lymphoceles, liquefied hematomas, seromas, urinomas, and bilomas typically occur after surgery, trauma, or infection at or near the site of inciting event. Histologically, there are two broad categories: (a) true cysts, which are lined by epithelium, or (b) pseudocysts lined by fibrous or granulation tissue without epithelium. Symptoms may arise if they are large and/or complicated by hemorrhage or infection. Percutaneous needle aspiration as well as catheter drainage with or without sclerotherapy are viable management options across a variety of anatomical locations in both adult and pediatric patients (2–5).

Percutaneous aspiration can be both diagnostic and therapeutic. In the event of a large-volume cyst, catheter drainage is typically more efficient and can be left in place for persistent drainage in the case of fluid reaccumulation. While cyst obliteration can occasionally be achieved via chronic drainage alone, sclerotherapy is a safe and effective option, especially if a cyst recurs after aspiration or drainage (6,7).

Sclerosants include povidone-iodine, tetracycline/doxycycline, bleomycin, cyanoacrylate, sodium tetradecyl sulfate, hypertonic saline, and fibrin sealant (e.g., TISSEEL [Baxter Healthcare, Westlake Village, CA]). Although no consensus exists on sclerosant of choice, ethanol is readily available, inexpensive, and well tolerated (2). More recently, management of lymphoceles also includes two lymphatic embolization techniques (8,9) (see Chapter 48).

Indications

1. Pain/discomfort: referred or localized
2. Secondary infection
3. Functional sequelae of mass effect
   a. Renal cysts—hematuria, collecting system compression, hypertension (2)
   b. Lymphoceles—leg swelling, thrombophlebitis, renal transplant dysfunction (7)
   c. Hepatic/peribiliary, renal, splenic cysts—biliary (jaundice/cholestasis) or bowel obstruction (constipation/early satiety)

Contraindications

Absolute
1. Communication with vital structures such as blood vessels, biliary system, pancreatic duct, or renal collecting system
2. Communication with the peritoneal cavity/retroperitoneum (particularly in cases of prior surgery)
3. Lack of a safe window for percutaneous access

Relative
1. Coagulopathy
2. Noncompliant patient (particularly if a drain is to be left in place for multisession therapy)

Preprocedure Preparation

1. Symptom/laboratory evaluation with imaging correlation
   a. Do patient symptoms (early satiety, urinary frequency, pain, etc.) correlate to site of known cystic lesion?
   b. Do laboratory abnormalities (hyperbilirubinemia, elevated serum creatinine, etc.) correlate to site of known cystic lesion?
2. Imaging
   a. Ultrasound, computed tomography (CT), and/or magnetic resonance (MR) imaging to characterize the lesion (simple vs. complex, soft tissue nodularity to suggest malignancy, vascularity). If lesion is large and/or poorly seen on ultrasound, obtain CT or MR imaging to fully characterize its extent and internal structure.
   b. Evaluate safety/possibility of percutaneous access, adjacent vital structures, and choose mode of imaging guidance. Because most symptomatic cystic lesions are large and fluid-filled, the majority are easily accessed under sonographic guidance.
   c. If cystic/necrotic neoplasm is suspected, reconsider drainage procedure and do not perform sclerosis. Drainage of cystic collections from tumor is occasionally performed for palliative purposes but *sclerosis should not be considered given risk to, and likely communication with, adjacent vital structures.*
3. Defining clinical expectations
   a. Clarify and communicate management plan to referring physician(s) as well as the patient. Multiple sessions are often required and the need for patient cooperation (e.g., postprocedural body position changes after sclerosant injection) should be emphasized.

b. The patient should be informed that he or she may have a drainage catheter during the course of treatment for which daily outputs should be recorded.

4. Routine interventional radiology (IR) preparation

a. Baseline laboratory values: coagulation status (partial thromboplastin time [PTT], prothrombin time [PT]/international normalized ratio [INR], platelet count), white blood cell (WBC) count (Is patient currently infected?). Correct coagulopathy/thrombocytopenia prior to drainage.

b. Except for aspirin therapy, stop anticoagulation prior to the procedure. Most cyst drainage procedures are low (superficial lesions) to moderate risk for bleeding.

c. If TISSEEL is to be used, the exceedingly rare risks of minor and serious allergic reactions and theoretical risk of viral transmission should be discussed with the patient before the procedure.

Procedure

Diagnosis

1. Initial aspiration/drainage can be done upon needle insertion without catheter placement (if easy access) or with catheter placement (if difficult access) to send fluid for laboratory evaluation (complete blood count [CBC], fluid creatinine/blood urea nitrogen [BUN], triglycerides, lymphocytes, cytology, and Gram stain/culture).

2. Urinomas may require aspiration/drainage for symptom management or to prevent superimposed infection. They should not contain lymphocytes or triglycerides but do exhibit creatinine concentrations greater than serum and equal to urine. Urinomas are not sclerosed; the underlying leak should be targeted for recalcitrant collections.

3. Seromas and lymphoceles are seen postoperatively and can require not only aspiration/drainage but recurrent collections may require sclerosis. Seromas should not contain lymphocytes or triglycerides while lymphoceles contain lymphocytes and possibly triglycerides (and chylomicrons).

4. Collections suspected of infection should be aspirated/drained in the setting of antimicrobial therapy. Sclerosis has been performed in certain circumstances, for example, hydatid cyst disease (10).

Aspiration and Drainage

1. Cyst drainage and/or sclerotherapy can be performed in an outpatient setting, either single-session or multisession treatment. Treatment of infected collections (such as in echinococcal disease) should be performed on inpatients only for prolonged monitoring.

2. It is worth attempting initial aspiration/drainage of a symptomatic cystic lesion without sclerosis until coincident cyst and symptom/sign recurrence has been established.

3. Either Seldinger or direct trocar technique may be used depending on operator comfort, and lesion size and location.

4. Ultrasound guidance is usually preferred (especially for clearly visualized superficial lesions). CT is useful for lesions difficult to visualize with ultrasound.

5. Upon establishing a safe percutaneous window to the lesion, initial access may be obtained with a coaxial micropuncture system or with an 18-gauge trocar needle.

6. If a drainage catheter is deemed necessary, for example, for larger collections or if long-term suction drainage is attempted, an 8- to 12-Fr all-purpose drainage catheter may be placed.

7. Persistent drainage (or recurrence of cyst and symptoms after drain removal) warrants consideration for sclerotherapy. Cross-sectional imaging with CT or ultrasound is recommended prior to therapy to reevaluate cyst characteristics/accessibility.

Sclerotherapy

1. Prior to sclerotherapy, a cystogram is performed to ensure the cyst is self-contained.
   a. Once confirmed, sclerotherapy can proceed. Multiple sclerotherapy sessions are generally required.
2. Procedural details
   a. Povidone-iodine: volume of 10% povidone-iodine (Betadine; Purdue Pharma, Stamford, CT) instilled equals half of the volume of fluid aspirated, not exceeding 100 mL. The catheter is then capped for 2 hours and the patient rotated 360 degrees, spending 15 minutes in each position (i.e., supine, right lateral decubitus, prone, left lateral decubitus). The catheter is then connected to gravity drainage (7).
   b. Dehydrated ethanol (95% to 99%): Procedural details are similar to povidone-iodine. Amount instilled is equal to half of the volume of fluid aspirated with a maximum of 100 mL in order to avoid ethanol toxicity. The catheter is capped and the patient rotated 360 degrees, spending approximately 5 to 10 minutes in each position. The ethanol should be completely aspirated before catheter removal. If pain is encountered during injection, 10 to 15 mL of 1% lidocaine can be instilled into the cyst cavity (2,7).
   c. Doxycycline: Doxycycline powder, 500 mg (AdvaCare, Suffern, NY) is reconstituted in 20 mL of normal saline and 5 mL of 1% lidocaine. The mixture is injected into the cyst cavity and the tube capped for 1 to 2 hours. The patient should be maneuvered to allow contact with the entire cyst wall. The sclerosant should then be aspirated (7,9).
   d. Fibrin sealant (TISSEEL VH; 5-mL, two-component kit): The cyst should be entirely aspirated to maximize wall contact. A-7 Fr, three-lumen central venous catheter (AK15703; Teleflex Arrow, Wayne, PA) can be used to deliver the fibrin sealant. A dual-lumen catheter will suffice but a single-lumen catheter is not compatible because the agents will polymerize in the catheter during delivery. The fibrin sealant is prepared per manufacturer's recommendations. The two syringes are warmed to a temperature of 37°C and the solutions are simultaneously injected through separate lumens of the catheter for a total of 10 mL. Eighty mg of gentamicin can be added to one of the syringes, but there is no evidence that this decreases the rate of postprocedural infection. The catheter is removed and the site massaged to limit leakage and maximize surface contact. Treatment with TISSEEL can be performed in one session followed by catheter removal. Repeat treatments in separate sessions can be performed if necessary.

Postprocedure Management

1. The patient should be monitored immediately postprocedure for 1 to 2 hours in an observation/holding area for hemodynamic stability and pain control (2 hours is advised if a drain is left in place).
2. Drain intolerance and/or marked pain should warrant inpatient management or drain removal. Typically, therapy is well tolerated without need for excessive pain control.
3. If a catheter is placed, the patient is instructed to record daily drain output for review upon a follow-up visit. Catheter dwell times can range from several days to weeks for sclerotherapy or even up to several months in some cases.
4. Catheter removal or cessation of sclerotherapy is considered when drain output is less than 10 to 20 mL per 24 hours. Drain evaluation is advocated prior to removal, either with CT or with contrast injection under fluoroscopy, to confirm cyst collapse and exclude drain malposition as a cause of decreased drainage.

Results

1. Drainage and sclerotherapy has proven efficacy in the management of symptomatic cystic lesions (2–4,7). Expected success rates:

    a. Simple renal cysts—93% to 98% volume reduction for single-session alcohol sclerosis

    b. Simple hepatic cysts—95% volume reduction (range 40% to 100%)

    c. Lymphoceles—percutaneous drainage success rate as high as 94% and sclerosis as high as 100% (2)

2. The size of the cyst likely affects success rates with larger cysts often proving more difficult to treat successfully (7).

3. Surgical treatment options exist, such as cyst marsupialization/deroofing; however, comparative studies generally show sclerotherapy to be as effective (1–4,7). Surgery may be considered in lesions difficult to access or lesions unsuccessfully treated with drainage/sclerotherapy.

4. Drainage and sclerotherapy is also an option when initial surgical management fails.

Complications

Major

1. Rare and can be minimized with appropriate planning of access route and careful evaluation prior to sclerosant instillation.

2. Absorption or unintentional intravascular injection of ethanol into the bloodstream can result in prolonged hypotension, increased pulmonary vascular resistance, or decreased level of consciousness/central nervous system (CNS) depression.

Minor

1. Catheter-related infections

2. Localized pain and/or tissue injury (e.g., renal: acute tubular necrosis; hepatic: tissue infarction, biliary strictures; peritoneal spillage: intense pain)

3. Cyst recurrence

R e f e r e n c e s

1. Lectures illustrative of various subjects in pathology and surgery. *Mon J Med Sci.* 1846; 6(66):419–425.

2. Cheng D, Amin P, Van Ha T. Percutaneous sclerotherapy of cystic lesions. *Semin Intervent Radiol.* 2012;29(4):295–300.

3. Long L, Cai-Chan C, Xin-Qiao Z. One-year results of single-session sclerotherapy with bleomycin in simple renal cysts. *J Vasc Interv Radiol* 2012;(23):1651–1656.

4. Akhan A, Dinconuln A, Madaffan S, et al. Ultrasound-guided percutaneous sclerosis of congenital splenic cysts using ethyl alcohol 96% and minocycline hydrochloride 10% a pediatric series. *J Pediatr Surg.* 2016;51(9):1480–1484.

5. Benzimra J, Ronot M, Fuks D, et al. Hepatic cysts treated with percutaneous ethanol sclerotherapy: time to extend the indications to haemorrhagic cysts and polycystic liver disease. *Eur Radiol.* 2014;24(5):1030–1038.

6. Wijnands TFM, Görtjes APM, Gevers TJG, et al. Efficacy and safety of aspiration sclerotherapy of simple hepatic cysts: a systematic review. *AJR.* 2017;208(1):201–207.

7. Mahrer A, Ramchandani P, Trerotola SO, et al. Sclerotherapy in the management of postoperative lymphocele. *J Vasc Interv Radiol.* 2010;21(7):1050–1053.

8. Baek Y, Won JH, Chang SJ, et al. Lymphatic embolization for the treatment of pelvic lymphoceles: preliminary experience in five patients. *J Vasc Interv Radiol.* 2016;27:1170–1176.

9. Hur S, Shin JH, Lee IJ, et al. Early experience in the management of postoperative lymphatic leakage using lipiodol lymphangiography and adjunctive glue embolization. *J Vasc Interv Radiol.* 2016;27(8):1177–1186.

10. Nayman A, Guler I, Keskin S, et al. A novel modified PAIR technique using trocar catheter for percutaneous treatment of liver hydatid cysts: a six-year experience. *Diagn Interv Radiol.* 2016;22(1):47–51.

55 Pulmonary Tumor Ablation

Bradley B. Pua, MD and Stephen B. Solomon, MD

Introduction

Thermal ablation of pulmonary tumors is an option for local tumor control for unresectable tumors. Radiofrequency ablation (RFA), first described in the lungs in 2000, has since been proven to be both feasible and efficacious in the treatment of lung cancers (1). Ablative techniques have been used to treat primary lung cancers, metastatic disease to the lungs, and in palliation for painful chest wall masses. Thermal ablative techniques include heat-based modalities such as RFA and microwave ablation (MWA) in addition to cold-based techniques such as cryoablation.

RFA utilizes frictional energy imparted by oscillating ions within tissue to heat and treat tumors. Cells undergo coagulation necrosis when heated to more than 54°C for more than 1 second. Therapeutic RFA strives to bring tissue temperatures to the range of 60°C to 100°C. Because this technology relies on tissue and electrical conduction, RFA can be difficult to apply in lung where air is a poor conductor.

The mechanism of cell death caused by MWA is similar to RFA. With microwave, a continuously oscillating microwave field targets polar molecules (predominately water), which align with this field resulting in increased kinetic energy and tissue temperatures. This does not require electrical conduction and therefore allows microwave energy to penetrate more effectively allowing for generation of a larger volume of heat surrounding each applicator.

Cryoablation causes cell death through cell membrane disruption from both intra- and extracellular ice crystal formation and subsequent release of intracellular material. Although cellular necrosis is related to tissue type, temperatures of −35°C to −20°C are usually required. Current cryoablation systems utilize the Joule–Thomson effect to induce these extreme temperatures. Gases (typically argon) are delivered at high pressures through an internal feed line into an expansion chamber in the cryoprobe; as the gas expands, a heat sink is created cooling the probe and surrounding tissues. As thermal conductivity is secondary to passive conduction, the probes' cooling capacity is related to the size of the cryoprobe.

Lung Cancer

Primary lung cancer is the leading cause of cancer death in the United States. Non–small cell lung cancer (NSCLC) represents 85% of these cancers, whereas small cell represents approximately 15%. Small cell lung cancers are generally more aggressive, and patients with this subtype generally present with extensive lymph node involvement and metastatic disease. Currently, this characteristic renders ablation of this tumor subtype to salvage therapy, with the mainstay of therapy being systemic chemotherapy and radiotherapy. Patients with NSCLC present much earlier, allowing these patients to be treated with local therapies such as surgery, stereotactic body radiotherapy (SBRT), and ablation. Currently, surgical therapy (lobar and sublobar resection) is considered as first line for treatment of early-stage lung cancer with SBRT and ablation reserved for patients who are not surgical candidates. Additional indications for treatment of NSCLC may include (a) salvage (poor or no response to chemotherapy, radiation, or surgery) or (b) a single growing focus of tumor in a patient with otherwise stable metastatic disease.

Treatment of metastasis in the lungs is still a much-debated topic. Treatment of limited metastatic disease with surgical metastasectomy has been validated retrospectively with improved actuarial survival seen if complete surgical excision (R0 resection) is achieved. Thermal ablation is an option for this subset of patients as well, and offers this patient population, who often may face additional future metastases, a lung function preserving treatment. There is mounting evidence to suggest the equivalence of thermal ablation for treatment of limited oligometastatic disease as compared to SBRT and surgical resection (2).

Indications

Biopsy-Proven Malignancy
1. Early-stage primary lung cancer
   a. Medically inoperable/refusing surgery
      (1) Limited pulmonary reserve (see "Preprocedure Preparation" section)
   b. Recurrence: after surgery, radiation, or chemotherapy
2. Limited metastatic disease
   a. Widely metastatic disease responding to systemic chemotherapy with a single focus that is not responding
3. Salvage therapy
   a. Prior radiation: local recurrence in postradiation bed
   b. Prior surgery: local recurrence in postsurgical bed
   c. Symptom palliation: usually pain

Contraindications

Absolute
1. Uncorrected coagulopathy
   a. Uncorrected laboratory abnormality
      (1) INR >1.5
      (2) Platelets less than 50,000 per μL
   b. Uncorrected bleeding diathesis
2. Bacteremia or active infection
   a. Postablated tissue can serve as a nidus for infection, which may result in abscess formation.

Relative
1. Tumors adjacent to vital organs
   a. Mediastinum, large blood vessels (aorta, main pulmonary artery), esophagus, and chest wall
   b. This is considered a relative contraindication; separation techniques (as described later) can be used to help create a buffer zone between tumor and neighboring vital structures.

Preprocedure Preparation

1. History and physical examination with attention to
   a. History of bleeding diathesis
   b. Concurrent cardiopulmonary compromise, which may affect choice of sedation.
      (1) Compromised pulmonary function may contraindicate surgical resection.
         (a) Pulmonary function tests may be transiently affected after ablation.
      (2) Ablation can be performed in the contralateral lung in a patient with prior pneumonectomy. Increased postprocedure monitoring is suggested such as routine overnight admission for observation.
   c. Pacemakers and metallic implants
      (1) Although RFA and MWA in patients with **pacemakers/defibrillators** have been reported, it is still recommended that these devices be deactivated during ablation of pulmonary tumors. Deactivation with a magnet over the pacemaker or defibrillator will remove sensing activity temporarily until the magnet is removed. Cryoablation may be utilized in these instances.

    (2) **Metal implants**, when small, can heat up due to the circuit created from the RFA probe to the grounding pad.

2. Team approach

    a. Treatment of patients with primary and metastatic tumors should be performed after discussion with the patient's multidisciplinary team.

      (1) Ideally, patients should be presented and discussed in a multidisciplinary setting, such as tumor board.

3. Preprocedure biopsy

    a. Lesions to be treated should generally be biopsy-proven malignancy.

      (1) Same session biopsy can be considered and appealing to some patients as compared to multisession SBRT.

      (2) To offset risk of biopsy hemorrhage obscuring nodule from adequate ablation targeting, placement of ablation probe/applicator can be performed first.

      (3) Some prefer biopsies be performed on a separate occasion because

        (a) Biopsy findings may alter management.

        (b) Potential of hemorrhage during biopsy may obscure lesion to be treated, thus decreasing effectiveness. A short interval between biopsy (~1 to 2 weeks) and ablation will allow these postbiopsy changes to resolve.

4. Preprocedure imaging and choice of guidance

    a. Preprocedure computed tomography (CT) and/or positron emission tomography (PET)/CT should be performed to assess stage, trajectory planning, and serve as baseline for follow-up.

    b. In the setting of treatment of primary disease, some advocate mediastinal staging with endobronchial ultrasound (EBUS).

    c. Guidance

      (1) CT: Vast majority of lung ablations will be performed under CT guidance.

      (2) Ultrasound (US): helpful in treatment of peripheral lung lesions or chest wall masses

      (3) CT fluoroscopy: has the advantage of real-time imaging during applicator placement

5. Factors affecting ablation effectiveness

    a. Tumors larger than 2 to 3 cm

    b. Proximity to large vessels may act as a heat sink limiting effectiveness

Procedure

1. Anesthesia

    a. Moderate sedation or general anesthesia with local anesthesia can be used

      (1) General anesthesia advantages

        (a) Airway control

        (b) Ventilation control (rate and tidal volume) can aid lesion targeting

        (c) Limited patient motion

2. Patient positioning

    a. Grounding pads (RFA)

      (1) Dispersive grounding pads should be placed in a well-prepared area, without hair/shaved, equidistant from target. Attention to proper placement before and during ablation will decrease potential risk of skin burns.

    b. Padding

      (1) It is important to place padding in areas with important neurovascular bundles.

        (a) Brachial plexus injuries have been reported in poorly positioned patients.

3. Antibiotics

    a. May be given within 1 hour before procedure to cover skin flora

      (1) No studies demonstrate the need for antibiotics. However, devitalized tissue may serve as a nidus for infection

Sagittal

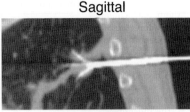

Coronals

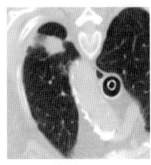

Preprocedure

FIGURE 55.1 • Radiofrequency ablation multitined applicator with tines deployed covering entire tumor. It is important to ensure that there is adequate coverage in multiple planes.

4. Positioning and access sites (similar to lung biopsies)
   a. Trajectory should limit number of interlobular fissures traversed
   b. Avoid bullae and cysts
   c. Avoid mediastinal structures and large vessels
5. Probe positioning
   a. Ideal probe positioning allows for postablative zone to cover tumor (Fig. 55.1)
      (1) Similar to surgery, the effective ablation zone should ideally cover 0.5 to 1 cm beyond the boundaries of the tumor.
      (2) Immediate postprocedure imaging shows *ground-glass opacity* in the ablated area. This region of ground-glass opacity has been associated with completeness of ablation.
         (a) One study suggests that postablation ground-glass opacity four times the original size of the tumor is predictive of complete ablation (3).
         (b) A minimum of 5-mm ground-glass opacity surrounding the tumor is suggested for complete ablation (4).
6. Ablating lung tissue
   a. Lung parenchyma is less thermally and electrically conductive as compared to liver.
   b. Power settings for RFA usually start at a lower wattage (~20 W) and gradually increase.
   c. Conductivity and therefore ablation times may be longer in lung tissue as compared to liver.

   Ablation settings vary by manufacturer: Probe selection varies by size of lesion to be ablated, location, and familiarity with system. Advantages of certain systems over others are controversial.

   Synergistic effects can be seen when multiple probes are combined allowing for more optimal ablation coverage. Consult manufacturer thermal maps.

Manufacturer thermal maps often underestimate in vivo ablation zones (5).

7. Additional techniques
  a. Overlapping probes
    (1) Can use more than one probe or ablate at multiple locations using a single probe when treating tumors larger than 3 cm.
  b. Separation techniques
    (1) For treatment of juxtapleural and paramediastinal lesions, an artificial pneumothorax can be created to separate the lesion from the aforementioned structures.
  c. Thermocouples
    (1) Thermocouples placed on the edge of the tumor or near sensitive structures can guide ablation device parameter choices.
8. Take advantage of imaging
  a. Routine use of three-dimensional (3D) reconstructions or planning software can help optimize probe placement.
9. Choice of ablation energy (RFA, microwave, or cryoablation)
  a. Microwave should be avoided with lesions <1 to 2 cm from the pleural surface. MWA zones abutting pleural surfaces are prone to bronchopleural fistula.
  b. A pretreatment short cycle of freeze and thaw (3-minute freeze, 3-minute thaw) may allow better ice ball formation when cryoablation is used secondary to enhanced conductivity of hemorrhage versus air.
  c. Cryoablation is often better tolerated in the patient who is undergoing the procedure under conscious sedation versus general anesthesia.

Postprocedure Management

1. Immediate postprocedure patient management
  a. Postprocedure CT to evaluate ablation zone, potential collateral damage, and assess for pulmonary hemorrhage or pneumothorax. If significant pneumothorax exists, a trial of aspiration of the air prior to removal of the ablation applicator can be performed.
  b. Procedure may be done on a same-day discharge basis, although overnight observation may be prudent in patients with multiple medical comorbidities.
  c. Postprocedure chest x-ray should be performed immediately after the procedure and 2 hours afterward. If patient is symptomatic, imaging should be performed earlier.
  d. Overnight stay
    (1) Pain control: Pain is usually well controlled with ibuprofen, with significant improvement by next day. Most patients are pain-free or with mild pain controlled with over-the-counter analgesics prior to discharge. Authors prefer ibuprofen 800 mg TID in the immediate postprocedure recovery period.
    (2) Chest x-ray should be performed prior to discharge to assess for late pneumothorax needing treatment or other complications.
  e. Chest tube: Chest tubes are placed in enlarging pneumothoraces and recurrent pneumothorax (if it recurs after initial aspiration).
    (1) Most symptomatic patients should receive chest tube.
    (2) Many chest tubes can be removed the day after the procedure.
2. Imaging follow-up
  a. CT
    (1) A new baseline contrast-enhanced CT is usually obtained in 1 to 3 months and a repeat CT obtained every 3 months to assess for local tumor recurrence.
    (2) Normal findings: ground-glass opacity surrounding the treated tumor that consolidates in 2 to 3 months

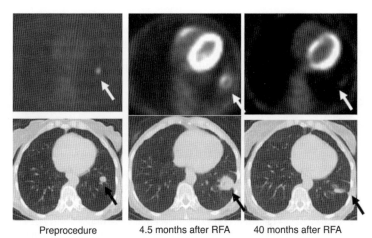

| Preprocedure | 4.5 months after RFA | 40 months after RFA |

FIGURE 55.2 • PET and CT follow-up imaging after RFA. Preprocedure imaging demonstrates a fluorodeoxyglucose (FDG)-avid lesion (*white arrow*) within the lung parenchyma (*black arrow*). Four and a half months after treatment, the lesion appears larger (*black arrow*) secondary to surrounding inflammatory changes with PET demonstrating a smooth, surrounding circular rim of FDG avidity (*white arrow*), which is an expected finding. Forty months after RFA, the treated lesion is smaller than the pretreatment lesion (*black arrow*) with no significant FDG activity within the tumor site (*white arrow*). Continued routine follow-up is needed to assess for an enlarging lesion or changes/increases in FDG activity.

3. Abnormal findings: enhancement
   a. New or irregular contrast enhancement in previously ablated areas in comparison to baseline study
   b. Magnetic resonance imaging (MRI): not usually used for follow-up secondary to poor lung visualization
   c. PET (Fig. 55.2)
      (1) Normal findings: Uniform rim of FDG low activity can be seen in the postablative region secondary to surrounding inflammatory tissue, which can remain for several months after therapy
      (2) Abnormal findings
         (a) Maximum *standardized uptake value* (SUV_{max}) of 3 or greater is suspicious (our clinical practice)
         (b) Increasing SUV on serial imaging

Results

1. Treatment of primary lung tumors
   a. RFA
      (1) Radiofrequency Ablation of Pulmonary Tumors Response Evaluation (RAPTURE) trial: prospective, multicenter, intention-to-treat clinical trial (6)—cancer-specific survival with NSCLC 92% at 1 year, 73% at 2 years (tumors less than 3.5 cm).
      (2) Simon et al. (7): with 5-year follow-up, overall survival (treated NSCLC) 78% at 1 year, 27% at 5 years (tumors less than 3.0 cm).
      (3) de Baère et al. (3): with 18-month follow-up, overall survival 76%; tumors less than 4.0 cm, patients with five tumors or less were treated.

b. Cryoablation
(1) Yamauchi et al. (8): with 29-month mean follow-up, overall survival 88% at 2 years, 88% at 3 years. Tumors treated—stage I NSCLC.
c. Microwave
(1) Wolf et al. (9): with mean 10-month follow-up, cancer-specific survival 83% at 1 year, 73% at 2 years, 61% at 3 years. Tumors treated included primary and metastatic cancers.
2. Treatment of metastasis
a. RFA
(1) RAPTURE (6): for colorectal metastasis, cancer-specific survival 93% at 1 year, 67% at 2 years.
(2) Simon et al. (7): for colorectal metastasis, overall survival 87% at 1 year, 57% at 5 years.
(3) de Baère et al. (3): with 18-month follow-up, overall survival 71%; tumors less than 4.0 cm, patients with five tumors or less.
(4) Petre et al. (10): for colorectal metastasis, 3-year progression free survival 77%; median survival from time of RFA 46 months.
b. Cryoablation—Callstrom et al. (2): local recurrence free response was 77.2% at 24 months; secondary local recurrence free response was 84.4% at 24 months.

Complications and Management

1. Pneumothorax
a. Risk of pneumothorax ranges (9% to 13%), pneumothorax requiring chest tube 3.5%
b. Rates of pneumothorax reported by larger studies
(1) RAPTURE (6): 19.7%
(2) Simon et al. (7): 28.4%
(3) de Baère et al. (4): 54%
2. Hemoptysis
a. Moderate hemoptysis in 3% of cases
b. Transient blood in sputum after ablation can occur; patients are counseled that this is self-limiting
3. Neuropathy
a. Paresthesias or pleuritic pain from treatment of juxtapleural tumors can occur.
(1) Although usually self-limiting with time, antiseizure medications such as pregabalin (Lyrica) or gabapentin (Neurontin) can be helpful.
b. Phrenic nerve injury from treatment of paramediastinal masses has been reported.
(1) Usually self-limiting, however, avoidance is preferred.
c. Brachial plexus injury: usually due to poor patient positioning or treatment of Pancoast lesions.
4. Pain
a. Patient-controlled analgesias (PCAs), NSAIDs or narcotics can be used the night of the procedure with the vast majority of pain either resolving or becoming significantly improved by the days after the procedure.
5. Others
a. Fever
b. Infection/abscess, *Aspergillus* in cavity
c. Bronchopleural fistula

References

1. Dupuy DE, Zagoria RJ, Akerley W, et al. Percutaneous radiofrequency ablation of malignancies in the lung. *AJR Am J Roentgenol.* 2000;174:57–59.

2. Callstrom MR, Woodrum DA, Nichols FC, et al. Multicenter study of metastatic lung tumors targeted by interventional cryoablation evaluation (SOLSTICE) *J Thorac Oncol.* 2020;15(7):1200–1209.
3. de Baère T, Palussière J, Aupérin A, et al. Midterm local efficacy and survival after radiofrequency ablation of lung tumors with minimum follow-up of 1 year: prospective evaluation. *Radiology.* 2006;240(2):587–596.
4. Anderson EM, Lees WR, Gillams AR. Early indicators of treatment success after percutaneous radiofrequency of pulmonary tumors. *Cardiovasc Intervent Radiol.* 2009;32(3):478–483.
5. Lyons GR, Winokur RS, Pua BB. Pulmonary cryoablation zones: more aggressive ablation is warranted in vivo. *Am J Roentgenol.* 2019;212(1):195–200.
6. Lencioni R, Crocetti, CR, et al. Response to radiofrequency ablation of pulmonary tumours: a prospective, intention-to-treat, multicentre clinical trial (the RAPTURE study). *Lancet Oncol.* 2008;9(7):621–628.
7. Simon CJ, Dupuy DE, DiPetrillo TA, et al. Pulmonary radiofrequency ablation: long-term safety and efficacy in 153 patients. *Radiology.* 2007;243(1):268–275.
8. Yamauchi Y, Izumi Y, Hashimoto K, et al. Percutaneous cryoablation for the treatment of medically inoperable stage I non-small cell lung cancer. *PLoS One.* 2012;7(3):e33223.
9. Wolf FJ, Grand DJ, Machan JT, et al. Microwave ablation of lung malignancies: effectiveness, CT findings, and safety in 50 patients. *Radiology.* 2008;247(3):871–879.
10. Petre EN, Jia X, Thornton RH, et al. Treatment of pulmonary colorectal metastases by radiofrequency ablation. *Clin Colorectal Cancer.* 2013;12(1):37–44.

56 Hepatic Tumor Ablation

Laura Crocetti, MD, PhD, EBIR, FCIRSE, Elena Bozzi, MD, and Roberto Cioni, MD

Introduction

The development of image-guided percutaneous techniques for local tumor ablation has been one of the major advances in the treatment of liver malignancies. Among these methods, radiofrequency (RF) ablation has been for a long time the primary ablative modality at most institutions. However, in the last decade, microwave (MW) ablation has been increasingly applied in clinical practice. Thermal ablation is accepted as the best therapeutic choice for patients with *very–early* and *early*-stage hepatocellular carcinoma (HCC) when liver transplantation or surgical resection is not a suitable option. In addition, thermal ablation is considered as a viable alternative to surgery for inoperable patients with limited hepatic metastatic disease, especially from colorectal cancer (CRC), in patients deemed ineligible for surgical resection because of extent and location of the disease or concurrent medical conditions. Cryoablation and nonthermal techniques such as irreversible electroporation (IRE) are applied in selected patient populations.

Indications

The indication for ablation of a liver tumor should come from multidisciplinary tumor board discussion and be clearly articulated in a concurrent manner by the interventional radiologist, oncologist, hepatologist, and liver surgeon, in order to select the best approach for the individual patient following the principles of precision medicine (1).

1. In patients with *very–early-stage HCC* (solitary small nodule less than 2 cm in diameter), image-guided tumor ablation is recommended as a first-line therapy even in surgical candidates. In patients with *early-stage HCC*, solitary HCC (less than 3 cm), or up to 3 nodules less than 3 cm, the choice of ablation as an

alternative to surgical resection is based on technical factors (location of the tumor), hepatic and extrahepatic patient conditions (1,2).

2. Patients with *early-stage HCC* as a neoadjuvant therapy before liver transplantation, as a "bridge" to prevent patient drop-out from the waiting list (1,2).

3. Patients with liver dominant *CRC oligometastases* (usually up to 5 metastases, less than 3 cm) in the following clinical scenarios (1,3):
   a. Patients "un-fit" for intensive chemotherapy protocols, candidates for supportive care
   b. "Fit" patients with initially resectable disease but poor lesion anatomical location or substantial comorbidities
   c. 'Fit' patients with initially nonresectable disease, as an adjunct to systemic therapy
   d. Selected patients with limited hepatic and pulmonary CRC metastatic disease may qualify provided that extrahepatic disease is deemed curable.

4. *Intrahepatic cholangiocarcinoma (iCCA):* single nodule ≤3 cm in nonsurgical patients (1).

5. Liver metastases from *neuroendocrine tumors (NETs)* as an alternative to systemic therapy in oligonodular disease (1).

6. Hepatic metastases from *other primary cancers.* Personalized approach, after multidisciplinary tumor board, tailored on features of the patient, of the disease and of liver sites (1).

Contraindications

Contraindications to ablative treatments are the following (1):

1. Tumor located <1 cm from the main biliary duct, due to risk of delayed stenosis of the main biliary tract
2. Significant ascites interposed along the applicator path
3. Exophytic location of the tumor when direct puncture of the tumor cannot be avoided due to the risk of tumor seeding and bleeding
4. Untreatable/unmanageable coagulopathy
5. Cardiac arrhythmias and the presence of a pacemaker if IRE is planned

Relative contraindications that can be managed to decrease complications rates (1):

1. Bilio-enteric anastomosis: the risk of hepatic abscesses is decreased by appropriate antibiotic prophylaxis. It is advised a regimen that includes oral levofloxacin 500 mg per day + oral metronidazole 500 mg twice daily beginning 2 days before and continuing for 14 days after ablation + neomycin 1 g and erythromycin base 1 g orally at 1, 2, and 11 PM on the day before ablation (1).
2. Superficial lesions may be treated with no-touch technique or laparoscopic approach
3. Gastrointestinal tract or gallbladder adjacent to the lesion to be treated can be safely displaced with hydro/gas dissection
4. Pacemaker/defibrillators may be protected during RF ablation and are not affected by MW ablation.

Preprocedure Preparation

1. Evaluate patient records, history, physical examination, and prior imaging studies to determine the indication and feasibility of ablation.
2. The interventional radiologist that will perform the ablation procedure needs to visit the patient as an outpatient clinic prior to the date of the procedure. The purpose of the visit is to describe the treatment that will be performed, including imaging ablation modality, benefits and risks, any ancillary procedures that may be required, and to obtain informed consent from the patient following national laws and institutional forms.

3. Preprocedural imaging—the tumor staging protocol must be tailored to the type of malignancy.
   a. In patients with HCC, the detection of a nodule by ultrasound (US) is usually followed by multidetector spiral computed tomography (CT) or dynamic magnetic resonance (MR), following the recommendations of the American Association for the Study of Liver Diseases (AASLD) and of the European Association for the Study of the Liver (EASL) (1).
   b. Patients with liver metastases should undergo CT or MR of the abdomen. Chest CT and positron emission tomography (PET)-CT are required to exclude or confirm extrahepatic metastatic disease (1).
4. Preprocedural laboratory testing
   a. Preprocedural laboratory test should include clotting function tests (platelet count, and international normalized ratio—see paragraph 5), full blood count and biochemistry tests evaluating liver and kidney function (1)
5. Evaluation of bleeding risk and correction of coagulopathy (4)
   a. Values of international normalized ratio less than 1.5 and platelet count greater than 50,000 per μL are required in order to proceed.
   b. When possible, antiplatelet/anticoagulation medications should be discontinued before the procedure. When cessation is problematic, risks and benefits should be carefully evaluated and patients informed of a potential increased risk of bleeding. It has to be taken into consideration that, in comparison to a biopsy, the applicator track can be coagulated during thermal ablation.
   c. Recommendations for bleeding risk evaluation and management in liver thermal ablation from the Society of Interventional Radiology (SIR), Canadian Association for Interventional Radiology and CIRSE are summarized in Table 56.1.

Procedure

1. Patients should be fasting for 4 to 6 hours prior to the procedure.
2. A peripheral venous access (18 to 20 gauge) should be obtained.
3. The routine use of prophylactic antibiotics is recommended although the risk of contamination is low, as the procedure is performed under sterile conditions. The large amount of necrotic material created during ablation poses a risk for bacterial seeding during percutaneous access, and the use of a single agent targeted to skin flora (e.g., cefazolin, 1 to 2 g IV) may be reasonable (1).
4. Thermal ablation is usually performed with the patient under intravenous sedation or general anesthesia, depending on operator or institutional preference. Local anesthesia is additionally provided by injecting 5 to 10 mL of local anesthetics (e.g., lidocaine) from the skin to the liver capsule along a specified insertion route. When general anesthesia is used, high-frequency jet ventilation might aid tumor targeting.
5. The goal of ablation is to produce a volume of necrosis that includes the ablation margin. This is the region ablated beyond the borders of the tumor to achieve complete tumor destruction. Ideally, it should measure 0.5 to 1.0 cm in its smallest width depending on tumor histotype (1).
6. At the end of the procedure, when a heat-based thermal ablation modality is used, coagulation of the needle track is performed to prevent bleeding and tumor seeding (1).
7. Technical considerations
   a. RF ablation
      (1) RF ablation induces thermal injury to tissue through electromagnetic energy deposition (frequency in the range of 375 to 500 kHz). With RF ablation, the patient is part of a closed-loop circuit that includes an RF generator, an electrode needle, and a large dispersive electrode

Table 56.1	Summary of Recommendations for Bleeding Risk Evaluation and Management in Liver Thermal Ablation from the Society of Interventional Radiology (SIR), Canadian Association for Interventional Radiology and CIRSE

Preprocedure Laboratory Testing

PT/INR	routinely recommended
Platelet count/Hemoglobin	routinely recommended
Fibrinogen	Recommended in patients with chronic liver disease
Management	
INR	correct to ≤1.5–1.8; correct to <2.5 in patients with chronic liver disease
Platelets	Transfusion recommended for count <50,000/µL transfusion recommended for count <30,000/µL in patients with chronic liver disease
Fibrinogen	Correct to >100 mg/dL in patients with chronic liver disease
Clopidogrel	Withhold for 5 days before procedure
Aspirin	Withhold for 3–5 days
Fractionated heparin	Withhold for 24 hours or up to two doses if therapeutic dose; withhold 1 dose if prophylactic
Warfarin	Withhold 5 days until target ≤INR 1.8; consider bridging for high thrombosis risk cases; if stat or emergent, use reversal agent

PT, prothrombin time; INR, international normalized ratio.
Modified from Hinshaw JL, Lubner MG, Ziemlewicz TJ, Lee FT Jr, Brace CL. Percutaneous tumor ablation tools: microwave, radiofrequency, or cryoablation—what should you use and why? *Radiographics.* 2014;34(5):1344–1362.

(grounding pad). An alternating electric field is created within the tissue of the patient. Because of the relatively high electrical resistance of tissue in comparison with the metal electrodes, there is marked agitation of the ions present in the target tissue that surrounds the electrode, as the tissue ions attempt to follow the changes in direction of alternating electric current. The agitation results in frictional heat around the electrode. The discrepancy between the small surface area of the needle electrode and the large area of the grounding pads causes the generated heat to be focused and concentrated around the needle electrode (5).

(2) The thermal damage caused by RF heating is dependent on both the tissue temperature achieved and the duration of heating. Heating of tissue at 50°C to 55°C for 4 to 6 minutes produces irreversible cellular damage. At temperatures between 60°C and 100°C, near immediate coagulation of tissue is induced, with irreversible damage to mitochondrial and cytosolic enzymes of the cells. At more than 100°C to 110°C, tissue vaporizes and carbonizes. For adequate destruction of tumor tissue, the entire target volume must be subjected to cytotoxic temperatures. Thus, an essential objective of ablative therapy is the achievement and maintenance of 50°C to 100°C temperature throughout the entire target volume for at least 4 to 6 minutes. However, the relatively slow thermal conduction from the electrode surface through the tissues increases the duration of application

to 10 to 20 minutes. To accomplish the increase in energy deposition into tissues, the RF output of all commercially available generators has been increased to 150 to 250 W.

(3) On the other hand, the tissue temperature should not be greater than 100°C to 110°C, so as to avoid carbonization with significant gas production that both serves as an insulator and diminishes the ability to effectively establish an RF field. After activation, automated programs, designed to modulate the released power relying on direct temperature measurement or on electrical measurement of tissue impedance, to avoid overheating and carbonization, run the generators.

(4) Another important factor that affects the success of RF thermal ablation is the heat loss through convection by means of blood circulation, the so-called heat sink effect. This may limit target volume and therefore the ability to ablate all viable tumor and produce an adequate tumor-free margin.

(5) One or multiple electrodes have to be inserted directly into the tumor to deliver RF energy current. Electrodes are coupled with RF generators and can be monopolar or bipolar, and they can have different designs (multi-tined expandable, internally cooled, perfused). There is no current evidence that one device is superior to the others. Similar results in term of technical success can be obtained by adjusting the time at target temperature and the number of overlapping ablations according to different device designs.

(a) Monopolar electrode: There is a single active electrode, with current dissipated at one or several return grounding pads.

(b) Bipolar electrode: There are two active electrode applicators, which have to be placed in proximity.

(c) Multi-tined expandable electrode: Multiple electrode tines that expand from a larger-needle cannula. They permit the deposition of this energy over a larger volume and ensure more uniform heating that relies less on heat conduction over a large distance.

(d) Internally cooled electrode: The electrode has an internal lumen, which is perfused by saline without coming into direct contact with patient tissues. They have been designed to minimize carbonization and gas formation around the needle tip by eliminating excess heat near the electrode.

(e) Perfused electrode: The tip of the electrode has small apertures that allow the fluid (usually saline) to come in contact with the tissue. Administration of saline solution during the application of RF current increases tissue conductivity and thereby allows greater deposition of RF current and increased tissue heating and coagulation (1).

b. MW ablation

(1) Electromagnetic microwaves heat matter by inducing an ultra–high-speed (between 900 MHz and 2,450 MHz) alternating electric field. Cell death in MW ablation is nearly identical to that observed in RF ablation. However, the mechanism of MW heating may have advantages in certain clinical applications. Polar molecules (primarily water) continuously realign with the oscillating MW field, effectively increasing kinetic energy and tissue temperature. In contrast to electric currents, microwaves radiate through all biological tissues, including those with high impedance to electric current, such as bone, lung, and charred or desiccated tissues. This allows microwaves to continuously generate heat in a much larger volume of tissue surrounding the applicator (5).

(2) As a result, MW energy can produce faster, hotter, and larger ablation zones in multiple tissue types compared with RF current. As a result, the advantage of MWA over RF ablation is that treatment outcome is less affected by vessels located in the proximity of the tumor.

(3) In addition, because MWA does not rely on an electrical circuit as does RF ablation, multiple applicators can be applied simultaneously.

(4) In the case of MW ablation, differences between devices are not related as much to the morphology of the applicators (which are, in all cases, straight needles without hooks), but rather to the following characteristics:

(a) MW frequency emission used are either 915 MHz or 2450 MHz;

(b) Antenna caliber varies between 11 gauge and 18 gauge

(c) Maximum available generator power varies between 60 W and 195 W, and a certain amount of power is lost between the generator and the antenna tip along the linking coaxial line. Due to this power loss, the maximum power at the antenna differs from the power at the generator.

(d) The number of antennas that can be used simultaneously with a single generator is 1 to 4. The simultaneous use of several applicators determines a more uniform, and larger ablation area.

(e) The methods of energy delivery (manual or automatic, continuous or pulsed) (1).

c. Cryoablation

(1) Cryoablation systems use the Joule–Thomson effect of expanding gases within a needle-like cryoprobe. As the cryogen (typically argon) moves from an internal feed line into an internal expansion chamber at the tip of the needle, it produces a heat sink near the antenna tip that cools the probe to temperatures of $-160°C$ or colder. Heat transfer from the tissue into the cryoprobe is governed by passive thermal diffusion (5).

(2) In liver tissue threshold for lethal cellular damage is $-40°C$. As a result, the surface area of the cryoprobe limits cooling efficiency; smaller cryoprobe diameters are associated with lower cooling capacity and, consequently, smaller ablation zones. Therefore, several cryoprobes are required to treat most tumors in clinical practice, and ablation times are typically 25 to 30 minutes.

(3) Cryoprobes size ranges from 17 to 8 gauge. In US, the ice ball is seen as hyperechoic line representing the proximal edge of the ice ball with posterior acoustic shadow. The ice ball is identified as a low attenuation (~0 HU) region on CT and signal void region on MRI.

(4) Cauterization of the needle track by means of thermal energy is available in the latest versions of some vendors' cryoprobes.

d. Irreversible electroporation

(1) IRE is a nonchemical, nonthermal image-guided ablation technique. IRE is a method to induce irreversible disruption of cell membrane integrity, by changing the transmembrane potential, resulting in cell death without the need for additional pharmacologic injury. IRE creates a sharp boundary between the treated and untreated area in vivo. This would suggest that IRE has the ability to sharply delineate the treatment area from the nontreated, and that treatment planning can be precisely performed according to mathematical predictions.

(2) Because IRE is a nonthermal technique, there appears to be complete ablation to the margin of blood vessels without compromising the functionality of the blood vessels. Therefore, issues associated with perfusion-mediated tissue cooling or heating (a significant challenge with thermal methods) are not relevant. IRE may be a treatment option for centrally located liver tumors with margins adjacent to major bile ducts where thermal ablation techniques are contraindicated.

(3) The procedure is technically challenging, requiring the placement of at least two needle electrodes parallel to each other at a distance of 1 to 2.5 cm and is more costly than RF and MW ablation.

(4) A number of contraindications exist, including cardiac arrhythmias and the presence of a pacemaker, and metallic objects such as surgical clips adjacent to the ablation margin can affect the predictability of the ablation zone (6).

(5) Imaging guidance/monitoring. Targeting of the lesion can be performed with US, CT, or MR imaging. The guidance system is chosen largely on the basis of operator preference and local availability of dedicated equipment such as fluoroscopy-CT, cone-beam CT or open MR systems.

(6) Robotics and image fusion software improve the precision of targeting and allow immediate assessment of the adequacy of ablative margins. This may improve the results of thermal ablation in terms of local control (7) (Fig. 56.1).

Postprocedure Management

1. After ablation, bed rest for 1 to 2 hours is advised.
2. Vital sign monitoring is performed in the recovery room. If vital signs are stable, blood count and liver function tests are not significantly changed, and no complications are noted the patient can be discharged the day after the procedure.
3. Tumor response evaluation
   a. CT and MR images obtained 4 to 6 weeks after treatment show successful ablation as a nonenhancing area with or without a peripheral enhancing rim (Fig. 56.2).
   b. The enhancing rim that may be observed along the periphery of the ablation zone appears as a relatively concentric, symmetric, and uniform process in an area with smooth inner margins. This is a transient finding that represents a benign physiologic response to thermal injury (initially, reactive hyperemia; subsequently, fibrosis and giant cell reaction). Benign periablational enhancement needs to be differentiated from irregular peripheral enhancement due to residual tumor that occurs at the treatment margin. Compared to benign periablational enhancement, residual unablated tumor often grows in scattered, nodular, or eccentric patterns (Fig. 56.2).
   c. Later follow-up imaging studies should be aimed at detecting the recurrence of the treated lesion (i.e., local tumor progression), the development of new hepatic lesions, or the emergence of extrahepatic disease (1).

Results

1. Hepatocellular carcinoma
   a. In patients with cirrhosis and very–early and early-stage HCC, the complete response rate of RF ablation is above 95%, with 5 years survival rates in 62% to 68% of cases (1,8).
   b. The small number of published randomized studies failed to show a statistically significant superiority of MW ablation in comparison to RF ablation in terms of the overall survival and disease-free survival. Superiority of MW ablation over RF ablation was not demonstrated in published metanalyses (1).
   c. A recently published series with correlation with histology after liver transplantation reported complete pathological response in 78% of HCC nodules <3 cm treated with a single treatment session and with reliable imaging findings (diagnostic accuracy: 89%). Ease of use, reproducibility and size of volumes of ablation, together with short procedural times make MW ablation widely used and often the preferred thermal ablation modality (9).
   d. There have been a limited number of studies comparing outcomes including overall survival and liver cancer-specific survival in patients treated with cryoablation or RF ablation. No significant difference in overall survival between RF ablation and cryoablation at 6 months has been demonstrated (1).
   e. Given the benefits of its nonthermal nature, IRE may broaden local ablative options for HCC, in particular where standard, local curative treatments are

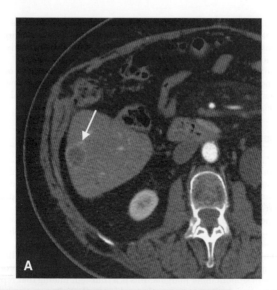

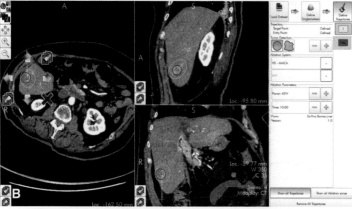

FIGURE 56.1 • Robotic-assisted MW ablation of small metastases from previously resected iCCA. Pretreatment CT shows the lesion as a small superficial hypodense nodule with hyperdense rim (**A**, *arrow*) in the arterial phase. During the planning phase with robotic assistance (CAS-One®, Cascination, Switzerland, CH) the intended ablation volume and the needle placement with respect to the liver surface are visualized (**B**, *red*, nodule; *green*, ablation volume according to device). (*continued*)

considered unsuitable due to risk of thermal injury or decreased efficacy due to heat-sink effect.

2. Colorectal hepatic metastases
   a. In patients with CRC liver metastases who are unfit for resection due to poor anatomical localization of the lesions or substantial comorbidities, ablation has been proven a viable alternative treatment. In cohort studies of nonsurgical patients treated with thermal ablation, the 5-year survival rates were in the range of 25% to 55% (1).

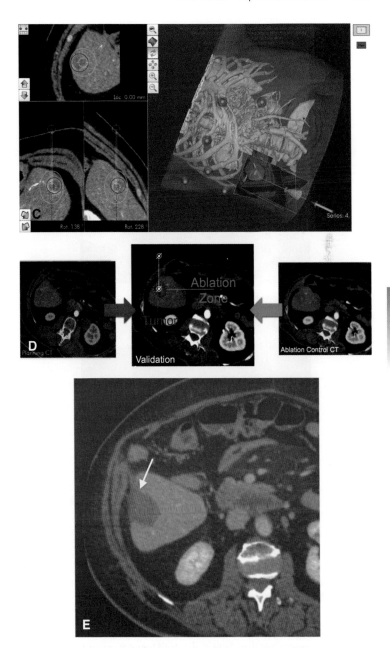

FIGURE 56.1 • (*Continued*) The needle access is visualized in 3D (**C**) and after treatment the adequacy of ablation volume is checked by fusion imaging (**D**). Follow-up CT performed 1 month after ablation shows complete response (**E**, *arrow*). (CAS-One®, Cascination, Switzerland, CH)

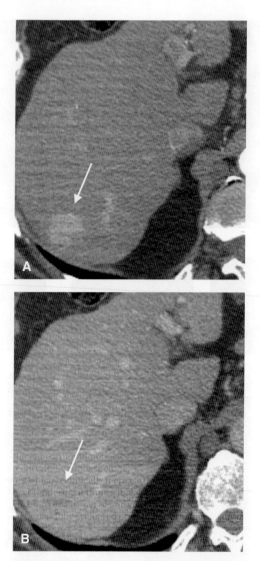

FIGURE 56.2 • CT-guided MW ablation of an early-stage HCC. Pretreatment CT obtained in the arterial (**A**, *arrow*) and the venous phase (**B**, *arrow*) shows the lesion with the typical radiological hallmarks of HCC nodule in segment 7. (*continued*)

b. Results comparable to surgery have been reached with RF ablation in solitary CRC metastases less than 3 cm in size, with tumor size representing one of the main limitations of ablative therapies (1).

c. In patients with oligometastatic disease, the phase II CLOCC trial compared chemotherapy alone versus chemotherapy with percutaneous or intraoperative RF ablation upfront in patients with up to 10 metastases. This trial

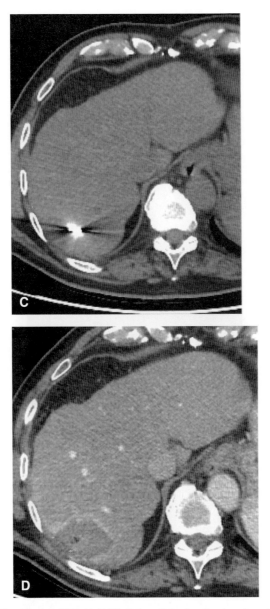

FIGURE 56.2 • (*Continued*) CT-guided MW ablation with two insertions is performed (HS AMICA®, Italy) with a wattage of 60 W for 7 minutes (**C**). After treatment contrast CT shows a large hypodense area covering the tumor as well as a cuff of surrounding liver parenchyma with peripheral hyperdense rim (**D**). (*continued*)

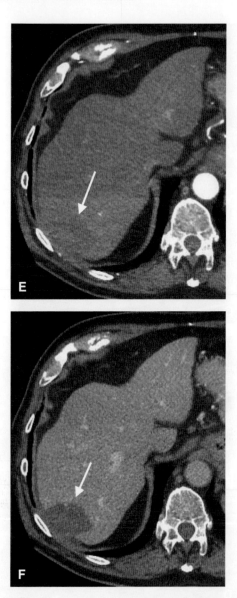

FIGURE 56.2 • (*Continued*) On CT images obtained in the arterial (**E**, *arrow*) and the portal venous phase (**F**, *arrow*) 1 month after treatment, the tumor is replaced by a nonenhancing ablation zone and complete response is confirmed. (HS AMICA®, Italy)

reported an improvement in both progression-free survival and overall survival. At the 8-year follow-up, progression-free survival was only 2% in the chemotherapy only arm, but 22.3% in the combined group with chemotherapy plus RF ablation. Overall survival was of 8.9% versus 35.9%, respectively (10).

   d. Several cohort studies have been published regarding the role of MW ablation in the treatment of CRC liver metastases. They reported a 3-,4- and 5-year overall survival for MW ablation between 35% and 79%, 35% and 58%, and 17% and 18% (1),

   e. Few series including small number of patients with CRC liver metastases ineligible for thermal ablation treated with IRE show complete response rate up to 74% to 96% and 26.5% 32.4 months survival after the procedure (6).

3. Other primary and secondary tumors

   a. iCCA—A recent meta-analysis evaluated 7 RF ablation studies including 84 iCCAs and reported pooled 1-, 3-, and 5-year overall survival rates of 82%, 47%, and 24% respectively. MW ablation was not associated with lower rates of local tumor progression when compared to RF in a study that reported a median overall survival of 23.6 months in patients treated for iCCAs with thermal ablation (1).

   b. Liver metastases from NETs—Patients submitted to RF ablation for liver metastases from NETs demonstrated a median survival of 10.3 to 11 years, with 5-year overall survival rate of 57% to 84% (1).

   c. Liver metastases from breast cancer—The results of a surgical series on breast metastasis resection shows that despite metastatic breast cancer being a systemic disease, local therapies have the potential to improve survival. In the case series, the median survival of patients with liver metastases treated with RF ablation was in the range of 30 to 60 months (1).

Complications

Overall grade 2 to 6 (or major) complication rate ranges from 2.2% to 3.1% (1).
1. Puncture-related complications
   a. Intraperitoneal bleeding (1%)
   b. Pneumothorax/hemothorax (0.1%)
   c. Tumor seeding along the needle tract (0.5%)
2. Thermal-related complications
   a. Bowel perforation (0.3%)
   b. Main portal vein thrombosis (0.1%)
   c. Liver abscess (0.3%)
   d. Bile duct stenosis and cholecistitis (0.1%)
3. Mortality (0.1% to 0.5%). The most common causes of death are sepsis, hepatic failure, colon perforation, and portal vein thrombosis

References

1. Crocetti L, de Baère T, Pereira PL, et al. CIRSE standards of practice on thermal ablation of liver tumors. *Cardiovasc Intervent Radiol.* 2020;43(7):951–962.

2. European Association for the Study of the Liver. EASL clinical practice guidelines: management of hepatocellular carcinoma. *J Hepatol.* 2018;69(1):182–236.

3. Van Cutsem E, Cervantes A, Adam R, et al. ESMO consensus guidelines for the management of patients with metastatic colorectal cancer. *Ann Oncol.* 2016;27(8):1386–1422.

4. Patel IJ, Rahim S, Davidson JC, et al. Society of Interventional Radiology Consensus Guidelines for the Periprocedural Management of Thrombotic and Bleeding Risk in Patients Undergoing Percutaneous Image-Guided Interventions-Part II: Recommendations: Endorsed by the Canadian Association for Interventional Radiology and the Cardiovascular and Interventional Radiological Society of Europe. *J Vasc Interv Radiol.* 2019;30(8):1168–1184.

5. Hinshaw JL, Lubner MG, Ziemlewicz TJ, et al Percutaneous tumor ablation tools: microwave, radiofrequency, or cryoablation–What should you use and why? *Radiographics.* 2014;34(5):1344–1362.

6. Meijerink MR, Ruarus AH, Vroomen LGPH, et al. Irreversible Electroporation to Treat Unresectable Colorectal Liver Metastases (COLDFIRE-2): A Phase II, Two-Center, Single-Arm Clinical Trial. *Radiology.* 2021;299:470–480.

7. Solbiati M, Muglia R, Goldberg SN, et al. A novel software platform for volumetric assessment of ablation completeness. *Int J Hyperthermia*. 2019;36(1):337–343.

8. Livraghi T, Meloni F, Di Stasi M, et al. Sustained complete response and complications rates after radiofrequency ablation of very early hepatocellular carcinoma in cirrhosis: is resection still the treatment of choice? *Hepatology*. 2008;47:82–89.

9. Crocetti L, Scalise P, Bozzi E, et al. Microwave ablation of very early and early-stage HCC: efficacy evaluation by correlation with histology after liver transplantation. *Cancers (Basel)*. 2021;13(14):3420. doi: 10.3390/cancers13143420

10. Ruers T, Van Coevorden F, Punt CJ, Pierie JE, Borel-Rinkes I, Ledermann JA, et al; European Organisation for Research and Treatment of Cancer (EORTC); Gastro-Intestinal Tract Cancer Group; Arbeitsgruppe Lebermetastasen und tumoren in der Chirurgischen Arbeitsgemeinschaft Onkologie (ALM-CAO); National Cancer Research Institute Colorectal Clinical Study Group (NCRI CCSG). Local Treatment of Unresectable Colorectal Liver Metastases: Results of a Randomized Phase II Trial. *J Natl Cancer Inst*. 2017;109(9).

57 Renal Tumor Ablation

Shilpa Reddy, MD, Joseph P. Erinjeri, MD, PhD, and Timothy W.I. Clark, MD, FSIR

Introduction

Cancer of the kidney accounts for approximately 4% of all malignancies in the United States. Although surgical extirpation remains the standard of care for small renal tumors, nephron-sparing techniques in the treatment of kidney cancer have made thermal ablation of renal tumors a viable alternative to both open and laparoscopic partial nephrectomy (PN).

Indications

T1a (≤4 cm) and T1b (<7 cm) renal masses in patients who:
1. Have comorbidities that preclude surgery or general endotracheal anesthesia
2. Require conservation of renal parenchyma (solitary kidney, renal insufficiency)
3. Have multiple tumors in the same kidney (Von Hippel–Lindau or Birt–Hogg–Dubé) where surgical extirpation would make renal reconstruction difficult
4. Have complex tumors where surgical resection would require an extended ischemia time
5. Prefer minimally invasive techniques over open or laparoscopic surgery
6. Prefer treatment over active surveillance of stable and/or small renal masses

Contraindications

Absolute
1. Uncorrectable coagulopathy (when international normalized ratio [INR] >1.5, platelet count <50,000 per μL).

Relative
1. Anatomic considerations
   a. Anteromedial masses without a safe percutaneous route to the lesion
   b. Masses proximal to ureter without ability to protect ureter from thermal injury
2. Contraindications to radiofrequency ablation (RFA)
   a. Hip prosthesis, which may act as an electrical conduit, increasing risk of skin burn

b. Pacemaker/defibrillator. Radiofrequency energy can interfere with pacer/defibrillator function. Some patients may be able to wear a magnet to deactivate the device and have it calibrated and reprogrammed after the procedure

Preprocedure Preparation

1. Clinical consultation
   a. Complete history and physical
   b. Laboratory studies including baseline hematocrit/hemoglobin, coagulation parameters (INR, platelet count), and renal function (creatinine, glomerular filtration rate [GFR]). A baseline hematocrit/hemoglobin should be obtained.
   c. Review of medications. For most patients, aspirin and other antiplatelet medications should be stopped 5 days before the procedure. However, in patients with prior coronary artery or vascular stents, it may be prudent to continue these medications to reduce the risk of stent thrombosis. Warfarin should be adjusted/stopped to an INR <1.5. Other anticoagulants should be withheld for at least 24 hours before the procedure.
2. Preprocedure imaging
   a. Contrast-enhanced computed tomography (CT) urogram provides optimal imaging, allowing for staging, characterization of the renal mass, and evaluation of the proximity of the mass to the collecting system and other vital structures (bowel, ureter, organs, nerves). Contrast-enhanced magnetic resonance imaging (MRI) is an alternative. Patients with GFR 30 to 60 mL/min/1.73 m^2 should undergo intravenous (IV) hydration (before contrast CT) or receive a decreased contrast dose (before MRI). Patients with GFR <30 mL/min/1.73 m^2 should not receive iodinated or group I or III gadolinium-based contrast agents. Although ultrasound imaging can clearly define the tumor and its relation to the collecting system and renal hilum, cross-sectional imaging provides a comprehensive survey of surrounding tissues, which can be helpful for treatment planning.
   b. Comparison with prior imaging should be performed to evaluate the growth rate of the lesion. Tumor size and growth rate of renal lesions are correlated with their malignant and metastatic potential. More than 40% of renal masses <1 cm are benign, 25% of renal masses <3 cm are benign (1).
   c. Typically, exophytic tumors can be treated more effectively, as perirenal fat acts as a thermal insulator that helps to maintain target temperature during ablation. Conversely, central lesions which are in close proximity to the collecting system or hilar vessels suffer from heat sink effects, which can limit the ability to reach target temperature throughout the lesion.
3. Biopsy. Overall diagnostic rate of renal mass biopsy is 92% (2). Sensitivity and specificity for biopsy of small renal masses are 98.7% and 99.2%, respectively (2). Up to 20% of biopsies of small renal masses result in diagnosis of benign tumors (1). Several cases exist when biopsy should be performed before proceeding with ablation to avoid unnecessary or ineffective procedures:
   a. Extrarenal malignancy (where the renal mass could represent metastatic disease rather than a primary renal malignancy)
   b. Suspected lymphoma
   c. Renal "mass" found in association with a urinary tract infection (where the mass could mimic an abscess or focal pyelonephritis)
4. Overnight fast, nil per os (NPO) for procedure
5. Informed consent
6. Device selection
   a. RFA. Both linear and multitined array (umbrella) applicators are available. Array applicators come in different geometries and can be deployed to different sizes, which allows the operator to tailor the ablation zone to the tumor size and shape. It is important to note whether an array "burns forward"

(from the tip to the undeployed applicator distally after deployment of the tines) or "burns backward" (from the tip to the undeployed applicator proximally after deployment of the tines). Linear probes may be simpler to use, since they do not require deployment of the tines, which can be difficult to deploy after the initial ablation due to change in the consistency of the coagulated renal tissue. With most radiofrequency devices, only one applicator can be used at a time. If the tumor is large, multiple serial ablations must be performed to ensure adequate coverage of the lesion.

   b. Cryoablation. The major technical advantage of cryoablation over RFA is that ablation zones can be monitored in real time with CT, MRI, or ultrasound. Two parameters can be varied in the selection of cryotherapy applicators to shape the ablation zone: (a) length of the active area of applicator, which affects the length of the cryoablated region or "ice ball," and (b) diameter of the shaft, which affects the axial diameter of the ice ball. Because multiple applicators can be placed simultaneously and the ablation zones coalesce, complex-shaped tumors can be targeted using a combination of different lengths and shaft diameter applicators.

   c. Microwave ablation. A needle antenna emits electromagnetic waves to surrounding tissue, which results in cytotoxic tissue heating. Case series on microwave ablation of small renal masses have shown early and intermediate results similar to other ablation modalities. Advantages of microwave ablation include achieving higher target tumor temperature with fewer probes as well as shorter procedural time.

   d. Emerging technologies. Preclinical and early phase trials are being conducted in new image-guided renal ablation modalities.

   (1) High-intensity focused ultrasound (HIFU). Ultrasonic energy is focused to produce high acoustic intensities in tissue, which results in cytotoxic heat generation due to absorption of the acoustic energy.

   (2) Irreversible electroporation (IRE). This nonthermal technique uses pulsed electrical fields to create permanent nanoscale defects or pores in the plasma membrane of cells resulting in cell death.

   (3) Laser ablation. Laser light applied directly to tissue results in cytotoxic tissue heating.

7. Antibiotics. Cefazolin IV (weight-based)

Procedure

1. Monitoring of vital signs for conscious sedation/anesthesia (electrocardiogram [ECG], blood pressure, pulse oximetry, and respiration)

2. Sedation/anesthesia. Thermal injury due to cold is associated with minimal pain, whereas thermal injury with heat can be considerably painful. Patients undergoing cryoablation generally tolerate the procedure with moderate sedation (fentanyl and midazolam), whereas patients undergoing RFA may require deep sedation or general anesthesia.

3. Patient positioning and approach. Patients are typically positioned prone. Prone positioning facilitates probe placement for lower pole, posterior lesions. For upper pole lesions, ipsilateral decubitus positioning deflates the ipsilateral lung, minimizing the risk of pneumothorax. Oblique supine positioning (ipsilateral up to 30 degrees) can be helpful for lateral lesions and can aid in displacing bowel medially away from the kidney. Supine transhepatic approaches have been described. For upper pole lesions, especially on the left, proximity to the lung and pleura can limit access options. An iatrogenic pneumothorax or pleural effusion can be created by insertion of a 22-gauge epidural needle into the pleural space, with infusion of air or 5% dextrose solution (D5W), respectively. A transpleural intercostal approach can then be performed for ablation. Prior to or immediately following ablation, a

small-bore chest tube should be inserted and placed to water seal. The chest tube can be removed the morning after the procedure after clamping trial and serial chest x-rays.

4. Ablation technique
   a. Scout imaging is obtained to localize the target. If necessary, contrast can be given to increase conspicuity of the target. The CT gantry can be angled on scout imaging to maintain longitudinal needle visualization during subcostal needle placement. The point of skin entry is determined based on the planned needle trajectory.
   b. The skin entry site is prepped and draped. The site is anesthetized with lidocaine. A small dermatotomy is made to facilitate needle placement.
   c. Biopsy (fine needle aspiration or core) can be performed, if tissue diagnosis of the lesion has not been performed previously.
   d. Under imaging guidance, the ablation probe(s) are placed. With cryoablation, multiple applicators may be placed simultaneously to ensure that the ice ball will encompass the lesion. With RFA, the electrode is first placed at one margin of the lesion, allowing subsequent electrode placements to create an overlapping ablation zone.
   e. Ablation
      (1) Cryoablation. After confirming needle placement(s), ablation is usually conducted with two freeze-thaw cycles (e.g., a 10-minute freeze, 8-minute thaw, and 10-minute refreeze). The diameter of the ice ball initially increases rapidly; cross-sectional imaging during the procedure may be performed at 3- to 5-minute intervals to minimize nontarget ablation. Cytotoxic intracellular ice formation in renal cells occurs best with rapid cooling below $-20°C$. Ice ball formation can be monitored in real time via CT (hypoattenuating ice ball) and MRI (hypointense ice ball). It should be noted that the edge of the ice ball marks the $0°C$ isotherm, and the $-20°C$ isotherm is deep to the ice ball margin. Therefore, to ensure cytotoxic target temperature within the lesion, the ice ball margin should exceed the margin of the lesion by at least 5 to 10 mm. Some operators utilize a thermocouple at the tumor margin to ensure that the target temperature at the margin of the lesion reaches $-20°C$. Following the freeze–thaw–freeze cycle, active thawing to $15°C$ should be performed before attempting to remove the applicator; the applicator should not be removed forcefully if it remains frozen to the lesion as renal fracture and bleeding can occur.
      (2) Radiofrequency ablation. After confirming needle placement (which may include deploying the multitined array prior to ablation), ablation is begun according to device protocol. Protocols usually involve at least 10 minutes of ablation, with temperature measurements during or immediately after ablation depending on the device. Protocols with impedance based end points utilize protocols with stepwise increases in power until maximal impedance, a surrogate marker for cytotoxic cellular change, is reached. During the ablation, the tines of the cluster are advanced periodically (according to device protocol) to allow for a larger volume of ablation. Care should be taken when advancing the tines with slight forward pressure on the shaft of the needle, as the increased firmness of the ablated tissue can lead to "backing out" of the needle and failure of the tines to advance through the previously ablated tissue. Cytotoxic coagulation necrosis occurs rapidly at temperatures of $60°C$ to $100°C$ (3). The area of the ablation zone cannot be directly monitored during RFA; however, ablated tissue becomes slightly lower in attenuation on CT due to tissue edema. The needle can be repositioned, and this process repeated with overlapping ablations until the lesion is adequately covered. In the event that the electrode is to be removed from the kidney for repositioning or following the last ablation, track ablation of intervening normal renal

parenchyma should be performed according to the device instructions. In general, the needle should be withdrawn to ensure a temperature within the tract of 80°C. Track ablation should be halted at least 1 cm from the skin surface to avoid skin burn.

f. Immediate postprocedure imaging should be performed following removal of the ablation probe to assess for immediate complications.

g. A sterile dressing is applied.

5. Special techniques to limit nontarget ablation

a. Ureteral stent placement. To protect the ureter and collecting system from thermal injury, retrograde ureteral stent placement can be performed cystoscopically for infusion of D5W through the renal collecting system, dissipating heat and minimizing injury. Dextrose is used rather than saline to minimize conduction effects during RFA.

b. Hydrodissection and pneumodissection (see Fig. 57.1A–C). Adjacent or intervening tissues (bowel, pancreas, adrenal, and spleen) can be displaced by infusion of D5W, carbon dioxide (CO_2), or air. A 22-gauge needle or sheath can be placed between the kidney and intervening structure, and D5W, CO_2, or air injected as needed to create a buffer of 1 to 2 cm. The choice of D5W or air is based on whether structures should be moved in a dependent or nondependent manner. If necessary, a large occlusion balloon (14 mm) can be inflated between the kidney and the adjacent structure to create a buffer between the lesion and tissue.

Postprocedure Management

1. Bed rest for 4 hours or until hematuria begins to clear.
2. Check vital signs every 15 minutes for 1 hour, every 30 minutes for 2 hours, every hour for 4 hours, and then every 8 hours.
3. Monitoring fluid input and output. Blood-tinged urine may be seen up to 48 hours after procedure. "Pink lemonade" appearance is typical.
4. Resume preprocedure diet.
5. Patients can be discharged the same day with low rate of rate of short-term readmission (4). If same-day discharge is planned, postprocedure observation is recommended for a minimum of 4 hours as the majority of bleeding complications will manifest within 4 hours (4). Overnight observation may be prudent in patients with larger treated tumors, underlying chronic renal insufficiency, or advanced age.
6. Imaging

a. CT or MRI at 1 to 3 months should be obtained to identify residual tumor from an incomplete ablation. Subtle enhancement can be seen in the periphery of the ablation zone on early imaging (which may represent inflammation) but is usually resolved by 6 months. Follow-up imaging every 3 to 6 months for the first year should be continued as surveillance for recurrent disease.

b. If the patient shows no residual enhancement over a 1-year period, longer imaging intervals (1 to 2 years) can be employed. Imaging follow-up after ablation is recommended for a minimum of 5 years and may be extended longer in patients with larger tumors at baseline, higher nuclear grade tumors, or history of multiple renal tumors. Imaging surveillance also includes chest imaging (radiograph or CT) annually to assess for pulmonary metastases. Additional imaging (e.g., bone scan) may be considered if clinically warranted by history and physical examination during the follow-up period.

Results

1. No randomized controlled trials have been performed to compare thermal ablation (RFA or cryoablation) to PN—the reference standard for treatment of T1 renal cancer.

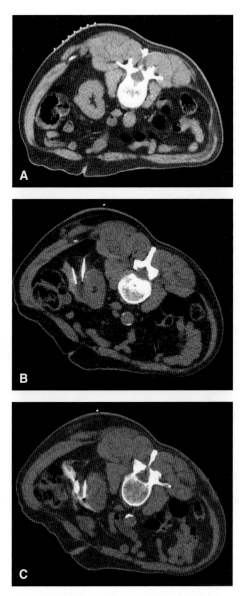

FIGURE 57.1 • **A:** Targeting: Scout CT in preparation of percutaneous ablation of a 1.2-cm left midpole exophytic clear cell carcinoma in a 72-year-old male with multiple comorbidities. Note proximity of descending colon. **B:** Hydrodissection: Following insertion of a 22-gauge Chiba needle into the intervening perirenal space, injection of saline with dilute contrast resulted in lateral displacement of the colon, enabling insertion of cryoablation probe. **C:** Ablation: Cryoablation was performed with two freeze-thaw cycles with ice ball engulfing renal tumor with adequate treatment margins during continued displacement of colon (note that although a single cryoprobe was sufficient here, most renal tumors require multiple cryoprobes to achieve a sufficient treatment margin).

2. Complete immediate response after ablation is seen in 96% of patients after a single treatment and in up to 99% of patients after two treatments (3,5).
3. Local recurrence free survival is similar between RFA, cryoablation, and PN for treatment of clinical T1a renal tumors (6). Risk factors for local recurrence include T1b or larger tumors, higher tumor nuclear grade, and clear cell RCC subtype on pathology (5,6).
4. Metastasis-free survival rates after RFA, cryoablation, and PN are 93%, 100%, and 99%, respectively, with a significant difference noted with RFA as compared with cryoablation and PN (7). Metastasis-free survival after cryoablation for T1b tumors is slightly lower as compared with PN (92% vs. 96%) but not statistically different (7).
5. Five-year cancer-specific survival is high across all modalities for treatment of T1a tumors (96%, 99%, and 100% for RFA, cryoablation, and PN, respectively) (8). Five-year cancer-specific survival after cryoablation for T1b tumors is lower as compared with PN (91% vs. 98%) (8).
6. Ablation may be associated with better preserved postprocedure renal function as compared with PN and RN, even in patients with compromised renal function (9,10). Overall, studies have shown no clinically significant change in baseline renal function after percutaneous ablation (9).

Lower overall periprocedural complications are reported after ablation as compared with PN (13% vs. 18%) (6). Major complications, Clavien–Dindo grade 3 and higher, are seen in 2.8% of patients after percutaneous ablation (3).

Complications

1. Bleeding: 20% to 30%, (majority Clavien–Dindo criteria grade <3) (3,4)
   a. Gross hematuria: Passage of clots is rare.
   b. Hematoma (subcapsular, extracapsular): Drainage is rarely helpful as bleeding will be tamponaded by the capsule. If severe, worsened renal function or hypertension can be seen (Page kidney).
2. Ureteral injury: <1%; Risk can be minimized by achieving at least a 1cm margin with hydrodissection or pneumodissection, or with pyeloperfusion (3).
3. Nerve injury: rarely reported (3,4).
4. Pneumothorax: Can occur with treatment of upper pole renal tumors (4).
5. Infection: rare; prophylactic antibiotics may minimize risk.
6. Nontarget ablation: rare if a 1-cm margin from vital organs, nerves, or bowel is maintained (3,4). It is important to note that the location of critical structures may change when comparing procedural and preprocedural imaging as well as intraprocedurally.

Management of Complications

1. Bleeding
   a. Hematuria. Gross hematuria can indicate damage to the renal collecting system. Even with passage of clots, hematuria usually resolves in 24 to 48 hours. Life-threatening bleeding may require arterial embolization. If a large amount of clot is seen, the urology service can be consulted, as the patient may benefit from bladder irrigation.
   b. Hematoma. Small subcapsular or extracapsular hematoma can be managed with serial hemoglobin measurement. Attention to follow-up creatinine levels and blood pressure is indicated as transient acute renal insufficiency can occur. Follow-up imaging to document resolution of the hematoma is typically not necessary. Life-threatening retroperitoneal hemorrhage may require arterial embolization.
2. Ureteral injury or urine leak. Small amounts of perirenal contrast on delayed follow-up imaging likely represents a small urine leak, which can resolve

spontaneously via urothelial healing. Large urinomas may require percutaneous drainage, as well as diversion, preferably with double-J ureteral stents. If the patient has an ileal conduit, a course of broad-spectrum antibiotics should be given, as the urinary tract is likely colonized and may lead to superinfection of the urinoma.

3. Infection. May require broadening of antibiotic coverage. Drainage may be required if perirenal abscess formation occurs.

4. Nerve injury. Numbness, paresthesias, or weakness can be self-limited. However, in some cases, sensory and motor deficits can persist.

5. Nontarget ablation. Ablation of the pancreas can result in pancreatitis while thermal ablation of the bowel can lead to bowel necrosis or perforation. NPO status and supportive care should be initiated. Surgical consultation should be considered because bowel repair or resection may be necessary on rare occasions.

6. Pneumothorax. Chest tube may be required if patient is symptomatic despite conservative management.

References

1. Frank I, Blute ML, Cheville JC, et al. Solid renal tumors: an analysis of pathological features related to tumor size. *J Urol.* 2003;170(6):2217–2220.

2. Marconi L, Dabestani S, Lam TB, et al. Systematic review and meta-analysis of diagnostic accuracy of percutaneous renal tumour biopsy. *Eur Urol.* 2016;69(4):660–673.

3. Aoun HD, Littrup PJ, Jaber M, et al. Percutaneous cryoablation of renal tumors: is it time for a new paradigm shift? *J Vasc Interv Radiol.* 2017;28(10):1363–1370.

4. Chen JX, Guzzo TJ, Malkowicz SB, et al. Complication and readmission rates following same-day discharge after percutaneous renal tumor ablation. *J Vasc Interv Radiol.* 2016;27(1):80–86.

5. Knox J, Kohlbrenner R, Kolli K, et al. Intermediate to long-term clinical outcomes of percutaneous cryoablation for renal masses. *J Vasc Interv Radiol.* 2020;31(8):1242–1248.

6. Yanagisawa T, Mori K, Kawada T, et al. Differential efficacy of ablation therapy versus partial nephrectomy between clinical T1a and T1b renal tumors: a systematic review and meta-analysis. Urologic Oncology: Seminars and Original Investigations. 2022;40(7):315–330.

7. Thompson RH, Atwell T, Schmit G, et al. Comparison of partial nephrectomy and percutaneous ablation for cT1 renal masses. *Eur Urol.* 2015;67(2):252–9.

8. Andrews JR, Atwell T, Schmit G, et al. Oncologic outcomes following partial nephrectomy and percutaneous ablation for cT1 renal masses. *Eur Urol.* 2019;76(2):244–251.

9. Wehrenberg-Klee E, Clark TWI, Malkowicz SB, et al. Impact on renal function of percutaneous thermal ablation of renal masses in patients with preexisting chronic kidney disease. *J Vasc Interv Radiol.* 2012;23(1):41–45.

10. Lippert JT, Lumberto RW, Thomas JC, et al. Incident CKD after radical or partial nephrectomy. *J Am Soc Nephrol.* 2018;29(1):207–216.

58 Musculoskeletal Biopsies, Aspirations, and Injections

Katherine Marchak, MD and Kristofer Schramm, MD

Biopsies

Introduction

Interventional radiologists play a critical role in characterization of bone and soft tissue lesions, both through imaging and biopsy. Percutaneous biopsy has supplanted surgical biopsy for most diagnoses as it is associated with lower cost, fewer complications, less frequent need for anesthesia, and less time in both the operating room and the hospital (1,2). The general techniques for musculoskeletal (MSK) biopsy are similar to those used for other soft tissue biopsies, but there are different instruments as well as considerations of biopsy tract that must be kept in mind when performing MSK biopsy. The way in which a musculoskeletal biopsy is performed has a profound impact on further care, and a collaborative approach with a multidisciplinary team is vital. Due to the risk of tract seeding associated with many sarcomas, proper planning of route of biopsy to allow a chance at limb salvaging surgery and reconstruction (3–5).

Indications

1. Diagnosis of a benign or malignant primary lesion of bone, muscle, or connective tissue
2. Confirmation of suspected metastasis
3. Isolation of microorganism in infection
4. Suspected metabolic bone disease (2)

Contraindications

Absolute
1. Bleeding diathesis
2. Incomplete imaging/staging prior to biopsy or uncertainty about the route of planned surgical excision (3)
3. Inaccessible sites (3)
4. Uncooperative patients
5. Known adverse reaction to a planned sedative or local medication, or inability to perform safe anesthesia

Relative
1. Pregnancy (for CT and fluoroscopic-guided procedures)
2. Overlying skin infection (2)

Preprocedure Preparation
1. Staging of lesion
   a. Single or multiple lesions
   b. If multiple, consider the site with the potential highest yield
2. Complete imaging of the lesion prior to biopsy
   a. MR imaging best delineates tumor boundaries and interfaces with myofascial compartments and neurovascular structures
   b. CT best demonstrates permeative bone destruction, erosion, and matrix calcification
   c. US or contrast-enhanced CT/MRI can allow differentiation of areas likely to have vascularity and therefore more likely to yield positive results from those that may be necrotic or cystic (4)

    d. Careful review of all imaging to exclude "do not touch" lesions (e.g., evolving myositis ossificans, traumatic apophyseal avulsion in a young adult)
3. Consultation with orthopedic oncologist for assessment of the biopsy tract and determination of possible definitive therapy
    a. Failure to consult with an orthopedic oncologist could result in unnecessary amputation, limited resection options, or limited reconstructive options
4. History: prior malignancy, prior interventions
5. Modality choice for guidance: CT, MRI, US or fluoroscopy
6. Device choice
7. Informed consent
8. Arrangement of periprocedural bed and nursing staff for monitoring
9. Patient should be NPO the day of procedure (2 hours for clear liquids, 8 hours for solids)
10. Arrangements should be made for patient postprocedure, to ensure they have a ride home or, if necessary, an overnight stay

Procedure

1. Patient preparation
    a. Intravenous access allows administration of intravenous analgesia (fentanyl) and sedation (midazolam) by nursing staff. General anesthesia is reserved for patients who have exceedingly high tolerance to narcotics or who cannot remain still/follow instructions during the procedure (3).
    b. Patient placed in a position which will be comfortable/maintained throughout the duration of the procedure. This position must also allow the optimal access to the biopsy route decided upon in preprocedural planning.
    c. The area to be accessed should be sterilized and draped.
2. Physician preparation
    a. Physicians should adhere to facility recommendations for sterile procedures including thorough hand washing, gowning, and gloving.
    b. A facial shield and eye protection are recommended.
    c. While setting up the sterile procedure tray, the use of a needle receptacle and devices which avoid the necessity of recapping are recommended.
3. Modality
    a. CT allows excellent spatial resolution and localization of osseous lesions. In addition, it is the modality of choice for deep soft tissue biopsy or biopsy adjacent to critical structures (2).
       (1) Preprocedural CT scan performed for precise localization of the lesion and planning of the entry point and pathway. This allows avoidance of neurovascular and visceral structures (1).
       (2) CT fluoroscopy images are reported to confirm the correct placement of the needle.
    b. Ultrasound (US) is the modality of choice for soft tissue lesions if the adjacent anatomy is readily identified. It can also be used for osseous lesions if there is a prominent soft tissue component.
       (1) US allows real-time visualization throughout the duration of the biopsy.
       (2) Doppler imaging allows the identification of vascular components of the lesion as well as adjacent vasculature.
       (3) Typically, a high-frequency linear array probe is used. In cases where the lesion is deep or the patient is obese, a lower-frequency probe may be used but the trade-off is lower spatial resolution (3).
    c. Fluoroscopic-guided biopsies are typically avoided unless the lesion is superficial with no surrounding vital structures. Poor soft tissue contrast limits utilization of this modality.
    d. Magnetic resonance imaging (MRI) is often not necessary but it does allow visualization of lesions that may not be well delineated by other modalities.

The major drawbacks are duration of the procedure, need for special open interventional MRI units for biopsy, and need for special MRI safe procedural equipment (i.e., nickel based needles) (2).

4. Biopsy procedural details
   a. The biopsy tract is planned. This may require placement of a grid for CT procedures. This allows calculation of the distance the biopsy needle will traverse so an appropriate length needle can be selected. The tract should be the shortest route available which violates as few anatomic compartments as possible. Care should be taken to avoid potential flaps, high-value muscles, joint spaces, bursae, and neurovascular planes.
   b. Local anesthesia is performed with lidocaine and/or bupivacaine. This is performed at the skin with a 25-gauge needle and also along the biopsy tract with a spinal needle. Good local anesthesia is paramount for successful biopsy, both within the soft tissues and periosteum.
   c. A skin incision is made in the longitudinal direction. This allows easier access for instruments, allows the surgeon to clearly see the puncture site utilized for the biopsy and requires a narrower soft tissue resection at the time of definitive surgery. Tattooing or site marking at the access site can be considered (5).
   d. The needle is introduced along the preplanned route under imaging guidance.
   e. The biopsy is taken.
      (1) Both osseous and soft tissue biopsies can be performed via cutting core needle biopsy if the lesion is soft or primarily soft tissue. These typically range in size from 12 to 20 gauge with 1- to 2-cm specimen length. These specimens preserve the architecture of the tissue and are therefore preferred over fine-needle aspiration (FNA) (2).
      (2) For sclerotic or firm lesions, 11- to 15-gauge trephine style needles (i.e., Jamshidi) can be utilized in order to obtain purchase through the lesion.
      (3) FNA does not preserve tissue architecture and therefore limits the histopathologic analysis to cytology only. This is generally inadequate for diagnosis of sarcomas. Therefore, FNA is typically reserved for very small lesions with adjacent critical structures, where a 1 cm core biopsy may risk inadvertent injury (2).
      (4) Biopsies should be done coaxially to allow multiple biopsies to be taken through the same access site.
      (5) Typically, an increased number of specimens increases diagnostic yield and at least three cores should be obtained. It is important to consult the pathologist to be sure that the proper number and type of samples are obtained.
      (6) Core needle samples from a sclerotic bone lesion will need decalcification for later sectioning.
   f. The needle is removed and pressure is placed over the puncture site in order to achieve hemostasis.
5. General approach tips
   a. Periosteum is highly sensitive. Adequate local anesthesia will prevent patient movement.
   b. Stabilize the access site.
   c. For bone biopsy, the approach should be orthogonal to the bone cortex. This aids in corticotomy and decreases the likelihood of slippage of the needle tip (1).
   d. Knowledge of compartmental anatomy is critical to avoid unnecessary added resection and to preserve options for limb salvaging reconstruction.
6. Biopsy approach tips by anatomic region
   a. Sacrum
      (1) The corridor lateral to the neural foramen is safe.
      (2) Avoid crossing the SI joint.

b. Iliac
   (1) Avoid the gluteus musculature if possible.
   (2) Consider a "straight down the barrel approach" through the anterior iliac wing.
   (3) Avoid traversing muscular attachment sites where possible.
c. Femoral head/neck
   (1) Tract should ideally be a lateral-to-medial approach.
   (2) Avoid traversing the gluteus and quadricep musculature.
   (3) Follow the alignment of the femoral neck. This avoids the femeroacetabular articular surfaces, joint capsule, greater trochanteric bursae, and the femoral neurovascular bundle.
d. Femoral shaft
   (1) Prone or steep oblique position is preferred.
   (2) Tract should ideally be a lateral-to-medial approach. An anterior approach will compromise the rectus femoris muscle. This approach avoids the sciatic nerve, femoral neurovascular bundle, excessive tract through the quadriceps and hamstring muscles, and minimizes flap compromise.
   (3) Consider internal rotation to optimize access.
e. Tibia/fibula
   (1) Supine positioning is ideal.
   (2) Utilization of internal and external rotation allows avoidance of muscular compartments.
   (3) Direct anteromedial approach is ideal for the tibia. Avoid a posterior approach which would compromise the calf musculature.
   (4) The common fibular nerve courses around the neck of the fibula and should be avoided.
f. Proximal humerus
   (1) Supine positioning is ideal
   (2) Consider external rotation of the arm to avoid the biceps tendon.
   (3) Approach through the anterior third of the deltoid as the deltoid is innervated posterior to anterior by the axillary nerve.
   (4) This approach avoids the cephalic vein, joint capsule, and biceps tendon.
g. Forearm
   (1) Positioning depends on the lesion site and route.
   (2) Radial head and neck are best approached through the lateral forearm.
   (3) Radial diaphysis is best approached from a lateral position to avoid the radial neurovascular bundle and the median nerve.
   (4) Distal radius is best approached from a direct lateral approach.
   (5) Distal ulna is best approached from direct medial position to avoid the extensor carpi ulnaris muscle and extensor compartment.
h. Sternum
   (1) Supine positioning is ideal with a steep lateral trajectory. This avoids the internal mammary vessels.
i. Ribs
   (1) Align the needle with the long axis of the rib to avoid the pleural space.
   (2) Target the soft tissue component.

Postprocedure Management

1. The patient is monitored depending on the amount of sedation and the institutional guidelines, often 2 hours. Following this observation period, the patient is typically ready to go home.
2. Vital signs are taken every 15 minutes for the first hour and then every 30 minutes thereafter. In addition, the puncture site is checked at the time of vital signs.
3. Intraprocedural imaging, photography, or skin tattooing can be utilized to document the tract taken in the setting of a planned reconstruction.

Results

1. Core needle musculoskeletal biopsy is highly successful, with diagnostic results in 91% to 97% of patients (3).
2. Biopsy accuracy is higher for malignant tumors than benign lesions (81.4% vs. 78%) (6).
3. Higher risk of nondiagnostic biopsy in the setting of necrotic or myxoid tumor.
4. Diagnostic yield of FNA is lower (72% to 87%) when used in isolation but may increase diagnostic yield when used as a complementary technique to core needle biopsy (7).

Complications

1. Bleeding and hematoma
2. Infection
3. Neural and vascular injury
4. Tumor seeding along the biopsy tract and recurrence within the biopsy tract can occur. This does not typically pose a problem if the tract is excised at the time of resection. However, if there is no consultation with the surgeon, the tract may limit the chance at limb-salvage surgery
5. Nondiagnostic biopsy

Management of Complications

1. Hematomas can be both avoided and minimized by compression and monitoring of the biopsy site.
2. Infection may require treatment with antibiotics.
3. Tumor seeding and tumor recurrence may result from a poorly planned procedural tract or lack of consultation with the oncologic surgeon. If this occurs, consultation after the procedure should occur with full disclosure of the procedural details. This may allow a different surgical approach or the use of radiotherapy and/or chemotherapy prior to resection.

Joint Injections and Aspirations

Introduction

Arthrography is an essential technique used for both aspiration of fluid in diagnosis of joint pathology as well as injection for diagnostic and therapeutic reasons. With significant advances in medical technology, there has been a parallel increase in the number and range of interventional MSK image-guided procedures. These can be performed under fluoroscopic, US, CT, or even MRI guidance.

Arthrocentesis is one of the most commonly performed MSK procedures as they are quick, inexpensive, and relatively straightforward to perform. This is defined as the puncture of a joint with subsequent aspiration of joint fluid. By using image guidance, essentially every major bursa and joint can be accessed.

In a similar fashion to arthrocentesis, a joint can be injected with material. This may be done for diagnostic reasons, with injection of contrast material for CT arthrography and MR arthrography. These allow better evaluation of the soft tissues of the joint, such as the menisci, labrum, and ligaments. In addition, joint injections may be done for therapeutic reasons, with the injection of corticosteroids, anesthetics, or hyaluronic acid (HA) for pain relief (8). HA induces normalization of the viscoelasticity of the synovial fluid and activation of the tissue regeneration of articular cartilage. Corticosteroids reduce the inflammation within joints. Local anesthetics are used for symptomatic relief of inflammatory conditions. These also play a diagnostic role in the preoperative evaluation of patients who may undergo arthroplasty (8).

Indications
1. Joint aspiration:
   a. Diagnosis of septic arthritis or crystal-induced arthropathies by synovial fluid analysis
   b. Diagnosis of bone or ligamentous injury by confirmation of blood within a joint
   c. Relief of pain by decompression of fluid or hemarthrosis
   d. Determination of whether a fistula or laceration communicates with a joint (9)
2. Joint injection:
   a. Diagnostic injection of contrast medium for MR or CT arthrography
   b. Therapeutic injection of medications for relief of pain

Contraindications
1. Joint aspiration:
   a. Absolute: inability to access the joint without traversing inflamed or infected tissues due to risk of infecting a previously sterile joint
   b. Relative: established bacteremia due to risk of infection spreading to a joint (9)
2. Joint injection: as above as well as allergy to any of the medications or contrast to be injected. In the setting of contrast allergy, air can be injected for diagnostic studies

Preprocedure Preparation

1. Review of pertinent history and allergies
2. Modality choice for guidance: CT, MRI, US, or fluoroscopy
3. Informed consent
4. Review of prior imaging if available
   a. If there is severe degenerative change such as osteophytes or overlapping of the normal bone structures, this is helpful to know prior to starting the procedure to plan for the appropriate modality as well as technique

Procedure

1. Patient preparation
   a. Patient placed in a position which will be comfortable/maintained throughout the duration of the procedure. This position must also allow optimal access.
   b. The area to be accessed should be sterilized and draped.
2. Physician preparation
   a. Physicians should adhere to facility recommendations for sterile procedures including thorough hand washing, gowning, and gloving.
   b. A facial shield and eye protection are recommended.
   c. While setting up the sterile procedure tray, the use of a needle receptacle and devices which avoid the necessity of recapping are recommended.
3. General procedure details
   a. Local anesthesia is performed with lidocaine of both the skin and deeper tissues.
   b. Using imaging guidance, the joint is accessed.
      (1) With fluoroscopic guidance, the tip of the needle should be superimposed over the hub. Upon contact with bone, the needle is slightly withdrawn and injection/aspiration performed.
      (2) Using US guidance, the needle should be introduced parallel to the transducer so that it can be accurately followed until it reaches the joint capsule, at which time injection/aspiration can be performed.

    c. The choice of needle for access depends on the joint, the patient's body habitus, and the anticipated fluid consistency to be injected/aspirated.

        (1) 3.5-in spinal needles are often used for hips and shoulders

        (2) 1.5-in needles may be used for superficial joint

        (3) Higher gauge needles (20 and above) are appropriate for injection

        (4) Smaller gauge needles may be needed for aspiration

    d. The radiologic joint space may not be readily accessible due to overlapping of normal bone structures or degenerative changes such as osteophytes. In this case, the articular recess can be targeted.

    e. For diagnostic injection using CT arthrography, the injectate should be iodinated contrast at a concentration of 240 mgI per mL. For MR arthrography, a dilution of 1/200 to 1/250 of gadolinium chelates in iodinated contrast of sterile saline (8).

    f. If pus is encountered, the joint should be decompressed and the referring provider immediately notified.

    g. Following appropriate aspiration or injection, the needle is removed and pressure is placed over the puncture site in order to achieve hemostasis. A sterile dressing is applied.

    h. Synovial fluid analysis should include a total cell count, differential leukocyte count, and culture. Crystal analysis can be performed if clinically indicated.

4. Details for specific joints

    a. Shoulder

        (1) Arm should be placed in external rotation.

        (2) Access the rotator cuff interval by targeting the upper medial quadrant of the humeral head.

        (3) Alternatively, the Schneider technique (straight AP approach at the junction of middle and lower thirds) can be used to directly access the glenohumeral joint space, but the subscapularis tendon and anteroinferior labrum are often perforated by the needle or impregnated with contrast by using this technique (8).

    b. Elbow

        (1) The radiocapitellar (lateral) approach is most common. A lateral view is obtained by having the patient lay prone or sit in a chair with the elbow in a flexed position.

        (2) The radiocapitellar joint is localized and directly accessed.

    c. Wrist

        (1) The patient should be placed with their palm down on the table.

        (2) To access the radiocarpal joint, the radioscaphoid articulation is identified. Access past the dorsal lip of the radius can be improved by caudocranial angulation of the needle or slight flexion of the wrist. Alternatively, the radiocarpal joint can be accessed via ulnar-sided injection at the triquetrium.

        (3) The distal radioulnar joint can be accessed by targeting the lateral aspect of the ulna.

    d. Hip

        (1) The hip is accessed from the lateral recess, either by medial (target the superior head–neck junction) or lateral (target the lateral aspect of the femoral neck) approaches.

        (2) The hip is placed in slight medial rotation (9).

    e. Knee

        (1) The lateral patellofemoral approach can be used with the knee in slight flexion to access the lateral aspect of the suprapatellar recess.

        (2) The anterior approach can be used with the knee in slight flexion to allow targeting of the lower aspect of the lateral femoral condyle.

    f. Ankle

        (1) The anterior recess or the ankle is best targeted just below the radiologic joint space with the ankle in slight plantar flexion.

g. SI joints
   (1) CT is typically used as it is challenging to access fluoroscopically.
   (2) Using CT, the patient is placed prone in the gantry and the inferior third of the joint space is accessed with a slight medial to lateral angulation to mirror the joint.
   (3) Using fluoroscopy, the patient is placed in prone oblique with the side to be accessed down and the needle is advanced into the inferior third of the joint.
   (4) A key structure to avoid is the sciatic nerve which is located anterior to the piriformis muscle at the same depth as the inferior portion of the SI joint.
h. Cervical facet joints
   (1) A posterior approach is safest to avoid neurovascular structures.
   (2) The patient should be positioned prone with the head rotated in the opposite direction. Target the inferior articular recess of the facet joint.
i. Lumbar facet joints
   (1) Physiologic lordosis is reduced by placing a pillow under the patient's abdomen. This allows access to the posteroinferior joint recess.
   (2) Target the apex of the inferior articular process until bone is contacted (9).

Postprocedure Management
1. The patient is observed for approximately 15 minutes after the procedure.
2. Instructions are given not to soak in water or a bath for the remainder of the day.
3. Limitations on activity are highly dependent on the individual and the joint for which arthrography was performed.
4. Instructions are given to not drive or operate heavy machinery for the remainder of the day.

Results
1. Image-guided aspiration of the joint is highly successful for diagnostic purposes.
2. In addition, image-guided injection of contrast or medications is similarly highly successful.
3. Severe degenerative changes with large osteophytes may limit ability to access the joint.

Complications
1. Bleeding or hematoma
2. Nontarget injection of medication
3. Infection
4. Transient weakness or paresthesia if an adjacent nerve is injected
5. Steroid side effects: glucose disturbance, insomnia, mood disturbance, transient decrease in immunity

Management of Complications
1. Hematomas can be both avoided and minimized by compression and monitoring of the biopsy site.
2. Infection may require treatment with antibiotics.

Soft Tissue Aspiration and Sclerosis

Introduction
Extremity fluid collections can be treated with image-guided percutaneous drainage with or without sclerotherapy. These collections include lymphoceles, hematomas, and abscesses. With advances in minimally invasive techniques, soft tissue collections can be accessed by US, CT, or fluoroscopy. Percutaneous aspiration allows diagnostic analysis and can also be therapeutic. When a collection is large or recurs, sclerotherapy can be used as an effective management strategy. The most

commonly used sclerosants are dehydrated ethanol, povidone-iodine, and doxy-cycline, although cyanoacrylate, hypertonic saline, acetic acid, fibrin sealant, and sodium tetradecyl sulfate can also be used.

Indications
1. Pain/discomfort
2. Secondary infection
3. Sequelae of mass effect (neurovascular compression, leg swelling)

Contraindications

Absolute
1. Communication with vital structures such as blood vessels
2. Lack of a safe percutaneous window

Relative
1. Coagulopathy
2. Noncompliant patient

Preprocedure Preparation
1. Review of pertinent history and allergies
2. Modality choice for guidance: CT, MRI, US, or fluoroscopy
3. Informed consent
4. Review of prior imaging if available
5. Routine labs (international normalized ratio [INR], platelet count, white blood cell count)

Procedure
1. Patient preparation
   a. Patient placed in a position which will be comfortable/maintained throughout the duration of the procedure. This position must also allow the optimal access.
   b. The area to be accessed should be sterilized and draped.
2. Physician preparation
   a. Physicians should adhere to facility recommendations for sterile procedures including thorough hand washing, gowning, and gloving.
   b. A facial shield and eye protection are recommended.
   c. While setting up the sterile procedure tray, the use of a needle receptacle and devices which avoid the necessity of recapping are recommended.
3. Aspiration and drainage
   a. Local anesthesia is performed with lidocaine of both the skin and deeper tissues. In addition, conscious sedation is administered, if necessary, for placement of drain. Typically, no conscious sedation is required for simple aspiration.
   b. Using imaging guidance, the soft tissue collection is accessed, either via the Seldinger or trocar technique. US is typically used for soft tissue collections due to real-time imaging guidance and ability to identify adjacent vascular structures. Fluoroscopy may also be used if a sinogram is to be performed.
   c. Aspiration should be performed to decrease intracavitary pressure and reduce the risk of bacteremia. Take care to not fully decompress the cavity if you are planning to place a drain.
   d. If the collection requires drain placement due to large size or suspected infection, a serial dilation is performed, and a pigtail catheter is placed. Typically, the catheter should range in size from 8 to 16 Fr. Following formation of the pigtail, the cavity should be decompressed.
4. Sclerotherapy
   a. Access to the cavity is obtained as above, including placement of a drain.

b. A cystogram is performed to ensure the cyst is self-contained. Once confirmed, sclerotherapy can begin.

c. Commonly used sclerosants
   (1) Povidone-iodine 10%: Instill a volume which is one-half of the volume aspirated, not exceeding 100 mL. Then cap the drain and have the patient rotate into different positions for approximately 2 hours before uncapping the drain and connecting it to gravity drainage.
   (2) Ethanol: Instill absolute alcohol in a volume of one-half of what was aspirated, not exceeding 60 mL. The solution should have a dwell time of approximately 10 minutes before aspiration. Take care to ensure catheter compatibility with ethanol given that ethanol can degrade the integrity of some catheters
   (3) Doxycycline: Reconstitute 500 mg of doxycycline powder into 20 mL of normal saline and 5 mL 1% alcohol. Instill this into the cavity, cap the drain for 2 hours and then connect it to gravity drainage.

d. Sclerotherapy is often required in multiple sessions to completely decompress the cavity.

e. Following appropriate aspiration and/or injection, the needle/catheter is removed and pressure is placed over the puncture site in order to achieve hemostasis. A sterile dressing is applied.

Postprocedure Management

1. The patient should be monitored postprocedurally according to whether or not they received sedation and institutional guidelines.
2. If a drain is left in place, it should be placed to gravity drainage. Catheter management consists of recording the output volumes and 5-mL saline flushes every 8 to 24 hours. Consider removal of the catheter when there is resolution of the fluid collection on imaging, the output falls to below 10 to 20 mL a day, and there is clinical improvement.
3. Drain evaluation should be considered prior to removal, either with CT or fluoroscopy, to ensure collapse of the collection and exclude malpositioning of the drain.

Results

1. Aspiration and drainage of soft tissue collections is often very successful.
2. Sclerotherapy success rates are estimated to be between 77% and 98% (10). The size of the cavity is associated with success rate, with larger cavities having lower success rate.

Complications

1. Infection
2. Absorption or unintended intravascular injection of the sclerosant into the bloodstream
3. Cyst recurrence
4. Bleeding and hematoma

Management of Complications

1. Infections may require treatment with antibiotics.
2. Cyst recurrence may require surgical management.
3. Hematomas can be both avoided and minimized by compression and monitoring of the biopsy site.

References

1. Gangi A, Guth S, Dietemann J, et al. Interventional musculoskeletal procedures. *Radiographics*. 2001;21ii.:e1–e1.

2. Daley N, Reed W, Peterson J. Strategies for biopsy of musculoskeletal tumors. *Semin Roentgenol.* 2017;52(4):282–290.
3. Le H, Lee S, Munk P. Image-guided musculoskeletal biopsies. *Semin Interv Radiol.* 2010;27(2):191–198.
4. Liu P, Valadez S, Chivers F, et al. Anatomically based guidelines for core needle biopsy of bone tumors: implications for limb-sparing surgery. *Radiographics.* 2007;27(1):189–205.
5. Errani C, Traina F, Perna F, et al. Current concepts in the biopsy of musculoskeletal tumors. *Scientific World J.* 2013;2013: 1–7.
6. Altuntas AO, Slavin J, Smith PJ, et al. Accuracy of computed tomography guided core needle biopsy of musculoskeletal tumours. *ANZ J Surg.* 2005;75(4):187–191.
7. Yang YJ, Damron TA. Comparison of needle core biopsy and fine-needle aspiration for diagnostic accuracy in musculoskeletal lesion. *Arch Pathol Lab Med.* 2004;128(7):759-764.
8. Masala S, Fiori R, Bartolucci D, et al. Diagnostic and therapeutic joint injections. *Semin Interv Radiol.* 2010;27(2):160–171.
9. Hansford BG, Stacy GS. Musculoskeletal aspiration procedures. *Semin Interv Radiol.* 2012;29(4):270–285.
10. Zuckerman DA, Yeager TD. Percutaneous ethanol sclerotherapy of postoperative lymphoceles. *Am J Roentgenol.* 1997; 169(2):433–437

59 Musculoskeletal (MSK) Ablation

Brandon M. Key, MD and Sean M. Tutton, MD, FSIR, FCIRSE

Introduction

Thermal ablation is technically feasible, safe, and efficacious for benign MSK tumors, pain palliation, and locoregional control of metastatic disease (1,2). Percutaneous ablation is minimally invasive with decreased morbidity and unique advantages compared to surgery or radiation (3). Choice of ablation modality is nuanced and requires consideration of lesion proximity to visceral organs, articular cartilage, nerves, and vessels as well as the evaluation of the cortical integrity within or surrounding the ablation zone. Mechanical stabilization with cement and/or screw fixation can also be performed as an adjunct to ablation to address biomechanical instability and added pain palliation (1,4,5).

Radiofrequency Ablation (RFA)

RFA is the gold standard for osseous heat-based ablation, however, it is limited by lesion size (<3 cm), heat sink, charring, and tissues with high impedance and low thermal conduction. RFA also precludes the use of nerve monitoring due to signal interference therefore its use should be limited when the ablation zone is in close proximity to motor nerves (6).

Microwave Ablation (MWA)

MWA produces similar tissue destruction (dielectric heating) as RFA however it is not limited by charring or bone conduction and thus allows for larger, although harder to predict, ablation zones in a shorter period of time (7). MWA should be utilized with caution near joints, ligaments, and nerves for risk of injury. MWA ablation does not interfere with nerve monitoring. Both RFA and MWA can desiccate tumor tissue leading to contraction which is helpful when there is tumor retropulsion (spine) and nerve compression (Fig. 59.1).

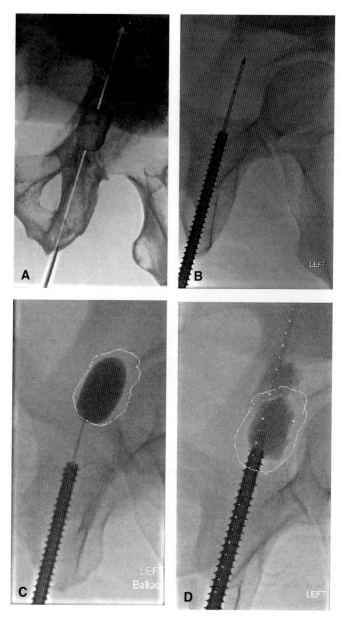

FIGURE 59.1 • **A:** Cone beam CT image with acetabular lesion segmented and planned guide pin trajectory. **B:** Short 8 mm fully threaded screw as a place holder to facilitate placement of a cryoablation probe. **C:** 15-mm kyphoplasty balloon insufflated within the ablation cavity. **D:** Osteoplasty via cement cannula through the screw with segmented tumor outlined in white.

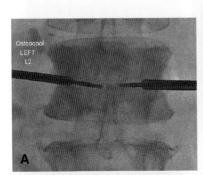

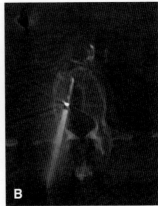

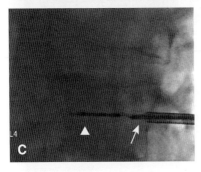

FIGURE 59.2 • **A:** Bipedicular access with RFA probes in place. **B:** CBCT image confirming position of RFA probe. The probe was slightly retracted prior to ablation. **C:** Unipedicular access with 10-g trocar. MWA antenna (*arrowhead*) and thermocouple (*arrow*).

Cryoablation (CA)

CA has the distinct advantage of ablation zone visualization through its cryogenic cooling of tissue which allows for sculpting of the ice ball and treatment of larger lesions (Fig. 59.2). CA is safer when utilized near joints, resulting in less cartilage and ligamentous damage, and has the added anesthetic effect during tissue cooling. CA does not interfere with nerve monitoring. Adjunctive cementoplasty following CA requires an extended active thaw cycle, delayed injection of cement to ensure thawed tumor, or staged procedure.

Combination Procedures

Patients with lesions at increased risk for fracture on imaging or a physical examination consistent with mechanical and/or a combination of tumoral and mechanical pain can be considered for adjunctive cementoplasty and potential percutaneous screw fixation (Fig. 59.3) (1,4,5).

Indications

1. Benign MSK tumors—osteoid osteoma, chondroblastoma, desmoids, and fibromatosis.
2. Palliation of painful metastatic bone and soft tissue lesions.
3. Locoregional control for oligometastatic disease—prostate, breast, and lung.

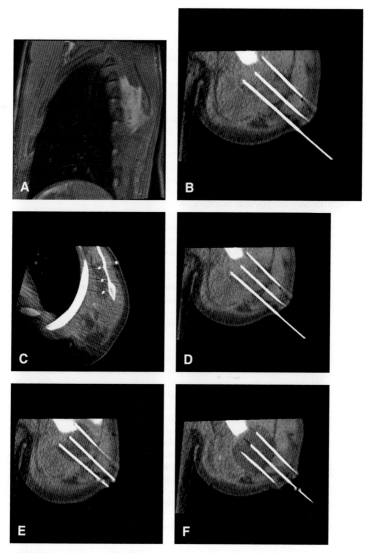

FIGURE 59.3 • **A:** Sagittal postcontrast T1 MR image of the left scapula demonstrating enhancing tumor. **B,C:** CT images demonstrating placement of cryoablation probes. **D–F:** Sequential CT images demonstrating growth of ice ball.

Contraindications

1. **Absolute**—Vital structures/organs in ablation zone, uncorrectable coagulopathy, active infection, and inaccessibility of target lesion via percutaneous approach.
2. **Relative**—Lesion proximity to joints, location within weight-bearing long bones and the proximity to neurovascular bundles.

Preprocedure Preparation

1. Patient evaluation
   a. Imaging
      (1) Preprocedural imaging obtained within 4 weeks of the planned procedure date.
      (2) CT, MRI, and/or PET—Depends on ablation target, intended goal of treatment, and plan for cementoplasty/screw fixation.
      (3) Identify critical structures within 1 to 1.5 cm of the intended ablation zone. Consider ablation modality selection and plan for protective techniques including hydrodissection, gas dissection, balloon displacement, and/or nerve monitoring.
      (4) Lesion characteristics—Osteoblastic lesions increase technical difficulty of probe/cannula placement, extent of lytic component may increase risk of fracture and necessitate combination cementoplasty or screw fixation.
   b. Preprocedure consultation/evaluation
      (1) History and physical examination
         (a) Emphasis on the physical examination for assessment of pain characteristics and correlation with imaging findings.
         (b) Patients with VAS of 4 or greater with solitary or oligometastatic disease and pain on physical examination correlating with imaging are most likely to benefit from intervention (3).
         (c) Differentiate mechanical versus tumoral versus combination. Patients with mechanical or combination pain should be considered for cementoplasty and/or screw fixation.
         (d) Functional assessment and risk of fracture scores can aid in the clinical decision-making process and/or serve as a measure for procedural efficacy, that is Musculoskeletal Tumor Society Rating Scale (MSTS), Spine Instability Neoplastic Score (SINS), Roland-Morris Disability Questionnaire (RMDQ), Mirels' Score for pathologic fracture risk, and Harrington Classification of periacetabular metastatic disease.
         (e) Radicular component—Preexisting radiculopathies should be documented and may be treated contemporaneously with epidural steroid injection.
      (2) Multidisciplinary consultation for coordination of treatment
         (a) Palliative care for goals of care and symptoms management.
         (b) Orthopedic oncology for assessing need for stabilization.
         (c) Radiation oncology for consolidating tumor after ablation.
      (3) Informed consent—risks, benefits, and alternatives should be discussed thoroughly with emphasis on nature of procedure (i.e., palliative, locoregional control, curative).
   c. Laboratory tests—INR (<1.5) and platelets (>50,000) obtained within 30 days.
   d. Procedural sedation
      (1) Location of ablation—If patient feedback during case is critical authors favor moderate sedation or MAC.
      (2) Straightforward ablation with low ASA is amenable to moderate sedation or monitored anesthesia care.
      (3) General endotracheal anesthesia is considered for complex, potentially long duration cases or when there are issues with positioning or airway.
2. Adjunctive procedural techniques
   a. Warm saline glove—sterile glove filled with warm saline place on the skin surface overlying the ablation zone.
   b. Displacement—create a 1.5 cm safety zone
      (1) Hydrodissection with D5 (RFA) or NS (MWA and CA) injected under CT or US.
      (2) Carbodissection—Carbon dioxide injected under CT guidance (epidural, perineural).

(3) CT-guided or endoscopic balloon catheter interposition.
   c. Nerve monitoring—Sensory and motor nerve monitoring (SSEP, EMG) utilized when ablation zone is near vital nerves. Cannot be used with RFA.
   d. Thermocouple—Temperature monitoring probe inserted adjacent to the ablation zone near vital structures to monitor for potential thermal injury.
   e. Access tools
      (1) Cannulas
         (a) 11 gauge—Primary access and working cannula.
         (b) 8 gauge—Accommodates Kirschner wires and allows for more working room under the detector and in the CT gantry during screw fixation cases.
      (2) Peel away sheaths—Maintain access when exchanging access cannula for ablation probe.
      (3) Power tools—Orthopedic power drills and Arrow OnControl powered bone access system allow for controlled access into sclerotic bone.
      (4) 2-lb mallet

Procedure

1. Standard preprocedure preparation applies with meticulous attention to sterile technique.
   a. Sterile covering of detector, x-ray tube, monitors, and Ioban sterile barrier appropriate when placing fixation hardware.
   b. Sterile water placed in warmer.
   c. Foley catheter for long cases with GETA.
2. Antibiotics—skin flora coverage.
3. Access and treatment should be planned off recent appropriate imaging.
   a. Access with 10- to 11-gauge diamond tip cannula to facilitate biopsy and subsequent ablation.
   b. CT fluoroscopy or CBCT with augmented fluoroscopy for real-time access.
      (1) Superficial structures afford use of US to allow real-time access.
   c. Sclerotic bone may require use of power drills.
   d. Small bones may necessitate "no touch" ablation technique with probe adjacent to lesion.
4. Ablation probe choice will depend on patient-specific parameters as detailed above.
   a. Ablation probes are 15 to 17 gauge regardless of energy type.
      (1) 8-Fr peel-away will allow exchange of biopsy and ablation probes while maintaining access.
      (2) Hydrodissection should be used liberally to protect skin and adjacent structures. 600 cc of fluid is easily absorbed by the tissues.
5. Stabilization/consolidation
   a. Cementoplasty is indicated when lesions are lytic or pathologic fracture is present.
   b. Cementoplasty can create a barrier to future tumor advancement.
   c. Live fluoroscopic or CT guidance required during injection to prevent leakage into joint, adjacent veins, or through a fracture line.

Postprocedure Management

1. Medications—Ketorolac (dose reduction in renal impairment), Decadron (post-RF and MW ablation), Tylenol, Gabapentin (neuropathic pain).
2. Recovery orders—Postop recovery time and admission dependent on extent of ablation/fixation. Most patients are discharged the same day or are admitted for 23 hours observation for overnight monitoring.
3. Pain management consult recommended for patients with preexisting high opioid tolerance.

4. Consider palliative care consult for best supportive care and symptom management.
5. Full admission for screw fixation cases for postoperative care.
6. Clinical follow-up occurs at 1, 3, 6, and 12 months. Routine imaging not necessary unless patient develops new or worsening symptoms.

Results

1. Adjunctive epidural steroid injections, nerve blocks, or neurolysis may improve overall outcomes.
2. Technical success rate of 96% to 100% and low incidence of significant adverse events or complication (8).
3. A 4- to 6-point decrease in pain score within 3 to 6 months with reduction in narcotic dose can be expected (3).
4. Percutaneous ablation in combination with cementoplasty and or screw fixation is effective and durable for pain palliation (4,8–10).

Complications

1. Thermal injury
   a. Skin—Displacement techniques and active monitoring of the ablation zone when lesions are near the skin surface may mitigate risk.
   b. Visceral organs.
   c. Nerves—Motor and/or sensory deficits. Mitigated via adjunctive displacement techniques, nerve monitoring, and mindful procedural planning.
   d. Connective tissue—Necrosis, accelerated degenerative changes, and/or joint pain.
2. Hemorrhage may occur in tissues along the tract or adjacent to the ablation zone. Cautery function available on select devices can reduce risk of hemorrhage.
3. Cement embolization/extravasation may result in pulmonary embolus, intraarticular leakage, nerve compression, and/or spinal canal narrowing with or without cord compression.
4. Infection.

Management of Complications

1. Symptomatic control dependent on tissue involved.
2. Skin and connective tissue injury may require grafting.
3. Infections are treated with antibiotics and rarely drainage.
4. Thermal neurapraxia may resolve spontaneously however persistent symptoms may necessitate treatment with NSAIDs and/or steroids. Adjunctive block/steroid injection may also provide symptomatic relief. Referral to physical/occupational therapy if injury limits patient mobility and or ADLs.
5. Cement extravasation may require neurosurgical or orthopedic intervention.

References

1. Lane MD, Le HBQ, Lee S, et al. Combination radiofrequency ablation and cementoplasty for palliative treatment of painful neoplastic bone metastasis: experience with 53 treated lesions in 36 patients. *Skeletal Radiol.* 2011;40(1):25–32. doi:10.1007/s00256-010-1010-5
2. Castañeda Rodriguez WR, Callstrom MR. Effective pain palliation and prevention of fracture for axial-loading skeletal metastases using combined cryoablation and cementoplasty. *Tech Vasc Interv Radiol.* 2011;14(3):160–169. doi:10.1053/j.tvir.2011.02.008
3. Kurup AN, Morris JM, Callstrom MR. Ablation of musculoskeletal metastases. *Am J Roentgenol.* 2017;209(4):713–721. doi:10.2214/AJR.17.18527

4. Hartung MP, Tutton SM, Hohenwalter EJ, et al. Safety and efficacy of minimally invasive acetabular stabilization for periacetabular metastatic disease with thermal ablation and augmented screw fixation. *J Vasc Interv Radiol*. 2016;27(5):682–688.e1. doi:10.1016/j.jvir.2016.01.142

5. Deschamps F, de Baere T, Hakime A, et al. Percutaneous osteosynthesis in the pelvis in cancer patients. *Eur Radiol*. 2016;26(6):1631–1639. doi:10.1007/s00330-015-3971-1

6. Kurup AN, Morris JM, Boon AJ, et al. Motor evoked potential monitoring during cryoablation of musculoskeletal tumors. *J Vasc Interv Radiol*. 2014;25(11):1657–1664. doi:10.1016/j.jvir.2014.08.006

7. Lubner MG, Brace CL, Hinshaw JL, et al. Microwave tumor ablation: mechanism of action, clinical results, and devices. *J Vasc Interv Radiol*. 2010;21(SUPPL. 8):S192. doi:10.1016/j.jvir.2010.04.007

8. Gennaro N, Sconfienza LM, Ambrogi F, et al. Thermal ablation to relieve pain from metastatic bone disease: a systematic review. *Skeletal Radiol*. 2019;48(8):1161–1169. doi:10.1007/s00256-018-3140-0

9. Tian QH, Wu CG, Gu YF, et al. Combination radiofrequency ablation and percutaneous osteoplasty for palliative treatment of painful extraspinal bone metastasis: a single-center experience. *J Vasc Interv Radiol*. 2014;25(7):1094–1100. doi:10.1016/j.jvir.2014.03.018

10. Pusceddu C, Sotgia B, Fele RM, et al. Treatment of bone metastases with microwave thermal ablation. *J Vasc Interv Radiol*. 2013;24(2):229–233. doi:10.1016/j.jvir.2012.10.009

60 Osteorestorative Techniques

**Alexios Kelekis, MD, PhD and
Dimitrios K. Filippiadis, MD, PhD, MSc, EBIR**

Overview

Bone metastatic lesions whether they are manifesting themselves as present or impeding osseous fractures, can result in severe pain, impairment of life quality, functional disability, and hospitalization (1,2). Traditional surgical repair is governed by higher complication rates and morbidity, longer recovery and hospitalization while it is related to a delay in systemic therapies due to the need for healing of the surgical incision. Percutaneous osteorestorative techniques include cement injection either solely performed or in combination with hardware including cannulated screws, peek (Polyether ether ketone) polymer implants, or other alternatives such as meshes of microneedles or Kirshner wires. These minimally invasive techniques apply advanced image guidance technology aiming for stabilization and structural support with subsequent pain reduction, functional restoration, and life quality improvement. The purpose of this chapter is to describe the most commonly applied osteorestorative techniques and the procedure itself. Advantages and disadvantages of different techniques and approaches will be addressed.

1. Introduction
   a. Pathologic or insufficiency as well as impeding fractures in cancer patients are related to the presence of one or more metastatic lesions, to bone weakening postradiation therapy or to cancer-related osteoporosis due to systemic therapies, nutritional deficiency, decreased mobility, and patient frailty (3,4).
   b. Vertebral spine, ribs, and pelvis are the most common locations of metastatic disease in the skeleton with multiple lesions being present in the vast majority of the cases; tumor subtype, metastatic burden, and response to systemic therapy govern prognosis in these patients.
   c. Pathologic or insufficiency fractures occur in approximately 20% to 40% while a significant number of patients are at risk for impending fractures. In

both cases the impaired osseous structural integrity results in pain, impairment of life quality, and functional disability (5,6).

d. All these patients should be discussed at a multidisciplinary tumor board with multimodality treatment plans being offered whenever possible; primary therapeutic goals should include pain improvement with or without functional improvement.

(1) Radiation therapy cannot provide fast and durable consolidation, furthermore, as a therapy it is related to increased risk of pathologic fracture due to resultant radiation-induced osteopenia and further bone weakening.

(2) Radical surgery is seldom indicated in multifocal metastatic disease; in addition, traditional surgical repair is governed by higher complication rates and morbidity, longer recovery, and hospitalization while it is related to a delay in systemic therapies due to the need for healing of the surgical incision.

2. Percutaneous osteorestorative techniques include cementoplasty, fixation with internal cemented screws (FICS) (Fig. 60.1) and augmented osteoplasty (Fig. 60.2 and Table 60.1) (6–8).

a. Standalone injection of poly-methyl methacrylate (PMMA) is a superb augmentation technique for locations such as spine where compression and tension forces of axial loading apply; in peripheral skeleton locations where shearing, torsion, and bending forces apply. PMMA is governed by moderate structural support capacity requiring additional reenforcement by hardware.

b. Apart from location, type of bone is also significant with cementoplasty being an efficacious treatment for fractures/defects of flat bones such as acetabular roof, femoral condyles, tibial endplates, or talus.

c. Whenever there is a need for resistance to tensile and torque stresses or a fracture/ osseous defect in the diaphysis of a long bone FICS or other augmented osteoplasty alternative should be proposed.

(1) At present application of cannulated screws in the peripheral skeleton and peek polymer implants in the femoral bone have been biomechanically tested and evaluated whereas other metallic hardware alternatives are only reported in case series with no bench evaluation.

(2) Presence of fractures as well as concerns for cement extravasation renders FICS an ideal approach for structural support and restoration of osseous integrity and stability.

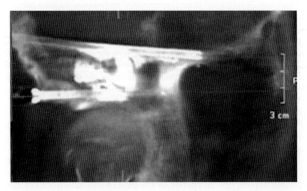

FIGURE 60.1 • A 68-year-old male patient with solitary hepatocellular carcinoma and a large-sized lytic metastasis involving the iliac bone and the acetabulum treated with percutaneous cryoablation followed by percutaneous fixation with internal cemented screws (FICS). Cone-beam computed tomography reconstruction post-FICS illustrating the two cannulated screws and the cement used for anchoring.

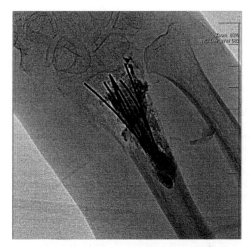

FIGURE 60.2 • A 64-year-old female patient with cholangiocarcinoma and multiple osseous metastases was treated for palliative pain reduction with augmented osteoplasty of the radius. Therapeutic session included microwave ablation followed by percutaneous insertion of a mesh of metallic microneedles followed by cement injection.

    d. Different types of bone involved and variety upon fracture morphology, location, and etiology demand a tailored patient as well as lesion-centered approach.
3. Combination percutaneous ablation + osteorestorative techniques (7)
    a. Whenever the therapeutic goal includes local tumor control
    b. Ablation of the target lesion will be combined with structural support and augmentation, required because of postablation bone necrosis and weakening.
    c. Polymerization of PMMA will produce an exothermic reaction with peak temperature transiently reaching 80°C.
    d. When prophylactic treatment for impeding pathologic fracture is considered surgical scores such as the Mirels' score for long bones or the Harrington (or the Levy) grading systems for the acetabulum can be used; in the remainder of the peripheral skeleton pain and significant cortical destruction could be considered as predictive factors of impeding fracture.

Table 60.1 Osteorestorative Techniques	
Percutaneous cementoplasty	Standalone cement injection into weakened bone aiming for internal trabecular consolidation, reduction periosteal nerve stimulation with subsequent pain reduction and functional restoration
Percutaneous fixation with internal cemented screws (FICS)	Metallic cannulated screws are inserted through small incisions across the fracture line or osseous defect followed by percutaneous cementoplasty
Percutaneous augmented osteoplasty	Cement injection is combined with implants or alternative metallic hardware such as meshes of microneedles or Kirshner wires.

(1) The Mirels' score evaluates presence of pain and lesion type, size, and site; any lesion with a score >9 is considered at high risk of fracture and stabilization should be considered.

e. Whenever a large-sized benign lesion such as aneurysmal bone cyst or osteoblastoma endangers osseous integrity due to size and associated cortical disruption cement injection can be combined with percutaneous ablation (or any other preferred technique).

(1) Due to the young age of patients (in the vast majority of these cases) and the lack of malignant substrate (therefore no need for the high temperatures produced by the exothermic reaction during PMMA polymerization) a synthetic bone graft substitute that consists of hydroxyapatite and calcium sulfate can be injected. These bone grafts promote de novo bone formation throughout the material which is fully remodeled into host bone within 6 to 12 months and combined with the graft's capacity to withstand loading, there is a significant reduction of fracture or nonunion risk.

4. Indications
   a. Painful osteolytic metastatic lesion
   b. Symptomatic osteoblastic metastases (if bone is not too dense or if fissures are present)
   c. Pathologic or insufficiency fracture in cancer patients
   d. Postablation augmentation for structural support due to bone necrosis and weakening
   e. Impeding fracture in cancer patients
   f. Benign bone lesions endangering osseous integrity due to size and associated cortical disruption (e.g., aneurismal bone cyst, osteoblastoma)

5. Contraindications
   a. Absolute contraindications to osteorestorative techniques include:
      (1) Presence of concomitant systemic or local infection
         (a) In the presence of infection, bone augmentation must be postponed until the patient undergoes a full antibiotic course, becomes afebrile and his or her laboratory workup illustrate normal white blood cell values and negative blood cultures.
      (2) Uncorrectable bleeding diathesis
         (a) Any kind of anticoagulation must be interrupted; duration of interruption is according the international guidelines for each medication
      (3) Allergy to cement or any other material used
      (4) Insufficient cardiopulmonary status to tolerate sedation
   b. Relative contraindications include:
      (1) Factors which technically increase the difficulty of the procedure without however rendering it impossible.
      (2) Presence of vessels, nerves or viscera in the expected trocar trajectory should be carefully evaluated prior to performance of any osteorestorative technique.
         (a) The Interventional radiologist should be familiar with nerve anatomy and function to diminish or avoid clinically consequential nerve damage.
      (3) Presence of sclerotic bone could require specific bone access devices (e.g., high-power electric drills) in order to achieve successful and accurate access.
      (4) Life expectancy <3 months and poor performance status.

6. Preprocedure preparation
   a. Therapeutic goal (local tumor control, pain palliation, stability of impeding fracture) should be clearly defined.
   b. Lesion location, size, and type along with the involved bone type are significant factors governing choice of specific osteorestorative technique.
   c. Same factors govern selection of specific materials (e.g., need for a high-power electric drill, length and type of cannulated screws).

d. A baseline CT scan will provide invaluable information concerning proper technique and material selection.

(1) Careful preoperative evaluation of the trocar's trajectory and its relation to structures at risk contributes to minimizing the risk of vascular, nerve, or visceral wounds.

e. Through review of patient's medical record should be performed in order to exclude anticoagulation, or infection or other disease which could increase the mortality and morbidity of the procedure.

f. Laboratory workup should include complete blood cell count, coagulation assessment, and screening of basic metabolic panel.

g. Electrocardiography, chest x-ray, and anesthesiologic evaluation are performed conforming to local practice guidelines.

h. In case of a patient with neuralgia, neurologic assessment can provide valuable information.

i. Ideally all anticoagulation drugs must be stopped; the duration of interruption is determined by societal guidelines specific to each medication.

j. In case of infection, osteorestorative techniques must be postponed until the patient completes a full antibiotic course, becomes afebrile and their laboratory workup demonstrates normal white blood cell values; ideally a percutaneous biopsy for culture would provide extra security.

k. Physical examination is critical for proper patient selection. The majority of oncologic patients will have more than one metastasis however, only symptomatic lesions should be treated. In case of painful metastatic lesions interventional radiologists should distinguish between mechanical and neuropathic pain in order to provide appropriate therapy.

l. Preoperative intravenous antibiotics should be administered 45 to 60 minutes prior to intervention.

7. Procedure

a. Using strict sterile technique, anesthesiology care, cardiovascular monitoring, and imaging guidance, direct access to the fracture/osseous defect target through normal bone is obtained using bone access needles.

b. In order to minimize risk of inadvertent vascular puncture and resultant bleeding specific corridors should be followed during trocar insertion; in addition, control scans (3D cone-beam CT or CT) during the procedure minimizes the risk of vascular, nerve, or visceral wounds.

c. Needle advancement can be performed using fluoroscopic guidance in multiple projections including anteroposterior, lateral and "gunsight" views, as well as cone-beam CT reconstructions.

d. In percutaneous cementoplasty, multiple bone access needles (2–3) per lesion can be placed, aiming to create sufficient coverage in medial/lateral and cranio/caudal orientation.

(1) An alternative to the original cementoplasty technique is the addition of balloon inflation in order to create a more contained space for cement injection; in theory this extra step decreases cement leakage offering a large-sized compact cement ball.

(2) Simultaneous injection of PMMA by two needles produces a more compact and solid block of cement, reducing radiation exposure and avoiding leakage from the first needle track (Fig. 60.3).

(3) In FICS, once the bone access needle is in position, a Kirshner wire is coaxially introduced over which the cannulated screw is inserted using a manual screwdriver or an electric drill.

e. Similar principles govern performance of any alternative osteorestorative technique mentioned in the literature. Cone-beam CT or standard CT scan is used to assess implant position posttreatment.

8. Postprocedure management

a. Patient remains in the hospital overnight and is then discharged.

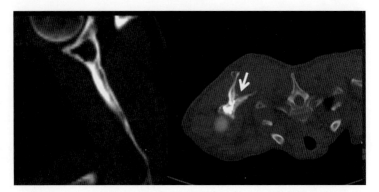

FIGURE 60.3 • A 58-year-old male patient with renal cell carcinoma and a lytic metastasis of the glenoid in the scapula (left image). Patient was treated with microwave ablation followed by percutaneous cementoplasty. Computed tomography axial scan (right image) illustrates cement distribution and filling of the lesion with a tiny extraosseous leakage along the needle tract.

   b. Depending on the location, type of bone and disease extent patient should remain confined to bed for the first 4 to 8 hours.

   c. Parenteral analgesics should be provided in order to avoid pain related to muscular injury during screw insertion.

   d. Intravenous antibiotics should be given during hospitalization and orally for an extra 5 days post discharge.

9. Results

   a. Differing success rates of the various techniques used determine how osteorestorative techniques are applied (8).

      (1) Percutaneous cementoplasty for lesions with a Mirels' score >9 results in significant pain reduction and functional restoration.

      (2) The technique is limited by a chance of posttherapeutic pathologic fracture in the range of 0% to 40.6% with lesion size and diameter of cortical defect being significant risk factors.

      (3) In cases of impending pathologic fractures FICS is a safe and durable preventive treatment with a 98% long-term consolidation efficacy rate.

      (4) Similar high success rates apply to application of FICS in cancer patients with osseous defects or fractures as well as in cases of pelvic fracture post high-energy trauma.

      (5) At the moment the scientific literature is limited to observational studies or case reports, and lack in depth in vitro biomechanical evaluation; however, the construct of cement mixed with a mesh of metallic microneedles (rebar concept) has been reported to provide long-term consolidations in case series with follow-up over 3 years.

10. Complications

   a. General risks and complications include pain, bleeding and arterial injury, neuralgia and nerve injury complications related to patient positioning, infection, misplacement or incomplete placement of the hardware used, material failure, cement leakage, and screw retraction (9).

   b. Muscle pain is most commonly seen as a result of muscular damage during screw positioning which causes tearing of the fibers along the path to the bone.

c. Arterial, nerve, or visceral injury may occur as a result of trocar injury. Similar to other percutaneous techniques caution should be taken when positioning the patient especially if he or she is under general anesthesia in order to avoid transient or permanent nerve injury.

d. Similar to traditional surgical approaches infection is a serious complication, especially when related to placement of a permanent implant; thus, all preventative measures, including strict local sterility and prophylactic antibiotics, should be followed according to existing guidelines.

e. Stripping of a screw head or breakage of a screw itself are rare complications especially when proper material selection is made in terms of thickness and diameter.

f. Cement leakages are very common especially with percutaneous cementoplasty with size of cortical defect and presence of a fracture being significant risk factors.

g. Complications and risk related to cancer stage and patient's performance status include tumor or fracture progression, bone failure, and muscle atrophy as well as venous thrombosis or pulmonary embolus.

11. Management of complications

a. Posttreatment muscle pain is more prominent during the first 48 hours thus nonopioid analgesics or patient-controlled analgesia (PCA) pump should be provided.

b. Bleeding is usually self-limited, however if there is persistent active extravasation due to arterial injury embolization or percutaneous thrombosis should be performed.

c. In order to avoid infection prophylactic antibiotics should be administered starting the morning of the procedure and lasting 5 days post; practice however, differs based on local habits.

d. If the procedure does not provide complete stability, supportive devices (crutches, walking cane, etc.) may be required for ambulation.

e. If there is dense bone, stainless steel screws are preferred over titanium in order to minimize chances of stripping of the screw head or breakage of the screw itself.

f. Similar to any other augmentation techniques involving cement application, injection of the polymer should be performed under continuous fluoroscopy in correct projections in order to minimize the risk of cement extravasation/leakage; additionally, high viscosity cements with long working times contribute to proper performance (10).

(1) Balloon inflation in order to create a contained space for low-pressure injection is another alternative

(2) Cement should anchor the screw in its final position over the fracture/osseous defect in order to avoid retraction.

References

1. Deschamps F, De Baere T. Cementoplasty of bone metastases. *Diagn Interv Imaging*. 2012; 93(9):685–689.
2. Deschamps F, de Baere T, Hakime A, et al. Percutaneous osteosynthesis in the pelvis in cancer patients. *Eur Radiol*. 2016;26(6):1631–1639.
3. Roux C, Tselikas L, Yevich S, et al. Fluoroscopy and cone-beam CT-guided fixation by internal cemented screw for pathologic pelvic fractures. *Radiology*. 2019;290(2):418–425.
4. Cazzato RL, Koch G, Buy X, et al. Percutaneous image-guided screw fixation of bone lesions in cancer patients: double-centre analysis of outcomes including local evolution of the treated focus. *Cardiovasc Interv Radiol*. 2016;39(10):1455–1463.
5. Yevich S, Odisio B, Sheth R, et al. Integrated CT-fluoroscopy equipment: improving the interventional radiology approach and patient experience for treatment of musculoskeletal malignancies. *Semin Interv Radiol*. 2018;35(4):229–237.

6. Yevich S, Tselikas L, Gravel G, et al. Percutaneous cement injection for the palliative treatment of osseous metastases: a technical review. *Semin Interv Radiol*. 2018; 35(4):268–280.

7. Kelekis A, Filippiadis D, Anselmetti G, et al. Percutaneous augmented peripheral osteoplasty in long bones of oncologic patients for pain reduction and prevention of impeding pathologic fracture: the rebar concept. *Cardiovasc Interv Radiol*. 2016;39(1):90–96.

8. Key BM, Scheidt MJ, Tutton SM. Advanced interventional pain management approach to neoplastic disease outside the spine. *Tech Vasc Interv Radiol*. 2020;23(4):100705.

9. Lea WB, Neilson JC, King DM, et al. Minimally invasive stabilization using screws and cement for pelvic metastases: technical considerations for the pelvic "screw and glue" technique. *Semin Interv Radiol*. 2019;36(3):229–240. doi: 10.1055/s-0039-1693982.

10. Filippiadis DK, Tselikas L, Bazzocchi A, et al. Percutaneous management of cancer pain. *Curr Oncol Rep*. 2020;22(5):43.

61 Musculoskeletal Pain and Palliative Procedures

Brandon M. Key, MD and Sean M. Tutton, MD, FSIR, FCIRSE

Spinal Injections

Introduction

Epidural steroid injections (ESIs) are the most widely used intervention for the treatment of spinal pain associated with sensory and or motor weakness secondary to disk herniations and/or neuroforaminal stenosis (1). Advances in imaging technologies have allowed for these injections to be performed accurately via multiple different approaches under fluoroscopy, computed tomography (CT), or cone-beam CT (CBCT).

Indications

1. Persistent radiculopathy secondary to herniated disk, spinal stenosis, axial lower back pain, and postlumbar surgery despite conservative medical therapy (1).
2. Diagnostic evaluation of back pain.

Contraindications

1. **Absolute:** INR ≥1.5, platelet count <50k, and active infection
2. **Relative:** Medication allergy, Plavix (requires a 5-day hold), and anticoagulants

Preprocedure Preparation

1. Patient evaluation
   a. Imaging: Review available cross-sectional imaging prior to procedure to determine ideal injection approach and identify potential obstacles to injection.
   b. Approaches (1)
      (1) Interlaminar: central/paracentral disk herniations
      (2) Transforaminal: foraminal or extraforaminal zone herniations
      (3) Caudal: postlaminectomy adhesions and spinal stenosis
   c. Imaging modality selection: Fluoroscopy versus CBCT versus CT depending on patient anatomy and operator preference. At our institution cervical injections are done under CT with adjunctive US as needed. Lumbar and sacral selective nerve root block (SNRB)/ESIs are typically performed with CBCT or fluoroscopy.

d. History and physical examination: Emphasis on the physical examination for assessment of pain characteristics and correlation with imaging findings.

e. Informed consent: Discussion of risks, benefits, and alternatives
   (1) Laboratory tests: INR and platelets within 30 days
   (2) Procedural sedation: Moderate sedation
      (a) Injectables
         i. Dexamethasone is used for all spinal injections at our institution due to concern for spinal ischemia with use of particulate containing steroids (2).
         ii. ESI maximum dose limited to 15-mg dexamethasone and no more than three ESIs in a 6-month period (3).
         iii. Preservative free lidocaine 1% or bupivacaine 0.25%
         iv. Contrast agent: Isovue-M 200

Procedure

1. **Cervical ESI**
   a. Performed primarily under CT guidance. US may be utilized in combination when the intended needle trajectory is near vasculature.
   b. Patient is positioned supine on the table and scout CT is obtained.
   c. A safe anterolateral trajectory targeting the anterior superior margin of the transverse process of the targeted level is determined based on imaging.
   d. Anesthetize the overlying skin with 1% lidocaine.
   e. Advance a 22- or 25-gauge spinal needle under direct image guidance down to the targeted transverse process.
   f. Walk the needle tip along anterior surface and into the foramen (Fig. 61.1).
   g. Inject 1-mL dilute Isovue-M 200 to confirm position within the epidural space.
   h. Inject anesthetic and steroid (Table 61.1).

2. **Lumbar Transforaminal ESI/Selective Nerve Root Block**
   a. Position the patient prone on the table.
   b. Prep and drape the lower back in usual sterile fashion.
   c. Angle the C-arm to obtain true AP view with the spinous process positioned midline between the pedicles. Angle the x-ray beam cranial or caudal until the beam is parallel to the disk space.
   d. Rotate the C-arm into an ipsilateral oblique position creating the "Scotty Dog" view (Fig. 61.2). For L5–S1 injections additional angulation must be considered to form a triangular window bordered by the transverse process of L5, the superior articulating process of S1, and the iliac crest.
   e. Anesthetize the skin with 1% lidocaine
   f. Advance a 22-gauge spinal needle under fluoroscopic guidance toward the inferolateral aspect of the pedicle and into the safe triangle (Fig. 61.2).

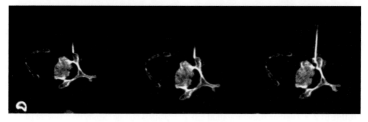

FIGURE 61.1 • Cervical epidural steroid injection. Sequential CT images demonstrating walking of the needle down the anterior aspect of the transverse process.

Table 61.1 Common Volumes and Dosages for Spinal Epidural Steroid Injections

	Cervical		Lumbar		
	Transforaminal	**Interlaminar**	**Transforaminal**	**Interlaminar**	**Caudal**
Contrast	IsoVue 200 M—1 mL	IsoVue 200 M—1–2 mL	IsoVue 200 M—1–2 mL	IsoVue 200 M—1–2 mL	IsoVue 200 M—1–2 mL
Anesthetic	Volume : 1 mL 0.25% Bupivacaine or 1% lidocaine	Volume : 1 mL 0.25% Bupivacaine or 1% lidocaine	Volume : 1 mL 0.25% Bupivacaine or 1% lidocaine	Volume: 1.5 mL 0.25% Bupivacaine or 1% lidocaine	Volume: 5 mL 0.25% Bupivacaine or 1% lidocaine
Steroid	Dexamethasone 10 mg	Dexamethasone 10 mg	Dexamethasone 10 mg	Dexamethasone 10 mg	Dexamethasone 10 mg

   g. Rotate to lateral view and advance the needle tip until the patient experiences discomfort in their typical pain distribution, or the needle tip reaches the posterior cortex of the vertebral body.

   h. Inject 1-mL dilute Isovue-M 200. Contrast should be seen tracking along the nerve root sheath and/or within the epidural space.

   i. Inject anesthetic and steroid (Table 61.1).

3. Interlaminar ESI

   a. Position the patient prone on the table.

   b. Prep and drape the lower back in usual sterile fashion.

   c. Angle the C-arm to target the interlaminar space.

   d. Anesthetize the overlying skin with 1% lidocaine.

   e. Advance a 22-gauge spinal needle under fluoroscopic guidance in AP and lateral projections until the tip reaches the midportion of the spinous process.

   f. Attach connecting tubing and a syringe filled with sterile saline to the needle hub.

   g. Under lateral fluoroscopy advance the needle slowly with light continuous pressure on the syringe plunger. A sudden loss of resistance will occur when the needle tip exits the ligament and enters the epidural space (Fig. 61.3).

   h. Inject 1-mL dilute Isovue-M 200 to confirm position within the epidural space.

   i. Inject anesthetic and steroid (Table 61.1).

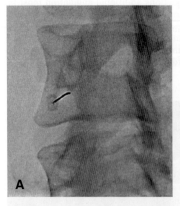 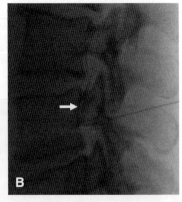

FIGURE 61.2 • Lumbar Transforaminal ESI. A: Ipsilateral oblique "Scotty Dog" view of L4 with the spinal needle entering the safe triangle. **B:** Lateral projection demonstrating contrast layering in the epidural space (*arrow*).

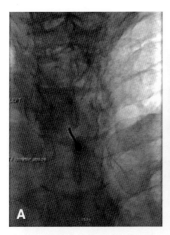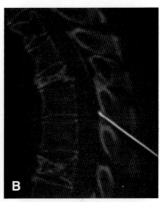

FIGURE 61.3 • **Thoracic interlaminar ESI. A:** AP projection of the thoracic spine with 22-gauge spinal needle projecting over the interlaminar space. **B:** CBCT demonstrating needle tip in the epidural space.

4. Caudal ESI
   a. Position the patient prone on the table.
   b. Prep and drape the lower back in usual sterile fashion.
   c. Locate the sacral hiatus via US, fluoroscopy, or palpation.
   d. Anesthetize the overlying skin with 1% lidocaine.
   e. Advance a 22-gauge spinal needle through the sacral hiatus with a steep cephalad angle.
   f. Attach connecting tubing and a syringe filled with sterile saline the needle hub.
   g. Advance the needle in the lateral projection with light continuous pressure on the syringe plunger. A sudden loss of resistance will occur when the needle tip passes through the sacrococcygeal ligament and into the epidural space (Fig. 61.4).
   h. Inject 1-mL dilute Isovue-M 200 to confirm position within the epidural space.
   i. Inject anesthetic and steroid with sufficient volume to propagate therapeutics to target level (Table 61.1).

Postprocedure Management

1. Postprocedure monitoring for at least 30 minutes prior to discharge.
2. Monitor for persistent anesthesia. Patient with persistent anesthesia should have voiding trial prior to discharge or bladder scan to assess for urinary retention.
3. Patients instructed to contact clinic should symptoms worsen after discharge.

Results (1)

1. Diagnostic blocks are effective within minutes and may provide up to 7 days of relief.
2. Mean duration of effect of therapeutic injections is 3 to 6 months. Patients may experience return of symptoms between the time local anesthetics have worn off and steroid takes effect.
3. TFESI > Interlaminar > Caudal approach yield greatest efficacy.

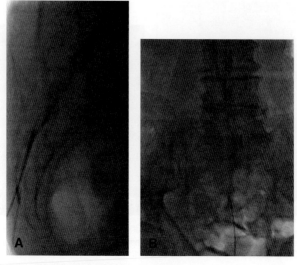

FIGURE 61.4 • Caudal epidural injection. A: Lateral projection of the sacrum with 22-gauge spinal needle traversing the sacral hiatus with contrast in the epidural space. **B:** AP projection of the sacrum demonstrating contrast in the epidural space extending cranially.

Complications
Hemorrhage, infection, transient headache, spinal ischemia, dural puncture, intrathecal injection, and/or transient lower extremity weakness, paresthesia, or autonomic dysfunction

Management of Complications

1. Symptomatic and supportive care
2. Antibiotics for infection
3. Epidural hemorrhage resulting in nerve root or cord compression and may require neurosurgical intervention

Palliative Nerve Blocks, Neurolysis, and Ablations

Ganglion Blocks/Neurolysis

Introduction
Sympathetic inputs from the celiac ganglia, superior hypogastric ganglia, and ganglion impar contribute to various abdominopelvic pain processes including malignancy related pain. Block/neurolysis of these ganglia can be safely preformed and profoundly impact a patient's quality of life, mental state, and ability to tolerate treatment (4). In addition, blockade of these ganglia may be utilized as an adjunct for periprocedural pain management.

Indications
1. Celiac plexus (5)
   a. Pain due to esophageal, pancreatic, hepatic, biliary, or retroperitoneal pathology
2. Superior hypogastric (6)
   a. Pain due to bladder, distal large bowel, or genital pathology
   b. Pain control prior to uterine artery embolization

3. Ganglion impar (7)
   a. Pain due to perineal, distal rectum, anus, distal urethra, vulva, scrotum, distal vaginal pathology, or coccydynia

Contraindications

1. **Absolute**—Uncorrectable coagulopathy, thrombocytopenia
2. **Relative**
   a. Somatic pain in the distribution of intended block/neurolysis
   b. Active infection at the site of injection
   c. Extensive tumor invasion obscuring relevant anatomy
   d. Celiac plexus specific—Abdominal aortic aneurysm, existing diarrhea, and bowel obstruction (5)

Preprocedure Preparation

1. Patient evaluation imaging
   a. Preprocedural cross-sectional imaging obtained ideally within 4 weeks of the planned procedure date
   b. Consultation/Evaluation
      (1) History and physical examination—Emphasis on the physical examination for assessment of pain characteristics and correlation with imaging findings
      (2) Informed consent—Discussion of risks, benefits, and alternatives
2. Laboratory tests—INR and platelets within 30 days
3. Procedural sedation—Moderate sedation

Procedure

1. Celiac plexus
   a. Anterior versus posterior approach and selection of imaging modality are patient and operator dependent
   b. Anterior antecural approach can be performed via CT, fluoroscopy, CBCT, and/or US with utilization of one or two needles. With a single-needle approach a Pakter needle (Cook Medical, Bloomington, IN) may be utilized to deliver anesthetic or alcohol to the contralateral ganglion if necessary
   c. Posterior antecural approach may be unilateral or bilateral. Various approaches include paravertebral, transaortic, transintervertebral disk, and direct tumor infiltration
   d. Position the patient and prep and drape in usual sterile fashion
   e. Anesthetize the overlying skin with 1% lidocaine
   f. Advance a 22-gauge Chiba needle to the antecrural space just inferior to the celiac axis (Fig. 61.5)
   g. Inject a small volume of dilute contrast to confirm proper antecrural needle position and to assess for adequate diffusion of contrast on both sides of the celiac axis and the anterior surface of the aorta. If there is inadequate coverage, then a Pakter needle be advanced coaxially to reach the contralateral ganglion or a second needle can be placed
   h. Injection
      (1) Diagnostic block—Inject 10-mL 0.5% bupivacaine
      (2) Neurolysis—Inject 6 mL of anesthetic agent with total of 30 to 40 mL of ethanol (30 mL for single needle and 20 mL per needle for bilateral access)
2. Superior hypogastric ganglion
   a. Anterior versus posterior approach and selection of imaging modality are patient and operator dependent. Anterior, posterior paravertebral, and posterior transintervertebral disk approaches under CT and fluoroscopy have been described in literature

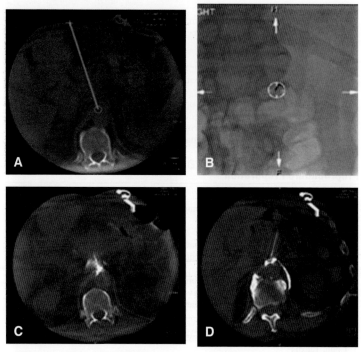

FIGURE 61.5 • Celiac Plexus Block. A: Anterior approach utilizing CBCT and iGuide (Siemens Healthcare AG, Forchheim Germany) for needle path planning. **B:** iGuide Bullseye view demonstrating needle advancement along the intended trajectory. **C,D:** CBCT performed after contrast injection confirming position of needle tip.

    b. Anterior with fluoroscopy and/or CBCT is the primary approach in the literature
    c. Prep and drape the patient's lower abdomen in usual sterile fashion
    d. Angle the C-arm to obtain true AP view of L5
    e. Angle the x-ray beam cranial or caudal until the beam is parallel to the disk space
    f. Anesthetize the overlying skin with 1% lidocaine
    g. Advance a 22-gauge Chiba needle under fluoroscopic guidance to the anterior cortex of the L5 superior endplate just to the **right midline**.
    h. Inject a small volume of dilute contrast in the lateral projection. Contrast should be seen layering in the prevertebral space (Fig. 61.6).
    i. Injection
        (1) Diagnostic block—6 mL 0.5% bupivacaine
        (2) Neurolysis—6-mL 0.5% bupivacaine and 15 mL of ethanol
    j. Return the C-arm to the AP position. Partially retract the needle
    k. Advance the needle under fluoroscopic guidance to the anterior cortex of the L5 superior endplate just to the left of midline
    l. Repeat steps 8 and 9.
3. Ganglion impar
    a. Transsacrococcygeal approach under fluoroscopic guidance is the dominant method in the literature.
    b. Position the patient prone on the table.

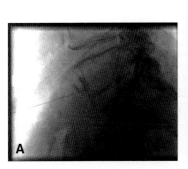
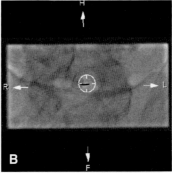

FIGURE 61.6 • **Superior hypogastric ganglion block. A:** Lateral projection demonstrating contrast in the prevertebral space at L5. **B:** AP projection of iGuide navigation for needle placement.

c. Prep and drape the lower back and upper gluteal cleft in normal sterile fashion.

d. Locate the sacrococcygeal junction in the AP projection.

e. Rotate the C-arm into the lateral projection to determine the appropriate craniocaudal trajectory.

f. Anesthetize the overlying skin with 1% lidocaine.

g. Advance a 22-gauge Chiba or 21-gauge micropuncture needle under AP and lateral fluoroscopy until the tip is just beyond the anterior margin of the sacrococcygeal junction.

h. Inject a small amount of contrast which should layer along the anterior surface of the sacrococcygeal junction and not diffuse laterally (Fig. 61.7).

i. Inject 4- to 6-mL 0.5% bupivacaine followed by 15-mL ethanol.

Postprocedure Management

1. Monitor for at least 2 hours prior to discharge if being performed as an outpatient.

2. Admit to observation if there are any immediate postprocedural complications.

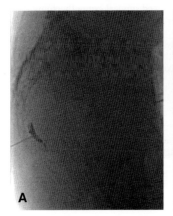
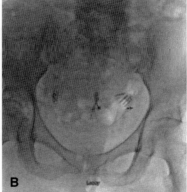

FIGURE 61.7 • **Ganglion impar block. A:** Lateral and (**B**) PA projections of the sacrum demonstrating a 21-gauge micropuncture needle traversing the sacrococcygeal junction with contrast appropriately layering anterior to the sacrococcygeal junction.

Results
1. Celiac plexus neurolysis (5)
   a. Major complication in less than 2%.
   b. 70% to 90% of patients have long lasting benefit regardless of approach.
   c. Reduces use of narcotic analgesics and drug-related side effects.
2. Superior hypogastric block/neurolysis (8)
   a. Neurolysis for malignancy-related pain demonstrates significant pain relief and reduction in opioid use in most patients.
   b. Block for UAE demonstrated 100% technical success rate with improved pain control post procedurally.
3. Ganglion impar (7)
   a. Cancer-related pain—VAS reduction up to 6 to 7 with reduction in opioid usage.
   b. Coccydynia—Equivocal efficacy, contemporary literature supports anesthetic in combination with steroid or thermocoagulation.

Complications

1. Autonomic dysfunction in region of targeted block/neurolysis
2. Celiac plexus—Back pain, transient diarrhea, and/or referred should pain, hypotension (5)
3. Superior hypogastric—Iliac artery, bladder, and/or bowel injury
4. Ganglion impar rectal injury, sciatic nerve impingement, and/or bladder, bowel, or sexual dysfunction (6)

Management of Complications

1. Symptomatic and supportive care
2. Fluid resuscitation for hypotension

Sympathetic Neurolysis (9)

Introduction
Lumbar sympathectomy was the mainstay of treatment of occlusive and vasospastic peripheral arterial disease prior to the development of contemporary endovascular and surgical procedures. Minimally invasive image-guided percutaneous lumbar sympathetic neurolysis has since replaced surgical sympathectomy, however it is only performed for cases of lower extremity pain when no available endovascular or surgical options remain.

Indications
1. Ischemic rest pain in patients with nonreconstructable arterial occlusive disease
2. Complex regional pain syndrome
3. Peripheral neuralgia
4. Vasospastic disorders

Contraindications
1. **Absolute**—INR ≥1.5, platelet count <50k, and active infection
2. **Relative**—Medication allergy and anticoagulants

Preprocedure Preparation
1. Patient evaluation
   a. Preprocedure consultation/evaluation
      (1) History and physical examination
      (2) Multidisciplinary approach is favored with involvement from vascular surgery and/or palliative care
      (3) Informed consent—Discussion of risks, benefits, and alternatives

2. Laboratory tests—INR and platelets within 30 days
3. Procedural sedation—Moderate sedation unless pain is severe and warrants monitored anesthesia care or general anesthetic.

Procedure
1. Position the patient prone on the table.
2. Prep and drape the lower back in usual sterile fashion.
3. Identify the ipsilateral L2 vertebral level.
4. Angle the C-arm to obtain true AP view with the spinous process positioned midline between the pedicles. Angle the x-ray beam cranial or caudal until the beam is parallel to the disk space.
5. Rotate the C-arm into an ipsilateral oblique position creating the "Scotty Dog" view.
6. Anesthetize the skin with 1% lidocaine approximately 7 cm lateral from midline.
7. Utilizing the ipsilateral oblique and lateral projections advance a 15-cm 20- to -22 gauge spinal needle inferior to the transverse process targeting the anterolateral aspect of the vertebral body.
8. Advance the needle tip to anterior margin of the vertebral body in the lateral projection.
9. Inject a small volume of contrast in the lateral projection. Contrast should layer longitudinally in the craniocaudal direction (Fig. 61.8).
10. Inject ~3-mL bupivacaine 0.5%.
11. Repeat for levels L3 and L4.
12. After all needles have been placed slowly inject 5-mL alcohol at each level.

Postprocedure Management
1. Postprocedure monitoring for minimum of 2 hours prior to discharge after neurolysis.
2. Frequent neurological examinations to monitor for nontargeted/neuraxial complication.

Results
1. Relief of ischemic rest pain is expected in 59% to 72%.
2. Greater symptomatic relief can be expected with patients with an ABI greater than 0.3.

Complications—Bleeding, genitofemoral neuralgia, neuraxial injury, and infection

Management of Complications

1. Symptomatic and supportive care
2. Antibiotics for infection
3. Epidural hemorrhage resulting in nerve root or cord compression and may require neurosurgical intervention

Peripheral Nerve Blocks (PNB) and Neurolysis

Introduction
A variety of peripheral nerve blocks can easily be performed for periprocedural pain control, pain palliation, or for diagnostic purposes. Most PNBs are performed quickly under US or fluoroscopic guidance with minimal risk to the patient. In addition, if pain relief is significant after a PNB, radiofrequency (RF) or cryoneurolysis can be performed for long-term pain palliation.

Indications
1. Periprocedural pain control
   a. Tibial blocks for foot procedures (AVMs, ablations)
   b. Interscalene block for upper extremity ablation, AV access interventions

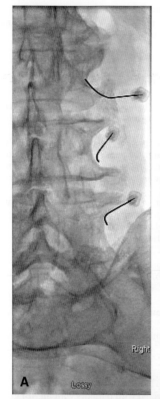

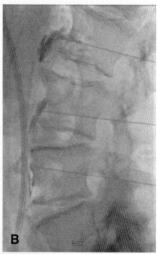

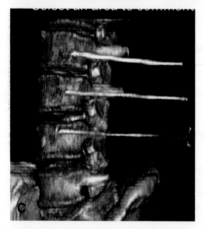

FIGURE 61.8 • Lumbar sympathetic neurolysis. A: AP and (**B**) lateral projections of L2–L4 demonstrating needle positioning for lumbar sympathetic neurolysis. Note contrast layering in the prevertebral space. **C:** 3D reconstruction demonstrating needle placement. (*continued*)

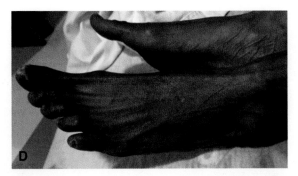

FIGURE 61.8 • (*Continued*) **D:** Postneurolysis photo of the patient's foot demonstrating hyperemia.

2. Pain syndrome in distribution of a peripheral nerve
3. Diagnostic block to confirm neurogenic source of pain

Contraindications
1. Absolute—None
2. Relative—Allergy to medication, coagulopathy, active infection

Preprocedure Preparation
1. Review relevant cross-sectional imaging
2. Patient evaluation
   a. Preprocedure consultation/evaluation
      (1) History and physical examination—Emphasis on the physical examination for assessment of pain characteristics and distribution
      (2) Informed consent—Discussion of risks, benefits, and alternatives
3. Laboratory tests—None
4. Procedural sedation—Most PNBs can be performed with no sedation. Utilization and depth of sedation determined by patient factors (e.g., severity of pain, difficulty positioning, anxiety)

Procedure (Figs. 61.9 to 61.11)
1. Position of the patient dictated by nerve targeted. Most can be done in supine position.
2. Prep and drape the target region in usual sterile fashion.
3. Anesthetize the overlying skin with 1% lidocaine.
4. Advance a 20- to 25-gauge needle under direct US, CT, or fluoroscopic guidance.
5. Inject a small volume of contrast as needed to confirm location.
6. Inject 4- to 6-mL bupivacaine around the targeted nerve targeting epineurium.
7. Neurolysis can be performed with 10 to 15 mL of ETOH however RF ablation or cryoneurolysis is more targeted.

Postprocedure Management
1. Recovery dependent on sedation utilized for the procedure.
2. Vascular examinations if block performed near an artery.

Results
1. Paresthesia/anesthesia in the distribution of targeted nerve for pharmacologic duration of the anesthetic utilized.
2. PNBs reduce the risk of perioperative complications via reduction in opioid-related adverse events (8).

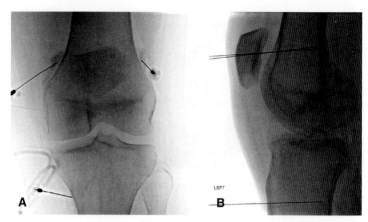

FIGURE 61.9 • Genicular Nerve Block. Useful for chronic knee pain. RFA ablation can be performed similarly if the patient responds to nerve block. **A:** AP projection of the knee demonstrating needles at the metadiaphyseal junctions of the distal femur bilaterally and proximal tibia medially. **B:** Lateral projection demonstrating needle tip projection over the posterior one-third of femur and tibia.

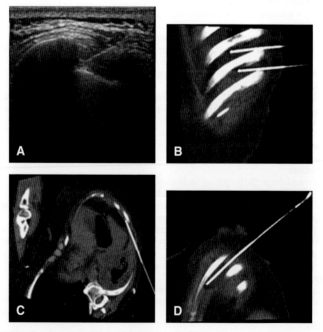

FIGURE 61.10 • Intercostal Nerve Block. Useful for chest wall pain, pleuritic pain, and other causes of thoracic dermatomal pain. **A:** US image of a 25-gauge needle appropriately positioned for intercostal nerve block with the tip at the undersurface of the rib. **B–D:** Multiplanar reformats of a no-touch technique of intercostal neurolysis.

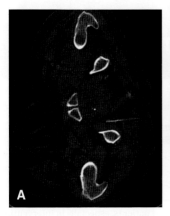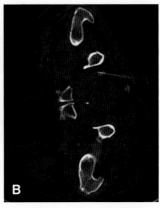

FIGURE 61.11 • Bilateral pudendal nerve block. Useful for pelvic pain conditions such as vaginal, penile, perineal, or scrotal pain. **A** and **B:** Axial CT images of 22-gauge Chiba needles in the pudenal canals, which are located caudal and medial to the ischial spine and medial to the obturator internus muscle.

Complications—Infection, hemorrhage, and/or pneumothorax (intercostal block/ablation)

Management of Complications
1. Symptomatic and supportive care
2. Antibiotics for infection

References

1. Shim E, Lee JW, Lee E, et al. Fluoroscopically guided epidural injections of the cervical and lumbar spine. *Radiographics.* 2017;37(2):537–561. doi:10.1148/rg.2017160043
2. Dietrich TJ, Sutter R, Froehlich JM, et al. Particulate versus non-particulate steroids for lumbar transforaminal or interlaminar epidural steroid injections: an update. *Skeletal Radiol.* 2015;44(2):149–155. doi:10.1007/s00256-014-2048-6
3. Schilling LS, Markman JD. Corticosteroids for pain of spinal origin. Epidural and intraarticular administration. *Rheum Dis Clin North Am.* 2016;42(1):137–155. doi:10.1016/j.rdc.2015.08.003
4. Ferreira F, Pedro A, Ganglion Impar neurolysis in the management of pelvic and perineal cancer-related pain. *Case Rep Oncol.* 2020;13(1):29–34. doi:10.1159/000505181
5. Kambadakone A, Thabet A, Gervais DA, et al. CT-guided celiac plexus neurolysis: a review of anatomy, indications, technique, and tips for successful treatment. *Radiographics.* 2011; 31(6):1599–1621. doi:10.1148/rg.316115526
6. Gunduz OH, Kenis-Coskun O. Ganglion blocks as a treatment of pain: current perspectives. *J Pain Res.* 2017;10:2815–2826. doi:10.2147/JPR.S134775
7. Scott-Warren JT, Hill V, Rajasekaran A. Ganglion impar blockade: a review. *Curr Pain Headache Rep.* 2013;17(1):306. doi:10.1007/s11916-012-0306-7
8. Midia M, Dao D. The utility of peripheral nerve blocks in interventional radiology. *Am J Roentgenol.* 2016;207(4):718–730. doi:10.2214/AJR.16.16643
9. Zechlinski JJ, Hieb RA. Lumbar sympathetic neurolysis: how to and when to use? *Tech Vasc Interv Radiol.* 2016;19(2):163–168. doi:10.1053/j.tvir.2016.04.008

SECTION V
INTRAPROCEDURAL PATIENT MANAGEMENT

62 Safety in IR

Rathachai Kaewlai, MD and
Hani H. Abujudeh, MD, MBA, FSIR, FACR, FASER

Introduction

Safety is paramount for both physicians and patients, especially in interventional radiology (IR) environment where invasive procedures are performed. Steps can be taken to minimize risks that include—but are not limited to—occupational health hazards, radiation and bleeding via a use of guidelines and standardized lists for periprocedural management. Society of Interventional Radiology (SIR) has issued multiple safety guidelines and toolkits, which are available on its website (1). In this chapter, authors discuss one of the most significant risks in IR—the wrong site, wrong procedure, and wrong patient errors (WSPEs). WSPEs—also termed "never events"—result in devastating injuries to the patient, attract negative media attention, undermine public confidence in the health care system, and devalue and demoralize physicians. These errors are generally rare (1 in 50,000 to 100,000 procedures) but more prevalent in procedures associated with laterality (2,3) and probably occur equally in nonsurgical interventions and surgical disciplines (4). They are frequently caused by *human factors* (such as competency assessment and staff supervision), *leadership* (such as priority setting and complaint resolution), and *failure in communication* (among staff, administration, and/or patients and families) (5). Organizational culture and steep hierarchical structures in the procedure room also play a role (3,6). To prevent such errors and improve patient safety, the Joint Commission (JC; effective 2004) requires the establishment of a *Universal Protocol* at all hospitals, ambulatory care, and office-based surgery facilities seeking accreditation. In 2008, the SIR published supplemental guidelines for fulfilling this requirement which are still considered up to date by the SIR Safety and Health Committee as of 2016 (7). The JC's latest revision of the Universal Protocol was effective January 1, 2010 (8). However, even in the Universal Protocol era, prevalence of WSPEs is still significant and unacceptable. Multifaceted strategy (Universal Protocol, WHO surgical safety checklist, medical team training, peer-learning opportunities) is required to eliminate these errors (9,10).

Universal Protocol

1. The Universal Protocol, a three-step process, includes multiple strategies to prevent WSPEs:
   a. Preprocedure verification
   b. Site marking
   c. Time-out
2. Each step in the Universal Protocol is complementary to the other and is intended to introduce redundancy to the practice of confirming the correct site, procedure, and patient (6).
3. Any step used alone is unlikely to reduce the incidence of WSPEs (6).

Indications

All surgical and nonsurgical invasive procedures that expose patients to more than minimal risk must have an indication.

1. JC defines "invasive procedures" as those involving "the puncture or incision of the skin, insertion of an instrument, or insertion of foreign material into the body. Invasive procedures may be performed for diagnostic or treatment-related purposes."
2. Common procedures such as peripherally inserted central catheters (PICCs) line insertion, as well as all central line and chest tube insertions, must fulfill the Universal Protocol requirement.

Exemptions to Universal Protocol

1. Routine "minor" procedures, relevant to IR are
   a. Puncture of small peripheral veins
   b. Peripheral intravenous line placement
   c. Insertion of a nasogastric tube or urinary bladder catheter
   d. Lithotripsy
   e. Performance of dialysis (does not include insertion of dialysis catheter)
   f. Minor procedure, posing minimal patient risk, whose need is discovered during a routine clinic visit, for example, drainage of a newly discovered seroma/cyst
2. Patient related
   a. Profoundly medically unstable patient
   b. Patient in cardiopulmonary arrest

Preprocedure Verification

1. Essentials
   a. The purposes of preprocedure verification are to ensure (a) availability of all relevant documents, information, and equipment prior to the start of the procedure; (b) understanding of the patient about the procedure to be performed; and (c) correct identification of the patient and procedure to be performed by all members of the operating or procedure area.
   b. Confirmation of *correct site, procedure, and patient* is made at every stage from the time of decision to perform the procedure to the time the patient undergoes the procedure. The verification may occur at more than one time and place before the procedure is performed.
   c. Verification should be performed with patient involvement, being awake and aware of the process, as much as possible.
   d. A standardized list can be used in the verification process. The list helps verify that all information, relevant documents, and necessary equipment are
      (1) Available prior to the start of the procedure
      (2) Correctly identified, labeled, and matched to the patient's identifiers
      (3) Reviewed and consistent with the patient's expectations and with the team's understanding of the intended patient, procedure, and site
2. When
   a. At the time the procedure is scheduled
   b. At the time of preadmission testing and assessment
   c. At the time of admission or entry to the facility for the procedure, whether elective or emergent
   d. Before the patient leaves the preprocedural area or enters the procedure room
   e. At any time, responsibility for care is transferred to any other member of the care team
3. How
   a. Patient identification (hospital wristband), proper labeling of patient-related items, and cross-confirmation by checking patient records, including imaging studies. This is done using a standardized list (previously called "checklist").

(1) A standardized list counteracts human failures of omission.

(2) A meaningful standardized list includes simple clearly defined information that physicians need and induces them to adhere to safety measures in daily practice.

(3) Successful safety standardized lists improve communication and consistency of care, decreasing complications and death rates. In a prospective, multinational trial involving 7,688 patients, the rate of any complication dropped from a baseline of 11% to 7%, and in-hospital mortality decreased from 1.5% to 0.8%, after standardized list implementation.

b. Standardized list

(1) Can be in paper, electronic, or other medium (e.g., wall-mounted board)

(2) Reviews and verifies that all items are available and accurately matched to the patient:

(a) Confirmation of *correct patient* by two identifiers: (a) If no identifying band on the patient, use full name and date of birth, and (b) if there is an identifying band on the patient, use full name and medical record number

(b) Confirmation of *correct procedure and site* by verbal/self-report by the patient or family member

(c) Reverification of correct procedure and site with history and physical examination note, nursing assessment note, or progress note

(d) Accurately completed and signed procedure consent form

(e) Verification of laboratory and radiology results (are in fact those of the patient; pay special attention to projections—anterior or posterior—in which images were obtained, so as to not confuse laterality), required blood products (properly matched and verified), implants, devices, and/or special equipment (sterile and not expired) needed for the procedure.

c. Consent process (see Chapter e-97)

(1) Consent must be obtained while the patient is awake and alert, prior to any sedation, and has the capacity to understand the details and implications of the procedure.

(2) Consent must be in a language that the patient understands (or employ an interpreter).

(3) Consent form should include a clear statement of the procedure to be performed and the site of the procedure.

(4) Consent form can be waived in emergency cases with a threat to life or limb.

Site Marking

1. Essentials

a. Site marking is required for any procedure involving an incision, percutaneous puncture, or insertion of an instrument before the procedure (see exemptions in the following text).

(1) At minimum, the site must be marked when there is more than one possible location for the procedure and performing the procedure in a different location could harm the patient (8).

(2) When both right- and left-sided structures are abnormal, the SIR recommends that skin marking be performed even if intraprocedural imaging is to be employed (7).

(3) Site marking for bilateral procedures (for identical procedure, team, and equipment) is recommended but not required by the JC.

b. Site to be marked must be unambiguous, clearly visible, and at or next to the procedure site. Nonprocedural site should not be marked unless necessary for some other aspect of care.

    c. Site marking takes place with the patient involved awake and aware, if possible.

    d. In specific circumstances (i.e., nonspeaking, comatose, or incompetent patients, children), the site-marking process should be handled similar to the informed consent process.

2. When

    a. The procedure site is initially marked before the patient is moved to the location where the procedure will be performed.

3. Exemption from site marking

    a. Interventional procedures for which there is no predetermined site of insertion (e.g., angiography, central line placement). This is because (7)

      (1) Side is irrelevant for the procedure and

      (2) Imaging guidance is an inherent part of the procedure.

      (3) For angiographic procedures, it is the opinion of SIR that vascular access is simply a means to provide a route to perform a procedure or to provide access to central veins. Skin marking at the vascular access is not needed. For angioplasty procedures, SIR recommends that the side (left or right) of intervention be confirmed with appropriate intraprocedural imaging.

    b. When technically or anatomically impossible or impractical to mark the site.

    c. Procedures that have a midline approach intended to treat a single, midline organ/lesion.

    d. Endoscopy without intended laterality.

    e. Patient refusal of site marking. The situation should be handled the same way (i.e., gentle explanation and documentation) as for any other refusal by a patient offered care, treatment, or services using organization's written, alternative process to ensure that the correct site is performed on. The Universal Protocol does not require that the procedure be canceled because the patient refuses site marking.

    f. Premature infants where there could be permanent tattooing of immature skin.

    g. For procedures in which site marking is not required, the other requirements of the Universal Protocol still apply.

4. Two-stage marking

    a. Spinal procedures

      (1) The general level of the procedure (cervical, thoracic, or lumbar) must be marked preoperatively.

      (2) If the procedure involves anterior versus posterior, or right versus left approaches, the mark must indicate this.

      (3) The exact interspace(s) to be treated should be precisely marked using standard intraprocedural radiographic marking technique.

5. Two-site marking

    a. When patient is having two procedures performed at different sites (i.e., regional anesthetic block prior to an interventional procedure), two separate marks are to be made.

6. Who performs site marking?

    a. The *interventionist*, as a licensed hospital-privileged practitioner, who will be performing the procedure should mark the site.

    b. Site marking can be delegated to another individual in limited situations: A *licensed practitioner*—such as a fellow, resident, advanced practice nurse, or physician assistant—can be delegated by an interventionist. This individual must be familiar with the patient, present, and actively involved during the procedure.

    c. Even when the site marking is delegated to another practitioner, the interventionist still remains responsible and accountable for all aspects of the procedure.

    d. Any delegation of responsibility for site marking must be consistent with applicable laws and regulations (7).

7. How

    a. Use a *sufficiently permanent marker* so that it is not removed during site preparation. Adhesive site markers should not be used as the sole means of marking the site (7).

    b. The mark must be *clearly visible after* the patient is in final on-table position, with the skin prepped and sterile draping in place.

    c. Types of mark

        (1) The Universal Protocol does not specify the type of mark but leaves the choice to the institution. However, the mark must be unambiguous and consistent throughout the institution.

        (2) The word *YES*, initials of the interventionist who will perform the procedure, or an arrow pointing to the site is generally used.

        (3) The cross (X) should not be used because this could denote a site that should not be operated upon and introduces ambiguity.

Time-Out

1. Essentials

    a. Time-out is a brief pause immediately before the procedure starts to *CONFIRM—correct site, correct procedure, correct patient!* The procedure is not started until all questions or concerns are resolved.

    b. It is an opportunity to

        (1) Identify any wrong site, wrong patient, or wrong procedure

        (2) Ensure correct patient positioning

        (3) Ensure availability of necessary instruments and equipment

        (4) Foster communication among team members

        (5) Clarify any inconsistencies or concerns from any team members

            (a) At minimum, the team members must agree on correct patient identity, correct site, and procedure to be performed.

            (b) The design and deployment of the time-out process is up to the individual institution. Documentation of adherence to Universal Protocol and the "time-out" process is mandatory.

2. When

    a. Immediately prior to the start of the procedure, after the patient is appropriately positioned, regardless of the venue—interventional suite, computed tomography (CT) suite, or at bedside with ultrasound guidance (7).

3. Who

    a. The interventionist (person who will perform the procedure) initiates time-out.

    b. The time-out *must not* occur without the individual performing procedure present.

4. How

    a. The time-out must be *verbal and interactive* with all team members involved in the procedure. The interventionist confirms:

        (1) Correct patient identity

        (2) Accurate and signed consent form

        (3) Agreement on the procedure to be done

        (4) Correct patient positioning

        (5) Correct side and site are marked

        (6) Relevant images and results are properly labeled and displayed

        (7) Appropriate antibiotic administration and/or fluids for irrigation

        (8) Special safety precautions due to patient's health and medication history

    b. During the time-out, all unnecessary activities (those that do not compromise patient safety) within the room are suspended.

    c. All team members must be in agreement before proceeding with incision or skin puncture.

Interventional Pre-Procedure Verification Form with Universal Protocol

1. Arrival *To be completed by the RSR or arriving Technologist.*

1. Confirmed patient identity	☐
2. Confirmed that patient has a scheduled appointment	☐
3. Confirmed patient has an MGH identification bracelet	☐
4. Falls assessment completed	☐

Signature/Title	Print Name	Date	Time

2. Pre-Procedure

To be completed by any staff member who is involved in the procedure. Areas in white may not apply.

1. Confirmed patient identity	☐	8. Verified that patient is alert and able to tolerate the procedure	☐
2. Confirmed planned procedure	☐	9. Patient has signed a completed consent form	☐
3. Reviewed diagnostic and radiology test results as required	☐	10. Women between the ages of 12-60 have been asked about possible pregnancy	☐
4. Confirmed that required blood products, supplies, etc. are present	☐	*If sedation or anesthesia is to be used*	
5. Reviewed patient medications	☐	11. Nursing assessment has been completed and reviewed	☐
6. Procedure site has been marked by radiologist or licensed practitioner*	☐	*If general anesthesia is to be used*	
7. Safety issues specific to the procedure (e.g. allergies, diabetes) have been reviewed	☐	12. Pre anesthesia assessment has been completed and reviewed	☐
		13. Anesthesia consent has been completed and signed	☐
Alternative site marking can be done		*If specimens are to be taken*	
		14. Confirmed specimen label(s)	☐

Signature/Title	Print Name	Date	Time

3. Time Out

To be completed by any staff member who is involved in the procedure. Areas in white may not apply.

1. Confirmed patient identity	☐
2. Team and patient have agreed upon procedure to be done	☐
3. Confirmed correct side, site, and position	☐
4. Administered pre-procedure antibiotics	☐

Signature/Title	Print Name	Date	Time

FIGURE 62.1 • Sample Universal Protocol checklist. (Adapted from MGH Radiology.)

    d. Time-out can be improved when the team (a) is aware of an ideal model of a good time-out, (b) has a culture to reward safety, (c) does not allow deviation from the standard time-out, and (d) constantly voices concerns and feedbacks.

5. Two time-outs

    a. When two or more procedures are to be performed on the same patient by separate teams, a complete time-out is performed before each procedure begins.

        (1) Example: epidural placement by anesthesiologist, followed by cesarean section by obstetrician.

(2) The exception is that when the same team is performing multiple components during a single procedure.
b. When hospital policy or law/regulation requires two separate consents.

Documentation

1. Documentation of Universal Protocol must be completed and included in patient's medical record.
   a. Adequate documentation includes one checkbox or a brief note regarding the successful completion of the time-out, located in a consistent location in the patient record. It is not necessary to individually document each step of time-out if the full content is specified elsewhere (policy, procedure manual, etc.).
2. Any team members directly involved in the procedure can complete the Universal Protocol documentation.
3. An example of Universal Protocol checklist is provided in Figure 62.1.

References

1. Society of Interventional Radiology. Steps toward physician and patient safety. https://www.sirweb.org/practice-resources/toolkits/quality-and-safety-toolkit/radiation-safety/ Accessed March 19, 2021.
2. Kwaan MR, Studdert DM, Zinner MJ, et al. Incidence, patterns, and prevention of wrong-site surgery. *Arch Surg.* 2006;141(4):353–358.
3. Seiden SC, Barach P. Wrong-side/wrong-site, wrong-procedure, and wrong-patient adverse events: are they preventable? *Arch Surg.* 2006;141(9):931–939.
4. Stahel PF, Sabel AL, Victoroff MS, et al. Wrong-site and wrong-patient procedures in the universal protocol era: analysis of a prospective database of physician self-reported occurrences. *Arch Surg.* 2010;145(10):978–984.
5. Sentinel event data: root causes by event type, 2004–2015. The Joint Commission Perspectives web site. http://info.jcrinc.com/rs/494-MTZ-066/images/Sentinel39.pdf. Accessed: March 19, 2021.
6. World Alliance for Patient Safety. World Health Organization web site. http://whqlibdoc.who.int/publications/2009/9789241598552_eng.pdf. Accessed November 15, 2014.
7. Angle JF, Nemcek AA Jr, Cohen AM, et al. Quality improvement guidelines for preventing wrong site, wrong procedure, and wrong person errors: application of The Joint Commission "Universal Protocol for Preventing Wrong Site, Wrong Procedure, Wrong Person Surgery" to the practice of interventional radiology. *J Vasc Interv Radiol.* 2008;19(8):1145–1151.
8. Facts about the Universal Protocol. The Joint Commission Web site. https://www.jointcommission.org/standards/universal-protocol/. Accessed July 2, 2022.
9. Adelman J, Chelcun J. Evidence-based safe surgical practices as adjuncts to the universal protocol. *Arch Surg.* 2011;146(4):489.
10. Higgins MCSS, Herpy JP. Medical error, adverse events, and complications in interventional radiology: liability or opportunity? *Radiology* 2021;298(2):275–283.

63 Sedation, Analgesia, and Anesthesia

John Crowe, MD and Marcus A. Lehman, MD, MBA

Introduction

The practice of vascular and interventional radiology often requires the use of medication to relieve anxiety, provide sedation, and minimize discomfort. Unfortunately, administration of local anesthetics, sedatives, and opioids can impose an additional element of risk to patients, mandating care in patient preparation, monitoring, and discharge from the radiology suite (1).

With growing complexity of care and patient acuity, hospital systems have found the benefit of including anesthesia services for many procedures that previously might have been done without them. Adding a preoperative assessment by anesthesia providers can also help mitigate risks and unexpected complications to care and workflow. At minimum, we strongly suggest reviewing sedation and anesthesia protocols and strategy with Anesthesiology providers to create a strong algorithm and standard work up for patients in the radiology suite.

Analgesia and Anesthesia: Options and Indications

1. **Local anesthesia.** Infiltration of skin and underlying tissues at procedural site. For brief diagnostic procedures where little discomfort is expected beyond the local puncture site in adult patients who are cooperative and tolerate the initial local anesthetic infiltration at the puncture site
2. **Local anesthesia with sedation.**
   a. **Local anesthesia with sedation provided by radiology care team**
      (1) Appropriate for most patients undergoing diagnostic and interventional procedures.
      (2) May still benefit from consultation with an anesthesiologist concerning the choice of medication and appropriate dosage in certain patient populations, for example, in patients during the first trimester of pregnancy.
   b. **Local anesthesia with sedation provided by anesthesia care team (monitored anesthesia care or MAC)**
      (1) With higher-risk, critically ill, or difficult patients. Often, difficult patients have a history of poor tolerance for invasive procedures, usually resulting from inadequate analgesia and sedation.
      (2) When intense analgesia or deep levels of sedation are require.
      (3) When procedure or positioning may compromise the airway.
      (4) When procedure may require or be facilitated by rapid raising or lowering of the systemic arterial pressure, such as for patients with AVMs.
      (5) Any situation where patient safety and procedural success would benefit from trained anesthesia personnel.
3. **Neuraxial or regional anesthesia.** Induction of segmental anesthesia and muscle relaxation with local anesthetics delivered by needle or catheter (e.g., spinal or epidural anesthesia).
   a. Neuraxial block via spinal or epidural is used when intense analgesia for the procedure and the postprocedural period is required, without the use of excessive opioid medication.
   b. When muscle relaxation is desirable or required.
4. **General anesthesia.** Induction and maintenance of a controlled state of unconsciousness characterized by a loss of protective airway reflexes, absence of response to painful stimuli, and inability to recall procedural events.

a. Appropriate for the uncooperative patient or the patient who refuses local or regional anesthesia, or who cannot tolerate the procedure otherwise.

b. When there is potential for airway obstruction as a result of the procedure or when airway patency or protection may be compromised by sedative medication.

Patient Evaluation

1. Preprocedural assessment:
   a. *NPO status.* Patient should be evaluated using the American Society of Anesthesiology's guidelines for NPO status. For instance, clear liquids may be ingested for up to 2 hours before procedures. A light meal (toast) may be ingested up to 6 hours before procedures, and everything else should have a minimum fasting time of 8 hours before procedures. While it may make it easier for patients to adhere to guidelines by telling them not eat anything after midnight the night before the procedure, other issues, such as blood sugar and patient comfort have to be considered, especially for procedures scheduled late in the day.
   b. *History and physical examination:*
      (1) Age. Advanced age alters dose requirements and elimination of many medications. For sedatives and analgesics, the elderly patient usually requires smaller increments and less frequent dosing intervals compared with younger adults. A reduction of 30% to 50% is a practical approach to initial dosing administration. Metabolism and drug elimination are both slowed in the elderly, which can result in excessive postprocedure sedation and delayed recovery (2). Elderly patients often require more extensive preparation for procedures, and they are at an increased risk for periprocedural complications because of significant concomitant medical disease and age-related impairment of cardiovascular, hepatic, and renal functions (2).
      (2) Cardiovascular disease. Coronary artery disease (CAD), congestive heart failure (CHF), cerebrovascular disease, insulin-dependent diabetes, and serum creatinine >2.0 are important factors associated with increased risk of perioperative cardiac complications. In addition, self-reported exercise ability remains an effective screening tool and is independently linked with the risk for adverse cardiovascular events, particularly a patient's ability to climb two flights of stairs. Well-controlled hypertension does not present an increased risk (3).
      (3) Pulmonary disease. Smoking is an important cause of perioperative respiratory morbidity and mortality. Before a procedure, cessation of smoking should be encouraged. Other important patient-related risk factors include poor exercise capacity, chronic obstructive pulmonary disease, and acute exacerbations of asthma (4).
      (4) Obesity. Recognition of associated comorbid issues is essential as the prevalence of obesity continues to rise. Obese individuals are at an increased risk for CAD, obstructive sleep apnea (OSA), hypertension, diabetes, and gastroesophageal reflux. In general, the risk will rise with increasing weight, especially with BMI >40, and often in a nonlinear fashion. Assessment of exercise tolerance may be difficult to assess secondary to body habitus. Limited pulmonary reserve and OSA contribute to the substantial risk of hypoventilation and obstruction caused by sedation. Practice guidelines by the American Society of Anesthesiologists may assist in determining the severity and appropriate perioperative management of patients with OSA (5). In addition, there are pharmacokinetic alterations in the obese patient. In general, the loading dose is based on the volume of distribution and maintenance dose on clearance; however,

in the obese population, published dosing information may not be appropriate (6). It has been suggested that dosing of medications, opioids in particular, should be based on lean body mass rather than actual weight (6). An experienced anesthesia provider should provide and monitor morbidly obese patients who require deep sedation.

(5) Hepatic disease. Reduced hepatic mass is associated with a decreased production of coagulation and drug-binding proteins (e.g., albumin). Initial doses of sedative and analgesic medications should be reduced because altered drug–protein binding can allow excessive "free" (i.e., unbound) drug to enter the central nervous system (CNS). In addition, drug metabolism can be markedly slowed, resulting in prolonged postprocedural sedation (2).

(6) Renal disease. Impairment of renal function will slow the ultimate elimination of many drugs, and although initial and maintenance doses may not require reduction, dosing intervals may need to be lengthened. The glomerular filtration rate (GFR) is the best laboratory metric available to determine overall measure of renal function (7). In patients with renal dysfunction, specific care should be exercised with administration of meperidine (Demerol since, its primary metabolite—normeperidine—can accumulate and lead to CNS stimulation, excitement, and seizures).

c. *Medication history.* Assessment of drug usage patterns and adverse reactions to medications are essential to the provision of safe patient care. Often, a drug effect or side effect (e.g., nausea) is described as an allergy. True allergic reactions to amide local anesthetics (lidocaine and bupivacaine) or benzodiazepines (diazepam and midazolam) are rare.

(1) Maintenance cardiovascular medication should be continued before the procedure. Attention should be given to the beneficial effects of continuing chronic perioperative β-blocker therapy, although starting this therapy immediately preoperatively may increase risk of complications and is no longer routine (3). Note that these can be given with sips of water while maintaining the patient in an otherwise fasted state.

(2) The insulin-dependent diabetic patient requires special consideration. Elective studies in these patients should be scheduled for early in the day. Often, half the usual morning dose of insulin is given and an infusion of 5% dextrose is begun on the day of the procedure. For lengthy procedures, frequent blood sugar determinations should be performed and an insulin infusion considered.

(3) In the elderly patient, adverse drug events from prescribed medications are common but often preventable. Meticulous care must be taken to review current medication list so that appropriate monitoring of the patient for adverse events can be performed. Specifically, cardiovascular, diuretic, nonopioid analgesic, oral hypoglycemic, and anticoagulant drugs are common medication categories associated with preventable adverse events (8).

2. Laboratory testing
   a. Overview. Preprocedural laboratory screening is expensive and often contributes little to patient care. When tests are ordered by protocol without specific indications, few significant abnormalities are found, and many of these determinations could be eliminated without measurably decreasing patient safety.
   b. Indications
      (1) Risk assessment for pregnancy (e.g., urine or serum beta human chorionic gonadotropin hormone [β-hCG])
      (2) Risk assessment for cardiovascular morbidity (e.g., electrocardiogram [ECG])
      (3) Risk assessment for hemorrhagic complications
      (4) Evaluation of hepatic and renal function

(5) Guide for preprocedural medical therapy (e.g., transfusion, electrolyte repletion, additional medical consultation)

Recommended Monitoring (Table 63.1)

1. Continuous monitoring by a physician or nurse is required during the entire procedure. The nurse evaluating patient responses to administered sedatives and analgesics may not be the person performing the procedure, but may assist with brief interruptible support measures. The responsible physician and registered nurse should be in constant attendance and have unrestricted immediate visual and/or physical access to the patient.
2. Their responsibilities include:
   a. Identify and confirm that the responsible physician for the procedure is immediately available.
   b. Maintain continuous IV access.
   c. Administer sedatives and analgesics as ordered by the responsible physician for moderate sedation.
   d. Monitor and document the patient's status.
   e. The registered nurse must sign the intraprocedure record and review the preprocedural sedation assessment.
   f. The dose, route, and time of administration of all drugs and agents administered should be documented at the time of their administration.
   g. Be capable of identifying and administering emergent intervention or activating such help if complications arise.
3. The following elements should be assessed and documented at least every 5 minutes and more often when the patient's condition warrants. During recovery, the frequency of assessments may decrease to every 15 minutes based on patient recovery course (9,10).
   a. Oxygen saturation (SpO_2)
      (1) The patient's presedation SpO_2 value must be recorded prior to the procedure.
      (2) Without exception or interruption, oxygen saturation is to be continuously monitored throughout the procedure.
   b. Respiratory rate
4. Concurrent with assessing respiratory rate, the person monitoring the patient must also assess the overall adequacy of the patient's airway and spontaneous ventilation, specifically seeking signs of airway obstruction and/or hypoventilation.

Table 63.1   Recommended Monitoring Parameters for Various Forms of Anesthesia

Parameter	Monitor	Anesthetic Option			
		Local Only	Local with Sedation	Regional	General
Circulation	BP	x	x	x	x
Cardiac rhythm	ECG	x	x	x	x
Oxygenation	Pulse oximeter	x	x	x	x
Respiratory depression	Respiration rate		x	x	x
Ventilation	$ETCO_2$		x	x	x
Temperature			x	x	x
Extent of block	Sensory level			x	

$ETCO_2$, end-tidal carbon dioxide.

a. End-tidal carbon dioxide ($ETCO_2$)
 (1) Without exception or interruption, $ETCO_2$ must be monitored throughout the procedure if sedation is given
 (2) $ETCO_2$ should be documented every 5 minutes during sedation and every 15 minutes during recovery from deep sedation until the patient reaches their preprocedure Aldrete Score.
b. Systolic and diastolic blood pressure
 (1) In children, the blood pressure monitoring interval may be adjusted by the individual needs of the patient and documented on the sedation-analgesia record. Administration of sedation should include knowledge of specialized parameters in this age group as well as resuscitative measures consistent with the care of a child.
 (2) Blood pressure should usually be checked within 2 to 3 minutes of administration of additional sedative-analgesic agent, unless it is clear the patient's status has not changed and/or measurement of blood pressure would otherwise disrupt the procedure.
c. Pulse (heart rate)
d. Level of consciousness (consider using the Richmond Agitation Sedation Score [RASS]), as well as the pain scale should be performed prior to sedation, in the event of a change in status and at the completion of the intended procedure.
e. The amount of oxygen being administered to the patient
f. All fluids (including blood) administered to the patient

Richmond Agitation Sedation Score (RASS)

+4	Combative, violent, danger to staff
+3	Pulling or removing tube(s) and/or catheters; aggressive
+2	Frequent nonpurposeful movement, "fights"/dissynchronous with the ventilator
+1	Anxious, apprehensive, but not aggressive
0	Alert and calm
−1	Awakens to voice >10 seconds
−2	Light sedation, briefly awakens to voice but for <10 seconds
−3	Movement or eye opening to voice but will not make eye contact
−4	No response to voice but responds to physical stimulation
−5	Cannot be aroused, no response to voice or physical stimulation

Required Resuscitation Equipment

1. In procedure room
 a. Pulse oximeter
 b. Blood pressure monitor
 c. Oxygen delivery systems, assorted size masks
 d. Oral and nasal airways, assorted sizes
 e. Cardiac monitor
 f. Oxygen delivery source capable of delivering 100% oxygen
 g. Positive pressure bag-valve and several size masks
 h. Equipment for continuous $ETCO_2$ monitoring
 i. Suction source, tubing, and appropriate selection of catheter sizes
 j. Yankaeur suction handle
 k. IV catheter in place
 l. IV solutions
 m. Medication labels
 n. Reversal agents: Naloxone and flumazenil

o. Electrical outlets with emergency power
p. Telephone
q. Crash cart immediately available, containing emergency airway equipment
2. In radiology suite
   a. Intubation equipment (e.g., laryngoscopes, endotracheal tubes)
   b. Defibrillator
   c. Advanced life-support medications (e.g., epinephrine, lidocaine, amiodarone, norepinephrine, and dopamine)
   d. Availability of assistive personnel with emergency airway management skills

Medication Prior to Procedure

1. **Guidelines**. The administration of medication prior to a procedure should never be routine. The choice of agent, dosage, and route of administration must be individualized. After oral and intramuscular (IM) administration, sufficient time (30 to 60 minutes) may be required for drug absorption to obtain desired effects. If continuous patient observation cannot be provided after an IM injection, IV administration of medication just prior to the procedure (with patient monitoring) is recommended. Medications used for sedation varies over time, regionally, and based on providers' experience with those medications. Ideally, providers choose a medication based on the available information, including but not limited to patient factors, plus length of, scope of, intensity of, requirements of, and painfulness of the procedure.
2. Below are some of the more frequently used drugs:
   a. Midazolam (Versed)
      (1) Indications: anxiolysis, induction of sedation, and amnesia
      (2) Dose/route of administration: 2 to 7 mg IM or 1 to 3 mg IV. Decrease dose by 25% to 50% when narcotics are given concurrently.
      (3) Adverse effects: profound sedation in patients over 70 years old. In patients aged 60 to 69 years, midazolam, 2 to 3 mg IM, is usually quite effective.
      (4) Effects may last beyond the timeline of shorter procedures.
      (5) Contraindication: first trimester of pregnancy, acute narrow-angle glaucoma
   b. Droperidol (Inapsine)
      (1) Indications: prevention and treatment of nausea and vomiting
      (2) Dose/route of administration: 2.5 to 5.0 mg IM or 0.625 to 1.250 mg IV
      (3) Adverse effects: prolonged sedation with IM administration, hypotension, extrapyramidal symptoms, and exacerbation of Parkinson disease
      (4) Contraindication: prolongation of corrected QT interval (QTc)
   c. Hydroxyzine (Vistaril)
      (1) Indications: prevention of nausea and vomiting, pruritus, anxiolysis
      (2) Dose/route of administration: 25 to 100 mg IM
      (3) Adverse effects: excessive sedation, dry mouth
      (4) Contraindication: narrow-angle glaucoma
   d. Diphenhydramine (Benadryl)
      (1) Indications: sedation, prophylaxis against contrast reaction
      (2) Dose/route of administration: 25 to 50 mg by mouth (PO), 25 to 50 mg IM, or 12.5 to 25 mg IV
      (3) Adverse effects: excessive sedation, dizziness, dry mouth, difficult urination, thickening of bronchial secretions
      (4) Contraindication: acute asthma, narrow-angle glaucoma
   e. Morphine sulfate
      (1) Indications: analgesia, sedation
      (2) Dose/route of administration: 2 to 10 mg IM or 1 to 3 mg IV

(3) Adverse effects: **respiratory depression**, hypotension, nausea, vomiting, itching, biliary spasm

f. **Fentanyl citrate** (Sublimaze)
   (1) Indications: analgesia
   (2) Dose/route of administration: 25 to 50 μg IV
   (3) Adverse effects: **respiratory depression**, bradycardia, nausea, vomiting, muscle rigidity, biliary spasm

g. **Nalbuphine hydrochloride** (Nubain)
   (1) Indication: analgesia, sedation
   (2) Dose/route of administration: 5 to 10 mg IM or 1 to 5 mg IV
   (3) Adverse effects: excessive sedation, nausea, vomiting, dizziness, limited analgesia, restlessness, reversal of analgesia produced by other opioids
   (4) Biliary tract: less elevation of biliary pressure than fentanyl and butorphanol

h. **Ketorolac** (Toradol)
   (1) Indication: analgesia without respiratory depression; can be used in combination with opioids
   (2) Dose/route of administration: 15 to 60 mg IM/IV
   (3) Adverse effects: reversible platelet dysfunction (24 to 48 hours after drug discontinuation), gastritis, peptic ulceration, and inhibition of renal autoregulation.
   Acute renal failure has been reported in patients following one dose of ketorolac because of its effect on renal autoregulation and therefore *must be used cautiously during procedures in which a high contrast–dye load is being administered* (11).

i. **Propofol (Diprivan)**
   (1) **Indication:** sedation for monitored anesthesia care, sedation with neuraxial anesthesia, induction and maintenance of general anesthesia, sedation of intubated, mechanically ventilated intensive care unit (ICU) patients.
   (2) **Dose/route of administration:** 1 to 2 mg per kg IV bolus for induction of general anesthesia; maintenance 25 to 200 μg/kg/min IV infusion depending on depth of sedation desired.
   (3) **Adverse effects:** hypotension, cardiovascular depression, apnea. Stinging at injection site. Anaphylactic reaction to emulsion; caution in egg and soy allergic patients. **Should be used only by providers able to rescue patients from deeper level of sedation than intended** (12).

j. **Dexmedetomidine (Precedex)**
   (1) Indication: sedation or supplemental sedation, often in the intensive care setting for intubated patients; maintains spontaneous respiration.
   (2) Dose/route of administration: 0.5 to 1.0 μg per kg IV over 10 minutes loading dose, followed by 0.2 to 1.0 μg/kg/h IV for up to 24 hours.
   (3) Adverse effects: bradycardia, hypotension.

k. **Prednisone**
   (1) Indication: prophylaxis against contrast reaction
   (2) Dose/route of administration: 50 to 75 mg PO the evening before and 1 to 2 hours prior to the examination
   (3) Adverse effects: hyperglycemia, hypertension, fluid retention

l. **Methylprednisolone** (Solu-Medrol [IV/IM], Medrol [PO])
   (1) Indication: prophylaxis against contrast reaction
   (2) Dose/route of administration: 32 mg PO the evening before and 1 to 2 hours prior to the examination
   (3) Adverse effects: hyperglycemia, hypertension, fluid retention

Techniques of Sedation, Analgesia, and Anesthesia During the Procedure

Local Anesthesia

1. **Indications:** anesthesia at puncture site
2. **Drug classification**
   a. **Amides:** lidocaine (Xylocaine), mepivacaine (Carbocaine), bupivacaine (Marcaine, Sensorcaine)
   b. **Esters:** chloroprocaine (Nesacaine), procaine (Novocaine)
3. **Choice of drug.** Most commonly used agents are amide local anesthetics. These local anesthetics are preferred over the esters because of increased potency, prolonged duration, and far fewer documented allergic reactions. For radiologic procedures, lidocaine (1% to 1.5%) is the most frequently used amide local anesthetic since it has a rapid onset of action and duration of 1 to 1.5 hours. However, both mepivacaine (1.0% to 1.5%) and bupivacaine (0.5%) provide longer durations of action (1.5 to 4 hours).
4. **Alkalinization of local anesthetics.** Subcutaneous (SQ) and intradermal infiltration of local anesthetics can be painful. However, alkalinization of local anesthetics (with the addition of sodium bicarbonate) can lessen the discomfort associated with skin and SQ infiltration (13). For lidocaine, 1 mEq of sodium bicarbonate is added to 10 mL of anesthetic. Alkalinization of bupivacaine is not recommended because even small amounts of sodium bicarbonate may result in precipitation of the local anesthetic.
5. **Injection technique and dosage.** Careful needle placement, aspiration prior to injection and after each 3 to 5 mL, and frequent patient observation during infiltration are required to avoid intravascular injections of local anesthetic. Rapid IV injection of local anesthetics can cause toxic manifestations. The total dose of lidocaine should not exceed 4 to 5 mg per kg (healthy adult), whereas bupivacaine doses should not exceed 3 mg per kg. A dose reduction of 30% to 50% is recommended in elderly patients and those with hepatic dysfunction and CHF, whereas maximum doses in the obese population should be based on lean body weight (6). Excessive local anesthetic doses, resulting in high serum concentrations, can result in prolonged lethargy following radiologic procedures, especially in the pediatric population.

Local Anesthesia with Sedation/Analgesia

1. Indications
   a. Anxious patient
   b. Procedures that produce discomfort distant from puncture site
2. Anesthesia consultation
   a. Extremes of age
   b. Hemodynamically unstable patient
   c. Severe cardiovascular or pulmonary disease
   d. Multiple maintenance medications (especially monoamine oxidase [MAO] inhibitors, chronic opioid use, heart failure medications, hypoglycemic agents)
   e. Pregnancy
3. Anesthesia attendance
   a. Critically ill patients
   b. Procedures that require intense analgesia or deep levels of sedation (e.g., difficult percutaneous biliary drainage or nephrostomy)
   c. Procedures or positioning that may comprise the airway
   d. Procedures that require or may be facilitated by close monitoring of the blood pressure and the ability to titrate vasoactive medications

4. Sedatives
   a. Midazolam: 0.5 to 2.0 mg IV every 30 to 60 minutes
   b. Diphenhydramine: 12.5 to 25.0 mg IV every 1 to 2 hours
5. Opioid analgesics
   a. Fentanyl: 25 to 75 µg IV every 15 to 60 minutes
   b. Morphine: 1 to 5 mg IV every 30 to 60 minutes
   c. Nalbuphine: 1 to 5 mg IV every 30 to 60 minutes
   d. Dilaudid: 0.5 to 1 mg IV every 2 to 3 hours
6. Biliary procedures. There may be an advantage to the use of nalbuphine for analgesia without marked elevations in biliary duct pressures and resistance to bile flow. IM or IV ketorolac can provide additional pain relief when used in combination with the nalbuphine, improving patient comfort during these procedures.
7. Coadministration of benzodiazepines and opioids. Extreme care must be exercised when administering these medications in combination. Hypoxemia and apnea may occur. Supplemental oxygen must be given to these patients, and personnel skilled in airway management must be available to attend these procedures (14).
8. Patient-controlled analgesia (PCA) and patient-controlled sedation (PCSA). This method of drug delivery can enhance patient satisfaction and decrease the total dosage needed to control acute pain. With PCA, the patient can self-administer small doses of opioid analgesic by means of a computer-controlled infusion by IV, SQ, or epidural route. In comparison to IM opioids given at "as-needed" intervals, self-administered doses provide more effective, sustained, and satisfactory analgesia (15). The PCA device is programmable to control dose delivered, time between doses (lockout interval), total dose limit over an hour or 4-hour period (4-hour maximum) and background continuous infusion. These parameters are adjusted to provide optimal patient comfort and safety. Nevertheless, side effects can occur including oversedation and respiratory depression. The PCA pump can also be used to provide sedation during surgical procedures under local or regional anesthesia (16). Drugs used for this technique include propofol, alfentanil, and fentanyl (Table 63.2). Using patient-controlled methods, midazolam and propofol have each been shown to provide sedation and amnesia for local anesthetic injection prior to dental surgery (16).
9. Nonpharmacologic considerations. Procedures performed while the patient is awake expose the subject to visual and auditory stimuli that may be anxiety provoking. Ear plugs or headset music may offer a relaxing distraction and provide a useful adjunct to a comprehensive sedation plan, decreasing sedative and analgesic requirements.

Table 63.2 Suggested Drugs and Intravenous Doses for PCA and PCSA (Adult 70 kg)

Drug	Intermittent Dose	Frequency (Lockout, min)	System	Usual Basal Infusion Rate
Hydromorphone	0.2–0.5 mg	6–10	PCA	0.2–0.5 mg/h
Meperidine	10–15 mg	6–10	PCA	15–50 mg/h
Morphine	1–2 mg	6–10	PCA	0.5–1 mg/h
Fentanyl	10–25 µg	2–5	PCA	25–50 µg/h
Alfentanil	0.01–0.03 mg	1–3	PCA	Not recommended
Propofol	5–20 mg	1–3	PCSA	Not recommended

PCA, patient-controlled analgesia; PCSA, patient-controlled sedation.

Neuraxial Anesthesia

1. Indications
   a. When intense analgesia for the procedure is required without use of excessive opioid medication
   b. Regional muscle relaxation
   c. Postprocedure pain management
2. Thoracic and lumbar epidural. Epidural anesthesia may be indicated for upper abdominal (hepatobiliary), renal, lower abdominal, or pelvic procedures (17).
   a. Suggested placement sites for radiologic procedures
      (1) Upper abdominal procedures at T4–L1
      (2) Renal procedures at T6–L1
      (3) Lower abdominal, pelvis, and lower extremities at T10–L3
   b. Choice and dosage of agents
      (1) The selection of the local anesthetic depends on the duration of the procedure. For long procedures (>2 hours), bupivacaine can be used, whereas lidocaine is best suited for shorter procedures.
      (2) The amount and area of anesthesia coverage can be adjusted throughout the procedure by intermittently dosing the epidural catheter. Postprocedure analgesia without muscle weakness can be provided by epidural opioid administration.
   c. Complications/side effects
      (1) Motor blockade
      (2) Hypotension
      (3) Pruritus
      (4) Urinary retention
      (5) Post dural puncture headache
      (6) Intravascular injection (epidural vein)
      (7) Intrathecal injection ("total" spinal)

General Anesthesia

1. Indications
   a. If procedure may compromise the patient's airway
   b. Highly anxious patients who refuse local anesthesia with sedation or regional anesthesia
   c. Patients who are unable to cooperate and potentially combative due to a mental disability or acute mental status
2. Disadvantages
   a. Risks are inherent to general anesthesia
   b. Need to arrange anesthesia coverage and transport of anesthesia equipment to the radiology suite
   c. Increased patient care costs
   d. Inhalational anesthetics have vasodilatory effects that reduce renal blood flow and glomerular filtration, which may increase the susceptibility to radiocontrast-induced nephropathy. Therefore, attention should be taken to adequately hydrate those patients that are anticipated to receive a significant volume of radiocontrast dye (18).

Other Procedural Considerations

1. **SCIP criteria.** The SCIP (Surgical Care Improvement Project) mandates periprocedural consideration of timely antibiotic dosing, glucose monitoring, and temperature monitoring and control (10). Additional equipment for dosing antibiotics and for active warming (fluid warmers, warming blankets) should be available and used as needed during procedures. Consideration for this equipment should be incorporated into the procedural planning, such as using active warming while in a scanner.
2. **Positioning.** During procedures involving sedation, a patient will not adjust body and limb position in response to reduced blood flow from compression for an

extended period. Patient's limbs and body parts should be positioned with this in mind, minimizing extreme flexion and extension of limbs and padding particularly susceptible areas, such as the ulnar nerve as it passes through ulnar groove behind the medial epicondyle of the humerus (19).

3. **Intensive care unit (ICU) patients.** ICU patients, some of who are already intubated and sedated, will present for interventional radiologic procedures. In such cases, the line is often blurred between moderate sedation and general anesthesia since sedative medications and airway devices are already in place. Many of these medications have the capability of a deeper level of sedation than desired, including general anesthesia with its concomitant hemodynamic and respiratory consequences. It is recommended that practitioners who are able to handle such consequences, as well as other complications of these medications and devices be engaged in the patient's management.

Postprocedure Management

1. **Monitoring.** Patient's vital signs should be monitored in a recovery area and observed for complications following interventional procedures performed with sedative/opioid medication, regional or general anesthesia. Of note, any patient who received naloxone or flumazenil at any time during or after sedation/analgesia shall have recovery monitoring for a minimum of 1 hour after administration of the last dose of reversal agent in recovery to assure the patient is continuously awake and alert.
2. **Discharge criteria for outpatients**
   a. Vital signs returning to preprocedural values and stable for 1 hour. Consider 1- to 2-hour additional time for OSA patients (5)
   b. Must be sufficiently recovered from sedative/hypnotic medications to allow ambulation with assistance
   c. Should return to baseline mental status
   d. Able to void and to tolerate oral fluids
3. **Discharge instructions for outpatients**
   a. Should be written and given to the responsible companion
   b. Expected problems should be listed
   c. Should have a telephone or beeper number to call for questions or complications
4. **Follow-up**
   a. Inpatient. All patients should be visited after an interventional procedure. A chart note documenting the effectiveness of sedation or anesthetic technique employed and any complications of the procedure is recommended. These comments can be invaluable in planning future interventional radiologic and surgical procedures.
   b. Outpatient. Outpatient follow-up is also important and can be accomplished via a telephone or mailed patient questionnaire.

References

1. Lind LJ, Mushlin PS. Sedation, analgesia, and anesthesia for radiologic procedures. *Cardiovasc Intervent Radiol.* 1987;10:247–253.
2. Lind LJ. Anesthetic management in surgical care of the elderly. *Oral Maxillofac Surg Clin North Am.* 1996;8(2):235–243.
3. Fleisher LA, Fleischmann KE, Auerbach AD, et al. 2014 ACC/AHA Guideline on perioperative cardiovascular evaluation and management of patients undergoing non-cardiac surgery. A Report of the American College of Cardiology/American Heart Association Task Force on Practice Guidelines *J Am Coll Cardiol.* 2014;64:e77–e137.
4. Smetana GW. Preoperative pulmonary evaluation. *N Engl J Med.* 1999;340:937–944.
5. Gross JB, Bachenberg KL, Benumof JL, et al. Practice guidelines for the perioperative management of patients with obstructive sleep apnea: a report by the American Society of

Anesthesiologists Task Force on Perioperative Management of patients with obstructive sleep apnea. *Anesthesiology*. 2006;104:1081–1093.

6. Casati A, Putzu M. Anesthesia in the obese patient: pharmacokinetic considerations. *J Clin Anesth*. 2005;17(2):134–145.

7. Stevens LA, Coresh J, Greene T, et al. Assessing kidney function—measured and estimated glomerular filtration rate. *N Engl J Med*. 2006;354(23):2473–2483.

8. Gurwitz JH, Field TS, Harrold LR, et al. Incidence and preventability of adverse drug events among older persons in the ambulatory setting. *JAMA*. 2003;289(9):1107–1116.

9. Tobin MJ. Respiratory monitoring. *JAMA*. 1990;264:244–251.

10. Specifications Manual for National Hospital Inpatient Quality Measures. https://manual.jointcommission.org/releases/archive/TJC2010B/SurgicalCareImprovementProject.html

11. Quan DJ, Kayser SR. Ketorolac induced acute renal failure following a single dose. *J Toxicol Clin Toxicol*. 1994;32(3):305–309.

12. Garnier M, Bonnet F. Management of anesthetic emergencies and complications outside the operating room. *Curr Opin Anaesthesiol*. 2014;27(4):437–441.

13. Ferrante FM, Steinbrook RA, Hughes N, et al. 1% lidocaine with and without sodium bicarbonate for attenuation of pain of skin infiltration and intravenous catheterization. *Anesthesiology*. 1991;75:A736.

14. Bailey PL, Pace NL, Ashburn MA, et al. Frequent hypoxemia and apnea after sedation with midazolam and fentanyl. *Anesthesiology*. 1990;73:826–830.

15. Etches RC. Patient controlled analgesia. *Surg Clin North Am*. 1999;79:297–312.

16. Torpe SJ, Balakrishnan VR, Cook LB. The safety of patient-controlled sedation. *Anaesthesia*. 1997;52(12):1144–1150.

17. Cousins MJ, Veering BT. Epidural neural blockade. In: Cousins MJ, Bridenbaugh PO, eds. Neural Blockade in Clinical Anesthesia and Pain Management. 3rd ed. Lippincott-Raven; 1998:243–322.

18. Brar SS, Shen AY, Jorgensen MB, et al. Sodium bicarbonate vs sodium chloride for the prevention of contrast medium-induced nephropathy in patients undergoing coronary angiography: a randomized trial. *JAMA*. 2008;300(9):1038–1046.

19. Winfree CJ, Kline DG. Intraoperative positioning nerve injuries. *Surg Neurol*. 2005;63(1):5–18.

64 Drug Administration

Denise Hegemann, BSN, RN, CRN

Preprocedural Considerations

All medication orders/administrations must be individualized considering patient's age, weight, medical and physical condition, anxiety level, allergy history, previous drug reactions, tolerance or abuse of drugs, lab data, and duration and type of procedure (1,2).

There are many steps and factors prior to medication administration, and more specifically, prior to sedation administration:

1. Obtain and document vital signs including oxygenation, American Society of Anesthesiologists Classification (ASA status), age, height, weight, past medical and surgical history, current medications, and allergies should be reviewed and documented prior to any medication administration. Comfort, anxiety, level of consciousness, and orientation should be assessed using hospital-based criteria (2,3).

2. One must consider, what are the sedation requirements for the procedure being performed? For example, is a local anesthetic such as lidocaine injection all that is required? Or does the patient require moderate sedation, deep sedation, or general anesthesia? (2,4)

a. Consultation with an anesthesiologist may be necessary in selected cases, such as when the patient has not tolerated or has failed sedation in the past; the patient is unlikely to tolerate the procedure with sedation alone; the patient has a history of difficult airway; or the patient is too critically ill (ASA status) to tolerate procedural sedation. If the patient is critically ill or will not be able to tolerate positioning, duration, or discomfort of the procedure, then an anesthesiology consult should be completed in order to evaluate the patient and provide direct care during the procedure (3).

b. The patient's nil per os (NPO) status needs to be addressed prior to any IV sedation administration. For any level of sedation above local anesthesia, the NPO requirements are usually anywhere from 2 to 8 hours. Check your institution's policies for further clarification on the requirements (2,4).

c. A licensed independent radiology provider (medical doctor, fellow, resident, physician's assistant, nurse practitioner) must evaluate the patient prior to the procedure. A focused history and physical examination including a heart, lung, and airway assessment must be obtained and documented prior to sedation administration. Current lab data, electrocardiograms (ECGs), and pertinent imaging studies should be reviewed as well. The practitioner, trained in procedural sedation and responsible for the patient's care and treatment, will discuss procedural sedation with the patient. Check your institution's policy for credentialing/certifications needed for moderate sedation administration (3).

3. A peripheral IV will be initiated, or an existing robust functioning access will be confirmed for the use of administering IV medications needed during the procedure. If any pertinent labs are needed prior to the start of the procedure, they can be drawn at the time of the IV start, or drawn separately by a phlebotomist.

4. Informed consent for the procedure and required sedation must be obtained and documented in the medical record prior to sedation administration. Informed consent should include discussion of the risks and benefits of the procedure and sedation, and alternative treatments. The patient's code status must be confirmed, and the reversal or continuance of a do-not-resuscitate (DNR)/do-not-intubate (DNI) status should be addressed, if in place.

In addition to sedation administration, there are other preprocedure medications and scenarios that may need to be addressed or considered.

1. Patients with a history of a contrast reaction may need premedication to prevent an adverse reaction or anaphylaxis to the contrast agent. A standard 13-hour prep prior to the procedure is preferred if it is an elective case. Elective procedures may be delayed or rescheduled in order for the patient to receive the full 13-hour prep. See Chapter 65 for additional information regarding contrast allergy premedication and treatment.

2. Antimicrobial prophylaxis for prevention of infections, may be required prior to puncture, prior to device deployment (i.e., stent), and/or prior to closure depending on the procedure and if any complications. The need for antimicrobial agents should be addressed in the timeout prior to the start of every procedure in order to verify if one is needed, and if so, to ensure the proper medication was ordered/given (5).

3. Antiemetics may be ordered in the preprocedure phase depending on the type of procedure being performed, and if additional nausea causing medications will be administered in the procedure (i.e., chemotherapy). Also, if the patient arrives to the facility nauseated, a preprocedure antiemetic (oral or IV) should be considered. Antiemetic prophylaxis may be recommended for patients who experience postprocedure/sedation nausea or vomiting as well (2).

4. Prior to the procedure date, a plan of care for anticoagulation use and bridging needs to be addressed by the procedural physician in cooperation with the physician or team that manages the anticoagulation for the patient. The duration of anticoagulation stoppage prior to the procedure or the need for bridging will depend on the procedure being performed and the initial indication for anticoagulation (6).

5. The need for hydration prior to the start of the procedure or during the postprocedure recovery should be considered. The patient's cardiopulmonary status should be assessed to determine tolerance if large volume or rates of fluid are to be administered, that is a CHF patient may not be able to tolerate a large volume of fluid.

Procedural Considerations

1. A qualified nurse (certified in administering procedural sedation) is assigned to one patient at a time for individualized care and monitoring during the period that the patient is in the procedural area. The procedure room must undergo a complete safety check prior to patient care. Emergency resuscitation equipment, supplies, and medications need to be readily available. All procedure areas must be equipped with the following (1):
   a. Resuscitation cart
   b. Defibrillator with multifunctional pads, paddles, and external pacemaker
   c. Full patient monitoring equipment including cardiac monitor, blood pressure monitor with a variety of sized cuffs, various oxygen delivery systems, pulse oximeter, capnography (if your institution requires), flashlight, stethoscope, thermometer.
   d. Various oral and nasopharyngeal airways, a bag-valve mask (BVM), and suction equipment.
   e. Medications including specific pharmacologic antagonists/reversal agents for the type(s) of sedation to be used, and contrast reaction kits or individual medications.
   f. All equipment must be inventoried and maintained on a regularly scheduled basis in conjunction with policies established by each institution.
2. A licensed independent provider (LIP) must be available upon the patient arrival to the procedure room, and if sedation medications are being administered.
3. Procedural sedation medications will be titrated to desired effect while maintaining adequate oxygenation and hemodynamic status (1,2,3).
   a. Blood pressure, heart rate and rhythm, respiratory rate, oxygenation and capnography (if your institution's policies require), and sedation levels should be monitored and documented at a minimum every 15 minutes (or per your institution's policies) during the procedure and for 30 minutes following the last dose of procedural sedation.
   b. Supplemental oxygen delivery is considered a medication. Orders must be written by a provider with parameters for oxygen use.
   c. Arterial hemodynamic monitoring may be used if indicated during selected procedures.
4. Additional medications may be used in the procedure areas depending on patient status and needs. Orders and medications may be needed intraprocedure for blood pressure control, anticoagulation, thrombolysis, etc. If prior to a procedure, it is known that a specific medication that is not normally used will be needed, order and verify the medication availability prior to procedure start.

Recovery and Postprocedure Care

During the recovery period and depending upon: the institution, the procedure performed, and the amount of procedural sedation, the physiologic parameters should be monitored at a minimum every 15 minutes, for 30 minutes, or until the patient reaches baseline physiologic status (prior to the administration of sedation).

Any patient receiving reversal agents requires a minimally extended recovery period of 2 hours following the last dose of reversal agents or until the patient reaches baseline as stated. Follow your institution's policies when using reversal agents (3).

Outpatients should be given written discharge instructions and on-call contact telephone numbers. A telephone follow-up is recommended at 24 hours in order to evaluate and correct, if needed, outcomes from the procedure or medications.

Table 64.1	**Abbreviations and Equivalents for Common Units**	
	Abbreviations	**Equivalents**
Microgram	μg	1,000 μg = 1 mg
Milligram	mg	1,000 mg = 1 g
Gram	g	1,000 g = 1 kg
Kilogram	kg	1 kg = 2.2 lb
Microdrop	μgtt	60 μgtt = 1 mL
Milliliter	mL	1,000 mL = 1 L

Five Rights of Medication Administration:
1. Right patient
2. Right medication
3. Right dose
4. Right route
5. Right time/frequency of administration

Dosage Calculations

Units (Table 64.1)
1. *Body weight* is measured in kilograms (kg).
2. *Drug concentration* is measured in micrograms per milliliter (μg/mL).
3. *Dosage* is measured in micrograms per kilogram (of body weight) per minute (μg/kg/min).

Calculating Infusion Doses
1. Dose in microgram per minute: dose (μg/kg/min) × body weight (kg)
2. Dose in milliliters per minute: dose (μg/min)/concentration (μg/mL)

References

1. Cornelis FH, Monard E, Moulin ME, et al. Sedation and analgesia in interventional radiology: where do we stand, where are we heading and why does it matter? *Diagn Interv Imaging.* 2019;100(12):753–762.
2. Johnson S, Sedation and analgesia in the performance of interventional procedures. *Semin Interv Radiol.* 2010;27(4):368–373.
3. Gross JB, Bailey PL, Collins RT, et al. Practice guidelines for sedation and analgesia by non-anesthesiologists. An Updated Report by the American Society of Anesthesiologists Task Force on Sedation and Analgesia by Non-Anesthesiologists. *Anesthesiology.* 2002;96(4): 1004–1017.
4. Practice guidelines for preoperative fasting and the use of pharmacologic agents to reduce the risk of pulmonary aspiration: application to healthy patients undergoing elective procedures. An Updated Report by the American Society of Anesthesiologists Task Force on preoperative fasting and the use of pharmacologic agents to reduce the risk of pulmonary aspiration. *Anesthesiology.* 2017;126:376–393.
5. Chehab MA, Thakor AS, Tulin-Silver S, et al. Adult and pediatric antibiotic prophylaxis during vascular and IR procedures: a Society of Interventional Radiology Practice Parameter Update endorsed by the Cardiovascular and Interventional Radiology Society of Europe and the Canadian Association for Interventional Radiology. *JVIR.* 2018;29(11):1483–1501.
6. Davidson JC, Rahim S, Hanks SE, et al. Society of Interventional Radiology Consensus Guidelines for the periprocedural management of thrombotic and bleeding risk in patients undergoing percutaneous image-guided interventions–Part I: Review of anticoagulation agents and clinical considerations: endorsed by the Canadian Association for Interventional Radiology and the Cardiovascular and Interventional Radiology Society of Europe. *J Vasc Interv Radiol.* 2019;30(8):1155–1167.

65 Contrast Media Reactions: Treatment and Risk Reduction

Michael A. Bettmann, MD, FSIR, FACR, FAHA

General Principles (1,2)

1. The radiologist should have the training, expertise, experience, and equipment to treat most (i.e., non–life-threatening) contrast media reactions without assistance.
2. Access to expertise and equipment for life-threatening reactions should always be readily available, including fully trained, advanced cardiac life support (ACLS)-certified personnel and full code cart, with accessible code team (1).
3. Everything needed to treat all reactions, from minor to acutely life-threatening, must be readily available and regularly updated (2,3). These include relevant medications (diphenhydramine, β-agonist inhalers, atropine, and epinephrine) and equipment (endotracheal tubes, laryngoscope, monitor, external pacemaker, and defibrillator). If not in the room, all this equipment must be located conveniently adjacent to the suite in which contrast is administered.
4. The response time to the treatment should be minimized (1). Not all contrast reactions present with a classical complex of signs and symptoms. Failure to consider and recognize that a patient is indeed having an adverse reaction may delay the appropriate treatment (3).
5. Three basic requirements for all patients:
   a. Know the patient.
   b. Recognize that there is a problem.
   c. Be prepared to deliver treatment and call for help quickly. (Know the ABCs of basic life support: Airway/Assessment, Breathing, and Circulation.)

Know the Patient

1. Before the procedure, inquire about prior exposure to iodinated contrast material, previous adverse reactions, and related relevant history.
   a. Does the patient have a history *of asthma?* If so, is the patient actively wheezing? On bronchodilators? Contrast media can provoke bronchospasm and worsen preexisting airway constriction.
   b. Does the patient have a strong history *of multiple and/or severe allergies?* This increases the risk of an adverse reaction to contrast agents.
   c. Does the patient have a history of *coronary artery disease* or other significant cardiac problem? Contrast material can compromise cardiac function (4,5).
   d. Is the patient being treated for *congestive heart failure?* Contrast material will increase the effective circulating volume and may cause pulmonary edema in poorly compensated patients.
   e. Are there any reasons why the patient may have *compromised renal function*? (see Chapter 66). This includes known renal dysfunction, bladder outlet obstruction, diabetes, and recurrent renal calculi or UTIs.
2. The radiologist performing the procedure should have knowledge of the patient's routine **medications**. Some medications may mask the symptoms of a contrast reaction.
   a. β-**Blockers** slow the heart rate and block the tachycardiac response to physiologic stress. β-Blockade blunts the effects of epinephrine (an α- and β-agonist), requiring increased doses to achieve similar physiologic effect. Once the β-blocker effect is overcome, an unopposed α-adrenergic effect of epinephrine predominates, with a marked increase in peripheral vascular resistance and a subsequent hypertensive response.

In addition, vasovagal reactions are characterized by hypotension and bradycardia. In patients on β-blocker therapy, an anaphylactoid reaction may be misjudged as a vagal reaction because of the absence of tachycardia.
b. Calcium channel blockers are frequently prescribed for hypertension, coronary insufficiency, and arrhythmias. They are peripheral vasodilators; correction of hypotension by fluid replacement may be more difficult due to persistent peripheral vasodilation.
c. Metformin, an oral hypoglycemic agent, can rarely lead to lactic acidosis, which is fatal in a high percentage of patients. The risk of lactic acidosis is increased in patients with compromised renal function (4). Updated guidance has lowered caution of metformin and contrast. The major concern is not contrast but depressed eGFR (see Chapter 66). In patients with a GFR <30 metformin should be discontinued at the time of the procedure and restarted after 48 hours if there is no compromise of renal function from the study performed.
d. NSAIDs are widely used. Some think that high-dose NSAID use may predispose to CIN, although there are no studies to support this concern.

Recognize That There Is a Problem

1. Look for the classical and more subtle signs that the patient is having an adverse reaction.
   a. First, talk to the patient and assess ABC status. Many "reactions" may simply be manifestations of *anxiety*, with resultant tachypnea and lightheadedness.
   b. *Dermal reactions:* Urticaria, pruritus, diffuse erythema, skin flushing. May only be seen if specifically looked for (6).
   c. "*Angioedema*" may present with increased production of tears, difficulty in swallowing, nasal congestion, or laryngeal edema with hoarseness. Facial edema may also occur, albeit rarely.
   d. *Bronchospasm* occurs almost solely in patients with *asthma*. It is characterized by dyspnea, sometimes tachypnea and *end-expiratory wheezing*. *Laryngospasm*, on the other hand, is less frequent and more concerning. It is characterized by *stridor or inspiratory wheezing*.
   e. Sudden *loss of consciousness* may have a CNS, cardiac, or pulmonary mechanism. It is crucial that vital signs be evaluated to try to distinguish the cause, so that appropriate treatment can be given immediately.
   f. *Vagal reactions* are characterized by lightheadedness, feelings of anxiety, diaphoresis, hypotension, and bradycardia. Full-blown *anaphylactoid reactions*, which are far less frequent than vagal reactions, are characterized by *hypotension, tachycardia* and, often, *loss of consciousness.*
   g. Other *mental status changes*, such as confusion, are rare, usually not related to a contrast agent, and most often due to sedation or other medication, or to a cerebral event.
2. All patients in an interventional lab should have continuous BP monitoring. With patients who receive contrast for CT-guided procedures or IV urography this is advisable but less stringent. The person in attendance (radiologist, RN, RT) will have to depend on the physical signs and the patient's symptoms to determine whether the patient is having an adverse reaction. At a minimum, then, close observation is always necessary.

Be Prepared to Deliver Treatment Quickly and Call for Help Early

Evaluate the situation, categorize the type of adverse reaction and patient status, and determine:
1. Is immediate treatment necessary and, if so, which specifically?
2. Is continued monitoring alone appropriate?

Regardless of whether the patient is monitored or treatment is started, re-evaluate the patient frequently and decide whether the situation is worsening, stabilizing, or improving. Always document as promptly and thoroughly as you can. Monitoring, with documentation, must be continuous until the reaction resolves.

Treatment of Adverse Reactions (Table 65.1)

1. Cutaneous
   a. Urticaria: Often but not always associated with pruritus—essentially always self-limited. Incidence increases if looked for (i.e., often is asymptomatic, covered by draping/gowns). Treat for symptoms, with diphenhydramine (Benadryl), 25 to 50 mg PO or IV. Caution patients not to drive after this treatment. **Not** a good predictor of a recurrent reaction, particularly not a more severe one.
   b. Generalized exanthem: Rare. May be associated with cardiovascular collapse (i.e., a severe, full-blown anaphylactoid reaction). Treat symptomatically—if

Table 65.1 **Treatment of Major Adverse Reactions**

Symptoms	Treatment (in Order of Increasing Severity)
Symptomatic urticaria	25–50 mg diphenhydramine IM or IV
Bronchospasm	1. Nasal oxygen, IV access, monitor ECG and oxygen saturation 2. β-Agonist inhaler (metaproterenol, terbutaline, albuterol) 3. Epinephrine 1:1,000, 0.1–1.0 mL SC *or* 4. Epinephrine 1:10,000, 1.0–3.0 mL IV
Laryngotracheal edema or symptomatic facial edema	1, 3, then 4 (NOT a β-agonist inhaler)
Pulmonary edema	1. Oxygen, IV access; monitor ECG and oxygen saturation 2. Elevate head; apply rotating extremity tourniquets 3. Furosemide 40 mg slow IV push—carefully monitor respiratory status, BP 4. Morphine 1–10 mg slow IV push
Vagal reaction (hypotension and bradycardia)	1. Monitor vital signs, ensure IV access 2. Elevate legs (more effective than Trendelenburg position) 3. Push IV fluids 4. As needed to stabilize BP and pulse, atropine 0.6–2.0 mg IV push (0.5-mg increments) 5. Crucial consideration to avoid significant complications is observation and treatment until vital signs return to baseline levels
Seizure	1. Diazepam 1–10 mg IV push, in 1-mg increments 2. Monitor vital signs 3. Obtain neurologic consultation
Cardiopulmonary arrest	1. Monitor vital signs and ECG 2. Ensure IV access 3. Ensure functional airway 4. Begin resuscitation 5. Call code team (*try to do 1–5 simultaneously*) 6. Epinephrine 1:10,000, IV 1–3 mL

associated with hypotension and tachycardia, will require epinephrine 1:10,000 IV.

c. Delayed: Incidence as high as 9%, but often not recognized, as these may occur 24 hours to 10 days postcontrast and are often ascribed to other causes, such as clopidogrel, warfarin, use of a new laundry detergent. Take various forms, but most often maculopapular rash. Tend to recur on exposure to a contrast agent, particularly with the same contrast agent; these appear to be uniquely T-cell immune-mediated. Rarely may be severe and life-threatening (i.e., Stevens–Johnson syndrome). Treat symptomatically, with topical steroids or, as needed, systemic steroids. Consider dermatology consult (6).

d. Contrast extravasation: Not usually a cause of major concern or complications, particularly with low osmolality contrast agents and limited volume. May be a concern in the pediatric age group, in diabetics with neuropathy or vasculopathy, or if volume of extravasation is very large. Treatment is symptomatic: cold or hot soaks early, rarely surgical consult for pressure release. Compartment syndrome is possible but almost never occurs (7).

2. Pulmonary
   a. Bronchospasm: Generally seen in patients with active asthma, rarely if ever in others. Treat as needed symptomatically. β-Agonist inhalers are usually sufficient, with monitoring of pulse oximetry and supplemental oxygen as needed. Occasionally, may need epinephrine (either 0.1 to 0.3 mL of 1:1,000 given subcutaneously or 1 to 3 mL of 1:10,000 given IV).
   b. Laryngospasm: Rare; may be a component of generalized edema. If symptomatic, treat with nonrebreather O_2 mask, IV epinephrine (1:10,000 dilution), and observe until symptoms and signs (i.e., stridor, inspiratory wheezing) resolve completely.
   c. Tachypnea: A not infrequent anxiety reaction. Generally not associated with any further signs or symptoms and requires only reassurance and occasionally sedation. Nasal O_2 may help.

3. Generalized systemic
   All such reactions, including diffuse erythema, should be considered potentially life-threatening. Patients should be observed and evaluated with the BLS ABCs.
   a. Vasovagal: More common than anaphylactoid reactions, may be hard to diagnose. Characterized by anxiety, diaphoresis, hypotension, and bradycardia. Not a true contrast reaction—usually related to general anxiety. Generally benign in course, but **MUST** *be followed and treated until full resolution.* Treatment: Raise legs (more effective than Trendelenburg position at increasing intravascular volume), IV fluids, atropine as needed (0.6 to 1.0 mg IV, repeat as needed).
   b. Respiratory: O_2 via nonrebreather mask, β-agonist (metaproterenol or similar) inhaler for bronchospasm, epinephrine SC (1:1,000, 0.1 to 0.3 mL) or IV (1:10,000, 1 to 3 mL) if bronchospasm is unresponsive and for laryngospasm/edema.
   c. Cardiovascular.
      (1) Vasovagal (see above): fluids, leg elevation, atropine (minimum 0.6 to 1.0 mg) IV.
      (2) Anaphylactoid: Characterized by hypotension, tachycardia, often loss of consciousness. Treatment is symptomatic: fluids, particularly if there is vascular compromise (e.g., severe hypotension), general vascular support; use epinephrine 1:10,000, 1 to 3 mL IV as needed. Call code team (better to call too early than too late!).
      (3) VT/ventricular fibrillation: Call code, initiate cardioversion.
      (4) Pulmonary edema: Again, may be caused not by the contrast per se but rather by acute cardiac decompensation with or without acute volume expansion. May be indicative of an acute myocardial infarction.

d. Seizures: Diazepam 1 mg IV in increments to effect, with careful monitoring of respiratory status.

4. Remember:
   a. Hypotension + bradycardia = vasovagal reaction.
   b. Hypotension + tachycardia = anaphylactoid or cardiac reaction. *Note:* If patient is on a β-blocker, tachycardiac response may be blunted or absent.
   c. Respiratory distress with a wet cough and pink frothy sputum = pulmonary edema. Consider: Is this patient having an acute myocardial infarction? Treat with O_2, rotating tourniquets, morphine, and furosemide.
   d. Corticosteroids and diphenhydramine have no role in the acute treatment of contrast reactions, due to both the pathophysiology of the reaction and the delayed action of these medications in an acute setting. The key treatments to consider are IV fluids, epinephrine, and atropine.
   e. Epinephrine is an extremely potent medication, with a relatively narrow toxic-to-therapeutic ratio. Use only with caution. Secondly, if needed, particularly with cardiovascular collapse, subcutaneous administration may not be effectively absorbed in a timely manner.

Prophylaxis for Contrast Media Reactions (8)

Most would consider a history of prior reaction to the same class of contrast media to be the highest risk factor for contrast reaction. Other risk factors include asthma, allergies to other substances, and some atopic conditions. Although there isn't level I evidence that prophylaxis prevents reactions in high-risk patients most centers do give premedication. The most common is the Modified Greenberger Protocol, prednisone 50 mg by mouth (PO) 13, 7, and 1 hour prior to contrast administration; the last dose is given in combination with either diphenhydramine (Benadryl) 50 mg intravenously (IV) or PO. Alternatives include the Lasser Protocol, 32 mg oral methylprednisolone 12 and 2 hours prior. Some add diphenhydramine 50 mg to the last dose. A further alternative for emergent situations uses 200 mg IV hydrocortisone immediately then every 4 hours prior to contrast administration with 50 mg IV diphenhydramine 1 hour prior.

References

1. Merchant RM, Topjian AA, Panchal AR, et al. Adult Basic and Advanced Life Support, Pediatric Basic and Advanced Life Support, Neonatal Life Support, Resuscitation Education Science, and Systems of Care Writing Groups. Part 1: Executive Summary: 2020 American Heart Association Guidelines for Cardiopulmonary Resuscitation and Emergency Cardiovascular Care. *Circulation*. 2020;142(16_suppl_2):S337–S357. doi: 10.1161/CIR.0000000000000918
2. Wang CL, Soloff EV. Contrast reaction readiness for your department or facility. *Radiol Clin North Am*. 2020;58(5):841–850. doi: 10.1016/j.rcl.2020.04.002
3. Jacquet GA, Hamade B, Diab KA, et al. The emergency department crash cart: a systematic review and suggested contents. *World J Emerg Med*. 2018;9(2):93–98. doi:10.5847/wjem.j.1920-8642.2018.02.002
4. Bush WH Jr. Treatment of acute contrast reactions. In: Bush WH Jr, Krecke KN, King BF Jr, et al., eds. Radiology Life Support. Oxford University Press, 1999:31–51.
5. Fleetwood G, MA. The effects of radiographic contrast media on myocardial contractility and coronary resistance in the isolated rat heart model. *Invest Radiol*. 1990;25(3):254–260.
6. Tasker F, Fleming H, McNeill G, et al. Contrast media and cutaneous reactions. Part 2: Delayed hypersensitivity reactions to iodinated contrast media. *Clin Exp Dermatol*. 2019;44(8):844–860. doi: 10.1111/ced.13991
7. Sonis JD, Gottumukkala RV, Glover M IV, et al. Implications of iodinated contrast media extravasation in the emergency department. *Am J Emerg Med*. 2018;36(2):294–296. doi: 10.1016/j.ajem.2017.11.012
8. Davenport MS, Cohan RH. The evidence for and against corticosteroid prophylaxis in at-risk patients. *Radiol Clin North Am*. 2017;55(2):413–421.

66 Contrast-Induced Nephropathy: Prevention and Management

Michael A. Bettmann, MD, FSIR, FACR, FAHA

Introduction

Contrast-induced nephropathy (CIN) may occur after administration of any iodine-based contrast agent. Although it rarely leads to the need for temporary or permanent renal replacement therapy, it is usually limited to a transient decrease in renal function, with return to or near baseline by 2 to 4 weeks. Clinically relevant CIN occurs essentially only in patients with a baseline compromise in renal function. CIN's importance is not the occasional need for renal replacement therapy (i.e., dialysis), but rather that its occurrence is associated with increased all-cause morbidity and mortality. The most widely used diagnostic criterion currently is an increase in serum creatinine (SCr) of 25% or 50% ≤48 hours after contrast administration. Many questions remain about the incidence and the pathophysiology, but studies have improved understanding of clinical relevance and approaches (1–3).

Pathophysiology

In the past, CIN was thought to be caused by alterations in blood flow to the kidneys, but this has been disproven, largely through the results of various studies on prophylaxis. CIN is now thought to be caused by alterations in the region of the thick ascending limb of the loop of Henle in the outer medulla, an area in which oxygen tension is normally borderline ischemic and lower than elsewhere in the tubules. It is likely that this area becomes hypoxic because of the effect of contrast administration. This leads to the formation of oxygen-free radicals and subsequent cellular damage. The precise reason for hypoxia is unknown; various theories have hypothesized a causative effect of hypertonicity, hyperviscosity, vascular spasm, and direct tissue toxicity (1,4).

Diagnosis

CIN is defined most often as a 25%, 50%, or, less relevantly, as a 0.5 mg per dL increase in SCr. The definitions used have sometimes even been changed to help support a hypothesis that is not statistically supported by the more common definitions. The estimated glomerular filtration rate (eGFR) is useful for better defining risk, but is not entirely accurate for defining incidence of CIN, for the three reasons: (1) SCr can vary fairly widely from day to day, thus significantly altering the calculated GFR; (2) creatinine rise lags behind an insult by as much as 1 to 3 days, so acute changes in renal function will not necessarily be reflected in the eGFR; and (3) although the actual risk of CIN is better defined by using an eGFR as derived from either the Cockroft–Gault or MDRD formula, both of which take age, gender, and body mass into account, neither formula has been completely validated in large populations over varying levels of renal function (5,6). Neither formula has been well validated for acute changes in renal function, nor have they been used extensively in studies of CIN.

Studies suggest that although the renal injury occurs fairly rapidly, serum creatinine may not rise for 24 to 48 hours. A more reliable measurement for acute renal injury is clearly needed (7). Cystatin C has been used in some studies, but its validation and availability remain unclear (8). For now, the best approach to making a clinically relevant diagnosis of CIN is to obtain a baseline serum creatinine and eGFR, followed in those at risk by a serum creatinine at 24 and/or 48 hours, with repeated measurements for 7 to 14 days if an initial elevation is seen. Although a rise in serum creatinine at 24 hours has been shown to be the single best predictor for CIN currently (9), due to normal day-to-day variations in serum creatinine, a single such measurement may be neither sufficiently sensitive nor sufficiently accurate.

Incidence

The incidence depends on risk factors, the definition of CIN, and perhaps, somewhat surprisingly, on route administration. All iodinated contrast agents are rapidly distributed throughout the intravascular space following injection. They are excreted by glomerular filtration without resorption or tubular excretion and have a T1/2 of less than an hour. The incidence of CIN approaches zero in patients with truly normal renal function or mild (stages 1 to 3a) chronic kidney disease. In patients with stage 3b or worse chronic kidney disease (GFR <45 mL/min/ 1.73 m^2), the incidence may be as high as 20% to 40%. Arriving at an accurate definition of incidence is difficult for other reasons as well: for example, particularly among hospitalized patients, there are many potentially nephrotoxic risk factors, including surgery, hypotension, CHF, and many medications. Many elderly patients with normal SCr have decreased renal function. GFR decreases with increasing age, as does muscle mass. As skeletal muscle is the source of SCr, in small elderly patients, normal SCr may actually correlate to a significant decrease in GFR. It is often difficult, therefore, to be certain that a specific occurrence of transient increase in SCr is actually solely or even primarily related to contrast administration (3,10,11).

Natural History

In most cases CIN develops with an increase in serum creatinine over days 1 to 7 after contrast administration, with a return to baseline renal function by 2 to 4 weeks. Development of end-stage renal disease is rare, even in patients with significantly compromised renal function (CKD Gr>3a) (3,10). The real concern, then, as shown in several large longitudinal studies (2,3), is that there is an increase in cardiovascular and all-cause major morbidity and mortality among those who develop CIN as compared to controls. It is rare that renal replacement therapy (either acute or chronic dialysis) is needed, on the order of 1% even in those at risk (9), and the incidence of major delayed morbidity/mortality varies as a function of associated risk factors, such as age and cardiovascular comorbidities (11).

Risk Factors

1. In patients with truly normal renal function (i.e., not just normal serum creatinine but also normal eGFR) the risk is very low, probably even absent. See the caveat below, however, regarding acute changes in renal function due to changes in renal perfusion.
2. Patients with preexisting renal dysfunction are at risk. Although it is logical to think that the risk increases with increasing CKD grade, it is not clear that this is true. The reason is that it is likely that numerous other risk factors play a role in the incidence and severity of CIN (e.g., nephrotoxic medications, poor cardiac output).
3. The risk is increased roughly by a factor of 2 in patients with diabetes mellitus (11). Again, the risk appears to be confined to those with a GFR ≤60 mL/min/1.73 m^2. This risk has been shown almost solely in patients with type I diabetes; the risk among the increasing population with type II diabetes is not clearly defined. There is likely to be an increased risk, as a function of the duration and severity of the diabetes.
4. Increasing age also is a risk factor, again only in those with compromised renal function. It is important to remember that renal function normally

decreases with age, as reflected in eGFR but NOT necessarily in serum creatinine.

5. Dehydration is thought to be a major risk factor. Many elderly patients are relatively dehydrated at baseline. Furthermore, it has unfortunately been a usual practice to keep patients NPO for 12 or more hours prior to procedures, thereby worsening dehydration. This is in large part done for forgotten reasons (perhaps related to the fear of nausea, vomiting, and aspiration after contrast administration). NPO status is generally not necessary, unless there are other overarching reasons. Even in patients who are to receive sedation, there is no need to avoid fluid intake for more than 3 to 4 hours prior to the procedure.

6. Poor renal perfusion is also a concern, and this may occur in the presence of heart failure, severe trauma with major blood loss, or other causes of hypotension or volume loss (e.g., major surgery). These situations may lead to an acute decrease in renal function that is not necessarily reflected in serum creatinine.

7. Various medications are thought to predispose to CIN. These include the aminoglycosides (known to be nephrotoxic), angiotensin-converting enzyme (ACE) inhibitors, beta blockers, and diuretics. To date, there is reason for caution with certain known nephrotoxins (aminoglycosides, certain chemotherapy drugs) but not with most drugs. Nonsteroidal antiinflammatory medications block prostacyclins that are important in intrarenal vasodilatation. In the presence of vasoconstriction, as in heart failure, high-dose NSAID use may precipitate renal failure. Vasoconstriction, however, is not thought to be a major factor in the etiology of CIN, so NSAID use in general is not likely an important factor in the development of CIN.

8. *Metformin* is a separate consideration. It is not directly nephrotoxic. There may, however, be a very rare incidence of associated lactic acidosis which can be fatal in up to 50%. Due to hepatic metabolism and renal excretion, the effect of metformin is prolonged in the presence of renal (or hepatic) failure. Metformin is, therefore, contraindicated in patients with severe hepatic disease or poor hepatic or renal perfusion (as in chronic CHF). Recommendations on stopping metformin before contrast administration have evolved and regulatory agencies have relaxed their concerns (12). The American College of Radiology Manual on Contrast Media, 2022 (13) recommends:

   a. In patients who are known to have GFR <30, or are undergoing arterial catheter studies that might result in emboli to the renal arteries, metformin should be discontinued at the time of the procedure and restarted after 48 hours if there is no compromise of renal function.

   b. In patients with no evidence of AKI and with eGFR ≥30 mL/min, there is no need to discontinue metformin either prior to or following the intravenous administration of iodinated contrast media, nor is there an obligatory need to reassess the patient's renal function following the test or procedure.

   c. Patients taking metformin are not at higher risk than other patients for post-contrast acute kidney injury.

9. Paraproteinemias such as multiple myeloma are also a separate concern. Renal failure related to these diseases occurs because of underlying dehydration, with resultant precipitation of protein in the renal tubules and consequent, often irreversible renal failure. The concern in these patients is not the contrast agents; use of contrast is safe as long as patients are well hydrated before, during, and after contrast administration.

Patient Preparation

Prior to contrast administration, it is important to determine whether or not there are any risk factors present, primarily underlying renal dysfunction. In generally healthy, younger individuals, this can be accomplished effectively by obtaining a good history. The crucial questions are:

1. Do you have diabetes?
2. Do you have kidney problems?
3. Do you have a history of kidney stones, urinary tract infections, or prostate or bladder problems?
4. What medicines do you take?

It is also important to evaluate patients for dehydration (skin turgor, blood pressure, history) and to try to achieve and maintain adequate intravascular volume, through both oral and parenteral hydration before, during, and after the administration of contrast.

Prophylaxis

There are currently no effective means of treating CIN after it has developed. There have, however, been major advances in prevention (14–16). The approach that is best supported by evidence and is most widely accepted is *hydration*. Studies suggest that:

1. IV hydration is more effective than oral (perhaps only because it is more reliable).
2. Normal saline is more effective than half normal saline.
3. 12 hours of NS is more effective than 4 hours.

The usual protocol, if feasible, is 12-hour prehydration with NS at 1 mL/kg/h, followed by continued hydration at the same rate during and after the procedure, for 6 to 12 hours. This regimen is obviously not practical for most outpatients. In these patients, oral hydration should be strongly encouraged and carefully explained, and IV hydration should be started as soon as possible. At least as importantly, dehydration should be avoided as much as possible, recognizing that patients may need to be NPO for 3 to 4 hours prior to sedation (depending on local standards).

Many other approaches to prophylaxis have been tried, essentially all in conjunction with some hydration protocol, with conflicting results. These include the use of furosemide (Lasix) (17), dopamine, fenoldopam (a dopamine agonist), atrial natriuretic peptide, a prostacyclin analog, salicylic acid, and statins (18). Theophylline is promising, but has a relatively narrow toxic-to-therapeutic ratio, making it difficult to use (19). Hemofiltration and acute hemodialysis have also been used, with mixed results, some associated risks, and substantial associated cost (20). In addition to saline hydration, the two most widely investigated and widely used prophylactic tools are n-acetyl cysteine (nAC) and sodium bicarbonate ($NaHCO_3$) hydration. nAC is most widely used in treatment of acetaminophen overdose.

1. nAC: There have been numerous studies of nAC as well as several large meta-analyses (18–20). The largest prospective randomized trial showed no benefit over placebo (21) but the bottom line is some physicians do feel nAC may be effective, with results dependent on timing, route of administration (oral vs. IV) and total dose. The usual dose of nAC has been 600 mg po twice on the day before and twice on the day of contrast administration. Four oral doses of 1,200 mg with the same dose schedule have been shown to be more effective (22). This double dose is justified because the medication is inexpensive, safe, gener ally well tolerated (but for an unappealing smell), and may be helpful.
2. $NaHCO_3$: This has been widely used but its efficacy remains unclear. Although early studies showed effectiveness, others show no benefit over saline (21). An additive effect with the use of both nAC and $NaHCO_3$ as compared to either alone has been suggested (23). The mechanism of action of $NaHCO_3$ is not known, but is thought to relate to preventing the development of a very acidic pH and consequent free radical formation and tissue damage in the tubules in the outer medullary region of the kidneys. As with nAC, $NaHCO_3$ is generally safe and well tolerated, inexpensive, fairly easy to use, and possibly effective (23,24). The most common protocol for use is three vials of $NaHCO_3$ (approximately 1,000 mEq) in

1,000 mL D_5W, given at 3 mL/kg for 1 hour before the procedure and then 1 mL/kg/h over 6 hours following the procedure.
3. Many other means of prophylaxis have been investigated. Some, including statin therapy, are promising (16,24) but their efficacy is not yet conclusively proven.

The Role of Specific Contrast Agents

The traditional high-osmolality contrast agents widely used in the past, are used only, and rarely, for nonvascular studies in the first world. They do not increase the risk of CIN in patients with normal renal function, but they do lead to a higher incidence in patients with underlying renal dysfunction. In one very large study, the incidence of CIN with high-osmolality (HOCA) versus low-osmolality (LOCA) agents was equal in patients with normal serum creatinine, slightly higher in patients with an elevated creatinine without diabetes, and much higher in patients with both elevated creatinine and diabetes (25). There has been an ongoing debate in the literature as to whether or not there is a difference in the incidence of CIN between most LOCA and the single available isotonic contrast agent, iodixanol (Visipaque, GE Healthcare, Princeton, NJ). Several studies have suggested that iodixanol is less nephrotoxic, while others have not shown a benefit. More recently, data seem to have accumulated that do confirm the benefit of iodixanol, although it may not be great (25–27). The major downside to the use of iodixanol is that it costs more. Consequently, it may be helpful to use iodixanol in patients with renal dysfunction (eGFR <60 mL/min/1.73 m^2), particularly if large volume contrast use (>100 mL) is anticipated.

Other Considerations

1. Patients on acute or chronic renal replacement therapy (hemodialysis, peritoneal dialysis).
   These patients do not appear to have an added risk from the nephrotoxicity of contrast agents. It should be kept in mind, however, that these patients usually have some residual renal function, and the more that is preserved, the lower the overall morbidity and mortality. It is important, therefore, to limit contrast volume as much as possible in these patients. Prophylaxis, other than hydration as possible, is not usually considered. Keep in mind, however, that increased intravascular volume is often a concern.
2. Patients with heart failure or poor cardiac output. Such individuals may be at increased risk both from volume overload and from poor renal perfusion that may lead to decreased renal function. The usual prophylactic approaches should be undertaken, again with the proviso that fluid volume may be a real concern.
3. The use of carbon dioxide as a contrast agent is considered safe (28), inexpensive and an effective, for certain intraarterial situations and is not nephrotoxic. Some (Group II) gadolinium-based contrast agents have been thought to cause nephrogenic systemic fibrosis in patients with chronic renal disease, particularly those with eGFR ≤30 mL/min/1.73 m^2. They may be a trigger rather than a cause, and the risk is low and likely not confined to those with renal dysfunction. Nonetheless, Gd-based agents should in general be avoided in patients with low eGFR (29,30).
4. Other causes of nephrotoxicity.
   As noted, there are many. This has led some to question whether or not CIN is a real clinical concern; there is little doubt that it occurs with intracardiac or other intraarterial use, but the incidence with IV use remains in question (31). While it is very likely that it does occur, comorbidities are so hard to exclude that this remains a real question. Regardless, whenever the administration of contrast is considered, it is important to answer three questions:

  a. Is contrast administration truly necessary?

  b. Are there risks that might predispose to worsening renal dysfunction? Medications, dehydration, CHF, surgery.

  c. Is prophylaxis a practical consideration?

The answers depend on the individual patient and clinical setting. Ultrasound or MRI may not be viable alternatives. In the presence of an acute, life-threatening trauma, it is usually not appropriate to delay a contrast-enhanced CT to allow for administration of prophylactic hydration and nAC. Finally, it is important to be aware that factors other than contrast administration, such as other medications or cholesterol emboli related to an angiographic or surgical procedure, may be the true cause of worsened renal function (32).

References

1. Bettmann MA. Contrast medium-induced nephropathy: critical review of the existing clinical evidence. *Nephrol Dial Transplant.* 2005;20(suppl 1):i12–i17.

2. Rihal CS, Textor SC, Grill DE, et al. Incidence and prognostic importance of acute renal failure after percutaneous coronary intervention. *Circulation.* 2002;105(19):2259–2264.

3. Mehran R, Dangas GD, Weisbord SD. Contrast-associated acute kidney injury. *N Engl J Med.* 2019;380(22):2146–2155. doi: 10.1056/NEJM

4. Vlachopanos G, Schizas D, Hasemaki N, et al. Pathophysiology of contrast-induced acute kidney injury (CIAKI). *Curr Pharm Des.* 2019;25(44):4642–4647. doi: 10.2174/13816128256 66191210152944

5. Michels WM, Grootendorst DC, Verduijn M, et al. Performance of the Cockcroft-Gault, MDRD, and new CKD-EPI formulas in relation to GFR, age, and body size. *Clin J Am Soc Nephrol.* 2010;5(6):1003–1009. doi: 10.2215/CJN.06870909

6. Inker LA, Schmid CH, Tighiouart H, et al. Estimating glomerular filtration rate from serum creatinine and cystatin C. *N Engl J Med.* 2012;367(1):20–29. doi: 10.1056/NEJMoa1114248. Erratum in: N Engl J Med. 2012 Aug 16;367(7):681. Erratum in: N Engl J Med. 2012 Nov 22;367(21):2060.

7. Khan MS, Bakris GL, Shahid I, et al. Potential role and limitations of estimated glomerular filtration rate slope assessment in cardiovascular trials: a review. *JAMA Cardiol.* 2022. doi:10.1001/jamacardio.2021.5151

8. Ferguson TW, Komenda P, Tangri N. Cystatin C as a biomarker for estimating glomerular filtration rate. *Curr Opin Nephrol Hypertens.* 2015;24(3):295–300. doi: 10.1097/MNH. 0000000000000115

9. Vanmassenhove J, Kielstein J, Jörres A, et al. Management of patients at risk of acute kidney injury. *Lancet.* 2017;389(10084):2139–2151. doi: 10.1016/S0140-6736(17)31329-6

10. Valdenor C, McCullough PA, Paculdo D, et al. Measuring the variation in the prevention and treatment of CI-AKI among interventional cardiologists. *Curr Probl Cardiol.* 2021;46(9):100851. doi: 10.1016/j.cpcardiol.2021.100851

11. Mehran R, Owen R, Chiarito M, et al. A contemporary simple risk score for prediction of contrast-associated acute kidney injury after percutaneous coronary intervention: derivation and validation from an observational registry. *Lancet.* 2021;398(10315):1974–1983. doi: 10.1016/S0140-6736(21)02326-6

12. https://www.fda.gov/drugs/fda-drug-safety-podcasts/fda-drug-safety-podcast-fda-revises-warnings-regarding-use-diabetes-medicine-metformin-certain.

13. American College of Radiology Manual on Contrast Media. 2022. https://www.acr.org/-/media/acr/files/clinical-resources/contrast_media.pdf.

14. Pistolesi V, Regolisti G, Morabito S, et al. Contrast medium induced acute kidney injury: a narrative review. *J Nephrol.* 2018;31(6):797–812. doi: 10.1007/s40620-018-0498-y

15. Faucon AL, Bobrie G, Clément O. Nephrotoxicity of iodinated contrast media: from pathophysiology to prevention strategies. *Eur J Radiol.* 2019;116:231–241. doi: 10.1016/j.ejrad.2019.03.008

16. Evidence review for preventing contrast-induced acute kidney injury: Acute kidney injury: prevention, detection and management. National Institute for Health and Care Excellence (NICE); 2019.

17. Hu M, Yan G, Tang H, et al. Effect of combining furosemide with standard hydration therapy on contrast-induced acute kidney injury following coronary angiography or intervention in a high-risk population. *Angiology.* 2021;72(2):138–144. doi: 10.1177/0003319720959968

18. Xinwei J, Xianghua F, Jing Z, et al. Comparison of usefulness of simvastatin 20 mg versus 80 mg in preventing contrast-induced nephropathy in patients with acute coronary syndrome undergoing percutaneous coronary intervention. *Am J Cardiol.* 2009;104(4):519–524.

19. Bagshaw SM, Ghali WA. Theophylline for prevention of contrast-induced nephropathy: a systematic review and meta-analysis [Review]. *Arch Intern Med.* 2005;165(10):1087–1093

20. Hölscher B, Heitmeyer C, Fobker M, et al. Predictors for contrast media-induced nephropathy and long-term survival: prospectively assessed data from the randomized controlled Dialysis-Versus-Diuresis (DVD) trial. *Can J Cardiol.* 2008;24(11):845–850.

21. Weisbord SD, Gallagher M, Jneid H, et al. Outcomes after angiography with sodium bicarbonate and acetylcysteine. *N Engl J Med.* 2018;378(7):603e14.

22. Briguori C, Airoldi F, D'Andrea D, et al. Renal insufficiency following contrast media administration trial (REMEDIAL): a randomized comparison of 3 preventive strategies. *Circulation.* 2007;115(10):1211–1217.

23. Recio-Mayoral A, Chaparro M, Prado B, et al. The reno-protective effect of hydration with sodium bicarbonate plus N-acetylcysteine in patients undergoing emergency percutaneous coronary intervention: the RENO study. *J Am Coll Cardiol.* 2007;49(12):1283–1288.

24. Su X, Xie X, Liu L, et al. Comparative effectiveness of 12 treatment strategies for preventing contrast-induced acute kidney injury: a systematic review and Bayesian network meta-analysis. *Am J Kidney Dis.* 2017;69(1):69–77. doi: 10.1053/j.ajkd.2016.07.033

25. Rudnick MR, Goldfarb S, Wexler L, et al. Nephrotoxicity of ionic and nonionic contrast media in 1196 patients: a randomized trial. The Iohexol Cooperative Study. *Kidney Int.* 1995;47(1):254–261.

26. Reed M, Meier P, Tamhane UU, et al. The relative renal safety of iodixanol compared with low-osmolar contrast media: a meta-analysis of randomized controlled trials. *JACC Cardiovasc Interv.* 2009;2(7):645–654.

27. Han XF, Zhang XX, Liu KM, et al. Contrast-induced nephropathy in patients with diabetes mellitus between iso- and low-osmolar contrast media: a meta-analysis of full-text prospective, randomized controlled trials. *PLoS One.* 2018;13(3):e0194330. doi: 10.1371/journal.pone.0194330

28. Hawkins IF, Cho KJ, Caridi JG. Carbon dioxide in angiography to reduce the risk of contrast-induced nephropathy. *Radiol Clin North Am.* 2009;47(5):813–825, v–vi. doi: 10.1016/j.rcl.2009.07.002

29. Woolen SA, Shankar PR, Gagnier JJ, et al. Risk of nephrogenic systemic fibrosis in patients with stage 4 or 5 chronic kidney disease receiving a group II gadolinium-based contrast agent: a systematic review and meta-analysis. *JAMA Intern Med.* 2020;180(2):223–230. doi: 10.1001/jamainternmed.2019.5284

30. Leyba K, Wagner B. Gadolinium-based contrast agents: why nephrologists need to be concerned. *Curr Opin Nephrol Hypertens.* 2019;28(2):154–162. doi: 10.1097/MNH.0000000000000475

31. Goulden R, Rowe BH, Abrahamowicz M, et al. Association of intravenous radiocontrast with kidney function: a regression discontinuity analysis. *JAMA Intern Med.* 2021;181(6):767–774. doi: 10.1001/jamainternmed.2021.0916

32. Quill IW. Atheroembolic renal disease: underdiagnosed and misunderstood. *Catheter Cardiovasc Interv.* 2007;70(6):789–790.

67 Noninvasive Physiologic Evaluation: Lower Extremity Arteries

Joseph F. Polak, MD, MPH, FAIUM, FACR

Segmental Pressure Measurements of the Lower Extremity: Ankle–Brachial Index and Stress Testing

Indications (1,2)

1. History of claudication
2. Clinical findings of arterial insufficiency
3. Prognostic indicator for healing of skin lesions of the toes or feet
4. Postoperative surveillance of infrainguinal bypass grafts (traditional)
5. Short- and long-term follow-up of endovascular interventions, including thrombolysis, balloon angioplasty, and endovascular stenting

Contraindications

1. Open wounds
2. Recent surgery
3. Bypass graft or stent at level of pressure cuff placement

Preprocedure Preparation

None

Procedure

1. **Segmental pressure:** Pressure cuffs are positioned around the upper and lower thigh and the upper and lower calf. The segments have been designated high thigh (HT), above-knee (AK), below-knee (BK), and ankle (A). Most commonly, cuffs of 10 to 12 cm in diameter with expandable bladders long enough to encircle the extremity are used. One thigh cuff is occasionally used.
2. Doppler signals are detected in either the dorsalis pedis or the posterior tibial artery.
3. Each blood pressure (BP) cuff is inflated and then in turn slowly deflated until a Doppler signal returns and is detected in the dorsalis pedis or posterior tibial artery. This is the segmental systolic pressure.
4. A systolic BP measurement is taken from both arms at the brachial artery. By convention, the higher of the two systolic pressure values is used to calculate the pressure index for both legs. A greater than 10 mm Hg difference in the brachial systolic pressures should prompt an investigation of the upper extremity arteries.
5. **Ankle–brachial index** (ABI): This is a ratio calculated by dividing the systolic ankle pressures by the systolic brachial pressure.
6. **Toe-Brachial Index (TBI):** The TBI is measured with photoplethysmography using a sensor and a toe pressure cuff (typically the great toe). Toe pressure is the reappearance of a photoplethysmography signal when the toe pressure cuff is deflated. The brachial pressure is measured as indicated above.

7. **Stress testing** is used to evaluate for the presence of claudication when the ABI is borderline (0.9 to 1.0) or near normal (>1.0).
   a. Stress testing is performed with the patient walking on a treadmill with a 12-degree incline, moving at 2 miles per hour. BP cuffs are placed on the ankles. Electrocardiogram (ECG) monitoring can be performed during the examination.
   b. The patient exercises for 5 minutes or until symptoms are reproduced. Sequential ankle and brachial pressures are measured at 30-second intervals for the first 4 minutes and then every minute until the pressure measurement returns to normal or to the preexercise level.

Postprocedure Management
None

Results
1. ABI (3–6)
   a. Normal: ABI ≥1.0 or slightly greater. Values ≥1.4 indicate noncompressible arteries
   b. Borderline: ABI ≥0.9 but <1.0
   c. Mild arterial disease: ABI = 0.7 to 0.9
   d. Moderate arterial disease: 0.5 to 0.7
   e. Severe arterial disease: 0.3 to 0.5
   f. Rest pain/very severe arterial disease: ABI <0.3
2. Prognosis for healing skin lesions of toes and feet: The probability of healing in diabetic and nondiabetic patients is listed in Table 67.1.
3. A drop of 15 to 30 mm Hg or greater in peak systolic pressure between the different segments is considered abnormal, indicating a significant lesion located between the two cuffs.
4. If the segmental BP at a particular level has a discrepancy of at least 20 mm Hg less than the opposite limb measured at the same level, a "horizontal" pressure gradient is present. This is indicative of a hemodynamically significant lesion proximal to the cuff of the extremity with the lower pressure.
5. A thigh (HT) pressure less than 20 mm Hg above the brachial pressure is considered abnormal and consistent with:
   a. Stenosis or occlusion of the aorta, iliac artery, or common femoral artery.
   b. Superficial femoral artery disease combined with stenosis or occlusion of the deep (profunda) femoral artery. The pulse volume recordings (PVRs) should help in the differential diagnosis (see the section on "Pulse Volume Recordings").
6. A normal TBI is 0.7 or greater. Mild disease is 0.5 to 0.7 and moderate disease is 0.1 to 0.5. A toe pressure in an absolute term of 20 mm Hg or less are indicative of poor wound healing. A toe pressure of >55 mm Hg indicates a good likelihood for wound healing.

Table 67.1 **Prognosis for Healing Skin Lesions of Toes and Feet**

	Probability of Healing (%)	
Ankle pressure (mm Hg)	Nondiabetic	Diabetic
Below 55	0	0
55–90	85	45
Above 90	100	85

Table 67.2 Clinical Categories of Chronic Limb Ischemia

Grade	Category	Typical Clinical Findings	Objective Criteria
	0	Asymptomatic, no hemodynamically significant disease	Normal results of treadmill stress test[a]
I	1	Mild claudication	Treadmill exercise completed. Postexercise ABI < 0.9. Postexercise AP >50 mm Hg but at least 25 mm Hg below baseline
	2	Moderate claudication	Symptoms between those of categories 1 and 3
	3	Severe claudication	Treadmill exercise cannot be completed; postexercise AP <50 mm Hg
II	4	Ischemic rest pain	Resting AP of ≤40 mm Hg; flat or barely pulsatile ankle or metatarsal plethysmographic tracing; toe pressure <30 mm Hg
III	5	Minor tissue loss: nonhealing ulcer, focal gangrene with diffuse pedal ischemia	Resting AP of <60 mm Hg; ankle or metatarsal plethysmographic tracing flat or barely pulsatile; toe pressure <40 mm Hg
	6	Major tissue loss: extending above transmetatarsal level, functional foot no longer salvageable	Same as for category 5.

[a]Five minutes at 2 mph on a 12-degree incline.
AP, ankle pressure.

7. A normal response to exercise is an unchanged or a slight elevation in the ABI. A decrease in ABI to 0.9 or lower is indicative of significant arterial disease. Disease severity is indicated by the drop in ABI and the time it takes for the pressures to return to pretest levels.
   a. Single level of disease: 2 to 6 minutes
   b. Multiple levels of disease: 6 to 12 minutes
   c. Severe occlusive disease: up to 30 minutes or longer
8. Ankle pressures during exercise and rest are used as objective criteria confirming the clinical categories of chronic limb ischemia (Table 67.2).
9. A decrease in the ABI of 0.15 or greater is considered a significant change.
10. An increase in the ABI of greater than 0.15 as a standalone criterion is defined as hemodynamic improvement. An increase of 0.10 if associated with categorical clinical improvement (see Table 67.2) is also defined as hemodynamic improvement.

Complications
None

Limitations and Artifacts
1. Diabetic patients typically can have a higher-than-expected ABI given the high prevalence of diffuse arterial wall calcification. This occurs because of the non-compressibility of the vessel. In some cases, the arteries are so rigid that pressure measurements cannot be obtained.

2. Pulsatile venous signals present in patients with congestive heart failure can be mistaken for arterial signals.
3. Extreme obesity may distort pressure measurements.
4. Absence of pedal Doppler signals because of severely diminished flow or complete occlusion may prevent measurements.

Pulse Volume Recordings

Indications
1. To complement pressure measurements in the evaluation of arterial disease
2. To help evaluate for the presence of compression syndromes such as thoracic outlet or popliteal entrapment syndromes
3. To help evaluate for the presence of arterial disease when noncompressible calcified arteries limit obtaining reliable pressure measurement
4. To help perform anatomical localization of hemodynamically significant peripheral vascular lesions

Contraindications
1. Open wounds
2. Recent surgery
3. Presence of arterial stents or bypass grafts at the location of a pressure cuff (relative contraindication)

Preprocedure Preparation
None

Procedure
1. Studies may be performed at rest or before and after exercise.
2. PVR cuffs are placed around the thighs, calves, and ankles of both legs.
3. The cuffs are inflated until a determined pressure (65 mm Hg) is achieved and with good apposition of the cuff to the skin.
4. The cuffs are calibrated so that a 1-mm Hg pressure change in the cuff provides a 20-mm chart deflection.
5. Cuff pressure changes are proportional to cuff volume changes, which are related to instantaneous limb volume changes.

Results (6,7)
1. Normal and abnormal pulse volume waves are shown in Figure 67.1.
2. PVR interpretation is mostly subjective.
3. PVR data have been classified into five categories (Table 67.3).
4. Pulse volume amplitudes have been found to remain highly reproducible in a given patient if the same cuff volumes and pressures are used. Significant changes correlate well with the appearance of significant occlusive vascular lesions.
5. Pulse volume amplitudes will vary with alterations in ventricular stroke volume, BP, vasomotor tone, and volume.
6. Exercise: The normal response to exercise is an increase in amplitude. Patients with occlusive arterial disease uniformly show a decrease in pulse volume at the ankle following exercise.
7. Other indications of significant arterial disease as indicated by the PVR contour include:
    a. Decrease in the rise of the anacrotic limb
    b. Rounding and delay in the pulse crest
    c. Decreased rate of fall of the catacrotic limb
    d. Absence of the reflected diastolic wave
8. Outcomes of PVR evaluation by PVR category are presented in Table 67.4.
    a. Rest pain can be evaluated to determine the likelihood that the pain is of vascular etiology.

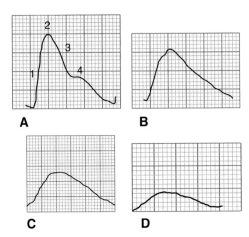

FIGURE 67.1 • Pulse volume recordings. **A:** Normal waveform demonstrating: (*1*) anacrotic rise, (*2*) pulse crest, (*3*) catacrotic decline, and (*4*) reflected diastolic wave following a notch. **B:** Loss of the dicrotic notch. **C:** Rounding of the peak and some rise time delay. **D:** Severe loss of upstroke and amplitude.

Table 67.3 **PVR Categories by Amount of Chart Deflection**[a]

| PVR Category | Chart Deflection (mm) | |
	Thigh and Ankle	Calf
1	>15[b]	>20[b]
2	>15[c]	>20[c]
3	5–15	5–20
4	<5	<5
5	Flat	Flat

[a]Raines J, Traad E. Noninvasive evaluation of peripheral arterial disease. *Med Clinics NA.* 1980;64(2):283–304.
[b]With reflected wave.
[c]Without reflected wave.

Table 67.4 **Outcomes by PVR Category for Rest Pain, Postexercise Pain, and Lesion Healing**

	Unlikely	Probable	Likely
Likelihood that rest pain is due to vascular etiology (diabetic and nondiabetic)	1–3	3, 4	4, 5
Likelihood that postexercise pain (from limiting claudication) is due to vascular etiology	2, 3	4	4, 5
Likelihood of lesion healing (diabetic and nondiabetic)	4, 5	3	1–3

b. Limiting claudication can be evaluated to determine the likelihood that exercise pain is of vascular etiology.

c. Lesion healing can be predicted according to PVR category (Table 67.4).

Complications
None

R e f e r e n c e s

1. Raines JK, Darling RC, Buth J, et al. Vascular laboratory criteria for the management of peripheral vascular disease of the lower extremities. *Surgery*. 1976;79(1):21–29.
2. Rose SC. Noninvasive vascular laboratory for evaluation of peripheral arterial occlusive disease: part II—clinical applications: chronic, usually atherosclerotic, lower extremity ischemia. *J Vasc Interv Radiol*. 2000;11(10):1257–1275.
3. Gerhard-Herman MD, Gornik HL, Barrett C, et al. 2016 AHA/ACC guideline on the management of patients with lower extremity peripheral artery disease: a report of the American College of Cardiology/American Heart Association Task Force on Clinical Practice Guidelines. *J Am College Cardiol*. 2017;69(11):e71–e126.
4. Rutherford RB, Becker GJ. Standards for evaluating and reporting the results of surgical and percutaneous therapy for peripheral arterial disease. *J Vasc Interv Radiol*. 1991;2(2):169–174.
5. Ahn SS, Rutherford RB, Becker GJ, et al. Reporting standards for lower extremity arterial endovascular procedures. Society for Vascular Surgery/International Society for Cardiovascular Surgery. *J Vasc Surg*. 1993;17(6):1103–1107.
6. Stoner MC, Calligaro KD, Chaer RA, et al. Reporting standards of the society for vascular surgery for endovascular treatment of chronic lower extremity peripheral artery disease. *J Vasc Surg*. 2016;64(1):e1–e21.
7. Darling RC, Raines JK, Brener BJ, et al. Quantitative segmental pulse volume recorder: a clinical tool. *Surgery*. 1972;72(6):873–877.

68 Duplex Ultrasound Imaging of Carotid and Peripheral Arteries

Joseph F. Polak, MD, MPH, FAIUM, FACR

Carotid Artery Disease

Indications
1. To detect the presence and degree of carotid artery stenosis in patients with neurologic symptoms
2. To evaluate individuals with carotid bruits
3. To detect recurrent stenosis following carotid endarterectomy or carotid stent placement
4. To monitor patients with known carotid stenosis for disease progression
5. To evaluate patients undergoing extensive cardiac procedures for significant asymptomatic carotid artery disease

Contraindications
Open wounds

Preprocedure Preparation
None

Procedure

1. Equipment: a 5 MHz or greater ideally 7 MHz or greater linear array transducer with color Doppler frequency of 3 MHz or more.
2. The examination is performed with the patient supine, head rotated away from the side being evaluated.
3. The transducer is placed in the transverse plane and moved from the low common carotid artery to above the bifurcation of the internal and external carotid arteries. This is used to survey carotid artery anatomy and identify key landmarks.
4. The transducer is placed longitudinally, parallel to the artery. The color Doppler window is angled 20 degrees in either direction or vertically depending on the angle between the transducer surface and the artery. The color Doppler velocity scale is typically set at 20 to 30 cm per second. The transducer is sequentially moved to evaluate the full length of the common carotid and internal carotid arteries. The external carotid artery is evaluated in its proximal portion.
5. The examination begins at the common carotid artery and includes Doppler tracings from the lower and upper common carotid artery; the external carotid artery; and the proximal, mid, and distal internal carotid arteries. Doppler velocity waveforms are obtained at sites of abnormal color signal (increased velocity). Doppler velocities are measured before, at, and just distal to the site of abnormal blood flow velocity. A velocity ratio is calculated from the peak systolic velocity (PSV) at the point of highest velocity in the internal carotid artery (ICA PSV) divided by the common carotid artery peak systolic velocity (CCA PSV) measured 2 to 4 cm proximal to the common carotid bulb.
6. Apparent absence of blood flow signals is confirmed with power Doppler imaging because it is more sensitive to low-velocity signals than color Doppler.
7. Following carotid endarterectomy, stent placement via femoral or carotid artery access, imaging should include the artery segment below the site of intervention, a thorough sampling of the area of intervention, and the artery segment downstream from the site.

Postprocedure Management
None

Results

1. The degree of carotid narrowing is estimated using Doppler velocity values (Fig. 68.1) calibrated against the degree of stenosis measured on arteriography according to the North American Symptomatic Carotid Endarterectomy Trial (NASCET) method (residual lumen at the stenosis compared to the ICA diameter distal to the stenosis) (1). Commonly accepted duplex ultrasound criteria for degree of stenosis are listed in Table 68.1, although there continues to be some debate on the correlation of measured values with degree of stenosis.
2. Very high-grade ICA stenoses can cause a decrease in velocities and a low-resistance pattern (tardus-parvus waveform) distal to the lesion. Color Doppler and power Doppler imaging are then used to confirm the presence of a very narrow residual lumen. Distinguishing between a subtotal occlusion and a total occlusion can be difficult and may require confirmation by magnetic resonance angiography or computed tomographic angiography (2).
3. Blood flow velocities can be moderately elevated for up to 1 year following *standard* carotid endarterectomy. Following patch endarterectomy, the lumen of the artery can be enlarged to the point that areas of blood flow stagnation can occur.
4. The presence of a carotid stent is often associated with an artificial increase in blood flow velocities. Grading of stent stenosis can be based on a velocity ratio greater than 2.7 or a PSV greater than 220 cm per second for a 50% stenosis and higher values such as a PSV of 340 cm per second for reintervention on a stenosis greater than 80% stenosis (3).

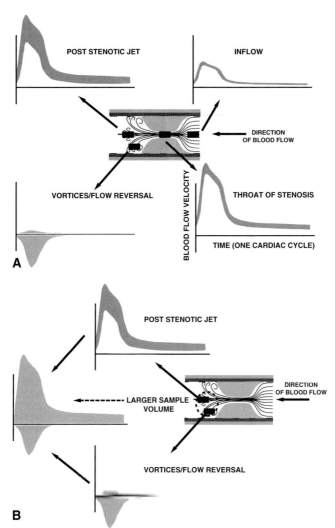

FIGURE 68.1 • A: Blood flow proximal to a high-grade stenosis is laminar. At the stenosis proper, all the red cells tend to travel at the same velocity (blunt flow profile or plug flow). The spectrum is therefore narrower than that sampled in the artery proximal to the stenosis, and it has a larger amplitude because all of the red cells must pass through the orifice. Distal to the stenosis, a more distinct jet of increased velocities develops surrounded by a zone of flow reversal. The jet is often asymmetric, hitting one or the other of the arterial walls rather than being directed toward the center of the artery. The zone of flow reversal is seen as a site where eddy currents cause the blood to flow back on itself. The jet will continue to dissipate energy as its effective radius grows. At the appropriate velocity/effective radius, turbulence will occur. **B:** Distal to the stenosis, it is possible to obtain a combination of forward- and backward-moving red cells. If the sample gate is large enough and placed at the interface between the zone of flow reversal and the velocity jet, a complex blood flow pattern will be registered. (Reprinted with permission from Polak JF. *Peripheral Vascular Sonography.* 2nd ed. Lippincott Williams & Wilkins; 2004.)

Table 68.1 Carotid Duplex Criteria for Carotid Stenosis (1)

Degree of Stenosis (%)	ICA Peak Systolic Velocity (PSV) (cm/s)	ICA /CCA PSV Ratio	ICA End-Diastolic Velocity (EDV)
Normal	<125	<2.0	<40
≥50%	125–229	2–4	>40
≥70%	≥230	≥4.0	>100
Near occlusion	Trickle flow	N/A	N/A
Occlusion	No detectable flow	N/A	N/A

Reprinted with permission from Grant EG, Benson CB, Moneta GL, et al. Carotid artery stenosis: gray-scale and Doppler US diagnosis—Society of Radiologists in Ultrasound Consensus Conference. *Radiology*. 2003; 229:340–346.

Complications

None

Peripheral Arterial Disease

Indications

1. To differentiate a stenosis from occlusion in symptomatic patients
2. To grade the degree of stenosis and determine the length of a lesion
3. To determine the length of an occlusion
4. To evaluate iatrogenic arterial injuries
5. To confirm the short-term technical adequacy of endovascular intervention
6. To perform the long-term follow-up of lesions following endovascular intervention
7. To evaluate peripheral aneurysms
8. Evaluate the suitability of radial arteries for arteriovenous (AV) fistula placement, harvesting or as an access site for endovascular procedures

Contraindications

Open wounds or ulcerations

Preprocedure Preparation

None

Procedure

1. Equipment: a 5 MHz or greater, ideally 7 MHz or greater, linear array transducer with color Doppler and pulsed Doppler frequencies of 3 MHz or more.
2. The examination is performed with the patient supine.
3. The transducer is placed longitudinally, parallel to the artery. The color Doppler window is angled 20 degrees in either direction or vertically depending on the angle between the ultrasound probe and the artery.
4. Above the knee evaluation: The examination begins at the common femoral artery and ends at the distal popliteal artery. The transducer is moved along the course of the superficial femoral artery, and all areas of abnormal color signal (increased velocity) are sampled with Doppler spectral analysis. A ratio is calculated from the PSV at the point of increased velocity divided by the systolic velocity measured in a segment 2 to 4 cm proximal to the site of blood flow abnormality.
5. Targeted examinations can be performed in the iliac and tibioperoneal arteries depending on the indication.
6. Sites of prior intervention (atherectomy, angioplasty, or stent placement) should be evaluated. Imaging should include the artery segment above the site of intervention, a thorough sampling of the area of intervention, and the artery segment downstream from the site.

7. Aneurysms are evaluated with and without color Doppler imaging. The diameter of the aneurysm and estimation of the amount of thrombus are made with gray-scale images (2). The proximal and distal extent of the aneurysm is documented, and the diameters of the vessel are recorded (outer wall to outer wall). Color Doppler imaging and Doppler spectral analysis are used to confirm flow within the aneurysm.

8. Pseudoaneurysms after iatrogenic injury are evaluated in a similar fashion. The channel from the artery to the aneurysm should be evaluated for length and width. Doppler waveforms sampled in the communicating neck typically show bidirectional flow in and out of the pseudoaneurysm sac, the so-called "to-and-fro" sign (Fig. 68.2).

9. Iatrogenic AV fistulas are evaluated with color Doppler to confirm the connection between the artery and vein and with Doppler waveform analysis to demonstrate the pulsatility in the draining vein and the low-resistance diastolic flow in the feeding artery. Pseudoaneurysms may be associated with AV fistulas.

10. A dissection will either have a discrete intimal flap in the vessel lumen or present as a stenosis or occlusion.

11. Use of a closure device can be associated with a pseudoaneurysm, stenosis, or occlusion at the site of placement. All can be evaluated with Doppler ultrasound imaging.

12. Radial artery diameter measurements are predictive of dialysis AV fistula failure (4). Prior to radial artery puncture, assessment for diameter, presence of a radial loop, and site of origin from the brachial artery should be confirmed.

Postprocedure Management
None

Results

1. The criteria for significant focal stenoses of greater than 50% diameter narrowing are increased color Doppler flow velocities and a corresponding doubling in the PSV (a PSV ratio greater than 2) (5,6). A PSV ratio above 3 corresponds to a stenosis above 75% lumen diameter narrowing. Accuracy has been estimated at approximately 90%.

2. Arterial ultrasound can be used to survey for the extent and severity of native atherosclerotic disease or in a targeted fashion.

3. Monitoring of arterial sites following angioplasty and stenting can be accurately done, but Doppler velocity thresholds need to be modified (7,8). A common systolic velocity threshold is ≥180 cm/s for 50% to 79% stenosis and ≥300 cm/s for a greater than 80% stenosis (7).

4. Popliteal aneurysms are evaluated with gray scale and color Doppler imaging. A relative diameter increase in the artery segment of 70% or more serves as a functional criterion for early aneurysm formation (ectasia). A very specific threshold of a 50% increase in diameter is considered a specific criterion for the presence of an aneurysm.

5. The ultrasound Doppler examination is considered the first-line study for the evaluation of iatrogenic arterial injuries such as pseudoaneurysms, AV fistulas, stenoses, occlusions, dissections, and closure device malfunctions.

Complications
None

Lower Extremity Bypass Grafts

Indications

1. To detect early stenotic lesions and allow for interventions that preserve graft patency using scheduled evaluations of saphenous vein bypass grafts in

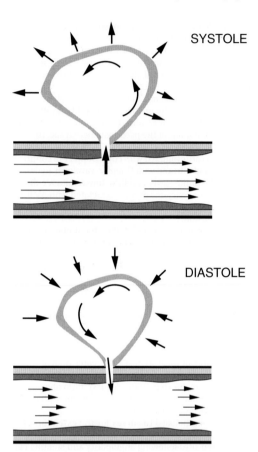

FIGURE 68.2 • The compliant nature of the soft tissues surrounding and containing a pseudoaneurysm explains the persistent flow pattern that is established within it and at its communication with the native artery. During systole, blood flows into the collection due to the relatively higher pressure in the artery lumen. Energy is stored in the collection as the surrounding soft tissues are compressed. During systole, the stored energy is released as the pressure within the artery becomes less than that generated by the elastic recoil of the soft tissues. This promotes flow into the artery. The swirling pattern of blood flow normally persists during the full cardiac cycle. A longer communicating channel will increase resistance to flow and disrupt the steady state responsible for setting up this constant motion. (From Polak JF. *Peripheral Vascular Sonography.* 2nd ed. Lippincott Williams & Wilkins; 2004, with permission.)

asymptomatic patients. Early stenoses due to fibrointimal hyperplasia can be detected with imaging during the first 2 years after the intervention. Additional yearly and biyearly examinations can be performed to evaluate for progression of atherosclerotic disease.

2. To confirm the source of *symptomatic* ischemic changes following bypass grafting by detecting area(s) of intragraft or anastomotic stenosis.
3. To detect persistent venous fistulas following in situ vein bypass graft placement.
4. Detect anastomotic stenoses in synthetic bypass grafts.

Contraindications
Open surgical wounds or ulcerations

Pre-Procedure Preparation
None

Procedure
1. Equipment: a 5.0 MHz or greater, ideally greater than 7 MHz, liner array transducer with Doppler frequency of 3 MHz or above. Color Doppler imaging is the key component of the study.
2. The transducer is held parallel to the graft while the proximal anastomosis is imaged. Presence of blood flow is confirmed both by color Doppler imaging and by Doppler waveform analysis.
3. The transducer remains oriented parallel to the graft conduit. The transducer is advanced in successive increments equal to the length of the probe. The color window is kept at a 20-degree angle to the graft lumen in order to enhance Doppler signals. The color scale is set to a maximal mean velocity between 20 and 40 cm per second in order to visualize blood flow patterns within the graft. Aliasing should be absent. The distal graft anastomosis is identified with color Doppler imaging and the Doppler waveforms sampled.
4. Doppler waveforms are sampled from any areas with abnormal color Doppler signals. Doppler velocity measurements are made every 10 cm even if color Doppler signals are normal.
5. Absence of color Doppler signals within the graft is confirmed with power Doppler imaging and Doppler waveform acquisition to confirm graft thrombosis.
6. Particular note is made of the PSV at the point of the graft with the smallest diameter.

Postprocedure Management
None

Results
1. The examination takes 20 to 30 minutes.
2. Doubling of the Doppler PSV at a site of abnormal color Doppler signal is considered indicative of a greater than 50% lumen narrowing. This method has a sensitivity of 95% and a specificity of 100%. Velocity ratios of 3 or above indicate a greater than 75% stenosis and a lesion likely to need intervention.
3. A PSV of less than 40 to 45 cm per second (9) or a decrease of greater than 30 cm per second compared to earlier evaluations should prompt further investigation for a stenotic lesion. These grafts usually fail within 3 to 9 months of the examination. However, this method is limited in large diameter grafts because they typically have low blood flow velocities.

Complications
None

References

1. Grant EG, Benson CB, Moneta GL, et al. Carotid artery stenosis: gray-scale and Doppler US diagnosis—society of radiologists in ultrasound consensus conference. *Radiology.* 2003;229(2):340–346.
2. Pellerito JS, Polak JF. Introduction to Vascular Ultrasonsongraphy. 7th ed. Elsevier; 2019.
3. Lal BK, Hobson RW II, Tofighi B, et al. Duplex ultrasound velocity criteria for the stented carotid artery. *J Vasc Surg.* 2008;47(1):63–73.
4. Parmar J, Aslam M, Standfield N. Pre-operative radial arterial diameter predicts early failure of arteriovenous fistula (AVF) for haemodialysis. *Eur J Vasc Endovasc Surg.* 2007;33(1):113–115.

5. Polak JF, Karmel MI, Meyerovitz MF. Accuracy of color Doppler flow mapping for evaluation of the severity of femoropopliteal arterial disease: a prospective study. *J Vasc Interv Radiol.* 1991;2(4):471–479.

6. Mittleider D. Noninvasive arterial testing: what and when to use. *Semin Intervent Radiol.* 2018;35(5):384–392.

7. Baril DT, Marone LK. Duplex evaluation following femoropopliteal angioplasty and stenting: criteria and utility of surveillance. *Vasc Endovascular Surg.* 2012;46(5):353–357.

8. Shrikhande GV, Graham AR, Aparajita R, et al. Determining criteria for predicting stenosis with ultrasound duplex after endovascular intervention in infrainguinal lesions. *Ann Vasc Surg.* 2011;25(4):454–460.

9. Tinder CN, Bandyk DF. Detection of imminent vein graft occlusion: what is the optimal surveillance program? *Semin Vasc Surg.* 2009;22(4):252–260.

69 Duplex Ultrasound of the Abdominal Vasculature

Ajay K. Singh, MD and Rathachai Kaewlai, MD

Introduction

Duplex ultrasound (DUS) examination is a noninvasive means for evaluating the anatomy and blood-flow dynamics of vascular aneurysms, stenoses, or occlusions. It can also guide the interventional radiologist during needle or catheter placement. Understanding the strengths and weaknesses of this modality is crucial for optimal clinical utilization. DUS provides real-time imaging and physiologic information without exposing the patient to ionizing radiation. This chapter describes six common indications for abdominal DUS related to vascular interventional procedures, namely, abdominal aortic aneurysms (AAAs), transjugular intrahepatic portosystemic shunts (TIPSs), liver transplantation, renal transplantation, and the interrogation of native renal and visceral arteries.

Abdominal Aortic Aneurysm

1. AAA is the most common large-vessel aneurysm encountered in vascular practice. In the United States, routine one-time ultrasound (US) screening is reimbursed for the diagnosis of AAA for men in the age group of 65 to 75 years, who are smokers or have first-degree relatives with AAA.

2. AAA is diagnosed when (a) there is a focal dilation, ≥3 cm or (b) the aortic diameter equals or exceeding 1.5 times its expected normal diameter (1). The majority of AAAs are infrarenal, fusiform, and "true" aneurysms caused by degenerative changes in the aortic wall.

3. Patients with AAA of 4.0 cm or less, 4.1 to 4.9 cm, and in men, 5.0 to 5.4 cm are advised to follow-up at 36, 12, and 6 months, respectively. An aneurysm 5.0 to 5.4 cm in women and ≥5.5 cm in both sexes requires intervention.

4. US is used to screen, confirm the diagnosis, and monitor the size of AAA (Fig. 69.1).
   a. In nonacute situation, 8 hours of fasting before abdominal DUS is required to reduce the amount of bowel gas.
   b. The abdominal aorta is interrogated from the level of aortic hiatus to the bifurcation with visualization of bilateral common iliac arteries. Due to the depth of the aorta from the anterior abdominal wall, a low-frequency curvilinear transducer is routinely used.

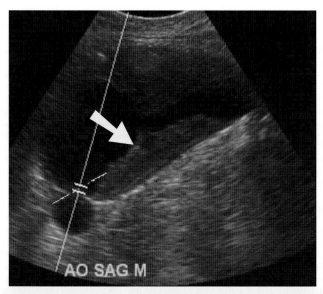

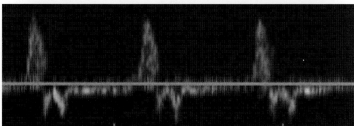

FIGURE 69.1 • Abdominal aortic aneurysm. Sagittal US view shows an aortic aneurysm with intraluminal thrombus (*arrow*). Spectral waveform is identified in the lumen of the aorta.

     a. The aorta and common iliac arteries are routinely measured in anteroposterior and transverse diameters from its outer to outer wall. The aorta is measured at the level of the diaphragm, superior mesenteric artery (SMA) origin, and just above the bifurcation. The distance from the renal artery or SMA origin to the most proximal extent of the aneurysm (nonaneurysmal proximal neck) is measured.

  5. Lifelong follow-up imaging of aortic grafts or stent grafts is mandatory for detecting possible complications, the two most frequent being endoleak and limb occlusion. Typical follow-up imaging after aortic stent-graft implantation is performed at 1 month. If there is no endoleak or sac expansion the next follow-up is at 12 months and then at every 1-year interval. If endoleak or sac expansion is detected at 1 month then imaging at 6 months post implant is recommended. In most institutions, computed tomographic angiography (CTA) is considered the gold standard for evaluation after AAA repair; however, DUS by experienced operators is helpful in patients who cannot receive iodinated contrast agents or wish to avoid radiation.

     a. Five types of endoleak include type I (poor sealing of either end of the stent with the native aortic wall), type II (retrograde filling of aneurysmal sac via an aortic branch), type III (leak through a defect or tear in the graft), type

IV (seepage of blood into aneurysmal sac due to graft porosity), and type V (significant expansion of the aneurysmal sac without visible leak).

b. Limb occlusion is recognized as a lack of flow in the limb(s) of the stent graft.

6. Compared with CTA, DUS has a wide range of sensitivity in detection of endoleak from 64% to 86% with a pooled sensitivity of 77% (2). An endoleak is identified on DUS as color flow outside the endovascular stent graft with a uniform, reproducible, color Doppler appearance that has spectral Doppler waveforms synchronous with the cardiac cycle.

7. Contrast-enhanced US (CEUS) overcomes limitation of US and DUS by providing better delineation of the AAA and detection of endoleak. It enhances characterization of endoleak with analysis of velocity and flow direction. Meta-analyses (2) reported pooled sensitivities and specificities of 89% to 98% and 86% to 88%, respectively. The European Federation of Societies for Ultrasound in Medicine and Biology currently recommends CEUS for detection and characterization of endoleak and follow-up of known endoleak (3).

Transjugular Intrahepatic Portosystemic Shunt

US is an extremely useful modality to evaluate the hepatic vasculature prior to and after TIPS placement.

1. Prior to the procedure, patency and flow in the portal, splenic, superior mesenteric, hepatic, and internal jugular veins are documented with DUS. The location of the portal vein bifurcation is assessed; undetected variant anatomy can increase the risk of portal vein perforation into the peritoneal cavity during the TIPS procedure.

2. After TIPS placement, DUS is routinely performed within 24 to 48 hours, at 3 months, and then at every 6 months to assess shunts patency and function. The TIPS stent appears as two parallel curvilinear lines, with corrugated appearance to the wall, connecting the hepatic and portal veins (Fig. 69.2). Although a typical

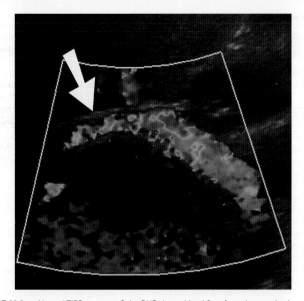

FIGURE 69.2 • Normal TIPS anatomy. Color DUS shows blood flow from the portal vein to the hepatic vein, in the TIPS (*arrow*).

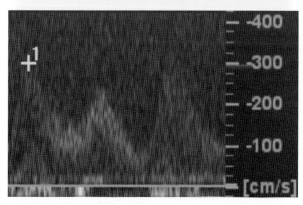

FIGURE 69.3 ▼ TIPS stenosis. Spectral Doppler wavoform shows elevated systolic velocity of 298 cm per second at the hepatic vein end of the TIPS (crosshairs), suggesting stenosis.

TIPS stent is 10 mm in diameter, its in vivo diameter is 8 to 9 mm due to surrounding hepatic tissue recoil (4). The portal venous and hepatic venous ends of the stent are normally slightly flared and should be within the lumen of hepatic and portal veins, respectively. PTFE-covered stents are routinely used and may contain some gas (air) that causes shadowing for several days until the gas is absorbed. The spectral waveform within TIPS is monophasic and slightly pulsatile. Normal peak systolic velocity (PSV) is similar throughout the shunt at 90 to 120 cm per second, but it should not be less than 50 to 60 cm per second.

3. Criteria for the diagnosis of TIPS (shunt) stenosis include (Fig. 69.3):
   a. Visible narrowing of the shunt
   b. Velocity less than 50 to 60 cm per second anywhere within the shunt
   c. Increase in a peak velocity of greater than 100 cm per second in the narrowed segment compared with a normal segment of the shunt

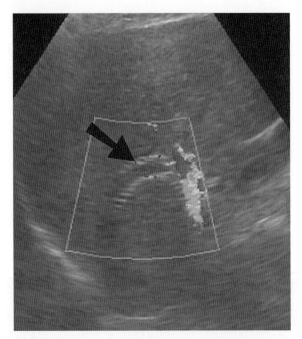

FIGURE 69.4 • TIPS occlusion. Color DUS shows lack of blood flow in the shunt (*arrow*).

    d. Continuous, nonpulsatile flow within the shunt
    e. Slow portal venous velocity of less than 30 cm per second
4. The use of fabric-covered stents has reduced prevalence of anatomic defects in TIPS, especially stenoses along the central portion of the TIPS.
5. TIPS occlusion (Fig. 69.4) is critical to identify, as it requires urgent corrective intervention (5). Suspicion of TIPS occlusion on DUS should be confirmed by CT or catheter angiography.

Liver Transplant Evaluation

Grayscale US is used for postoperative evaluation of liver transplantation to identify a hematoma, fluid collections, hepatic infarction, or biliary obstruction. Duplex scanning is used to confirm patency of hepatic arteries, portal veins, hepatic veins, and inferior vena cava (IVC).

1. Baseline DUS is performed within 24 to 48 hours of liver transplantation (6).
    a. A normal hepatic artery has a sharp systolic upstroke with high continuous diastolic velocity and a resistive index (RI) of 0.5 to 0.8. The systolic acceleration time is less than 0.1 second. In an early postoperative period, RI may be elevated (greater than 0.8) secondary to reperfusion edema. On the other hand, decreased RI or tardus-parvus waveform in this period should raise a suspicion for proximal thrombosis or stenosis (7).
    b. A normal portal vein is easier to visualize because of its large size (Fig. 69.5). Beware not to confuse an anatomic reduction of vessel caliber at the portal vein anastomosis with stenosis. This occurs due to size discrepancy between the donor and recipient portal veins. Normal portal venous flow is hepatopetal with a velocity of less than 50 cm per second.

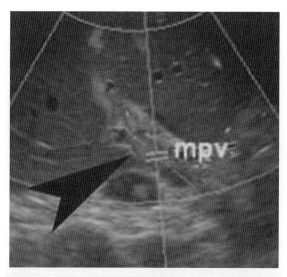

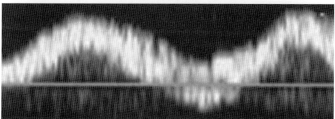

FIGURE 69.5 • Portal vein spectral Doppler waveforms. A normal portal venous (*arrowhead*) has flow with an undulating waveform. *mpv*, main portal vein.

    c. Normal hepatic veins and IVC have a multiphasic flow pattern due to cardiac pulsation.

2. Vascular complications of liver transplantation

    a. Thrombosis of the hepatic artery typically occurs within the first 6 weeks to 3 months of surgery. DUS can diagnose hepatic arterial thrombosis with a sensitivity of 60% to 80% (6), manifested by an absence of arterial signal in the hepatic artery and its branches. Actual thrombus may be visualized on grayscale US.

    b. Stenosis of the hepatic artery usually occurs at the anastomotic site and is characterized by a high PSV (greater than 200 cm per second or three times of prestenotic segment) at the point of stenosis with poststenotic turbulence. The intrahepatic arteries may show tardus-parvus waveform, a low RI of less than 0.5, and delayed systolic acceleration time of greater than 0.1 second.

    c. Pseudoaneurysm (PSA) of the hepatic artery may be seen on grayscale US as a round anechoic fluid collection adjacent to the hepatic artery (6) (Fig. 69.6). Intrahepatic PSAs are commonly related to biliary interventions, but extrahepatic PSAs raise a possibility of mycotic infection. If it is not thrombosed, a to-and-fro pattern waveform is seen within the aneurysm on DUS.

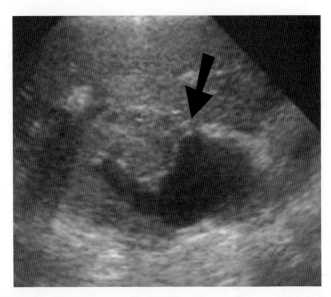

FIGURE 69.6 • Fusiform aneurysm of the common hepatic artery. US shows a complex cystic lesion at the porta hepatis (*arrow*). Color DUS (not shown) revealed blood flow in the aneurysm with thrombus at the wall (*right of arrow*).

d. Stenosis of the portal vein usually occurs at the donor–recipient anastomosis. Focal narrowing of portal vein, aliasing, and increased flow velocity at the site of stenosis are typical findings on DUS. When the velocity gradient increases three- to fourfold relative to a prestenotic segment, it is considered to be hemodynamically significant (6). Thrombosis of the portal vein is characterized by lack of flow.

Renal Transplant Evaluation

1. Similar to liver transplant evaluation, grayscale US and DUS are used in postoperative period to identify peritransplant fluid collection, hydronephrosis, patency and flow direction of renal artery, anastomosis, renal vein, and evaluation of intrarenal arteries.
2. Vascular complications of renal transplantation (8)
   a. Renal artery stenosis frequently occurs at the anastomotic site, approximately 3 to 12 months after transplantation. It is characterized by a high velocity (greater than 250 cm per second or 1.8 times of external iliac artery) and focal aliasing at the point of stenosis. The intrarenal artery may show tardus-parvus waveform and a low RI.
   b. Renal artery thrombosis/infarction can occur from the main renal artery to segmental arteries. There is no parenchymal flow of the entire transplant kidney on DUS if the main renal artery is completely occluded. Segmental lack of parenchymal flow can be more difficult to detect. Power Doppler or CEUS improves the detection rate.
   c. Renal vein thrombosis is a rare complication. It often occurs within 2 weeks after transplantation. A combination of direct visualization of thrombus in the main renal vein, lack of flow, or reversed diastolic flow is diagnostic on DUS.

3. Vascular complications after interventional procedures (8)
   a. Arteriovenous fistula (AVF) commonly occurs after percutaneous biopsy of the transplant. There is focal turbulent high-velocity and low-resistive waveforms with tissue reverberation artifact. On grayscale US, no hypoechoic pocket is visualized unlike PSA. More than 70% of iatrogenic AVFs will regress spontaneously.
   b. PSA appears as a round or oval anechoic/hypoechoic structure on grayscale US with swirling motion (yin-yang sign) on DUS. Connection of the sac to the artery and width/length of the PSA neck should be assessed.

Renal Artery Evaluation

1. Normal renal arteries have a low-resistance waveform pattern with a broad systolic phase and continuous forward flow throughout diastole. PSV, acceleration time, and RI are obtained at origin, proximal, mid, and distal portions of each renal artery. Intrarenal arterial waveforms and RI are assessed within the segmental arteries in the upper pole, midportion, and lower pole of the kidneys.
2. Approximately 20% to 30% of patients referred for Doppler evaluation are considered inappropriate subjects due to technical reasons including obesity or arterial calcifications (9).
3. Renal artery stenosis (Fig. 69.7) is manifested on DUS as an increase in PSV of greater than 180 to 200 cm per second, renal/aortic ratio (PSV at stenotic portion divided by that of the aorta at the renal artery origin) of greater than 3.3 or 3.5, prolonged acceleration time of more than 0.07 seconds, and poststenotic flow disturbance. Dampening of intrarenal arterial waveform (tardus parvus) is an indirect sign suggestive, but not specific, of renal artery stenosis.

Visceral Artery Evaluation

1. Doppler examination of the splanchnic arteries is a useful method to diagnose stenoses and follow-up patients after intervention.
   a. Abdominal aorta is measured at the level of mesenteric arteries for baseline velocities (PSV). PSVs of normal adults are between 70 and 100 cm per second. PSVs are subsequently obtained at the origins, proximal and midsegments of the celiac artery, SMA, and IMA.
   b. The normal celiac artery shows (end-organ) low vascular resistance that does not differ before and after meals.
   c. The normal SMA shows a high intestinal vascular resistance in a preprandial state (Fig. 69.8). There is a triphasic waveform with a peak systolic component, low diastolic flow, and end-systolic reversal flow. There is significantly increased SMA flow in the postprandial period with increased systolic velocity, end-diastolic velocity, and loss of its flow reversal.
   d. Stenosis (Fig. 69.8) is primarily diagnosed on US as elevation of PSV, mesenteric artery/aortic PSV ratio (MAR) and presence of tardus-parvus waveforms. Focal area of luminal narrowing, color flow aliasing, poststenotic turbulence, and presence of collateral vessels are helpful secondary signs.
2. Threshold of hemodynamically significant stenosis of the celiac artery is a PSV of greater than 200 cm per second and MAR of greater than 3 to 3.5.
3. In the SMA, a PSV of 275 cm per second or greater is correlated with significant stenosis, with a sensitivity of 89% to 100% and a specificity of 92% to 98% (10). An MAR of 3 to 3.5 or greater is suggestive of a significant SMA stenosis.
   a. If all three vessels (celiac artery, SMA, IMA) show increased PSVs, this might be due to a high-output state. On the other hand, low PSVs of all three vessels are suggestive of low-output state. High PSV of the entire course of a vessel might be compensatory flow due to occlusion/stenosis of adjacent mesenteric arteries.

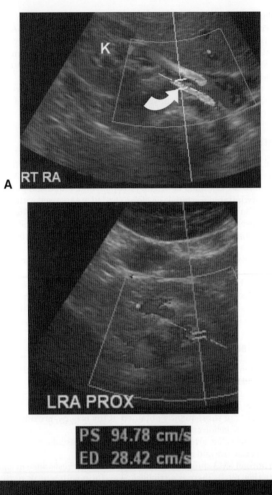

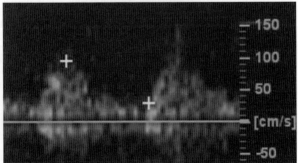

FIGURE 69.7 • Renal artery stenosis. **A:** Color DUS along axis of the vessel shows renal artery (*curved arrow*) located adjacent to renal vein. There is a suggestion of narrowing closer to its origin. **B:** Spectral Doppler (cross-sectional orientation) of renal artery origin shows *pulsus parvus et tardus* pattern secondary to an osteal stenosis. *K,* kidney.

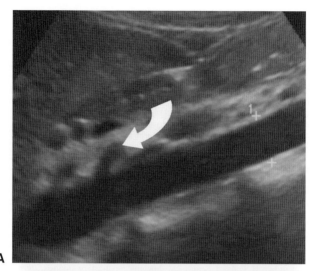

A

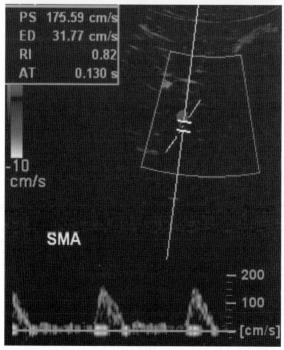

B

FIGURE 69.8 • Superior mesenteric artery with a hemodynamically nonsignificant stenosis.
A: Grayscale US shows the SMA (*curved arrow*) arising off the proximal abdominal aorta.
B: Spectral Doppler waveform shows PSV of 176 cm per second and delayed systolic upstroke.
The SMA-to-aortic systolic velocity ratio (2.2) was less than 3, so it does not meet the criterion for
a hemodynamically significant stenosis.

References

1. Chaikof EL, Dalman RL, Eskandari MK, et al. The Society for Vascular Surgery practice guidelines on the care of patients with an abdominal aortic aneurysm. *J Vasc Surg.* 2018;67(1):2–77.e2

2. Gummadi S, Eisenbrey JR, Lyshchik A. A narrative review on contrast-enhanced ultrasound in aortic endograft endoleak surveillance. *Ultrasound Q.* 2018;34(3):170–175.

3. Piscaglia F, Nolsøe C, Dietrich CF, et al. The EFSUMB guidelines and recommendations on the clinical practice of contrast enhanced ultrasound (CEUS): update 2011 on non-hepatic applications. *Ultraschall Med.* 2012;33(1):33–59.

4. Brehmer WP, Saad WE. Dysfunctional transjugular intrahepatic portosystemic shunt: anatomic defects and Doppler ultrasound evaluation. *Ultrasound Clin.* 2013;8(4):125–135.

5. Colombato L. The role of transjugular intrahepatic portosystemic shunt (TIPS) in the management of portal hypertension. *J Clin Gastroenterol.* 2007;41(Suppl 3):S344–S351.

6. Ackerman SJ, Irshad A, Lewis M. Update on the role of sonography in liver transplantation. *Ultrasound Clin.* 2014;9:641–652.

7. Garcia-Criado A, Gilabert R, Salmeron JM, et al. Significance of and contributing factors for a high resistive index on Doppler sonography of the hepatic artery immediately after surgery: prognostic implications for liver transplantation recipients. *AJR Am J Roentgenol.* 2003;181:831–838.

8. Zarzour JG, Lockhart ME. Ultrasonography of the renal transplant. *Ultrasound Clin.* 2014;9:683–695.

9. Moukaddam H, Pollak J, Scoutt LM. Imaging renal artery stenosis. *Ultrasound Clin.* 2007;2:455–475.

10. Lim HK, Lee WJ, Kim SH, et al. Splanchnic arterial stenosis or occlusion: diagnosis at Doppler US. *Radiology.* 1999;211:405–410.

70 Color Doppler and Ultrasound Imaging of Peripheral Veins

Joseph F. Polak, MD, MPH, FAIUM, FACR

Veins of the Lower Extremity

Indications

1. To evaluate patients with acute onset of lower extremity swelling or pain, raising the clinical suspicion of acute deep vein thrombosis (DVT).

2. To monitor the veins of high-risk, asymptomatic patients. The definition of "high-risk" is extensive and includes elderly, bedridden, following surgery (especially following hip replacement or neurosurgical procedures), or after trauma.

3. To establish a baseline study following the completion of anticoagulation. This will permit the detection of recurrent episodes of DVT or onset of venous reflux.

4. To evaluate patients with dyspnea and suspected pulmonary embolism, although the diagnostic yield is low.

5. To monitor in-hospital quality control programs aimed at the prophylaxis of DVT, particularly in high-risk groups of patients.

6. Mapping of the great and small saphenous veins prior to operative or endovascular procedures.

7. Detection and segmental analysis of venous reflux in patients with
   a. Varicose veins
   b. Recurrent varicose veins after intervention
   c. Cutaneous ulceration
   d. Serious venous stasis symptoms with or without subcutaneous induration

Contraindications

Relative
1. Difficulty of the examination is a function of body habitus and the transducer used (5.0 MHz or above)
2. Wounds at sites to be surveyed
3. Pain at site to be evaluated

Preprocedure Preparation
1. No patient preparation is needed.
2. Intensive care patients can be examined with portable units.
3. Equipment
   a. Inferior to the inguinal ligament, high-resolution grayscale imaging with a linear array transducer equipped with color Doppler and duplex imaging capability. Grayscale frequency of at least 5 MHz, ideally above 7 MHz, with Doppler frequency of 3 MHz or above. Color Doppler imaging and Doppler waveform analysis are used for evaluating blood flow patterns.
   b. A sector or curved array transducer is used above the inguinal ligament, in the iliac veins, and inferior vena cava (IVC). Imaging and Doppler frequencies are lower than in the extremities. The gain is set so that the lumen of a normal vessel is free of internal echoes. The accompanying artery is used as a reference.
   c. Color Doppler imaging and Doppler waveforms are used to confirm venous obstruction and confirm the presence of nonobstructive thrombus and also used to detect venous reflux.
   d. Tilt tables or reclining stretchers held in reverse Trendelenburg position (feet down) can help to evaluate poorly mobile patients and patients with venous reflux.

Detection of Deep Vein Thrombosis

Procedure
1. **Compressibility** of the vein walls is the most important criterion to exclude the presence of acute thrombus (Figs. 70.1 to 70.3).
   a. Interrogation of the veins begins at the level of the inguinal ligament, roughly at the groin crease, and continues to include the calf veins.
   b. Examination of the femoral veins: The patient is positioned supine with the leg to be examined in slight external rotation. The patient's head/torso may be elevated 15 to 20 degrees (or placed in reverse Trendelenburg) to facilitate venous filling. The examination includes Doppler interrogation of the common femoral and femoral veins, including the proximal portion of the great saphenous vein at the sapheno–femoral junction just below the inguinal ligament.
   c. The transducer is held transverse to the axis of the vein and centered on the vein segment as pressure is applied on the skin to compress the vein walls. The walls of a normal vein segment collapse and appose together with minimal pressure. Failure to fully compress the vein indicates intraluminal thrombus.
   d. The compression maneuver is performed along the length of the vein by having the operator displace the transducer every 2 to 3 cm staying centered on the vein and then pressing on the skin.
   e. The femoral vein may be difficult to compress as it passes through the adductor canal. This can be the site of a false-positive study; adjunctive imaging with color Doppler imaging can help evaluate the patency of the venous segment or confirm the presence of a thrombus.
   f. The sapheno–femoral junction may be difficult to compress. This area should be carefully examined because thrombus in the great saphenous vein near

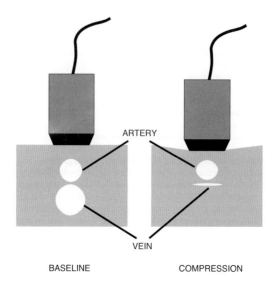

ARTERY

VEIN

BASELINE   COMPRESSION

FIGURE 70.1 • The compression maneuver is performed with the transducer held transverse to the vein. Pressure is applied to the surface of the skin through the transducer. This is transmitted to the deeper structures and causes the vein walls to collapse. On real-time imaging, repeating this maneuver causes the vein to wink. The maneuver shown here was applied to the femoral vein, which lies deep to the artery. The artery should not deform before the vein. On rare occasions, we have seen the artery collapse before the vein in patients with a prominent sartorius muscle. Reorienting the transducer more medially on the inside of the leg and repeating the compression maneuver then led to a normal response. (Reprinted with permission from Polak JF. *Peripheral Vascular Sonography.* 2nd ed. Lippincott Williams & Wilkins; 2004, with permission.)

the femoral junction may propagate into the common femoral vein, thereby becoming a deep vein thrombus.

g. The popliteal vein is examined with the leg slightly flexed. Alternatively, the patient can be imaged prone with the calf elevated approximately 30 degrees, with a towel or pillow beneath the shin to prevent spontaneous collapse of the vein. The patient can also be examined in the decubitus or prone positions.

h. The popliteal vein is compressed from the adductor hiatus to the level of the calf veins.

i. The transducer is rarely placed over the anterior compartment to evaluate the paired anterior tibial veins. Isolated thrombosis of the anterior tibial veins is very rare.

j. The paired posterior tibial and peroneal veins are in the posterior compartment and can be found by displacing the transducer medially and posterior to the tibia. The posterior tibial artery and accompanying paired veins lie medial and posterior to the tibia. The peroneal artery and accompanying veins are located deeper on top of the fibula.

k. The paired gastrocnemius veins accompany the gastrocnemius artery in the gastrocnemius muscle. Compressibility is mainly used for the diagnosis of thrombosis.

l. The muscular (mostly soleal) veins lie within the deep muscles of the calf and typically communicate with the peroneal and posterior tibial veins. Compressibility is mainly used for the diagnosis of thrombosis.

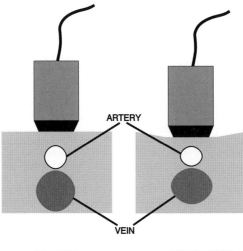

BASELINE   COMPRESSION

FIGURE 70.2 • Abnormal compression ultrasonography is defined as a failure to appose the walls of the deep vein while pressure is applied onto the skin through the transducer. Sufficient pressure is exerted to the extent that the artery wall deforms slightly. An ancillary finding to the presence of DVT is distention of the vein. The additional presence of echogenic material in the vein lumen reinforces the diagnosis. (Reprinted with permission from Polak JF. *Peripheral Vascular Sonography.* 2nd ed. Lippincott Williams & Wilkins; 2004, with permission.)

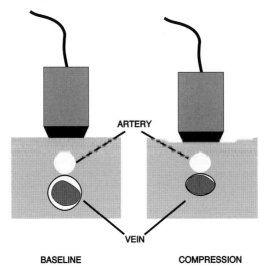

BASELINE   COMPRESSION

FIGURE 70.3 • Compression ultrasonography will also detect the presence of partly obstructing thrombus. There is failure for the walls of the vein to completely oppose during the compression maneuver. The vein is not distended. An echogenic structure need not be visualized in the vein lumen. (Reprinted with permission from Polak JF. *Peripheral Vascular Sonography.* 2nd ed. Lippincott Williams & Wilkins; 2004, with permission.)

    m. Compression of the calf veins may require more force than in the popliteal and femoral regions depending on body position. A noncompressible, often dilated, vein segment is diagnostic of venous thrombosis.

2. **Doppler waveforms** are used to evaluate:

    a. Spontaneous venous blood flow. Doppler signals are easily detected in large veins but detection of blood flow may require squeezing the calf to augment venous return in smaller veins.

    b. Respiratory phasicity: cyclical variation in venous blood flow measured in the common femoral vein that parallels the respiratory cycle. Continuous, monophasic low-velocity venous blood flow is compatible with proximal (pelvic or above) venous obstruction.

    c. Venous augmentation: a transient increase in blood flow velocity caused by distal compression of the calf and emptying of blood from the calf veins. A normal response indicates the absence of occlusion between the point of distal compression and the location of the transducer.

3. **Color Doppler imaging** is helpful when results of compression ultrasound are indeterminate or the examination is compromised by technical factors such as large patient size, previous episodes of DVT, or pain with attempted compression.

    a. The color gain and sensitivity are set to enhance the detection of low-velocity blood flow.

    b. Evaluation of the lower extremity veins is performed in the transverse and longitudinal planes.

    c. The study is considered positive for thrombus when a loss of color Doppler signal is seen in the vessel lumen and negative if the lumen is filled with color Doppler signals.

    d. Chronic DVT can cause a narrowed, irregular color lumen with wall thickening or the presence of numerous venous collateral channels.

4. **Thrombus visualization** within the lumen of the vein is the most specific criterion for the presence of DVT. It may be difficult when the echogenicity of fresh thrombus is close to that of blood. Therefore, fresh thrombus may escape detection if only grayscale imaging is used.

Postprocedure Management

Patients with positive calf vein thrombosis who are not treated with anticoagulation should be followed at a 5- to 7-day interval to identify the propagation of thrombus into the popliteal vein (1). Similarly, high-risk patients with a negative above-the-knee study should have a repeat study at 5 to 7 days in order to detect the 20% of calf vein thrombus cases that can extend into the popliteal (above-the-knee) vein (1).

Results

1. Compression ultrasound (not including calf veins) has high sensitivity and specificity when originally correlated with the findings of ascending venography. Its diagnostic value is based on outcomes analysis and the low rate of DVT recurrence following a negative venous ultrasound examination (2,3).

2. Calf vein imaging requires an additional 10 to 20 minutes of examination time.

    a. In symptomatic patients with isolated calf vein symptoms and negative above-the-knee ultrasound studies, the accuracy of calf vein imaging is very high (above 95%) (4).

    b. The sensitivity for detecting isolated calf vein thrombus in hospitalized asymptomatic and high-risk groups is highly variable, ranging from 13% to 85%.

3. Studies that include the full length of the lower extremity have high accuracy when outcomes are evaluated at 3 months (3,4).

4. Two-point examinations (common femoral and popliteal vein compression only), if negative, should be repeated 5 to 7 days later (1).

Complications (Rare)

Dislodgment of blood clot during compression causing pulmonary embolism is very rare.

Saphenous Vein Mapping Prior to Infrainguinal Bypass Procedures (5–7)

1. Equipment: linear array transducer with grayscale frequency above 5 MHz, preferably above 7 MHz, and Doppler frequency of 3 MHz or above
2. Place the limb to be scanned in a dependent position to maximize distention. The examination is performed with the patient standing or in 15- to 30-degree reverse Trendelenburg position with the knee slightly flexed (6,7).
3. Begin the examination at the sapheno–femoral junction just below the inguinal ligament with the transducer in transverse orientation. Grayscale imaging is mostly used, and color Doppler is added as needed.
4. Keep the great saphenous vein centered beneath the transducer, which is kept perpendicular to the skin surface. Follow the course of the vein, and, if needed, use a marker to draw the path of the vein on the skin surface. Note the vein diameter, any duplication/tributaries, varicosities, and any abnormal-appearing valves. Compression examination is performed to confirm vein patency.
5. The same procedure may be used for the small saphenous vein, which originates laterally at the ankle and most frequently joins the popliteal vein at the popliteal fossa. Communication with the vein of Giacomini can be important in endovascular treatment so should be noted.
6. Proximal compression can be used to distend the veins (6).

Results

1. Mapping of the great saphenous vein reveals several anatomic variations: complete double venous system, branching double system, and the standard single medial dominant trunk in the thigh with an anterior dominant vein in the calf.
2. Good estimates of vein diameters are obtained in most cases (7).

Detection and Segmental Evaluation of Venous Reflux

1. Equipment: greater than 5 MHz, preferably above 7 MHz, grayscale imaging transducer with pulsed and color Doppler frequencies of 3 MHz or above
2. The upper leg is examined with the patient standing, ideally on a step stool with some means of support such as a chair or orthopedic walker. An alternative is a stretcher in 15- to 30-degree reverse Trendelenburg. The calf can be examined with the patient sitting, either with the leg dangling or supported by the examiner's thigh.
3. The sapheno–femoral junction is identified and the Doppler sample gate placed in the common femoral vein just above it and the response to a Valsalva maneuver is recorded. There should be minimal reversal of blood flow.
4. The Doppler response is then recorded in various venous segments following augmentation either by compressing the calf by hand or using an automated inflator. The cuff is inflated for 1 to 3 seconds; the presence of reflux is evaluated following cuff deflation. The duration of retrograde blood flow is recorded. Normal reversal of blood flow can last up to 0.5 to 0.7 seconds.
5. Recordings are made in the upper common femoral, the proximal femoral, the proximal deep femoral, the distal femoral, and the upper popliteal and lower popliteal veins. It is also performed for the great saphenous vein 4 cm from the sapheno–femoral junction, the great saphenous vein in the distal thigh and the upper calf. Other veins that may be studied depending on the clinical situation are the small saphenous vein just below the sapheno–popliteal junction and the calf veins.
6. Grayscale imaging is used to locate the perforating veins (perforators). The transducer is displaced in the transverse plane along the superficial veins. The perforators course deep into the fascia and are difficult to identify if they

are normal. Their evaluation includes sampling of the direction of blood flow (normal is from the skin into the deep veins) and measuring their diameter (normal is <2 mm; incompetent veins are almost always present when the diameter reaches 3 mm).

7. Because the status of the deep veins is often unpredictable from the physical examination or clinical presentation, a complete examination of the deep and superficial veins is recommended. The status of the deep system can have profound effects in directing treatment of superficial venous reflux disease.

Postprocedure Management
None

Results
1. Normal reversal of blood flow (reflux) is <0.5 seconds in the superficial system but can be up to 1 second in the popliteal vein (8).
2. Venous incompetence can be segmental. This knowledge and careful evaluation of the affected segments permit more targeted surgical and percutaneous interventions.
3. Superficial vein reflux and perforator incompetence contribute to the pathogenesis of venous ulceration and both are easily documented by ultrasound.
4. Grayscale imaging and color Doppler imaging have been used to guide endovenous ablation, delimit injection sites for venous sclerotherapy, and evaluate the success of such treatments.

Complications
None

Veins of the Upper Extremity

Indications
1. Unexplained swelling of the upper extremity
2. Suspicion of venous thrombosis associated with a central venous catheter (9)
3. Pre- and intraprocedure assessment endovascular clot treatment
4. Mapping prior to surgical or endovascular dialysis fistula creation
5. To evaluate patients with dyspnea and suspected pulmonary, although the diagnostic yield is low

Contraindications
None

Preprocedure Preparation
None

Procedure
1. The patient is positioned supine or in slight Trendelenburg position to distend the upper extremity veins. The jugular and subclavian veins are examined with the patient's arm at his or her side; axillary and brachial veins are examined with the patient's arm slightly abducted, palm directed upward. The examiner is positioned either at the patient's head or side.
2. Equipment: 5.0 MHz or above, preferably above 7 MHz, linear array transducer with color and pulse wave Doppler capability (3 MHz or above). Color Doppler is used intermittently during the examination because the presence of thrombus causes a flow defect.
3. The examination begins at the jugular vein in the mid to upper neck. The vein is easily identified next to the carotid artery. The vein is compressed. Color Doppler confirms patency of the vein. Doppler waveforms are used to confirm the presence of cardiac pulsatility and of cyclical respiratory variation. The vein is imaged in both longitudinal and transverse orientations.

4. In the transverse orientation, the transducer is swept down the jugular vein to the clavicle. The common carotid artery–brachiocephalic artery junction is encountered first. Then, caudal to the artery, the junction of the jugular vein–brachiocephalic vein–subclavian vein is found. To reach this level, the transducer may have to be acutely angled caudal and pressed into the supraclavicular fossa. This area is examined for the presence of thrombus, and a color Doppler image is recorded.

5. The medial aspect of the upper arm is scanned with color Doppler and grayscale ultrasound. Compression examination is performed as far into the axilla as can be reached. An infraclavicular approach is used to image the segment of the axillary and subclavian vein not seen in the previous orientations.

6. While imaging over the subclavian vein in transverse orientation, the patient is asked to sniff vigorously. A normal response is a decrease in vein diameter.

7. The presence of venous catheters is documented as well as their effect on the blood flow dynamics within the vein.

Postprocedure Management
None

Results (10)

1. Compression examination, augmentation, and respiratory variation are lower than in the evaluation of the lower extremity. Cardiac pulsatility is a good indicator of central vein patency.

2. There is good accuracy when results of venous ultrasound are compared to venography.

Complications
None reported

R e f e r e n c e s

1. Bernardi E, Camporese G, Büller HR, et al. Serial 2-point ultrasonography plus D-dimer vs whole-leg color-coded Doppler ultrasonography for diagnosing suspected symptomatic deep vein thrombosis: a randomized controlled trial. *JAMA*. 2008;300(14):1653–1659.

2. Cornuz J, Pearson SD, Polak J. Deep venous thrombosis: complete lower extremity venous US evaluation in patients without known risk factors—outcome study. *Radiology*. 1999;211:637–641.

3. Schellong SM, Schwarz T, Halbritter K, et al. Complete compression ultrasonography of the leg veins as a single test for the diagnosis of deep vein thrombosis. *Thromb Haemost*. 2003;89(2):228–234.

4. Simons GR, Skibo LK, Polak JF, et al. Utility of leg ultrasonography in suspected symptomatic isolated calf deep venous thrombosis. *Am J Med*. 1995;99(1):10–17.

5. van Dijk LC, Wittens CH, Pieterman H, et al. The value of pre-operative ultrasound mapping of the greater saphenous vein prior to 'closed' in situ bypass operations. *Eur J Radiol*. 1996;23(3):235–237.

6. Hoballah JJ, Corry DC, Rossley N, et al. Duplex saphenous vein mapping: venous occlusion and dependent position facilitate imaging. *Vasc Endovascular Surg*. 2002;36(5):377–380.

7. Cruz CP, Eidt JF, Brown AT, et al. Correlation between preoperative and postoperative duplex vein measurements of the greater saphenous vein used for infrainguinal arterial reconstruction. *Vasc Endovascular Surg*. 2004;38(1):57–62.

8. Labropoulos N, Tiongson J, Pryor L, et al. Definition of venous reflux in lower-extremity veins. *J Vasc Surg*. 2003;38:793–798.

9. Luciani A, Clement O, Halimi P, et al. Catheter-related upper extremity deep venous thrombosis in cancer patients: a prospective study based on Doppler US. *Radiology*. 2001;220(3):655–660.

10. Pater, Payal, Braun C, Patel, Parth, et al. Diagnosis of deep vein thrombosis of the upper extremity: a systematic review and meta-analysis of test accuracy. *Blood Advance*. 2020;4(11):2516–22.

71 Magnetic Resonance Angiography

Nanda Deepa Thimmappa, MD and Martin R. Prince, MD, PhD, FACR

Introduction

Just as with conventional angiography, it is essential to learn all aspects of the operation of magnetic resonance imaging (MRI) equipment to select the appropriate imaging coil and sequences. It is important to evaluate patients prior to imaging in order to determine the specific clinical issues that need to be addressed, and to assess how cooperative the patient is likely to be with suspending respiration and remaining still for the scans. It is especially critical to determine the extent of vascular anatomy to be examined because it does not necessarily correspond to the traditional organ-based magnetic resonance (MR) anatomical regions. Technologists are not always familiar with the regions of coverage required for vascular studies and may need guidance from the radiologist about the anatomy of interest.

Preprocedure Preparation

1. **Safety screening:** Before accepting a patient for MRI, do a quick check for the major contraindications (e.g., pacemakers, cochlear implants, and brain aneurysm clips). The technologist must screen for other less frequent contraindications, including metallic foreign bodies in the orbits and certain medical implants. Most surgical clips outside the brain, orthopedic hardware, stents, coils and vena cava filters, especially if nonferromagnetic and remote from the imaging site, do not generally pose a safety hazard, but they may create artifacts if included in the imaging field.

2. **Gadolinium deposition and nephrogenic systemic fibrosis (NSF):** For many years we have been checking the glomerular filtration rate (GFR) (visit www.MDRD.com for GFR calculator) prior to using gadolinium-based contrast agents (GBCAs). However, nearly all of the linear GBCA which had greatest risk of NSF have been withdrawn from the market and the macrocyclic GBCA are believed to have negligible if any risk of NSF so there is less concern about using GBCA in renal compromised patients (1). Two linear GBCAs which are still on the market, gadobenate dimeglumine and gadoxetate both have protein binding and substantial biliary excretion which also seems to reduce risk of NSF. If GFR <30 mL per minute, avoid high GBCA doses and consider noncontrast magnetic resonance angiography (MRA) techniques. Patients in acute renal failure should *not* receive Gd until the serum creatinine recovers toward normalcy or hemodialysis is instituted. Outpatients should be asked if they are on dialysis or about to begin dialysis. All dialysis patients should have their MR scheduled for just prior (within 24 hours) to the next dialysis treatment session. Macrocyclic agents include gadobutrol (Gadavist, Bayer, Berlin, Germany), gadoteridol (ProHance, Bracco, Princeton, NJ) or gadoterate meglumine (Dotarem, Guerbet, Bloomington, IN or Clariscan, GE Healthcare, Oslo, Norway). Agents with biliary excretion in addition to renal excretion including gadobenate dimeglumine (MultiHance, Bracco, Princeton, NJ) and gadexetate disodium (Eovist, Bayer, Berlin, Germany).

3. **Clothing:** Ideally, patients should arrive for their MRI appointments wearing MR safe clothing which have no metal zippers, clasps, hooks, or buttons or other metallic features. This way the patient can minimize their time indoors at the MR facility and avoid the dressing room to reduce COVID-19 risk. If there is any

uncertainty about wearing metal, however, remove all clothing (including bras) with *metallic components* such as zippers, snaps, etc. *Have the patient wear a hospital gown.* Remove hairpins and metallic jewelry. Nonmagnetic gold and silver rings should not be removed so they do not get lost, but they should not be near or within the field of interest. If there is a question about safety, metallic paraphernalia should be tested with a small hand magnet to verify they are nonmagnetic. Otherwise remove.

4. **Sedation:** Patients with *claustrophobia* will benefit from being scanned in a larger, 70 cm bore diameter MRI scanner. Alternatively diazepam (Valium) 5 to 10 mg by mouth (PO) or lorazepam (Xanax) 1 to 2 mg PO taken 20 to 30 minutes prior to MR scanning. The patient should not be given the sedative until arriving at the scanner in case the facility is behind schedule. Sedated patients need a responsible adult escort to go home.

5. **Intravenous (IV) lines**
   a. For gadolinium-enhanced MRA (Gd-MRA), a right arm IV access is preferred because this provides the most direct route to the central circulation. It is acceptable to use a small-gauge IV access (minimum 22 gauge or high flow 24 gauge) in the antecubital fossa, hand, or wrist. However, if the IV access is tenuous, consider using a nonionic, low-osmolar Gd contrast preparation to avoid potential pain caused by extravasation of high-osmolar ionic Gd preparations. Nonionic contrast tends to be of lower viscosity since ionic GBCA dissociate into positively and negatively charged species thereby doubling the number of particles in solution.
   b. For hand injection of GBCA, consider using sufficiently long tubing to easily reach into the MRI scanner bore and contain the entire GBCA bolus so that the injection of flush will advance the GBCA into the patient in one continuous push. If you have to switch from a GBCA syringe to saline flush syringe in the middle of the injection there may be a gap in the bolus which will create a ringing artifact on the images. Caution is urged with power injectors because they are prone to misadministration, extravasation, and a greater risk to the patient in the event of a contrast reaction compared to hand injection because the pump is activated remotely from the control room.

6. **Coil selection:** Coil selection has to be optimized because the choice determines the available field-of-view (FOV) and the signal-to-noise ratio (SNR)—both of which significantly affect image quality. Because of the complexity of coil selection, many radiologists leave this up to the discretion of the technologist. However, it is important to be aware of the basic *coil selection principles* because technologists will generally pick the coil that makes the examination easiest to perform instead of one that produces the highest image quality.
   a. Use the smallest possible coil that still covers the anatomy of interest.
   b. Choose coils that are used routinely and are reliable such as the head, knee, torso, and body coils or large FOV arrays of multiple small coils packed together with high density such as the air coil to TIM system. Keep in mind that circumferential coils with birdcage construction (head, body, and knee coils) tend to have the most homogeneous sensitivity to MR signal and are less likely to produce confusing bright or dark spots on the images.
   c. When using coil arrays, make sure all elements are working properly. One bad element can reduce vascular signal locally giving the false impression of disease.

Procedure

It is essential to keep the examination time as short as possible so that the patient is able to tolerate holding still for the entire examination. Try to keep the total imaging time below 25 minutes so that the examination can be completed within 45 minutes.

1. Protocols
   a. Scout sequences: When selecting protocols for MRA examinations, it is useful to start with a large-FOV, low-resolution, 3-plane scout sequence to guide the prescription of subsequent smaller FOV sequences confined to the vascular anatomy of interest (2–4).

      (1) Single-shot fast spin echo (SSFSE) (General Electric, Milwaukee, WI) *or* half-Fourier acquisitions with single-shot turbo-spin echo (HASTE) (Siemens, Erlangen, Germany) are also useful as "black blood" scout sequences.

      (2) Three-plane ungated steady state free precession (SSFP) is a very useful "bright-blood" localizer because it has high SNR and yet is fast enough to minimize motion artifact and cover a large FOV with multiple slices in a short time.

   b. Multiplanar images: Take advantage of the multiplanar imaging capability of MRI to optimize visualization of anatomy in as many different orientations as possible. For this reason, try to have at least one sequence in each cardinal plane: axial, coronal, and sagittal.

   c. Contrast mechanisms: MRI has numerous contrast mechanisms that can be optimized to see anatomy and pathology in various ways. Some of the most popular contrast mechanisms for MRA studies include:

      (1) T1-weightd (T1-W): high SNR with black blood—note the black blood effect can be accentuated with longer TE up to 20 msec and make sure not to use gradient moment nulling which reduces flow-relate spoiling of the blood signal.

      (2) Proton density: higher SNR than T1-W and black blood

      (3) T2-weighted (T2-W): tumors, inflammation, and other lesions are bright, whereas fast flowing blood is black. Slow flowing blood in hemangiomas or slow flow vascular malformations may be bright. This sequence is usually performed with fat saturation.

      (4) Short T1 inversion recovery (STIR): like T2-W with fat saturation but without the degradation due to field inhomogeneity. Veins and especially vascular malformations are typically very bright due to slow flow.

      (5) SSFSE or HASTE: These sequences are immune to motion artifacts but they may have slice misregistration so in the chest and abdomen try to get the whole stack of slices in a single breath hold.

      (6) SSFP: High SNR, bright-blood MRA—prone to artifacts especially at larger FOV but the small FOV renal MRA implementations (InHance, timeslip, Native TrueFISP, B-Trance) are often excellent. Keep the TR short (<4 msec) to maximize SNR.

      (7) Three-dimensional (3D) Gd-MRA: provides a robust bright-blood MRA sequence similar to conventional angiography—least prone to artifacts.

      (8) Time-of-flight (TOF): bright-blood MRA sequence—subject to flow and motion artifacts. ECG gating reduces artifacts due to arterial pulsation. Requires gradient moment nulling. For peripheral arteries use a 1-cm sat gap when using saturation

      (9) Cine-SSFP: SSFP images acquired multiple times during the cardiac cycle and displayed as a movie to show variations between systole and diastole. Greats for imaging the heart.

      (10) Phase contrast-MRA (PC-MRA): allows quantification of intraluminal blood flow and demonstrates flow disturbances. The latest version which measures flow in all directions as it varies from systole to diastole for an entire 3D volume of interest is known as 4D-flow.

      (11) Arterial spin labeling: blood is excited proximal to the region of interest (ROI) and imaged after flowing into the ROI.

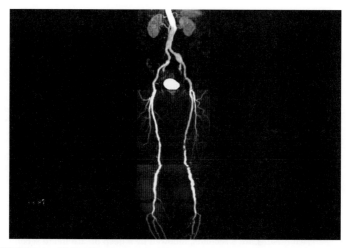

FIGURE 71.1 • 3D Gd-MRA demonstrating bilateral common iliac and popliteal artery aneurysms.

(12) Fresh blood imaging (Delta flow, native Space, Trance): images gated to systole are subtracted from images gated to diastole to show arteries without Gd.

(13) "TimeSlip" (InHance, B-Trance, native trueFISP): good for renal arteries in patients with fast blood flow. Gd injection is not necessary.

(14) QISS (Quiescent Interval Slice-Selective) noncontrast MRA: A large FOV, robust, ECG-gated SSFP-based MRA technique optimized for imaging peripheral arteries.

2. MRA pulse sequences

   a. 3D Gd-MRA: This is the most robust sequence for evaluating vascular anatomy and pathology. Figure 71.1 is a 3D Gd-MRA study from the abdominal aorta to the proximal calf region. The image illustrates the ability of the technique to demonstrate bilateral common iliac and popliteal artery aneurysms. 3D Gd-MRA is performed similarly to CT angiography by acquiring a 3D-spoiled gradient echo (SPGR) pulse sequence during the arterial phase of a contrast bolus (5) or Time Resolved Imaging of Contrast KineticS (TRICKS) during arterial and venous phases. Use the shortest possible repetition time (TR) and echo time (TE), while being careful not to make the bandwidth (BW) too high. A flip angle of about 30 degrees is good for the peak arterial phase but should be lower for venous and equilibrium phases when Gd concentration has diminished. The bolus duration should equal half the scan duration—timed for maximum arterial Gd concentration "opacification" to coincide with acquisition of center of k-space. The contrast dose should not exceed 0.1 mL per kg in any patient at risk of NSF (GFR <30). More advanced, state-of-the-art MR scanners generally can produce high-quality MRA with lower Gd doses. *Bolus timing for long acquisitions:* For long acquisitions, lasting more than 100 seconds, timing is easy because errors of 10 to 15 seconds are small relative to the total scan duration.

      (1) Use sequential ordering of k-space, so that the center of the k-space is collected during the middle of the acquisition.

      (2) Begin injecting the Gd just after initiating imaging. Finish the injection just after the midpoint of the acquisition, being careful to maintain the maximum injection rate for the approximately 10 to 30 seconds prior

to the middle of the acquisition. This will ensure a maximum arterial enhancement during the middle of the acquisition, when central *k-space* data are collected.

(3) To ensure full use of the entire dose of contrast agent, it is useful to flush the IV tubing with 20 mL of normal saline.

b. *Bolus timing for fast (breath-hold) scans:* For fast scans, less than 30 seconds in duration, contrast agent bolus timing is more critical and challenging. This is because timing errors of 15 seconds can ruin a fast breath-hold scan. There are several approaches to determining the optimal bolus timing for these fast scans. The simplest, although least successful approach, is to guess on the basis of patient's age, cardiac status, presence of aortic aneurysmal disease, and location of the IV access.

(1) For a *breath-hold scan,* lasting 30 to 40 seconds, of a reasonably healthy patient with an IV in the antecubital vein, a delay of approximately 10 to 12 seconds is appropriate. Therefore, in this scenario, begin the injection, and then 10 seconds later, start imaging while the patient suspends breathing. If there is no convenient clock available to time this delay, take advantage of the natural rhythm of the patient's respiration. One deep breath in followed by a deep breath out takes approximately 4 seconds. Two breaths are 8 seconds, followed by a deep breath in (10 seconds), which represents the optimum delay between start of injection and beginning of scanning.

(2) If a patient is older and has a history of cardiac or aortic aneurysm, add one or two extra breaths to the delay. Also, if the IV site is in the wrist, add an extra breath to the delay.

(3) Alternatively, if the patient is a marathon runner or you are injecting via a central line, it may be suitable to use only 1.5 breaths of delay, or 6 seconds.

(4) A fast injection is necessary to keep the contrast agent as a concentrated bolus. However, if the injection is too vigorous, it may rupture the vein causing extravasation of the contrast agent. Injecting by hand gives an adequate flow rate while minimizing risk of extravasation.

c. *Other bolus timing techniques:* More sophisticated, reliable, and precise techniques for determining the contrast travel time are also available. These include:

(1) Using a test bolus to precisely measure the contrast travel time (6).

(2) Using an automatic pulse sequence (7) that monitors signal in the aorta and then initiates imaging after contrast is detected arriving in the aorta (fluoroscopic triggering or automatic triggering).

(3) Imaging so rapidly that bolus timing is unimportant, for example, time-resolved MRA (8,9). These techniques are increasingly popular and are known as 3D TRICKS, TWIST, and Keyhole. Advanced methods of oversampling the center of *k*-space which allow for 3D volumes to be acquired at subsecond temporal resolution are developing rapidly including Vastly undersampled Isotropic Projection Reconstruction (VIPR) and spiral LAVA.

d. TOF: The bright-blood effect acquired with this sequence can be maximized by:

(1) Acquiring images perpendicular to the vessel of interest (usually in the axial plane).

(2) Using thin slices.

(3) Using a sufficiently long TR so there is time for inflow of fresh, unsaturated spins between pulses (typically 10 msec per 1 mm of slice thickness).

(4) Using gradient moment nulling (flow compensation).

(5) Pulsatility artifact can be minimized by electrocardiogram (ECG) gating or reducing the flip-angle.

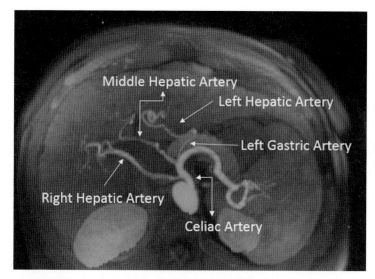

FIGURE 71.2 • Axial high-resolution dynamic spiral LAVA (3D SPGR) sequence showing variant hepatic arterial anatomy. The right hepatic artery is replaced to the celiac trunk, the left hepatic is replaced to the left gastric, and the middle hepatic artery supplying segment 4 arises separately from celiac artery.

e. SSFP: This bright-blood sequence has revolutionized vascular imaging by utilizing "rewinder" gradients that obtain residual signal from each pulse and superimpose it on the signal of the next pulse. This builds up the signal over multiple pulses to attain high SNR. Because blood is a fluid with long T2, high SNR can be accumulated over many pulses without requiring inflow of unsaturated spins. Accurate "rewinding," requires a short TR (<4 msec) and good field homogeneity. It may not work in the setting of metal clips and other susceptibility sources. Image quality is improved with a localized shim of the magnetic field over the ROI. SSFP sequences can be used to acquire fast two-dimensional (2D) ungated localizer scans or, with gating, to show vascular pulsation and flow variation over a cardiac cycle. In a 3D "breath-hold" or navigator mode, SSFP is useful for coronary artery imaging. An ECG-gated 2D version, quiescent interval single shot (QISS), is excellent for imaging peripheral vascular disease.

f. PC: By adding additional gradient activity to the basic TOF technique, it is possible to obtain a phase shift that is proportional to velocity and then to reconstruct phase images in which signal intensity is proportional to velocity. This technique can be implemented in various ways, all of which require setting a velocity encoding value (VENC) to the estimated velocity of blood flow in the artery of interest.

g. TimeSlip (InHance, native trueFISP, B-TRANCE): In this technique, an inversion pulse is applied to an axial slab encompassing the kidneys. When background tissues reach the null point, signal is readout using segmented gradient echo, SSFP, or other techniques. The long inversion times, typically 800 to 1,400 msec, allow ample time for the inflow of unsaturated blood into the imaging volume. Extending the inversion slab inferior to the kidneys help to suppress venous signals entering from below. More recent implementations allow two inversion volumes which can be positioned to cover each entire kidney and the inferior vena cava (IVC) below the renal arteries to further enhance inflow (Fig. 71.2).

h. Double inversion recovery (DIR) is a T1-W black blood MRA sequence with breath holding and ECG gating. The inversion time is set to around 650 msec so that blood will be at the null point and appear black on the images. Because the R–R interval is about the same duration as the optimal inversion time, the inversion pulses can be given after a first ECG trigger and the readout performed on a second ECG trigger one R–R interval later. The first inversion pulse is applied to the entire volume of tissue within the coil while the second inversion pulse is applied to the slice being imaged. In this way, the slice being imaged receives 360 degrees (no effect) while all blood outside the imaging slice has a 180-degree inversion. Readout occurs after all in-slice blood has been replaced by nulled out-of-slice blood. DIR provides fine details of the boundary between the lumen and the vessel wall, and is especially useful for identification of subtle dissection flaps. DIR is usually a breath-holding technique with one image per acquisition. A more advanced version using a smaller inversion pulse can be performed within a single R–R interval to double the acquisition speed.

i. LAVA (liver accelerated volume acquisition, also VIBE, THRIVE) is a bright-blood technique that combines contrast-enhanced, multiphase imaging with high-resolution, large-coverage, zero-filling interpolation, and uniform fat suppression. It is based on a 3D SPGR pulse sequence. LAVA acquires a stack of overlapping slices with high in-plane resolution in one breath hold. The usual protocol repeats this acquisition three or more times. To shorten the duration of breath holding, parallel imaging is used with partial Fourier data filling and short TR/TE. The lower flip angle, typically 10 to 15 degrees allows for greater tissue visualization compared to standard 3D contrast MRA acquired at higher flip angles. It is particularly useful in imaging both the lumen and wall of arteries and the features of aneurysms, for example, presence of thrombus, sac diameter, and so forth. It is also particularly useful for post-Gd venous imaging where there is greater dilution of Gd contrast into the entire blood pool, for example, in identifying deep vein thrombosis (DVT) in the legs.

j. Fresh Blood Imaging, Native Space, TRANCE, Deltaflow: A 3D, non–contrast-enhanced MRA application for peripheral arterial imaging. It is based on cardiac-gated, 3D fast-spin echo and acquires two echoes, one in diastole and the other in systole. Slow arterial flow during diastole results in bright arteries in the diastole images, while faster arterial flow during systole results in dark arteries in the systole images. A subtraction of the systole images from diastole images provides arterial-only images with excellent suppression of venous and background signal. Interleaved acquisition and parallel imaging with optimized k-space trajectory helps reduce motion misregistration and improve vessel visualization, respectively. In addition, the use of partial Fourier and coronal plane acquisition allows for considerably reduced scan time.

3. Postacquisition image processing

a. Zero padding: This is an excellent method of increasing reconstructed image resolution via interpolation. It involves filling out peripheral lines of k-space data with zeroes prior to performing the Fourier transform. Although no additional time is required for data collection, the Fourier transform will reconstruct more images with a smaller spacing. For example, with twofold zero padding, if the partition thickness is 3 mm, the Fourier transform will reconstruct additional images that also have a 3-mm slice thickness but at 1.5-mm spacing with 50% overlap. This helps eliminate volume-averaging artifact and creates smooth visualization of small vessels on the reformatted maximum intensity projection (MIP) images. If available, twofold zero padding in the slice direction is recommended.

b. MR digital subtraction angiography (MRDSA): Image contrast can be improved by digital subtraction of precontrast image data from dynamic,

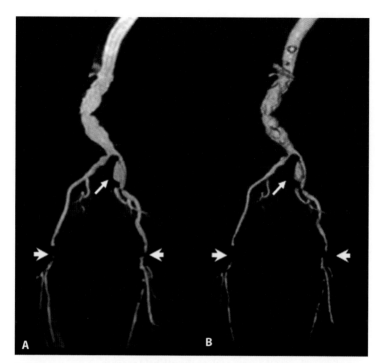

FIGURE 71.3 • Maximum intensity projection (**A**) and volume rendered (**B**) images demonstrate a tortuous aorta with a left common iliac artery aneurysm (*arrow*). *Arrowheads* show focal atherosclerotic stenosis in common femoral arteries, and there is a severe focal stenosis of left internal iliac artery origin as well as proximal left superficial femoral artery stenoses.

arterial-phase, or venous-phase image data. This subtraction can be performed either slice by slice or prior to the Fourier transform by using a complex vector subtraction method. The improvement in contrast achieved with DSA may reduce the Gd dose required. However, there must be no change in the patient position between the precontrast and dynamic contrast-enhanced imaging. This requirement for no motion is easily met in the pelvis and legs, which can be sandbagged and strapped down. It is more difficult to achieve this in the chest and abdomen, where respiratory, cardiac, and peristaltic motions are more difficult to avoid. More recently, removal of the brightest background tissue signal, fat, has been accomplished using Dixon and other fat-water separation methods (LAVA flex).

c. Multiplanar reconstructions: One approach to performing a subvolume MIP is to first load the entire 3D volume of arterial-phase image data into the computer workstation 3D analysis program. Display a coronal MIP image of the entire volume, an axial reformation, and an oblique view. On the coronal view, move the tracker location icon cranially and caudally while watching the axial reconstruction window to find the renal arteries. Display this subvolume of sagittal data as a MIP (Fig. 71.3). Make this oblique MIP thick enough to encompass most of the aorta. Be certain to align the axis of the subvolume MIP so that it is parallel to the origin of the vessel. Although the entire length of the vessel may not be seen on this image, it will be an accurate representation of the vessel's origin, with no overlap from the aorta. This may then be repeated by moving the tracker icon on the axial image and watching the oblique view to create a sagittal view of the celiac and superior mesenteric arteries. This will show the celiac and superior and inferior mesenteric arteries as well as the anterior and posterior margins of the aorta, to best advantage.

   d. Volume rendering: This is a method of 3D visualization in which tissues can have different degrees of transparency allowing visualization through overlying structures. It gives more of a 3D perspective than is possible on MIPs (see Fig. 71.3).

Standard MRA Examinations (see also Appendix D for Common Protocols)

1. **Aortic arch and carotids:** stroke, transient ischemic attack (TIA), great-vessel anatomy, anomalies
   a. Coil: A neurovascular coil extending caudally, low enough to the chest to include the aortic arch, is ideal if available. If a neurovascular or head–neck coil is not available, use a torso array coil with elements placed anterior and posterior to the upper chest and neck.
   b. Axial 2D TOF imaging with superior saturation to suppress veins
   c. Axial T1-W with fat saturation (optional for carotid dissection)
   d. Coronal 3D Gd-MRA (arch to skull base)
2. **Thoracic aorta:** Rule out dissection, aneurysm, embolic source, coarctation, aortitis, and great-vessel anatomy/anomalies, pre/postop.
   a. 3-plane ungated SSFP localizer
   b. Axial black blood DIR – SSFSE/HASTE can be faster but with lower resolution
   c. Sagittal cine-SSFP, oblique view of aortic arch (candy cane view), about 5 to 6 slices will cover the aorta, with *one* breath hold per slice.
   d. Coronal cine-SSFP of ascending aorta, including aortic valve
   e. Axial cine-SSFP in-plane view of aortic valve—identifies bicuspid and stenotic valves
   f. Coronal 3D Gd-MRA with ECG gating
      i. To look for thoracic outlet syndrome, this can be performed as a coronal time resolved MRA with the arms elevated over the head using a half dose and enough phases to see venous enhancement (~20 at 5 seconds temporal resolution). Then repeat the time resolved MRA with the arms along the patient's sides.
   g. Post-Gd coronal and axial LAVA to look for adventitial enhancement in vasculitis. DWI may also be useful to assess Aortitis activity.
3. **Pulmonary artery:** embolism, arteriovenous (AV) fistula, aneurysm, and pulmonary hypertension
   a. 3-plane SSFP locator
   b. Coronal 3D Gd-MRA of both lungs (single injection)
   c. Post-Gd axial and coronal LAVA/VIBE
4. **Abdominal aorta (aneurysm):** preoperative, pre–stent-graft, to monitor diameter, dissection
   a. 3-plane SSFP of SSFSE localizer: use large FOV (48 cm)
   b. Coronal 3D Gd-MRA (see Fig. 71.1)
   c. Post-Gd axial and coronal LAVA
5. **Renal artery:** Transplant donor/recipient, hypertension, renal failure, postoperative, and preangioplasty mapping of arterial anatomy
   a. Timeslip, InHance, Native trueFISP, B-Trance—noncontrast renal MRA
   b. Coronal 3D Gd-MRA
   c. Axial 3D PC imaging of renal arteries. Adjust VENC based on age and renal function—higher (50 to 60 cm per second) in younger patients with normal

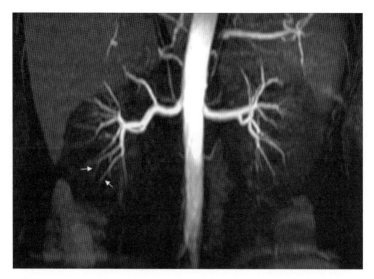

FIGURE 71.4 • Maximum intensity projection images of the non–contrast-inhance sequence showing renal artery and their branches up to third and fourth order (*arrows*).

renal function and lower (30 cm per second) in patients >60 years old and with GFR <60.

   d. Delayed coronal 3D SPGR imaging of collecting system, ureters, and bladder (MR urogram). Images can be improved with IV administration of Lasix (10 mg).

6. Mesenteric artery: mesenteric ischemia, preoperative mapping of mesenteric vascular anatomy, pre- or postliver transplantation. Use renal artery protocol (above), add MR-cholangiopancreatography (MRCP) as well as post-Gd axial and coronal LAVA.

7. Celiac and hepatic arteries: pre-SIRT (Selective Internal Radiation Therapy) Mapping for radioembolization. Use a high temporal resolution dynamic 3D fast spoiled gradient echo dynamic MRI sequence using spiral encoding in the imaging plane and Cartesian encoding along the slice direction (Fig. 71.4). Post-Gd axial and coronal LAVA.

8. Peripheral MRA: claudication, rest pain, nonhealing ulcer, and prior free-flap repair.

   a. QISS or other noncontrast MRA method

   b. Time-resolved MRA of symptomatic foot and calf

   c. 3D bolus-chase MRA from diaphragm to ankle, using blood pressure cuffs on thigh inflated to 50 to 60 mm Hg to reduce venous contamination

9. Veins of the extremities for DVT (10)

   a. Keep legs warm, with multiple blankets as needed, to maximize flow to legs; consider elevating ankles to enhance venous return.

   b. Use three-plane ungated SSFP localizers and axial 2D TOF to image from above the iliac crest to below the knee. Do this in at least two acquisitions per station to avoid acquiring poor-quality images at the inferior and superior extent of the image volume.

      (1) Any region that has an intraluminal filling defect should be further imaged with SSFP or 2D PC MRA, with superior-to-inferior flow encoding, to determine if a filling defect on TOF is real or a flow artifact. Adjust VENC (velocity encoding value) as follows: pelvis, 40 cm per second; thigh, 30 cm per second; calf, 20 cm per second.

(2) To distinguish between acute and chronic venous thrombosis, axial T2 (with fat saturation) and LAVA (3D T1 with fat saturation) post-Gd are helpful. Acute thrombosis stimulates a perivenous inflammatory response that is bright on T2-W images and enhances with Gd contrast.

(3) Dynamic TRICKS: Twenty phases is typically performed to see both arterial and venous phases.

(4) Post-Gd axial and coronal LAVA, matrix size 512×192, with 3 to 5 mm slices, can be especially helpful in identifying subtle DVTs. Gadobenate dimeglumine has longer intravascular half-life than other GBCA making it especially well suited for imaging veins.

References

1. https://www.acr.org/Clinical-Resources/Contrast-Manual. Accessed July 1, 2022.
2. Kuo AH, Nagpal P, Ghoshhajra BB, et al. Vascular magnetic resonance angiography techniques. *Cardiovasc Diagn Ther.* 2019;9(Suppl 1):S28–S36.
3. Westbrook C, Talbot J. *MRI in Practice Clinical Magnetic Resonance Angiography.* 5th ed. Wiley Blackwell; 2018.
4. Vessie EL, Liu DM, Forster B, et al. A practical guide to magnetic resonance vascular imaging: techniques and applications. *AnnVasc Surg.* 2014;28(4):1052–1061.
5. Prince MR, Grist TM, Debatin JF. *3D Contrast MR Angiography.* 3rd ed. Springer-Verlag; 2003.
6. McRobbie DW, Moore EA, Graves MJ, et al. *MRI: From Picture to Proton.* 3rd ed. Cambridge University Press; 2017.
7. Ludwig DR, Shetty AS, Broncano J, et al. Magnetic resonance angiography of the thoracic vasculature: technique and applications. *Magn Reson Imaging.* 2020;52(2):325–347.
8. Zanardo M, Sardanelli F, Rainford L, Monti CB, et al. Technique and protocols for cardiothoracic time-resolved contrast-enhanced magnetic resonance angiography sequences: a systematic review. *Clin Radiol.* 2021;76(2):156.e9–156.
9. Agrawal MD, Spincemaille P, Mennitt KW, et al. Improved hepatic arterial phase MRI with 3-second temporal resolution. *J Magn Reson Imaging.* 2013;37(5):1129–1136.
10. Lombardi P, Carr JC, Allen BD, et al. Updates in magnetic resonance venous imaging. *Semin Intervent Radiol.* 2021;38(2):202–208.

72 Computed Tomographic Angiography
Michael L. Martin, BMSc, MD, FRCPC

As with catheter-directed angiography and MR angiography, prior to imaging, it is essential to evaluate the patient to determine the appropriateness of the examination, address any clinical issues that might impact the study, select the area to be imaged, and assess how cooperative the patient is likely to be. Technologists not familiar with the regions of coverage or bolus timing issues germane to vascular studies will need guidance from the radiologist.

Choice of Appropriate Modality

1. CT angiography has become the mainstay of noninvasive arterial imaging in most clinical scenarios for which arterial imaging is necessary. However, knowledge of,

and expertise with, other noninvasive modalities including ultrasound and MR angiography will allow optimization of imaging strategies for individual patients (1).

2. Use MRA instead of CTA when
   a. There is greater local experience with MRA
   b. Patient is allergic to iodinated contrast
   c. There is a desire to avoid ionizing radiation
   d. Excessive vascular calcification is anticipated or observed
   e. Endoleak is suspected and the patient has an MR compatible stent-graft. Consider MRA when a questioned endoleak is occult to other imaging modalities (2)

Preprocedure Preparation

1. Contrast associated acute kidney injury (CA-AKI): Acutely and chronically ill patients requiring arterial imaging will frequently have multiple risk factors for CA-AKI. Therefore, determination of eGFR and avoidance of dehydration are essential. Screening guidelines and interventions to mitigate CA-AKI are dealt with in Chapter 66.

2. Clothing: The patient should remove all clothing with metallic components from the area to be examined.

3. Sedation: Sedation is rarely necessary. If given, sedated patients need a responsible adult escort post examination.

4. Intravenous (IV) lines: Right arm IV access is preferred when evaluation of the thoracic aorta, proximal arch branch arteries, or the pulmonary arteries is required. The site of IV access and the size of cannula are chosen to allow an injection rate of at least 4 mL per minute. Our standard procedure for most examinations is a 20-gauge cannula in the right antecubital fossa.

Procedure (see Appendix E for Common CTA Protocols)

This chapter will describe general principles. Sample protocols are summarized in Appendix E however scanner-specific protocols will need to be developed for each examination (3,4). CTA of all vascular beds can be performed with most modern CT scanners without additional hardware. Automated tube current modulation is recommended to decrease radiation dose and to optimize image quality (5). While acquisition protocols may vary between scanners, generally all territories can be scanned with isotropic voxel acquisition, allowing for multiplanar reconstruction and volumetric reconstruction. Pulsation artifact in the ascending aorta can be largely eliminated using cardiac-gating techniques.

1. Scanning protocol
   a. Scout sequence: A digital radiograph topogram is performed to define scanning area and to provide a level for contrast detection for bolus triggering.
   b. Occasionally a nonenhanced acquisition through a territory of interest is performed. This is typically used to depict arterial wall calcification, intramural hematoma, or to improve detection of subtle GI hemorrhage in GI bleeding studies.
   c. Test-bolus (if bolus triggering is not used).
   d. CTA acquisition. Imaging of the territory of interest is performed during maximum opacification of arteries of interest.
   e. Delayed phase acquisition. This optional acquisition may be useful in certain circumstances, including assessment for endoleak, to depict GI hemorrhage, for improved depiction of distal vessel in cases of slow runoff, and for assessment of venous structures.

2. Contrast injection (6)
   a. The time course and intensity of arterial enhancement are determined by the rate and duration of injection. They are adjusted depending on the vascular bed to be studied.

   b. One to 1.5 g of iodine injected per second usually results in adequate arterial enhancement of an average-sized patient. Body weight–based adjustments to the injection flow rate and volume are recommended if patient weighs more than 90 kg or less than 60 kg.

   c. Typically, a two-phase intravenous injection is used with a power injector: Iodinated contrast is followed with a normal saline "chaser" to achieve more uniform arterial enhancement over time.

3. Contrast bolus timing (7,8)

   a. Image acquisition must occur when opacification of target vessels is sufficient for luminal assessment and is timed to coordinate with arterial opacification after intravenous contrast injection (contrast transit time).

   b. The variability of contrast transit time can be compensated for by using:

      (1) A test bolus injection—10 mL of contrast is injected and serial images are acquired every second, without table movement, with the ROI on the artery of interest immediately proximal to the area to be examined. A contrast enhancement curve is generated and the peak opacification time calculated.

      (2) Bolus triggering techniques—automated detection of bolus arrival and triggering of scan acquisition.

   c. Depending on the regional to be scanned, the scan delay (the interval between the start of contrast injection and the beginning of scan acquisition) is the set to equal the contrast medium transit time or is chosen at a predefined interval after the contrast medium transit time.

4. Postacquisition image processing (3,9,10)

   Stored images from the examination should include at least one series of 2D cross-sectional images. Interpretation of the CT angiographic study is performed primarily through the review of these images. Axial reconstructed data with an effective slice thickness of 2.5 mm is typically adequate for thoracic, abdominal, and peripheral imaging. Submillimeter reconstructed data sets are helpful for small vessel evaluation such as in the peripheral upper or lower extremity arteries, intracranial region, or occasionally renal arteries.

   Advanced image reconstruction images are used mostly to confirm findings seen on cross section, further evaluate complex lesions or tortuous vascular segments, and summarize findings for referring clinicians. Optimally a standardized set of reformatted images is created for each examination type, including at least one series mimicking conventional angiography.

   a. Maximum intensity projection (MIP) images: The MIP algorithm stacks pixels with attenuation values above an arbitrary threshold from a set of slices into a composite image. The resulting images are similar to a nonsubtracted catheter angiogram unless osseous structures are removed from the data set prior to the creation of the MIP image.

   Limitations

      (1) Image generation is time consuming if bones must be removed manually from the data set.

      (2) Vessels may be inadvertently removed in the bone removal process, creating potential for misdiagnosis.

      (3) The vessel lumen may be obscured by dense mural calcification or stents, especially in small vessels.

   b. Volume rendering: Images are rendered of several MIP frames in which the viewpoint is slightly changed from one to the other, thus creating the illusion of 3D volume. 3D rendering provides a visually efficient display allowing fast interactive exploration of the large data sets of CTA. One can use interactive selection of the appropriate viewing angles to expose relevant vascular segments. Adjustment of the opacity transfer function allows blending in or carving out of vascular detail.

Limitations

(1) Stents or calcifications essentially preclude assessment of the vessel lumen.

(2) Most PACS workstations do not display the color information in high-resolution grayscale monitors.

c. Multiplanar reformations: Sagittal and/or coronal reformatting is especially helpful in pulmonary and aortic examinations, and oblique MPRs are useful for carotid CTA. Simultaneous viewing of orthogonal projections in heavily calcified or stented vessels can be a useful means of assessing the vascular lumen. Curved planar reformats (CPRFs), also called "centerline" reconstructions, are longitudinal cross sections along a predefined vascular centerline. CPRFs are another useful technique for evaluation the lumen in stented or heavily calcified vascular segments.

Limitations: CPRFs work well in normal or minimally diseased vessels but can fail in segments that are severely diseased.

References

1. Mittleider D. Noninvasive arterial testing: what and when to use. *Semin Interv Radiol.* 2018;35(5):384–392.

2. Picel AC, Kansal N. Essentials of endovascular abdominal aortic aneurysm repair imaging: postprocedure surveillance and complications. *AJR Am J Roentgenol.* 2014;203(4): 358–372.

3. Fleischmann D, Chin AS, Molvin L, et al. Computed tomography angiography: a review and technical update. *Radiol Clin N Am.* 2016;54 (1):1–12.

4. Cook TS. Computed tomography angiography of the lower extremities. *Radiol Clin N Am.* 2016;54(1):115–30.

5. Kalra MK, Maher MM, Toth TL, et al. Techniques and applications of automatic tube current modulation for CT. *Radiology.* 2004;233(3):649–657.

6. Fleischmann D. Use of high-concentration contrast media in multiple-detector-row CT: principles and rationale. *Eur Radiol.* 2003;13 (5):M14–M20.

7. Bae KT. Intravenous contrast medium administration and scan timing at CT: considerations and approaches. *Radiology.* 2010;256(1):32–61.

8. Fleischmann D, Rubin GD. Quantification of intravenously administered contrast medium transit through the peripheral arteries: implications for CT angiography. *Radiology.* 2005; 236(3):1076–1082.

9. Lell MM, Anders K, Uder M, et al. New techniques in CT angiography. *RadioGraphics.* 2006; 26(Suppl 1):S45–S62.

10. Rubin GD, Leipsic J, Joseph Schoepf U, et al. CT angiography after 20 years: a transformation in cardiovascular disease characterization continues to advance. *Radiology.* 2014; 271(3):633–652.

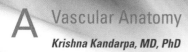

A Vascular Anatomy

Krishna Kandarpa, MD, PhD

Pulmonary Artery Segmental Branches

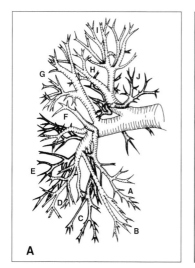
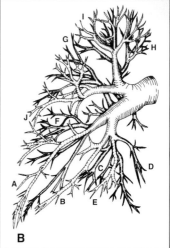

A **B**

FIGURE A.1 • Right pulmonary artery in right anterior oblique (**A**) and left anterior oblique (**B**) projections. A, Right middle lobe (RML) medial segment; B, right lower lobe (RLL) anterior basal segment; C, RLL lateral basal segment; D, RLL posterior basal segment; E, RLL medial basal segment; F, RML lateral segment; G, RLL superior segment; H, right upper lobe (RUL) posterior segment; I, RUL apical segment; J, RUL anterior segment. (Courtesy of S. J. Singer, MD.)

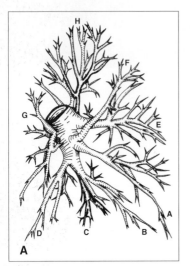
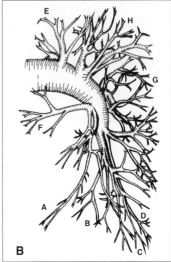

FIGURE A.2 • Left pulmonary artery in right anterior oblique (**A**) and left anterior oblique (**B**) projections. A, Lingular inferior segment; B, left lower lobe (LLL) anteromedial basal segment; C, LLL lateral basal segment; D, LLL posterior basal segment; E, left upper lobe (LUL) anterior segment; F, lingular superior segment; G, LLL superior segment; H, LUL apical-posterior segment. (Courtesy of S. J. Singer, MD.)

Abdominal Aorta

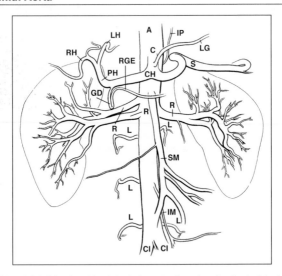

FIGURE A.3 • Labeled drawing of the abdominal aorta and branches. *Arteries:* A, abdominal aorta; C, celiac; LG, left gastric; IP, inferior phrenic; S, splenic; CH, common hepatic; GD, gastroduodenal; RGE, right gastroepiploic; PH, proper hepatic; RH, right hepatic; LH, left hepatic; R, renal; SM, superior mesenteric; IM, inferior mesenteric; L, lumbar; CI, common iliac. (From Dyer R. *Handbook of Basic Vascular and Interventional Radiology.* Churchill Livingstone; 1993:65, with permission.)

Common Locations of Abdominal Aortic Branches

Celiac artery	T12–L1, interspace (anterior aortic wall)
Superior mesenteric artery	Mid-L (anterior aortic wall)
Renals	Upper border of L2 (lateral aortic walls)
Inferior mesenteric artery	L2–L3 interspace (anterolateral wall)
Artery of Adamkiewicz	From intercostal or lumbar artery; T8–L4 (usually on left); injection of normal saline (NS) or contrast may cause transverse myelitis

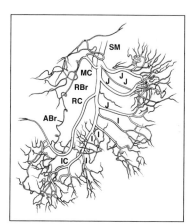

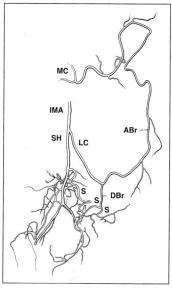

FIGURE A.4 • Labeled drawing of the superior mesenteric artery and branches. *Arteries:* SM, superior mesenteric; MC, middle colic; RBr, right branch of middle colic; RC, right colic; J, jejunal; I, ileal; IC, ileocolic; ABr, ascending branch of right colic. (From Dyer R. *Handbook of Basic Vascular and Interventional Radiology.* Churchill Livingstone; 1993:100, with permission.)

FIGURE A.5 • Labeled drawing of the inferior mesenteric artery. *Arteries:* IMA, inferior mesenteric; LC, left colic, SH, superior hemorrhoidal; MC, middle colic (filled retrogradely); ABr, ascending branch left colic; DBr, descending branch left colic; S, sigmoid. (From Dyer R. *Handbook of Basic Vascular and Interventional Radiology.* Churchill Livingstone; 1993:108, with permission.)

Suggested Readings

Delaney D. *Netter's Surgical Anatomy and Approaches.* 2nd ed. Elsevier; 2020.

Geschwind J, Dake, M. *Abrams' Angiography: Vascular and Interventional Radiology.* 3rd ed. Wolters Kluwer; 2013.

Arteries of the Pelvis

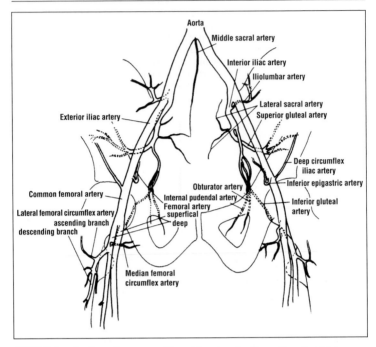

FIGURE A.6 • Arteriographic anatomy of the pelvic and proximal femoral branches. (From Johnsrude IS, Jackson DC, Dunnick NR. *A Practical Approach to Angiography.* 2nd ed. Little, Brown and Company; 1987, with permission.)

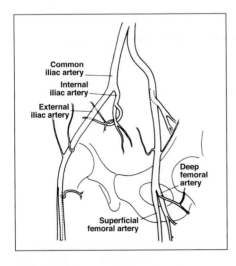

FIGURE A.7 • Right posterior oblique projection. The right common iliac and left common femoral bifurcations are better outlined in this projection. The origin of the left deep femoral artery branch (profunda femoris) may be hidden on the anteroposterior projection. With the patient in the supine position, elevate the symptomatic side to uncover hidden pathology in the profunda femoris. (From Johnsrude IS, Jackson DC, Dunnick NR. *A Practical Approach to Angiography.* 2nd ed. Little, Brown and Company; 1987, with permission.)

Collateral Pathways in Aortoiliofemoral Occlusive Disease

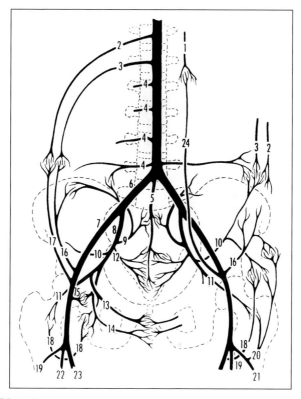

FIGURE A.8 • Schematic diagram of the major potential parietal pathways of collateral circulation demonstrated in aortoiliofemoral occlusive disease. *Arteries:* 1, superior epigastric; 2, intercostal; 3, subcostal; 4, lumbar; 5, middle sacral; 6, common iliac; 7, external iliac; 8, internal iliac; 9, iliolumbar; 10, superior gluteal; 11, inferior gluteal; 12, lateral sacral; 13, obturator; 14, internal pudendal; 15, external pudendal; 16, deep iliac circumflex; 17, superficial iliac circumflex; 18, medial femoral circumflex; 19, lateral femoral circumflex; 20, lateral ascending branch; 21, lateral descending branch; 22, profunda femoris; 23, superficial femoral; 24, inferior epigastric. (From Figley MM, Muller RF. The arteries of the abdomen, pelvis, and thigh. I. Normal roentgenol anatomy, II. Collateral circulation in obstructive arterial disease. *Am J Roentgenol Radium Ther Nucl Med.* 1957;77:296–311, with permission, © by the American Roentgenology Society.)

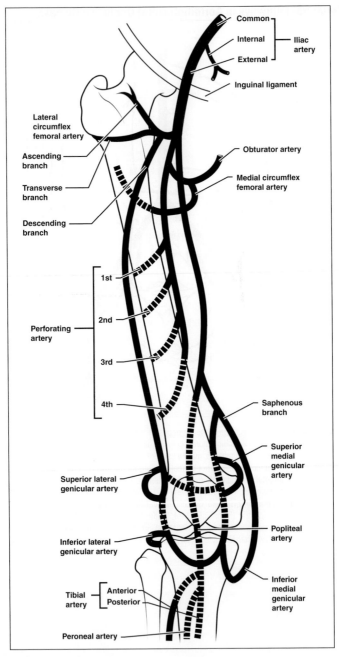

FIGURE A.9 • A composite drawing of the normal anatomy of the femoral artery, its branches, the distal runoff arteries, and the potential collateral vessels.

Common Collateral Pathways

Circuit	Collaterals
SFA occlusion	PFA to popliteal
Common iliac to IMA	IMA to hemorrhoidals to internal iliac to external iliac
SMA to IMA	Midcolic to left colic artery and vice versa (via marginal artery of Drummond; arc of Riolan)
Celiac to SMA	Pancreatic-duodenal
Subclavian artery occlusion	Intercostals to distal subclavian artery
Lower abdominal aorta or aortic bifurcation occlusion	Lumbar arteries to internal iliac (via iliolumbar and superior gluteal branches) or external iliac artery (via deep iliac circumflex or inferior epigastric arteries)
	SMA or IMA to internal iliac artery (via hemorrhoidal and vesicular or rectal arteries)
	Internal mammary to external iliac artery (via superior and inferior epigastric arteries)

SFA, superficial femoral artery; PFA, profunda femoris artery; IMA, internal mammary artery.

Suggested Readings

Delaney D. *Netter's Surgical Anatomy and Approaches.* 2nd ed. Elsevier; 2020.

Geschwind J, Dake, M. *Abrams' Angiography: Vascular and Interventional Radiology.* 3rd ed. Wolters Kluwer; 2013.

Arteries of the Upper Extremity

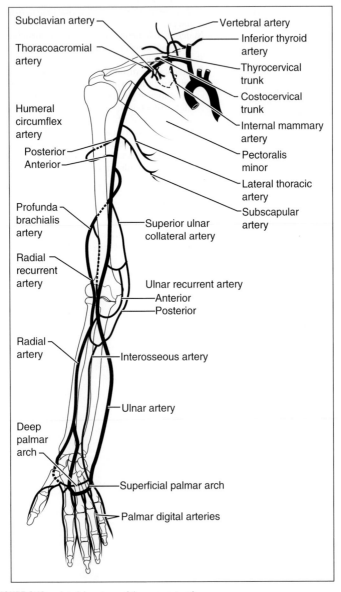

FIGURE A.10 • Arterial anatomy of the upper extremity.

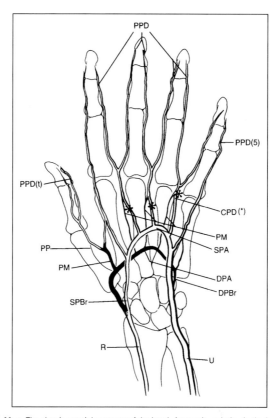

FIGURE A.11 • The classic arterial anatomy of the hand. Anatomic variation in the hand vasculature is commonplace. R, radial artery; DPA, deep palmar arch; PP, princeps pollicis artery; PPD(t), proper palmar digital artery (thumb) from deep palmar arch; U, ulnar artery; SPA, superficial palmar arch; CPD, common palmar digital arteries (from superficial arch); PM, palmar metacarpal arteries (from deep arch); PPD, proper palmar digital arteries; PPD(5), proper palmar digital artery (fifth finger) from superficial arch; SPBr, superficial palmar branch (from ulnar artery); DPBr, deep palmar branch (from radial artery). (From Dyer R. *Handbook of Basic Vascular and Interventional Radiology*, Churchill Livingstone; 1993:132, with permission.)

Intracranial Arteries

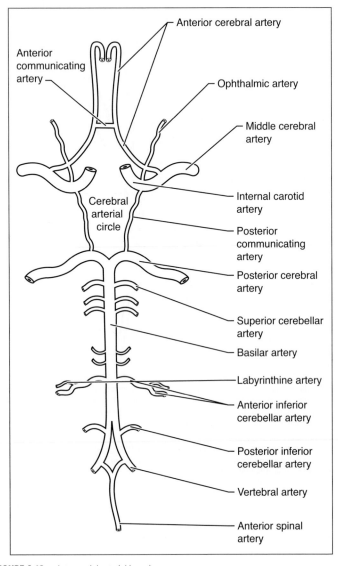

FIGURE A.12 • Intracranial arterial branches.

B Nursing Checklist

*Evelyn P. Wempe, MBA, MSN, ARNP, ACNP-BC, AOCNP, CRN,
DéAnn O. McNamara, MS, ACNP-BC, CRN, and
Krishna Kandarpa, MD, PhD*

Preprocedure Nursing Evaluation Checklist

Outpatient phone screen ☐   Patient chart review ☐

Labs ☐   H&P ☐   Signed requisition ☐

Patient name _____ MRN _____

Home phone # _____ Cell phone # _____

Planned procedure _____

Date _____ Arrival time _____

If ☐ TBA or ☐ Labs needed, patient is instructed to report/register in Admissions 30 minutes early.

☐ Patient or responsible person giving interview _____

COMMUNICATION: Patient able to speak and understand ENGLISH ☐ Yes ☐ No

Primary language _____

INTERPRETER services ☐ Yes ☐ No Confirm # _____

CONSENT: Patient legally competent to give CONSENT? ☐ Yes ☐ No

If no, who will accompany patient to give CONSENT? _____

Relationship to patient _____ Phone # _____

TRANSPORTATION: Ride and caregiver (stay if necessary) arranged? ☐ Yes ☐ No

Transitional Care Facility or Rehab (if applicable)

Name _____ Phone # _____

Outside facility EKG, Labs, H&P, reviewed ☐ Yes ☐ No

Patient will be transported by ambulance? ☐ Yes ☐ No

AMBULANCE Company _____ Phone # _____

ALLERGIES & CONTRAST REACTIONS:

Any known drug allergies? ☐ Yes ☐ No

Specify: _____

CONTRAST REACTION: History of contrast reaction? ☐ Yes ☐ No

If yes, what kind of reaction? _____

IR/radiologist notified of PRIOR contrast reaction _____

Plan for current contrast administration: _____

OTHER PRECAUTIONS ☐ Yes ☐ No

Specify: _____

MEDICATION LIST: Reviewed with patient ☐ Patient bringing home medications ☐

Patient taking an ANTICOAGULANT: ☐ Yes ☐ No

Patient instructions provided: ☐ Yes ☐ No

Is patient DIABETIC? ☐ Yes ☐ No

Is patient on Glucophage and undergoing a contrast study? ☐ Yes ☐ No

If yes, instructions provided: ☐ Yes ☐ No

Is patient on insulin? ☐ Yes ☐ No

If yes, instructions given? ☐ Yes ☐ No

ANESTHESIA

DIFFICULT AIRWAY ☐ Yes ☐ No

PONV ☐ Yes ☐ No

Previous head/neck surgery ☐ Yes ☐ No

Respiratory problems _____

History with sedation agents: _____

Medications for pain or anxiety ☐ Yes ☐ No

Medication/doses _____

SLEEP APNEA: Does patient have a history of sleep apnea? ☐ Yes ☐ No

If yes, patient instructed to bring BIPAP machine? ☐ Yes ☐ No

Weight _____ Height _____

Do you have difficulty breathing when lying flat? ☐ Yes ☐ No

Claustrophobia ☐ Yes ☐ No

Arrange anesthesia support ☐ Yes ☐ No

Anesthesia consult ☐ Yes ☐ No

VENOUS ACCESS CASES:

Does patient have history of central venous catheter? ☐ Yes ☐ No

☐ RIGHT SIDE ☐ LEFT SIDE ☐ BILATERAL TYPE:

_____

TUBES/DRAINS/LINES: Foley, ostomy, etc. _____

INTERNAL/EXTERNAL DEVICES:

List: _____

LABWORK:

Is patient's creatinine >1.3 AND undergoing a contrast study? ☐ Yes ☐ No

If yes, name of MD/PA notified _____

Is platelet count >50 K and INR ≤1.5? ☐ Yes ☐ No

Are labs current and within acceptable range for the procedure ordered?
☐ Yes ☐ No

If radioembo/chemoembo-preprocedure LFT's ordered ☐

Transjugular liver biopsy: Obtain order for CBC and clot to BB ☐

Nephrostomy or biliary drain capping ☐ Check with MD to order necessary labs ☐

LMP if applicable _____

TRANSFUSION:

If blood products are needed prior to procedure, name of
person notified _____

Plan, if needed, to address issue: _____

POSTPROCEDURE CARE:

Does patient currently have home care services? ☐ Yes ☐ No

Is home care needed postprocedure? ☐ Yes ☐ No

If yes, name and phone # of person contacted: _____

Plan _____

Recent travel _____

Anything else you would like to share about your personal health history/status?

_____

PATIENT INSTRUCTIONS:

☐ NPO *6 hours* before the procedure except for sips of clear liquids to take oral
medications.

☐ Avoid bringing valuables, jewelry, or money to the hospital. Wear comfortable
clothing.

☐ Take all regular oral antihyperglycemics, cardiac, antihypertensives, antianxiety,
and pain meds.

☐ Patient reminded to bring medication list and/or bottles of any medications
necessary during stay.

☐ Patient understands procedure process including possibility of extended wait
or delay.

☐ Length of time expected to be in hospital.

☐ DIRECTIONS TO hospital/family waiting area.

Website information for further information related to the hospital, maps,
parking options, hotels, etc. Patient given telephone number to contact IR nurse
with any questions or concerns:

PPE complete ☐ Date _____ RN completing PPE _____
Comments _____

C Hemodynamic Monitoring and Cardiovascular Pressures

Michael G. Flater, RN

Hemodynamic monitoring is an essential component of cardiopulmonary and peripheral angiographic procedures and provides assessment of hemodynamic status by direct intracardiac, intravascular, and pulmonary arterial pressure (PAP) monitoring. Right heart pressure analysis is often performed during cardiac catheterization and pulmonary angiography. Systemic arterial pressure is analyzed during cardiac catheterization and in the angiographic evaluation of the peripheral vasculature, particularly when a stenosis is present. Identification of characteristic pressure waveforms and analysis of the component deflections can provide the angiographer with valuable information about cardiac output, ventricular function, valvular function, pulmonary function, and fluid volume status.

See e-book for overview and monitoring set-up.

Right Heart Catheterization

Right heart pressures are most frequently obtained using flow-directed, balloon-tipped catheters. Common insertion sites include the internal jugular vein, subclavian vein, brachial vein, and femoral vein. Meticulous aseptic technique is essential to minimize the potential for nosocomial infection. Fluoroscopic visualization is recommended.

Technique

1. Flush the catheter lumen; purge all air from the system using a heparinized isotonic solution.
2. Verify balloon integrity: Submerge the catheter tip in solution and inflate the balloon; inspect for leaks or defects such as eccentricity.
3. Obtain venous access; insert an introducer sheath.
4. Advance the catheter to the central venous system. Inflate balloon with 1.5 mL of carbon dioxide. Although many operators prefer the accessibility of room air, the balloon should never be inflated with air when the catheter is used in a child, or when intracardiac or intrapulmonary shunting is suspected.
5. Advance the catheter to the right atrium (RA).
   a. Continue to advance the catheter with the balloon inflated; the RA is approximately 40 cm from the femoral insertion site.
   b. Deflate the balloon and record phasic and mean RA pressure.
6. Advance the catheter to the right ventricle (RV).
   a. Inflate the balloon and advance the catheter across the tricuspid valve; tricuspid regurgitation may impede this maneuver.
   b. Position the catheter at a nonarrhythmogenic site within the RV apex; the RV apex is approximately 50 cm from the femoral insertion site.
   c. Deflate the balloon and record phasic RV pressure.
7. Advance the catheter to the pulmonary artery (PA).
   a. Inflate the balloon.
   b. Apply counterclockwise torque to the catheter until the balloon is directed superiorly toward the RV outflow tract.
   c. Withdraw the catheter slowly.
   d. Advance the catheter using the RV systolic ejection wave to assist in directing the balloon across the pulmonic valve.

(1) Deep inspiration by the patient may facilitate this maneuver.
(2) Monitor the electrocardiogram (ECG) for right bundle branch block.
   (a) In the patient with underlying left bundle branch block, complete heart block may ensue.
   (b) Prophylactic placement of a temporary ventricular pacing catheter in patients with left bundle branch block may be prudent.
   (c) Emergent placement of a temporary ventricular pacing lead may be necessary should complete heart block occur.

8. Advance the catheter to the pulmonary capillary wedge (PCW) position.
   a. Continue to advance the catheter with the balloon inflated (approximately 65 cm from the femoral insertion site) until the catheter is no longer free in the PA and a discernible change in the pressure waveform is observed. Avoid excessive damping of the pressure waveform.
   b. Record phasic and mean wedge pressures with the balloon inflated.
   c. Deflate the balloon and withdraw the catheter 3 to 5 cm to the main PA.
   d. Record phasic and mean PA pressures.

9. The practice of recording right heart pressures can be expedited by introducing the catheter into the venous system, inflating the balloon, and advancing the catheter directly to the PCW position. The right heart pressures are continuously recorded as the balloon is deflated, and the catheter is slowly withdrawn to the RA, pausing in the main PA and again in the RV for the duration of the selected chamber recording. The transducer is opened to atmospheric pressure at the beginning and again at the end of the recording to verify the accuracy of the recording. This technique is not used when it is necessary to exchange the catheter over a wire for selective catheter placement in the pulmonary vasculature or when continuous pulmonary pressure monitoring is desired.

Complications

1. Segmental pulmonary infarction
   a. May result from distal migration of the catheter tip to the peripheral pulmonary vasculature and spontaneous catheter tip wedging
   b. May result from air embolization to the distal pulmonary vasculature following rupture of the balloon in the PA, right heart, or venous system

2. PA perforation
   a. May result from prolonged balloon inflation.
      (1) Balloon inflation times should be minimal.
      (2) Limit the number of pulmonary capillary wedge pressure (PCWP) measurements and limit the inflation time to two respiratory cycles or 10 to 15 seconds.
      (3) There is a higher risk for PA perforation in female patients who are elderly, anticoagulated, hypothermic, or have pulmonary hypertension.
   b. May occur following overdistention of the vessel.
      (1) The balloon should not be inflated above the recommended volume as overdistention of the vessel may result in vascular trauma.
      (2) PAP should be monitored prior to balloon inflation to verify that the catheter is in the PA and has not migrated distally.
         (a) Discontinue balloon inflation on recognition of the transition from a PAP to a PCWP trace.
         (b) If the catheter balloon inflates with less than 1.5 mL of gas, deflate the balloon and withdraw it 1 to 2 cm before reinflating.
      (3) Fluoroscopic evaluation of catheter position is recommended.
   c. Monitor the patient for signs and symptoms of PA perforation.
      (1) Hemoptysis
      (2) Pain
      (3) Respiratory distress

3. Embolization
   a. May result from catheter microthrombus formation and consequent migration to the distal pulmonary vasculature. PA catheters should be flushed regularly or continuously (3 to 6 mL per hour) with a heparinized isotonic solution to minimize thrombus formation.
   b. Risk of thrombosis increases with long-term use of indwelling central catheters.
   c. May result from iatrogenic introduction of air into the venous circulation with migration to the distal pulmonary vasculature. Injection of <2 mL of air into the right heart or PA, as may occur with balloon rupture, usually does not result in adverse sequelae in adults without right-to-left shunting. The system must be purged of air prior to forward flushing into the venous circulation.
4. Cardiac arrhythmias
   a. May occur during catheter insertion and removal.
   b. May result from retrograde migration of the catheter tip into the RV following balloon deflation.
   c. ECG monitoring is essential from insertion to removal of the catheter.
      (1) Transient premature ventricular depolarizations are predominant.
      (2) Lethal ventricular arrhythmias may result.
      (3) Right bundle branch block may result.
      (4) Complete heart block may result, especially in the patient with underlying left bundle branch block.
5. Infection, sepsis, and endocarditis
   a. A risk of nosocomial infection exists with any invasive procedure.
   b. The risk may be substantially decreased by using proper aseptic technique during preparation, vascular access, and insertion and manipulation of the catheter.
      (1) Shaving and preparation of the puncture site with an antimicrobial agent (i.e., 1% povidone-iodine solution)
      (2) Proper handwashing
      (3) Use of sterile garments and gloves is essential.
6. Perforation of the heart or great vessels: A rare complication that may be avoided by ensuring that the balloon is inflated prior to advancement of the catheter through the heart.
7. Pneumothorax: A rare complication that has been reported following vascular access via the internal jugular and subclavian vein approaches.

Right Heart and Pulmonary Artery Pressure Waveforms

1. **Right atrium**
   a. **Pressure:** mean RA pressure = 0 to 8 mm Hg
   b. **Waveform analysis** (Figs. C.1 and C.2)
      (1) **a wave:** RA contraction (follows the ECG P wave by approximately 80 msec)
      (2) **x descent:** RA relaxation and downward movement of the atrioventricular (A-V) junction
      (3) **c wave:** upward movement of the tricuspid valve toward the RA at the onset of RV systole (follows the a wave by a period equal to the ECG PR interval). This deflection is not always present (best visualized in the presence of ECG PR interval prolongation).
      (4) **v wave:** passive venous filling of the RA during RV systole, while the tricuspid valve is closed (occurs at the end of the ECG T wave). The peak of the v wave occurs at the end of RV systole when the tricuspid valve is closed.
      (5) **y descent:** rapid atrial emptying following the opening of the tricuspid valve

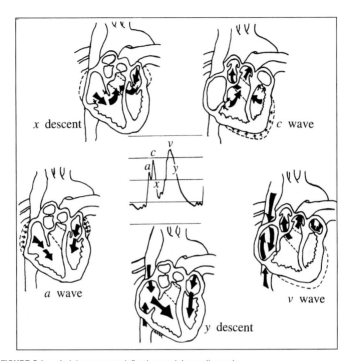

FIGURE C.1 • Atrial component deflections and the cardiac cycle.

2. Right ventricle

a. Pressure: RV pressure = 15 to 30/0 to 8 mm Hg

(1) Right ventricular end-diastolic pressure (RVEDP) equals RA pressure because they essentially form a common chamber during diastole when the tricuspid valve is open.

(2) RVEDP does not equal RA pressure in the presence of tricuspid valve disease.

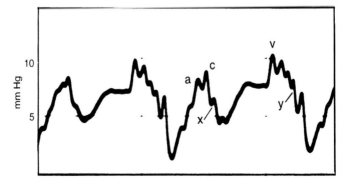

FIGURE C.2 • Right atrial pressure tracing.

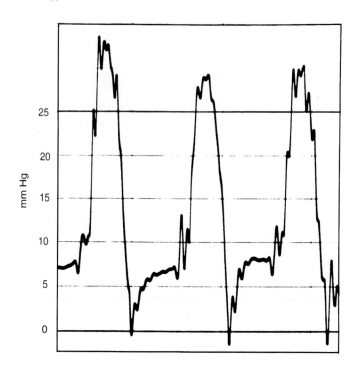

RV pressure

FIGURE C.3 • Right ventricular pressure tracing.

b. **Waveform analysis** (Fig. C.3)
  (1) **Isovolumetric contraction**
    (a) The onset of RV systole occurs at the peak of the ECG R wave.
    (b) The rapid upstroke of the systolic component is a result of RV contraction against closed tricuspid and pulmonic valves.
  (2) **Ejection**
    (a) RV pressure exceeds PAP, the pulmonic valve opens, and blood is ejected into the PA.
    (b) Rapid ejection phase occurs from the opening of the pulmonic valve to the peak of RV systolic pressure.
    (c) Reduced ejection phase follows from the peak of RV systolic pressure to the closure of the pulmonic valve.
  (3) **Isovolumetric relaxation**
    (a) As the pressure in the PA exceeds that of the RV, the pulmonic valve closes.
    (b) Isovolumetric relaxation follows, and the negative waveform deflection continues.
    (c) The opening of the tricuspid valve marks the end of isovolumetric relaxation and the onset of RV diastole.
  (4) **Rapid ventricular filling** occurs from the opening of the tricuspid valve until diastasis is achieved. Rapid negative deflection results from RV relaxation.

    (5) Reduced ventricular filling/diastasis
       (a) Slow filling of the RV occurs until systole and is distinguished by a gradual rise in RA and RV pressures and RV volume.
       (b) The static baseline is inscribed because RV and RA pressures are equal throughout the phase.
       (c) RVEDP is measured at the peak of the ECG T wave.
3. Pulmonary artery
  a. Pressure: PAP 5 15 to 30/4 to 12 mm Hg; mean PA pressure 5 9 to 18 mm Hg
    (1) PA systolic pressure equals RV systolic pressure because they essentially form a common chamber during systole when the pulmonic valve is open.
    (2) PA systolic pressure does not equal RV systolic pressure in the presence of pulmonary valve disease.
  b. Waveform analysis (Fig. C.4)
    (1) Systole
       (a) The rise in PAP occurs as blood is ejected from the RV into the PA.
       (b) The peak of the systolic wave occurs during the ECG T wave.
       (c) The RV and PAP continue to increase until the RV begins to relax.
    (2) Diastole
       (a) The RV and PAP decrease until the pressure in the PA exceeds that of the RV and the pulmonic valve closes. This produces the dicrotic notch, which marks the onset of RV isovolumetric relaxation.
       (b) Pressure continues to fall until RV contraction occurs and the cycle repeats.
4. Pulmonary capillary wedge
  a. Pressure: mean PCWP = 2 to 10 mm Hg

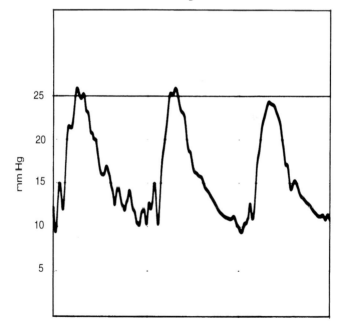

PA pressure

FIGURE C.4 • Pulmonary artery pressure tracing.

(1) Inflating the balloon occludes a small branch of the PA and permits the retrograde transmission of the left atrial (LA) pressure wave through the pulmonary vasculature.

(2) PCWP equals LA pressure when there is no obstruction between the PA and the LA throughout the cardiac cycle.

(3) PCWP equals pulmonary artery diastolic pressure (PADP) because they are at equilibrium during diastole.

(4) PCWP does not equal PADP during certain conditions, including increased pulmonary vascular resistance (PVR), positive end-expiratory pressure (PEEP) ventilation, and diffuse pulmonary disease states.

(5) PCWP will not reflect LA pressure under certain conditions, including increased alveolar pressure as is generated with PEEP ventilation, pulmonary venous obstruction, pulmonary venoconstriction, pulmonary hypertension, LA myxoma, and cor triatriatum sinistrum.

b. **Waveform analysis** (Figs. C.1 and C.5)

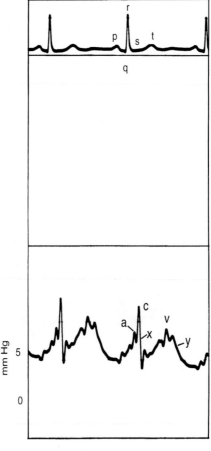

PCW pressure

FIGURE C.5 • Pulmonary capillary wedge pressure tracing.

(1) **a wave:** LA contraction (follows the ECG P wave by approximately 240 msec).

(2) **x descent:** LA relaxation and downward movement of the A-V junction.

(3) **c wave:** upward movement of the mitral valve toward the LA at the onset of LV systole (follows the a wave by a period equal to the ECG PR interval). This deflection is not always present (best visualized in the presence of ECG PR interval prolongation).

(4) **v wave:** passive venous filling of the LA during LV systole while the mitral valve is closed (occurs after the inscription of the ECG T wave). Peak of the v wave occurs at the end of ventricular systole when the LA is maximally filled.

(5) **y descent:** rapid LA emptying following the opening of the mitral valve.

Left Heart Catheterization

Aortic (Ao) and LV pressures are commonly recorded using a pigtail catheter. The coiled primary curve of the pigtail reduces the potential for endomyocardial and vascular trauma (i.e., perforation of the heart or great vessels), resists recoil during high-flow contrast injection, and decreases the incidence of ectopic ventricular depolarizations. Its multiple side-hole design allows diffuse opacification of a large chamber with a high volume of angiographic contrast material while reducing the potential for myocardial or intimal staining.

Technique
1. Flush the pigtail catheter with a heparinized isotonic solution prior to its introduction into the arterial system.
2. Consider systemic anticoagulation, especially in cases where a guidewire will be in prolonged contact with the blood (i.e., crossing a stenotic Ao valve), or when a protracted procedure time is anticipated or realized.
3. Because of its circular design, the pigtail catheter is advanced over a guidewire to the central aorta using fluoroscopic guidance.
4. Remove the guidewire and flush the catheter with care.
5. Record phasic and mean Ao pressure.
6. Advance the pigtail catheter to a nonarrhythmogenic position in the LV. A moderately to severely stenotic Ao valve may obstruct progression to the LV, requiring use of a guidewire to traverse the annulus.
7. Remove the guidewire and flush the catheter with care.
8. Record phasic LV pressure, scaled so that the vertical axis (amplitude) includes the full excursion of the LV pressure waveform (e.g., 0 to 200 mm Hg). Some operators will also record LV pressure at a fast sweep speed (e.g., 100 mm per second), scaled so that the vertical axis includes only the diastolic component of the waveform (e.g., 0 to 40 mm Hg), to facilitate accurate measurement of left ventricular end-diastolic pressure (LVEDP).
9. When mitral or submitral stenosis is suspected, record simultaneous LV and PCWP at a fast sweep speed (e.g., 100 mm per second), scaled so that the vertical axis includes only the diastolic components of the LV pressure waveform (e.g., 0 to 40 mm Hg) (Fig. C.6). This will facilitate accurate measurement of the mitral transvalvular pressure gradient, which may be used to calculate the mitral valve area (i.e., using the Gorlin or Hakki equations).
   a. Retrograde transmission of the LA pressure wave through the pulmonary vasculature to the site of PA balloon occlusion results in a delay in the upstroke of the PCWP waveform. Use of the PCWP without adjustment for this delay results in overestimation of the mitral transvalvular pressure gradient and underestimation of the mitral valve area. This time delay is a function of PVR and can be adjusted by horizontal phase shift (superimposition

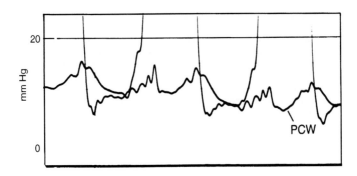

LVEDP and PCW superimposed

FIGURE C.6 • Left ventricular end-diastolic pressure tracing and pulmonary capillary wedge tracing superimposed.

of the LV and PCW waveforms) to improve accuracy in the measurement of the mitral transvalvular gradient.

b. Simultaneous recordings of LA and LV pressure waveforms may be accomplished using a pigtail catheter inserted through a sheath placed in the LA via atrial transseptal puncture. Transseptal catheterization is a complex procedure requiring specialized training and meticulous technique and is associated with perforation and embolic risks that preclude routine use.

10. When Ao or subaortic stenosis is suspected, simultaneous LV and systemic arterial pressures should be recorded at a fast sweep speed (e.g., 100 mm per second), scaled so that the vertical axis includes the full excursion of the LV pressure waveform (e.g., 0 to 200 mm Hg) (Fig. C.7). This will facilitate accurate measurement of an Ao transvalvular pressure gradient, which may be used to calculate the Ao valve area (i.e., using the Gorlin or Hakki equations).

a. Anterograde transmission of the Ao pressure wave through the systemic vasculature results in a delay in the upstroke of the systemic arterial pressure waveform. Use of the systemic arterial pressure without adjustment for this delay results in overestimation of the Ao transvalvular pressure gradient and underestimation of the Ao valve area. The delay time is a function of systemic vascular resistance (SVR) and can be adjusted by a horizontal phase shift (superimposition of the Ao and systemic arterial waveforms) to improve accuracy in the measurement of the mitral transvalvular gradient.

b. The distance of the systemic arterial cannula from the Ao valve will result in peripheral augmentation of the systemic peak systolic and pulse pressures, which will artifactually overestimate the Ao pressure gradient and underestimate the Ao valve area.

c. A single catheter pullback (from LV to Ao) while continuously recording catheter pressure will provide sequential recordings of LV and Ao pressure waveforms, obviating the need for overshoot correction.

d. Use of a dual-lumen pigtail catheter positioned across the Ao valve will allow simultaneous recordings of Ao and LV pressures without delay.

e. The operator may insert a 4-Fr pigtail in the LV through a 7-Fr 60-cm catheter (fitted with a Tuohy–Borst adapter) that has been positioned in the Ao arch to allow simultaneous recordings of Ao and LV pressures without delay.

(1) Prior to recording pressures, assure that the Tuohy–Borst adapter has been tightened to prevent blood loss and to avoid loss of wave energy from fluid volume escaping the closed system.

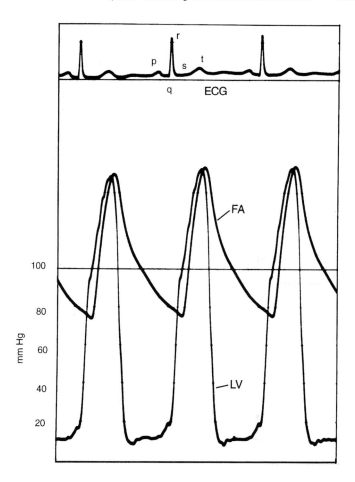

LV pressure with
systemic arterial (FA)
pressure superimposed

FIGURE C.7 • Left ventricular pressure tracing with systemic arterial (FA) tracing superimposed.

(2) Check the manufacturer specifications (i.e., internal diameter [ID] of the outer catheter and outer diameter [OD] of the inner catheter) to determine coaxial compatibility.

(3) Vigilance must be exercised in maintaining luminal patency in a coaxial catheter system. Disruption of laminar flow around the inner catheter promotes luminal stasis and increased thrombogenicity.

Complications

1. Embolization

   a. May result from catheter or guidewire microthrombus formation and consequent embolization to the brain, viscera, or extremities. Arterial catheters should be flushed regularly or continuously (3 to 6 mL per hour) with a heparinized isotonic solution to minimize thrombus formation. Guidewire contact with blood should be limited. Guidewires should be carefully wiped upon removal.

b. May result from fragmentation of intracardiac or intravascular thrombi. Exercise careful technique to minimize this risk. Risk is increased in patients with known arteriosclerotic disease, valvular stenotic disease, heart failure, LV aneurysm, recent myocardial infarction with suspected mitral thrombus, atrial fibrillation, or hypercoagulability; systemic anticoagulation is recommended to minimize this risk.

c. May result from iatrogenic introduction of air into the arterial circulation with migration to the brain, viscera, or extremities. The system must be purged of air prior to forward flushing into the arterial circulation.

2. Cardiac arrhythmias
    a. May occur during catheter insertion and removal. ECG monitoring is essential during catheter and wire manipulations within the LV.
    b. Transient premature ventricular depolarizations are predominant. Some lethal arrhythmias or left bundle branch or fascicular block may result. Complete heart block may result in the patient with underlying right bundle branch block.

3. Infection, sepsis, and endocarditis
    a. A risk of nosocomial infection exists with any invasive procedure.
    b. The risk may be substantially decreased by using proper aseptic technique during preparation, vascular access, and insertion and manipulation of the catheter.
        (1) Shaving and preparation of the puncture site with an antimicrobial agent (i.e., 1% povidone-iodine solution)
        (2) Proper handwashing
        (3) Use of sterile garments and gloves is essential.

4. Perforation of the heart or great vessels: a rare complication; the pigtail catheter design minimizes this risk.

Left Heart and Aortic Pressure Waveforms

1. **Left ventricle**
    a. **Pressure:** LV pressure 5 100 to 140/3 to 12 mm Hg
        (1) LVEDP is an indicator of LV function. Changes in left ventricular end-diastolic volume (LVEDV) affect LVEDP. LVEDP affects myocardial fiber length during end-diastole (preload) and reflects the compliance of the LV myocardium, and therefore, the LA pressure necessary to fill the ventricle just prior to systole.
        (2) LVEDP equals LA pressure, which equals PCWP when there is no obstruction between the PA and the LV while the mitral valve is open during diastole (Fig. C.6).
        (3) PCWP will not reflect LVEDP under certain conditions, including mitral valve disease, increased alveolar pressure as is generated with PEEP ventilation, pulmonary venous obstruction, pulmonary venoconstriction, pulmonary hypertension, LA myxoma, and cor triatriatum sinistrum.
        (4) LV systolic pressure equals Ao systolic pressure when there is no obstruction between the LV and the aorta while the Ao valve is open during LV systole.
        (5) LV systolic pressure will not equal Ao systolic pressure in the presence of Ao stenosis or hypertrophic obstructive cardiomyopathy (asymmetrical septal hypertrophy; idiopathic hypertrophic subaortic stenosis).
    b. **Waveform analysis**
        (1) **Isovolumetric contraction**
            (a) The onset of LV systole occurs at the peak of the ECG R wave.

(b) The rapid upstroke of the systolic component is a result of LV contraction against closed mitral and Ao valves.

(2) **Ejection**

(a) LV pressure exceeds Ao pressure, the Ao valve opens, and blood is ejected into the aorta.

(b) Rapid ejection phase occurs from the opening of the Ao valve to the peak of LV systolic pressure.

(c) Reduced ejection phase follows from the peak of LV systolic pressure to the closure of the Ao valve.

(3) **Isovolumetric relaxation**

(a) As the pressure in the aorta exceeds that of the LV, the Ao valve closes.

(b) Isovolumetric relaxation follows, and the negative waveform deflection continues.

(c) The opening of the mitral valve marks the end of isovolumetric relaxation and the onset of LV diastole.

(4) **Rapid ventricular filling** occurs from the opening of the mitral valve until diastasis is achieved. Rapid negative deflection results from LV relaxation.

(5) **Reduced ventricular filling/diastasis**

(a) Slow filling of the LV occurs until systole and is distinguished by a gradual rise in LA and LV pressures and LV volume.

(b) The static baseline is inscribed as LV and LA pressures are equal throughout the phase.

(c) LVEDP is measured at the peak of the T wave.

2. **Central aorta**

a. **Pressure:** Ao pressure = 100 to 140/60 to 90 mm Hg; mean Ao pressure = 70 to 105 mm Hg

(1) Systemic arterial systolic pressure equals Ao systolic pressure, which equals LV systolic pressure, while the Ao valve is open during LV systole.

(2) These pressures may not be equal in the presence of Ao valve disease, Ao disease, or peripheral arterial disease.

b. **Waveform analysis** (Figs. C.7 and C.8)

(1) **Systole**

(a) The rise in Ao pressure occurs as blood is ejected from the LV into the aorta and distally to the systemic vasculature.

(b) This occurs during the ECG T wave.

(c) The LV and Ao pressures continue to increase until the LV begins to relax.

(2) **Diastole**

(a) The LV and Ao pressures decrease until the pressure in the aorta exceeds that of the LV and the Ao valve closes. This produces the dicrotic notch, which marks the onset of LV isovolumetric relaxation.

(b) Pressure continues to fall until LV contraction occurs and the cycle repeats.

Clinical Significance of Waveforms

Right Atrial Pressure

1. Mean = 0 to 8 mm Hg

a. Elevated

(1) RV failure

(2) Pericardial effusion/tamponade

(3) Acute ventricular septal defect (VSD)

(4) Tricuspid stenosis

(5) Pulmonary embolus

(6) Pulmonary hypertension

(7) Hypervolemia

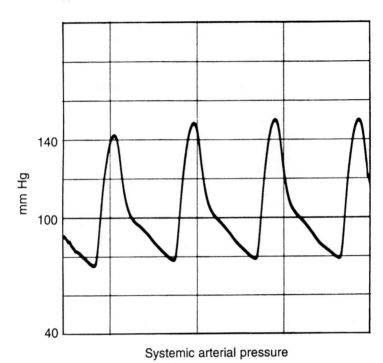

Systemic arterial pressure

FIGURE C.8 • Systemic arterial pressure tracing.

    b. Elevated on inspiration (Kussmaul sign)
      (1) RV infarct
      (2) Tricuspid insufficiency
      (3) Constrictive pericarditis
    c. Decreased: hypovolemia/dehydration
    d. Decreased on inspiration: pericardial effusion
    e. Equalization of RA and LA pressures (PCWP)
      (1) Severe atrial septal defect (ASD)
      (2) Constrictive/restrictive cardiomyopathy
    f. Equal to or exceeding PCWP: acute RV infarct
    g. Dissociation of atrial and ventricular waveform components: Ebstein anomaly
      (atrialization of the RV)
2. a wave = 2 to 8 mm Hg
    a. Absent
      (1) Atrial fibrillation
      (2) Atrial flutter
      (3) Atrial standstill
    b. Elevated
      (1) Increased resistance to RV filling
      (2) Pulmonary hypertension
      (3) Tricuspid stenosis
      (4) Decreased RV compliance
      (5) Constrictive pericarditis
      (6) Tricuspid insufficiency

(7) Pulmonic stenosis
(8) RV hypertrophy
c. Cannon waves (regular): atrial contraction against a closed tricuspid valve
(1) Nodal rhythms
(2) A-V node reentrant tachycardia
d. Cannon waves (irregular): A-V dissociation and wave summation (shortened diastole)
(1) Wide complex tachycardia (highly suggestive of ventricular tachycardia [VT])
(2) Complete heart block
(3) Ventricular pacing
e. Cannon waves (single): ventricular ectopy
f. Mechanical flutter waves: atrial flutter (approximately 300 beats per minute)
3. x descent—prominent
a. Pericardial effusion
b. RV infarct
c. Volume expansion therapy
4. v wave—large
a. Tricuspid insufficiency
b. Constrictive pericarditis
c. ASD
d. Atrial fibrillation
e. Hypervolemia
5. y descent
a. Prominent/rapid
(1) Tricuspid insufficiency
(2) Constrictive pericarditis
(3) RV infarct
(4) Volume expansion therapy
b. Attenuated/absent: pericardial effusion

Right Ventricular Pressure
1. Peak systolic = 15 to 30 mm Hg
a. Elevated
(1) Pulmonary hypertension
(2) Pulmonic stenosis
(3) VSD
b. Decreased
(1) Congestive heart failure (CHF)
(2) Pericardial tamponade
(3) Hypovolemia
2. End-diastolic = 0 to 8 mm Hg
a. Elevated
(1) RV failure
(2) Chronic CHF
(3) Pulmonary insufficiency
(4) Constrictive pericarditis
(5) Pericardial tamponade
(6) Hypervolemia
b. Decreased
(1) Tricuspid stenosis
(2) Hypovolemia
c. Square root sign (early rapid diastolic dip with a mid-diastolic plateau)
(1) Constrictive pericarditis
(2) Restrictive cardiomyopathy

    (3) Moderate-to-severe RV failure
    (4) Bradycardia (artifactual)
  d. Equalization (RVEDP and PADP within 4 mm Hg)
    (1) Restrictive constrictive cardiomyopathy
    (2) Shock
  e. a wave—attenuation/absence
    (1) Tricuspid stenosis
    (2) Tricuspid insufficiency (with decreased RV compliance)
    (3) Atrial fibrillation
    (4) Atrial flutter
    (5) Atrial standstill

Pulmonary Arterial Pressure
1. Mean = 9 to 17 mm Hg
2. Peak systolic = 15 to 30 mm Hg
  a. Elevated
    (1) Increased pulmonary flow: left-to-right (L-R) shunt
    (2) Increased PVR
      (a) Parenchymal pulmonary disease
      (b) Pulmonary stenosis
      (c) Pulmonary embolus
      (d) Primary or secondary pulmonary hypertension
    (3) Increases with PCWP, pulmonary venous pressure, LA pressure, or LVEDP
      (a) Mitral stenosis
      (b) Mitral insufficiency
      (c) LV failure
  b. Decreased
    (1) Hypovolemia
    (2) Pulmonic stenosis
    (3) Ebstein anomaly
    (4) Hypoplastic right heart syndrome
    (5) Tricuspid stenosis
    (6) Tricuspid atresia
3. Diastolic = 4 to 14 mm Hg
  a. PADP > mean PCWP: primary pulmonary disorder (PADP–PCWP) >6 mm Hg
  b. PADP < mean PCWP: acute mitral insufficiency

Pulmonary Capillary Wedge Pressure/Left Atrial Pressure
1. Mean PCWP = 2 to 12 mm Hg
  a. Elevated
    (1) Mitral stenosis
    (2) Mitral insufficiency
    (3) LV failure
    (4) LV hypertrophy
    (5) Decreased LV compliance
    (6) Increased PVR
    (7) "Overwedged" catheter
    (8) During negative pressure phase of PEEP/continuous positive airway pressure ventilation
    (9) Hypervolemia
  b. Decreased: hypovolemia
  c. Equalization of PCWP/LA and RA pressures
    (1) Severe ASD
    (2) Constrictive/restrictive cardiomyopathy
2. a wave = 3 to 10 mm Hg
  a. Absent

      (1) Atrial fibrillation
      (2) Atrial flutter
      (3) Atrial standstill
   b. Elevated—increased resistance to LV filling
      (1) Systemic hypertension
      (2) Mitral stenosis
      (3) Mitral insufficiency
      (4) Ao stenosis
      (5) LV hypertrophy
   c. Cannon waves (regular)—atrial contraction against a closed mitral valve
      (1) Nodal rhythms
      (2) A-V node reentrant tachycardia
   d. Cannon waves (irregular): A-V dissociation and wave summation (shortened diastole)
      (1) Wide complex tachycardia (highly suggestive of VT)
      (2) Complete heart block
      (3) Ventricular pacing
   e. Cannon waves (single): ventricular ectopy
   f. Mechanical flutter waves: atrial flutter (approximately 300 beats per minute)
3. v wave—elevated
   a. Mitral insufficiency
   b. Atrial fibrillation
   c. Constrictive pericarditis
   d. Hypervolemia
4. y descent
   a. Prominent
      (1) Mitral insufficiency
      (2) Constrictive pericarditis
   b. Attenuated/absent: pericardial effusion

Left Ventricular Pressure
1. Peak systolic = 100 to 140 mm Hg
   a. Elevated
      (1) Systemic hypertension
      (2) Ao stenosis
      (3) Ao insufficiency
   b. Decreased
      (1) Hypovolemia
      (2) CHF
      (3) Pericardial tamponade
2. End-diastolic = 3 to 12 mm Hg
   a. Elevated
      (1) LV failure
      (2) LV hypertrophy
      (3) Decreased LV compliance
         (a) Ao insufficiency
         (b) Constrictive pericarditis
         (c) Pericardial tamponade
         (d) Endocardial fibrosis
   b. Decreased
      (1) Hypovolemia
      (2) Mitral stenosis
   c. Square root sign (early rapid diastolic dip with a mid-diastolic plateau)
      (1) Constrictive pericarditis
      (2) Restrictive cardiomyopathy

    (3) Moderate-to-severe LV failure
    (4) Bradycardia (artifactual)
  d. a wave—attenuation/absence
    (1) Severe Ao insufficiency
    (2) Mitral stenosis
    (3) Mitral insufficiency
    (4) Atrial fibrillation
    (5) Atrial flutter
    (6) Atrial standstill

Aortic Pressure/Systemic Arterial Pressure
1. Mean = 70 to 105 mm Hg
2. Peak systolic = 100 to 140 mm Hg
  a. Elevated
    (1) Systemic hypertension
    (2) Ao sclerosis
    (3) Elevated catecholamine states
    (4) Anxiety
  b. Decreased
    (1) Ao stenosis
    (2) Decreased cardiac output
    (3) Shock
3. Diastolic = 60 to 90 mm Hg; elevated: systemic hypertension
4. Pulse pressure
  a. Wide
    (1) Systemic hypertension
    (2) Ao insufficiency
    (3) Large L-R shunt
      (a) Patent ductus arteriosus
      (b) Aortopulmonary fistula
      (c) Truncus arteriosus communis
      (d) Perforated sinus of Valsalva aneurysm
  b. Narrow
    (1) Ao stenosis
    (2) CHF
    (3) Pericardial tamponade
    (4) Shock
  c. Arterial pulsus bisferiens (spiked)
    (1) Ao insufficiency
    (2) Hypertrophic obstructive cardiomyopathy (asymmetrical septal hypertrophy; idiopathic hypertrophic subaortic stenosis)
  d. Pulsus paradoxus (>10 mm Hg decrease in systolic pressure on inspiration): pericardial tamponade
  e. Pulsus parvus et tardus (weak pulse that rises and falls slowly): Ao stenosis
  f. Pulsus alternans (alternating weak/strong arterial pressure)
    (1) CHF
    (2) Cardiomyopathy

Respiratory Effects

Variation in intracardiac and pulmonary pressures may result with changes in intrathoracic pressure.
1. All pressures: There may be cyclical variation in the amplitude of both the phasic and mean tracings of the systemic, ventricular, and PA pressures. The amplitude of pressure may be accentuated in the presence of significant pulmonary disease

or severe heart failure or during mechanical ventilation. Pressures should be measured at end-expiration, with the patient off ventilator, if possible.

a. Spontaneous respiration effects a decrease in intracardiac and intravascular pressures upon inspiration.

b. Positive pressure ventilation effects an increase in intracardiac and intravascular pressures upon inspiration.

c. Mixed mechanical and triggered or spontaneous breaths (e.g., intermittent mandatory ventilation, controlled mandatory ventilation) may present a challenge in determining end-expiration. Manual palpation of chest rise and fall during real-time hemodynamic monitoring and recording may be advantageous.

2. Atrial pressures: Mean RA, mean LA, and PCWP pressures decrease on inspiration. The a and v waves and x and y descents are prominent during inspiration.

Suggested Readings

Barash PG, Cullen BF, Stoelting RK, eds. *Clinical Anesthesia*. 8th ed. Wolters Kluwer; 2017.

Kern MJ, Lim MJ, Goldstein JA, eds. *Hemodynamic Rounds: Interpretation of Cardiac Pathophysiology from Pressure Waveform Analysis*. 4th ed. Wiley; 2018.

Moscucci M, ed. *Grossman and Baim's Cardiac Catheterization: Angiography and Intervention*. 8th ed. Wolters Kluwer; 2020.

Sorajja P, Lim MJ, Kern MJ, eds. *The Cardiac Catheterization Handbook*. 7th ed. WB Saunders; 2019.

D Common Magnetic Resonance Angiography Protocols

Nanda Deepa Thimmappa, MD and Martin R. Prince, MD, PhD, FACR

	Aortic Arch and Carotids	Thoracic Aorta	Abdominal Aorta	Peripheral MRA
Common Indications	Great-vessel anatomy, anomalies, stroke, TIA	Dissection, aneurysm, aortitis, embolic source, coarctation, pre/postop	Preoperative, pre–stent graft, aneurysm, dissection, follow-up	Claudication, rest pain, nonhealing ulcer, and prior free-flap repair
Sequences	Axial 2D TOF Axial T1-W FS Coronal 3D Gd-MRA	Axial SSFP and black blood DIR Sagittal cine-SSFP (candy cane) Coronal cine-SSFP Cine SSFP in aortic valve plane Coronal 3D Gd-MRA with ECG gating Post-Gd coronal and axial LAVA	Coronal 3D Gd-MRA Post-Gd axial and coronal LAVA	Time-resolved MRA of symptomatic foot and calf. 3D bolus-chase MRA from diaphragm to ankle with inflated blood pressure cuffs on thigh to reduce venous contamination

MRA, magnetic resonance angiography; TIA, transient ischemic attack; AV, arteriovenous; SIRT, selective internal radiation therapy; DVT, deep vein thrombosis; 2D, two-dimensional; TOF, time-of-flight; T1-W, T1-weighted; FS, fat saturated; 3D Gd-MRA, three-dimensional gadolinium MRA; SSFP, steady-state free precession; DIR, double inversion recovery; ECG, electrocardiogram; LAVA, liver acquisition with volume acquisition; MR, magnetic resonance; MRCP, MR-cholangiopancreatography; FISP, fast imaging with steady-state precession; SSFSE, single-shot fast-spin echo.

Pulmonary Artery	Renal Artery	Mesenteric Arteries	Celiac and Hepatic Arteries	Venous Imaging
Embolism, AV fistula, aneurysm, pulmonary hypertension	Transplant donor/recipient, hypertension, renal failure, preangioplasty mapping of arterial anatomy, postoperative follow-up	Mesenteric ischemia, preoperative mapping of mesenteric vascular anatomy, pre- or postliver transplantation	Pre-SIRT mapping for mapping pre-radioembolization	DVT, stenosis. To distinguish between acute and chronic venous thrombosis
Coronal 3D Gd-MRA of both lungs (single injection) Post-Gd axial and coronal LAVA.	Noncontrast renal MRA (Timeslip/InHance/Native trueFISP, B-Trance) Coronal 3D Gd-MRA. Axial 3D PC Coronal 3D SPGR (+/– Lasix 10 mg or 2 glasses fluids) of collecting system (MR urogram)	3D MRCP Timeslip, InHance, Native trueFISP Coronal 3D Gd-MRA Post-Gd coronal and axial LAVA	Axial/Coronal SSFSE Dynamic high temporal resolution LAVA (e.g., spiral/radial LAVA). Post-Gd coronal/axial LAVA	Axial 2D TOF- > Intraluminal filling defect: SSFP or 2D PC MRA Dynamic TRICKS Pre/Post Gd axial/coronal LAVA Axial T2 FS

E Computed Tomographic Angiography

Michael L. Martin, BMSc, MD, FRCPC

Commonly Used Protocols for Standard Computed Tomographic Angiography Examinations

The studies described are performed on a GE Revolution CT 160-mm detector scanner (GE Healthcare, Waukesha, WI). Omnipaque 300 contrast (GE Healthcare, Oslo, Norway) or equivalent and automated dose modulation is used for all **computed tomography (CT)** angiography studies. For all studies, a 30-mL "chaser" of saline is given at the completion of contrast injection at the same rate as contrast administration.

Please note that imaging protocols are machine-specific. Alternative protocols should be available from CT vendors. Numerous online sources for imaging protocols are available.

Study	Indication	Range
Arch to vertex	Carotid stenosis, dissection, FMD, vascular malformation	Lesser curve of aortic arch to cranial vertex
Pulmonary artery	Pulmonary embolism, AV fistula	Thoracic apex to inferior costophrenic angle
Whole aorta	Dissection, aneurysm, acute thoracic aortic syndrome, aortitis, embolic source	Thoracic apex to groin
Thoracic aorta	Follow-up study of known thoracic aortic pathology	Thoracic apex to inferior costophrenic angle
Abdominal aorta	Aneurysm, mesenteric ischemia	Apex of diaphragm to groin
Renal arteries	Hypertension	Diaphragm to iliac crest
GI bleeding study	Acute GI bleeding	Apex of diaphragm to groin
Post-EVAR (thoracic aorta)	Evaluation following endovascular aneurysm repair	Thoracic apex to inferior costophrenic angle
Post-EVAR (abdominal aorta)	Evaluation following endovascular aneurysm repair	Apex of diaphragm to groin
Lower extremity	Claudication, limb-threatening ischemia, evaluation for free flap graft	Apex of diaphragm to toes
Upper extremity	Chronic or acute ischemia, penetrating trauma	Affected arm above head, lesser curve of aortic arch to fingertips
DIEP assessment	Preoperative planning	Xiphoid to pubic symphysis

FMD, fibromuscular dysplasia; AV, arteriovenous; N/A, not applicable; GI, gastrointestinal; EVAR, endovascular aortic aneurysm repair; IV, intravenous; DIEP, deep inferior epigastric artery perforator.

Contrast	Trigger	Scan Delay	Additional Phases
100 mL at 5 mL/s	Automated trigger off ascending aorta—100 HU	4 s	N/A
100 mL at 5 mL/s	Automated trigger off main pulmonary artery—115 HU	7 s	N/A
120 mL at 4 mL/s	Automated trigger off ascending aorta—100 HU	5 s	Noncontrast through same range for suspected acute thoracic aortic syndrome
90 mL at 4 mL/s	Automated trigger off ascending aorta—100 HU	5 s	N/A
90 mL at 4 mL/s	Automated trigger off aorta at T12—100 HU	15 s	Venous phase at 60–90 s postcontrast for acute intestinal ischemia
90 mL at 4 mL/s	Automated trigger off aorta at T12—100 HU	12 s	N/A
120 mL at 4 mL/s	Automated trigger off aorta at T12—100 HU	15 s	Noncontrast and venous phase at 60 s through same range
90 mL at 4 mL/s	Automated trigger off ascending aorta—100 HU	5 s	Optional noncontrast through endograft ± 60 s postcontrast through endograft
90 mL at 4 mL/s	Automated trigger off aorta at T12—100 HU	15 s	Optional noncontrast through endograft ± 60 s postcontrast through endograft
120 mL at 4 mL/s	Automated trigger off aorta at T12—100 HU	17 s	N/A
120 mL at 4 mL/s IV in unaffected arm	Automated trigger off ascending aorta—100 HU	6 s	N/A
120 mL at 4 mL/s	Automated trigger off aorta at T12—100 HU	15 s	N/A

F Contrast Media Table

Class	Generic Name	Trade Name/ Company	Availability
High Osmolality Ionic	sodium and/ or meglumine diatrizoate	Renografin/Bracco	Yes
		Hypaque/GE Medical	
	sodium iothalamate	Conray/Liebel-Flarsheim	Yes
Low osmolality Ionic	sodium–meglumine ioxaglate	Hexabrix/Guerbet	Not in USA
Low osmolality monomeric	Ioversol	Optiray/Guerbet	Phasing out in USA
	Iohexol	Omnipaque/GE Healthcare	Yes
	Iopamidol	Isovue/Bracco	Yes
	Iopromide	Ultravist/Bayer	Yes
	Ioxilan	Oxilan/Guerbet	No longer available
	iobitridol	Xenetix/Guerbet	Not available in USA
Low osmolality dimeric	Iodixanol	Visipaque/GE Healthcare	Yes
	Iotrolan	Isovist/Bayer	Not marketed widley

Iodine Concentration, mg/mL	Osmolality, mOsm/kg	Viscosity, CPS at 37°C
141–370	633–1940	10.5
200–400	100–2100	4
320	602	7.5
160–350	355–702	5.5
240–350	520–844	10.4
200–370	413–796	9.4
300–370	605–780	10
300–350	585–695	8.1
250–350		
270–320	290	11.8
300	320	8.1

Table G.1 Randomized Controlled Trials Comparing Endarterectomy with Stenting in Symptomatic Patients with Carotid Stenosis

Trial, Year (Reference)	Patients	Key Features	Death or Any Stroke	OR (95% CI)	Comments
CAVATAS-CEA, 2001 (1)	504	Multicenter; patients of any age with symptomatic or asymptomatic carotid stenosis suitable for CEA or CAS	CEA: 25/253 (9.9%) CAS: 25/251 (10.0%)	$P =$ NS in original article; OR not reported	Follow-up to 3 y; relatively low-stent use (26%) in CAS group
SAPPHIRE, 2004 (2)	334	Multicenter randomized trial of patients with ≥80% asymptomatic carotid stenosis (70%) and ≥50% symptomatic carotid stenosis (30%)	CEA: 9.3% symptomatic patients CAS: 2.1% symptomatic patients	$P = .18$	Terminated prematurely because of a drop in randomization
EVS-3S, 2006 (3)	527	Multicenter; patients with symptomatic carotid stenosis >60% within 120 d before enrollment suitable for CEA or CAS	CEA: 10/259 (3.9%) CAS: 25/262 (9.6%)	RR = 2.5 (1.2–5.1), $P = .01$	Study terminated prematurely because of safety and futility issues; concerns about operator inexperience in the CAS arm and nonuniform use of embolism protection devices

	N				
SPACE, 2006 (4)	1,183	Multicenter; patients >50 years old with symptomatic carotid stenosis >70% in the 180 d before enrollment	Primary end point of ipsilateral ischemic stroke or death from time of randomization to 300 d after the procedure; CEA: 37/584 (6.3%) CAS: 41/599 (6.8%)	1.19 (0.75–1.92)	Study terminated prematurely after futility analysis; "concerns about operator inexperience in the CAS arm and nonuniform use of embolism protection devices"
EVA-3S, 4-y follow-up, 2008 (5)	527	Multicenter, randomized, open, assessor-blinded, noninferiority trial. Compared outcome after CAS with outcome after CEA in 527 patients who had carotid stenosis of at least 60% that had recently become symptomatic	Major outcome events up to 4 y for any periprocedural stroke or death: CEA: 6.2% CAS: 11.1%	HR for any stroke or periprocedural death 1.77 (1.03–3.02) P=.04 HR for any stroke or death 1.39 (0.96–2.00) P=.08 R for CAS vs. CEA 1.97 (1.06–3.67) P=.03	A hazard function analysis showed 4-y differences in cumulative probabilities of outcomes between CAS and CEA were largely accounted for by the higher periprocedural (within 30 d of the procedure) risk of stenting compared with endarterectomy. After the periprocedural period, the risk of ipsilateral stroke was low and similar in the two treatment groups

(continued)

Table G.1 Randomized Controlled Trials Comparing Endarterectomy with Stenting in Symptomatic Patients with Carotid Stenosis (*Continued*)

Trial, Year (Reference)	Patients	Key Features	Death or Any Stroke	OR (95% CI)	Comments
SPACE 2-y follow-up, 2008 (6)	1,214	Patients with symptomatic, severe carotid artery stenosis (70%) were recruited to this noninferiority trial and randomly assigned with a block randomization design to undergo CAS or CEA	Intention-to-treat population: Ipsilateral ischemic strokes within 2 y, including any periprocedural strokes or deaths: CAS: 56 (9.5%) CEA: 50 (8.8%) Any deaths between randomization and 2 y: CAS: 32 (6.3%) CEA: 28 (5.0%) Any strokes between randomization and 2 y: CAS: 64 (10.9%) CEA: 57 (10.1%) Ipsilateral ischemic stroke within 31 d and 2 y: CAS: 12 (2.2%) CEA: 10 (1.9%) Per-protocol population: Ipsilateral ischemic strokes within 2 y, including any periprocedural strokes or deaths: CAS: 53 (9.4%) CEA: 43 (7.8%) Any deaths between randomization and 2 y: CAS: 29 (6.2%) CEA: 25 (4.9%) Any strokes between randomization and 2 y: CAS: 61 (11.5%) CEA: 51 (9.8%) Ipsilateral ischemic stroke within 31 d and 2 y: CAS: 12 (2.3%) CEA: 10 (2.0%)	Intention-to-treat population: Ipsilateral ischemic strokes within 2 y, including any periprocedural strokes or deaths: $HR = 1.10 (0.75–1.61)$ Any deaths between randomization and 2 y: $HR = 1.11 (0.67–1.85)$ Any strokes between randomization and 2 y: $HR = 1.10 (0.77–1.57)$ Ipsilateral ischemic stroke within 31 d and 2 y: $HR = 1.17 (0.51–2.70)$ Per-protocol population: Ipsilateral ischemic strokes within 2 y, including any periprocedural strokes or deaths: $HR = 1.23 (0.82–1.83)$ Any deaths between randomization and 2 y: $HR = 1.19 (0.83–1.73)$ Ipsilateral ischemic stroke within 31 d and 2 y: $HR = 1.18 (0.51–2.73)$	In both the intention-to-treat and per-protocol populations, recurrent stenosis of 70% was significantly more frequent in the CAS group than the CEA group, with a life table estimate of 10.7% vs. 4.6% ($P = .0009$) and 11.1% vs. 4.6% ($P = .0001$), respectively

Study	N	Description	Results	Notes
SAPPHIRE 3-y follow-up, 2008 (7)	260	Long-term data were collected for 260 individuals; included symptomatic carotid artery stenosis of at least 50% of the lumina diameter or an asymptomatic stenosis of at least 80%	Stroke: CAS: 15 (9.0%) CEA: 15 (9.0%) Ipsilateral stroke: CAS: 11 (7.0%) CEA: 9 (5.4%) Death: CAS: 31 (18.6%) CEA: 35 (21%) Note: Data were calculated using $n = 167$ for both groups because breakdowns of CAS and CEA for $n = 260$ were not given	Stroke: $P = .99$ (−6.1–6.1) Death: $P = .68$ (−10.9–6.1)
ICSS, 2010 (8)	1,713	Multicenter study. In the study, the degree of carotid stenosis was 70–99% in 69% of stent patients and in 91% of endarterectomy patients. Study patients had >50% carotid artery stenosis measured by the NASCET criteria	120-d follow-up data: CAS: 72/853 (8.5%) CEA: 40/857 (4.7%)	OR not available HR = 1.86 (1.26–2.74) $P = .001$	Primary outcome was 3-y rate of fatal or disabling stroke in any territory; interim results have been provided for 120-d rate of stroke, death, or procedural MI

(*continued*)

Table G.1 Randomized Controlled Trials Comparing Endarterectomy with Stenting in Symptomatic Patients with Carotid Stenosis (*Continued*)

Trial, Year (Reference)	Patients	Key Features	Death or Any Stroke	OR (95% CI)	Comments
CREST, 2010 (9)	2,502	The study included 1,321 symptomatic patients and 1,181 asymptomatic patients. Symptomatic patients in the study had ≥50% carotid stenosis by angiography, ≥70% by US, or ≥70% by CTA or MRA. Asymptomatic patients had carotid stenosis (patients with symptoms beyond 180 d were considered asymptomatic) ≥60% by angiography, ≥70% by US, or ≥80% by CTA or MRA	Any periprocedural stroke or postprocedural ipsilateral stroke: Symptomatic: CAS: 37 (5.5 ± 0.9 SE) CEA: 21 (3.2 ± 0.7 SE) Any periprocedural stroke or death or postprocedural ipsilateral stroke: Symptomatic: CAS: 40 (6.0 ± 0.9 SE) CEA: 21 (3.2 ± 0.7 SE)	Any periprocedural stroke or postprocedural ipsilateral stroke: Symptomatic: $P = .04$ Any periprocedural stroke or death or postprocedural ipsilateral stroke: Symptomatic: $P = .02$	The risk of composite primary outcome of stroke, MI, or death did not differ significantly among symptomatic and asymptomatic patients between CAS and CEA

| ICSS, 2015 (10) | 1,713 | Multicenter study. In the study, the degree of carotid stenosis was 70–99% in 89% of stent patients and in 91% of endarterectomy patients. Study patients had >50% carotid artery stenosis measured by the NASCET criteria | Median of 4.3-y follow-up. Events: Fatal or disabling strokes: CAS: 52/853 (6.1%) CEA: 49/857 (5.7%) Any stroke: CAS: 119/853 (13.9%) CEA: 72/857 (8.4%) | 5-y cumulative risk HR = 1.71, 95% CI 1.28–2.30, $P <$ .001; per-protocol population, 5-y cumulative risk 8.9% vs. 5.8%, 1.53, 1.02–2.31, $P =$ .04 | Any stroke was more frequent in the CAS group than in the CEA group were mainly nondisabling strokes. The distribution of modified Rankin scale scores at 1 y, 5 y, or final follow-up did not differ significantly between treatment groups. Long-term functional outcome and risk of fatal or disabling stroke are similar for stenting and endarterectomy for symptomatic carotid stenosis |

CI, confidence interval; OR, odds ratio; RR, risk reduction; SE, standard error.
Adapted with permission from Brott TG, Halperin JL, Abbara S, et al. 2011 ASA/ACCF/AHA/AANN/AANS/ACR/ASNR/CNS/SAIP/SCAI/SIR/SNIS/SVM/SVS guideline on the management of patients with extracranial carotid and vertebral artery disease: executive summary: a report of the American College of Cardiology Foundation/American Heart Association Task Force on Practice Guidelines, and the American Stroke Association, American Association of Neuroscience Nurses, American Association of Neurological Surgeons, American College of Radiology, American Society of Neuroradiology, Congress of Neurological Surgeons, Society of Atherosclerosis Imaging and Prevention, Society for Cardiovascular Angiography and Interventions, Society of Interventional Radiology, Society of NeuroInterventional Surgery, Society for Vascular Medicine, and Society for Vascular Surgery. Developed in collaboration with the American Academy of Neurology and Society of Cardiovascular Computed Tomography. *J Am Coll Cardiol.* 57(8):1002–1044.

Table G.2 Trials Comparing Endarterectomy with Stenting in Asymptomatic Patients with Carotid Stenosis

Trial, Year (Reference)	Patients	Key Features	Death or Any Stroke	P Value	Comments
SAPPHIRE, 2004 (2)	334	Multicenter randomized trial of patients with >50% symptomatic carotid stenosis (58%) or >80% asymptomatic carotid stenosis (42%) with one or more comorbidity criteria[a] (high–surgical risk group)	Asymptomatic: CEA: 10.2%[b] CAS: 5.4%[b] Combined: CEA: 9.8%[b] CAS: 4.8%[b]	.2	Terminated prematurely because of a drop in randomization
SAPPHIRE, 2008 (7)	334	Multicenter randomized trial of patients with >80% asymptomatic carotid stenosis (70%) and ≥50% symptomatic carotid stenosis (30%)	SAPPHIRE 3-y data Stroke: CEA: 15/167 CAS: 15/197 Death: CEA: 35/167 CAS: 31/167	Stroke: .99 Death: .68 (or not reported)	No significant difference could be shown in long-term outcomes between patients who underwent CAS with an EPD and those who underwent CEA

| CREST, 2010 (9) | 2,502 | The study included 1,321 symptomatic patients and 1,181 asymptomatic patients. Symptomatic patients in the study had ≥50% carotid stenosis by angiography, ≥70% by ultrasound, or ≥70% by CTA or MRA. Asymptomatic patients in the study had carotid stenosis (patients with symptoms beyond 180 d were considered asymptomatic) ≥60% by angiography, ≥70% by US, or ≥80% by CTA or MRA | Any periprocedural stroke or postprocedural ipsilateral stroke: Asymptomatic: CAS: 15 (2.5 ± 0.6 SE) CEA: 8 (1.4 ± 0.5 SE) Any periprocedural stroke or death or postprocedural ipsilateral stroke: Asymptomatic: CAS: 15 (2.5 ± 0.6 SE) CEA: 8 (1.4 ± 0.5 SE) | Any periprocedural stroke or postprocedural ipsilateral stroke: Asymptomatic: .15 Any periprocedural stroke or death or postprocedural ipsilateral stroke: Asymptomatic: .15 | The risk of the composite primary outcome of stroke, MI, or death did not differ significantly among symptomatic and asymptomatic patients between CAS and CEA |

EPD, embolic protection device; OR, odds ratio; SE, standard error.

[a]Criteria for high risk as discussed previously.

[b]Death, stroke, and MI.

Adapted with permission from Brott TG, Halperin JL, Abbara S, et al. 2011 ASA/ACCF/AHA/AANN/AANS/ACR/ASNR/CNS/SAIP/SCAI/SIR/SNIS/SVM/SVS guideline on the management of patients with extracranial carotid and vertebral artery disease: executive summary: a report of the American College of Cardiology Foundation/American Heart Association Task Force on Practice Guidelines, and the American Stroke Association, American Association of Neuroscience Nurses, American Association of Neurological Surgeons, American College of Radiology, American Society of Neuroradiology, Congress of Neurological Surgeons, Society of Atherosclerosis Imaging and Prevention, Society for Cardiovascular Angiography and Interventions, Society of Interventional Radiology, Society of NeuroInterventional Surgery, Society for Vascular Medicine, and Society for Vascular Surgery. Developed in collaboration with the American Academy of Neurology and Society of Cardiovascular Computed Tomography. J Am Coll Cardiol. 57(8):1002–1044.

References

1. Ederle J, Bonati LH, Dobson J, et al. Endovascular treatment with angioplasty or stenting versus endarterectomy in patients with carotid artery stenosis in the carotid and vertebral artery transluminal angioplasty study (CAVATAS): long-term follow-up of a randomised trial. *Lancet Neurol*. 2009;8(10):898–907.

2. Yadav JS, Wholey MH, Kuntz RE, et al. Protected carotid-artery stenting versus endarterectomy in high-risk patients. *N Engl J Med*. 2004;351(15):1493–1501.

3. Mas JL, Chatellier G, Beyssen B, et al. Endarterectomy versus stenting in patients with symptomatic severe carotid stenosis. *N Engl J Med*. 2006;355(16):1660–1671.

4. Ringleb PA, Allenberg J, Brückmann H, et al. 30 Day results from the SPACE trial of stent-protected angioplasty versus carotid endarterectomy in symptomatic patients: a randomised non-inferiority trial. *Lancet*. 2006;368(9543):1239–1247.

5. Mas JL, Trinquart L, Leys D, et al. Endarterectomy versus angioplasty in patients with symptomatic severe carotid stenosis (EVA-3S) trial: results up to 4 years from a randomised, multicentre trial. *Lancet Neurol*. 2008;7(10):885–892.

6. Eckstein HH, Ringleb P, Allenberg JR, et al. Results of the stent-protected angioplasty versus carotid endarterectomy (SPACE) study to treat symptomatic stenoses at 2 years: a multinational, prospective, randomised trial. *Lancet Neurol*. 2008;7(10): 893–902.

7. Gurm HS, Yadav JS, Fayad P, et al. Long-term results of carotid stenting versus endarterectomy in high-risk patients. *N Engl J Med*. 2008;358(15):1572–1579.

8. Ederle J, Dobson J, Featherstone RL, et al. Carotid artery stenting compared with endarterectomy in patients with symptomatic carotid stenosis (International Carotid Stenting Study): an interim analysis of a randomised controlled trial. *Lancet*. 2010;375(9719): 985–997.

9. Brott TG, Hobson RW II, Howard G, et al. Stenting versus endarterectomy for treatment of carotid-artery stenosis. *N Engl J Med*. 2010;363(1):11–23.

10. Bonati LH, Dobson J, Featherstone RL, et al. Long-term outcomes after stenting versus endarterectomy for treatment of symptomatic carotid stenosis: the International Carotid Stenting Study (ICSS) randomised trial. *Lancet*. 2015;385(9967): 529–538.

INDEX

Italic page numbers indicate online-only chapters. Page numbers followed by f and t indicate figures and tables, respectively.